GRAY'S
ANATOMY REVIEW

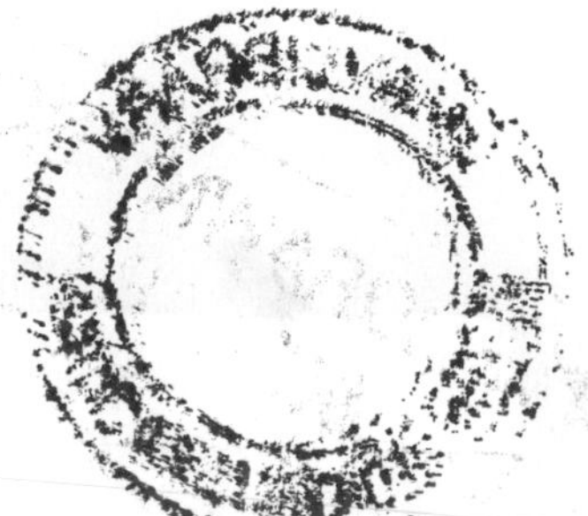

GRAY'S ANATOMY REVIEW

SECOND EDITION

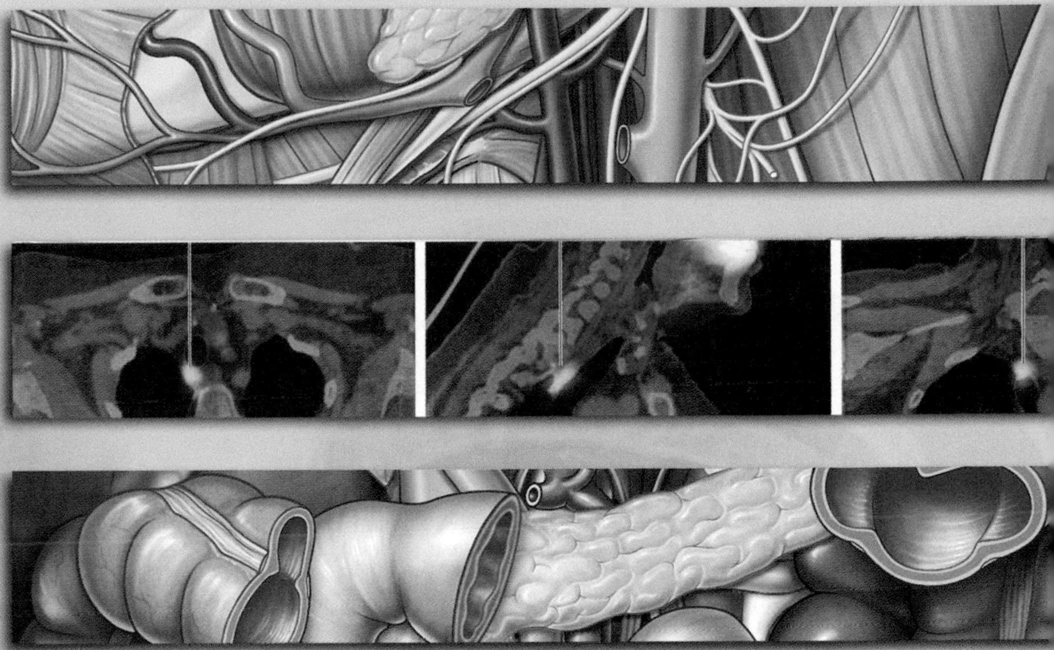

Marios Loukas, MD, PhD
Professor, Department of Anatomical Sciences
Dean of Basic Sciences
St. George's University School of Medicine
Grenada, West Indies

R. Shane Tubbs, MS, PA-C, PhD
Professor of Anatomy
Children's of Alabama
Birmingham, Alabama;
Department of Anatomical Sciences
St. George's University
Grenada, West Indies;
Centre of Anatomy and Human Identification
University of Dundee
Dundee, United Kingdom

Peter H. Abrahams, MBBS, FRCS(ED), FRCR, DO(Hon), FHEA
Professor Emeritus of Clinical Anatomy
Institute of Clinical Education
Warwick Medical School
University of Warwick
Coventry, United Kingdom

Stephen W. Carmichael, PhD, DSc
Professor Emeritus of Anatomy and Orthopedic Surgery
Mayo Clinic
Rochester, Minnesota

ELSEVIER

ELSEVIER

1600 John F. Kennedy Blvd.
Ste. 1800
Philadelphia, PA 19103-2899

GRAY'S ANATOMY REVIEW, SECOND EDITION **ISBN: 978-0-323-27788-4**

Notices

Knowledge and best practice in this field are constantly changing. As new research and experience broaden our understanding, changes in research methods, professional practices, or medical treatment may become necessary.

Practitioners and researchers must always rely on their own experience and knowledge in evaluating and using any information, methods, compounds, or experiments described herein. In using such information or methods they should be mindful of their own safety and the safety of others, including parties for whom they have a professional responsibility.

With respect to any drug or pharmaceutical products identified, readers are advised to check the most current information provided (i) on procedures featured or (ii) by the manufacturer of each product to be administered, to verify the recommended dose or formula, the method and duration of administration, and contraindications. It is the responsibility of practitioners, relying on their own experience and knowledge of their patients, to make diagnoses, to determine dosages and the best treatment for each individual patient, and to take all appropriate safety precautions.

To the fullest extent of the law, neither the Publisher nor the authors, contributors, or editors, assume any liability for any injury and/or damage to persons or property as a matter of products liability, negligence or otherwise, or from any use or operation of any methods, products, instructions, or ideas contained in the material herein.

International Standard Book Number: 978-0-323-27788-4

VP Global Medical Education Content: Madelene Hyde
Senior Content Strategist: Jeremy Bowes
Content Development Specialist: Lauren Boyle
Publishing Services Manager: Patricia Tannian
Senior Project Manager: John Casey
Design Direction: Julia Dummitt

Printed in Canada

Last digit is the print number: 9 8 7 6 5 4 3 2

To my daughter, Nicole, my son, Chris, and my wife,
Joanna, for their continuous support and love

ML

To Kevin, Kendall, and Logan Tubbs—
the perfect family

RST

To "Lucy in the Sky with Diamonds," who puts
up with my early mornings and late nights—
For all the descendants of "Papi and Lulu"

PA

To Susan Stoddard and Allen Carmichael

SC

PREFACE

Rote memorization of anatomic facts has been the cardinal feature of exhaustive, and exhausting, courses in human anatomy for many generations of students in medicine, dentistry, and other allied health science programs. Often, little distinction was made between the wheat and the chaff, and little attention was given to the practical, clinical application of the data. In the face of the modern explosion of information and technical advances in the medical sciences, *Gray's Anatomy for Students* was conceived and written as a clinically oriented, student-friendly textbook of human anatomy. The authors, Richard L. Drake, A. Wayne Vogl, and Adam W. M. Mitchell, have provided a sound basis for student learning and understanding of both normal and altered human anatomy in the clinical setting.

Gray's Anatomy Review was designed for use by students after they have read the textbook and is in keeping with the objectives of a course that uses this textbook. The questions, answers, and explanations in this book are intended to serve multiple purposes for students in various programs.

1. This review provides a thought-provoking source for study by students in preparation for examinations in various programs of gross anatomy.
2. To avoid pointless memorization by the student, all the questions are framed within clinical vignettes that guide the student toward practical applications of the textual material.
3. The multiple-choice, single-best-answer format of the questions is designed to facilitate student review in preparation for the USMLE and similar qualifying examinations.
4. The explanations of the answers emphasize the critical importance of understanding normal and dysfunctional human anatomy.
5. Student understanding is further enhanced by critical examination of alternative, incorrect answers that students might be tempted to choose.
6. Finally, the review provides a succinct distillation of the plethora of facts in clinical anatomy, assisting the student's learning and understanding of important concepts in the practice of medicine, irrespective of the student's career choice.

The questions in this review are correlated with the following textbooks:

- *Gray's Anatomy for Students*, ed 3, by Richard L. Drake, A. Wayne Vogl, and Adam W. M. Mitchell
- *Netter Atlas of Human Anatomy,* ed 6, by Frank Netter
- *McMinn's and Abrahams' Clinical Atlas of Human Anatomy,* ed 7, by Peter H. Abrahams, Jonathan D. Spratt, Marios Loukas, and Albert N. Van Schoor

Each answer is referenced to pages in Gray's *(GAS)*, Netter's *(N)* and McMinn's *(McM)*.

For the embryology chapter we have correlated the clinical vignettes with *Before We Are Born: Essentials of Embryology and Birth Defects*, ed 8, by Keith L Moore, TVN Persaud, and Mark G. Torchia.

We have incorporated or adapted many drawings, full-color illustrations, and radiographic images in an attempt to accelerate the learning process and to enhance understanding of both the anatomy and the clinical applications. The primary sources on which we have drawn for illustrative material are from *McMinn's and Abrahams' Clinical Atlas of Human Anatomy.*

ACKNOWLEDGMENTS

A clinical review book is the work not only of the authors but also of numerous scientific and clinical friends and colleagues who have been so generous with their knowledge and given significant feedback and help. This book would not have been possible were it not for the contributions of the colleagues and friends listed below.

A very special group of medical students, members of the Student Clinical Research Society at the Department of Anatomical Sciences at St. George's University, helped enormously with the completion of this project through their comments and criticism of each chapter as part of the advisory board of this book.

Advisory Board
Nkosi Alvarez *(Neck)*
Meha Bhargava *(Pelvis and Perineum)*
Liann Chin Casey *(Lower Limb)*
Rana Chakrabarti *(Upper Limb)*
Ramya Chitters *(Embryology)*
Monica Dandapani *(Abdomen)*
Piyumika De Silva *(Upper Limb)*
Uta Guo *(Embryology)*
Rich Hajjar *(Abdomen)*
Roland Howard *(Lower Limb)*
Lijo C. Illipparambi *(Upper Limb)*
Theofannis Kollias *(Upper Limb)*
Jun Lee *(Back)*
Olivia Lu *(Lower Limb)*
Prateek Mathur *(Head)*
Spiro Mavromatis *(Neck)*
Lewis Musoke *(Lower Limb)*
Anastasiya Nelyubina *(Pelvis and Perineum)*
Georgia Paul *(Pelvis and Perineum)*
Tony Sadek *(Thorax)*
Shanojan Thiyagalingam *(Back)*
David Thornton *(Abdomen)*
Randy Tigue *(Head)*
Ryan Uyan *(Thorax)*
Lindsey Van Brunt *(Head and Neck)*
Danielle Van Patten *(Head and Neck)*

The following professors from the Department of Anatomical Sciences at St. George's University have also been very helpful with their comments and criticism as part of the advisory board:

Emanuel Baidoo, MD
Feisal Brahim, PhD
Kathleen Bubb, MD
Danny Burns, MD, PhD
James Coey, MBBS
Maira Du Plessis, MSc
Francis Fakoya, MD, PhD
Deon Forrester, MD
Iketchi Gbenimacho, MD
Rachael George, MD
Robert Hage, MD, PhD
Robert Jordan, PhD
Ahmed Mahgoud, MD
Ewarld Marshall, MD
Vid Persaud, MD, PhD
Kazzara Raeburn, MD
Ramesh Rao, MD
Vish Rao, PhD
Deepak Sharma, MD
Alena Wade, MD

Dr. Anthony D'Antoni, PhD, Clinical Professor and Director of Anatomy at The City College of New York (CUNY), has always been a great friend and colleague. His continuous support, comments, criticism, and enthusiasm have contributed enormously to the completion of this project.

We are especially thankful to Ms. Madelene Hyde, publisher at Elsevier, for her invaluable insights, advice, and encouragement.

The authors would also like to thank Jeremy Bowes and Lauren Boyle, our developmental editor, and all the team at Elsevier for guiding us through the preparation of this book.

The authors thank the following individuals and their institutions for kindly supplying various clinical, operative, endoscopic, and imaging photographs:

Dr. Ray Armstrong, Rheumatologist, Southampton General Hospital, Southampton, and Arthritis Research Campaign

Professor Paul Boulos, Surgeon, Institute of Surgical Studies, University College London Medical School, London

Professor Norman Browse, Emeritus Professor of Surgery, and Hodder Arnold Publishers, for permission to use illustrations from *Symptoms and Signs of Surgical Disease,* 4th edition, 2005.

Mr. John Craven, formerly Consultant Surgeon, York District Hospital, York

Professor Michael Hobsley, formerly Head of the Department of Surgical Studies, The Middlesex Hospital Medical School, London

Mr. Ralph Hutchings, photographer for Imagingbody .com

Mr. Umraz Khan, Plastic Surgeon, Charing Cross Hospital, London

Professor John Lumley, Director, Vascular Surgery Unit, St. Bartholomew's and Great Ormond Street Hospitals, London

Dr. J. Spratt, Consultant Radiologist, University Hospital of North Durham

Dr. William Torreggiani, Radiologist, The Adelaide and Meath Hospital, Tallaght, Dublin

Miss Gilli Vafidis, Ophthalmologist, Central Middlesex Hospital, London

Mr. Theo Welch, Surgeon, Fellow Commoner Queens' College, Cambridge

Professor Jamie Weir, Department of Clinical Radiology, Grampian University Hospitals Trust, Aberdeen, Scotland, and editor of *Imaging Atlas of Human Anatomy,* 3rd edition, Elsevier, 2003.

CONTENTS

Bonus Online-Only Content—To see a list of objectives for each question in the book, activate your title on www.StudentConsult.Inkling.com using the pin code on the inside front cover

1 BACK

INTRODUCTION

First Order Question

1 A 35-year-old man is admitted to the emergency department after a severe car crash. After examining the patient the emergency medicine physician concludes that the serratus anterior muscle is damaged. Which of the following nerves innervates the serratus anterior muscle?

- ▢ **A.** Long thoracic
- ▢ **B.** Axillary
- ▢ **C.** Spinal accessory
- ▢ **D.** Dorsal scapular
- ▢ **E.** Thoracodorsal

Explanation

A: The long thoracic is the only nerve that innervates the serratus anterior. The axillary nerve innervates the deltoid, the spinal accessory nerve innervates the sternocleidomastoid and trapezius, the dorsal scapular nerve supplies the rhomboid muscles and levator scapulae, and the latissimus dorsi is the muscle supplied by the thoracodorsal nerve.

First Order Question

2 A 35-year-old man is admitted to the emergency department after a severe car crash. After examining the patient the emergency medicine physician concludes that the serratus anterior muscle is damaged. Which of the following functions does the serratus anterior muscle serve?

- ▢ **A.** Adducts scapula
- ▢ **B.** Depresses ribs
- ▢ **C.** Protraction and rotation of scapula
- ▢ **D.** Elevation of scapula
- ▢ **E.** Adducts, extends, and medially rotates arm

Explanation

C: The functions of the serratus anterior are protraction and rotation of the scapula. The rhomboid major and minor adduct the scapula, the serratus posterior inferior depresses the lower ribs, the levator scapulae elevates the scapula, and the latissimus dorsi adducts, extends, and medially rotates the arm.

Second Order Question

3 A 35-year-old man is admitted to the emergency department after a severe car crash. After examining the patient the emergency medicine physician concludes that the serratus anterior muscle is damaged. Which of the following functions will the patient most likely be unable to perform?

- ▢ **A.** Retraction of the scapula
- ▢ **B.** Elevation of the scapula
- ▢ **C.** Depression of the scapula

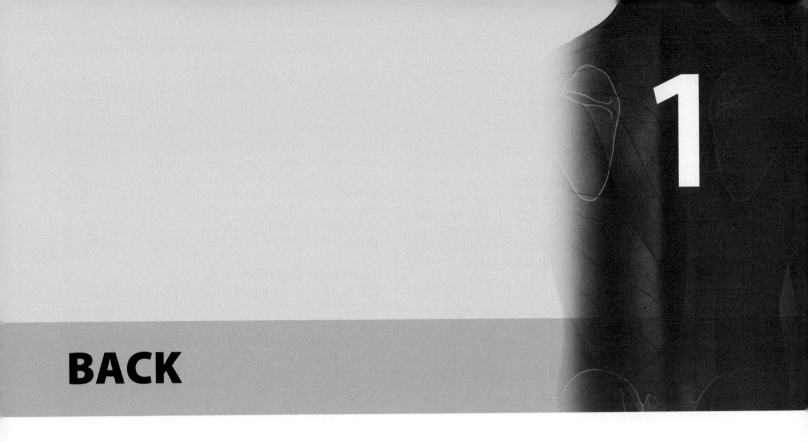

- ▢ **D.** Protraction of the scapula
- ▢ **E.** Medial rotation of the scapula

Explanation
D: The serratus anterior muscle pulls the scapula forward (protraction) over the thoracic wall. Elevation of the scapula is carried out mainly by the trapezius and levator scapulae muscles while depression is performed primarily by the lower fibers of the trapezius. Different muscles contribute to the movement of the scapula such as the serratus anterior, trapezius, levator scapulae, rhomboids, and pectoralis minor.

Second Order Question

4 A 35-year-old man is admitted to the emergency department after a severe car crash. During physical examination of the patient the emergency medicine physician observes a winged scapula. Which of the following muscles is most likely injured?

- ▢ **A.** Levator scapulae
- ▢ **B.** Serratus anterior
- ▢ **C.** Trapezes
- ▢ **D.** Rhomboid major and minor
- ▢ **E.** Serratus posterior superior

Explanation
B: The serratus anterior muscle pulls the scapula forward (protraction) and keeps the costal surface of the scapula closely opposed to the thoracic wall, preventing "winging" of the scapula. The levator scapulae elevates the scapula. The trapezius muscle is a powerful elevator of the shoulder and also rotates the scapula during reaching overhead. The rhomboid major and minor elevate and retract the scapula.

Second Order Question

5 A 35-year-old man is admitted to the emergency department after a severe car crash. While performing the physical examination the emergency medicine physician observes a winged scapula. Which of the following nerves is most likely injured?

- ▢ **A.** Long thoracic
- ▢ **B.** Axillary
- ▢ **C.** Spinal accessory
- ▢ **D.** Dorsal
- ▢ **E.** Thoracodorsal

Explanation
A: The long thoracic nerve innervates the serratus anterior muscle, which protracts and upwardly rotates the scapula. Persons with injury to this nerve will have their scapulae protrude on their back like a wing. The axillary nerve supplies the deltoid and teres minor muscles. The deltoid abducts, flexes, and extends while the teres minor laterally rotates the arm. The spinal accessory nerve is responsible for supplying the trapezius and sternocleidomastoid muscles. The trapezius elevates and upwardly rotates the scapula while the sternocleidomastoid flexes and pulls the chin upward to the opposite side. The dorsal scapular nerve supplies the rhomboid major and minor muscles and are responsible for retraction of the scapula. The thoracodorsal nerve supplies the latissimus dorsi muscle, which adducts, medially rotates, and extends the arm.

Third Order Question

6 A 35-year-old man is admitted to the emergency department after a severe car crash. The emergency medicine physician examines the patient and observes what is shown in Figure 1-1. Which of the following nerves is most likely injured?

- ▢ **A.** Long thoracic
- ▢ **B.** Axillary
- ▢ **C.** Spinal accessory
- ▢ **D.** Dorsal
- ▢ **E.** Thoracodorsal

Explanation
A: The long thoracic nerve innervates the serratus anterior muscle, which protracts the scapula, holds the

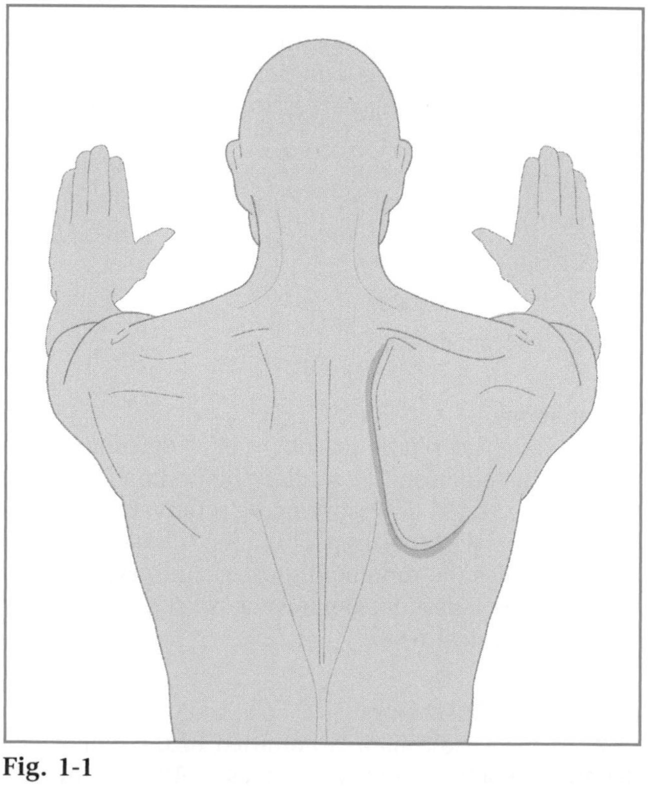

Fig. 1-1

scapula close to the thoracic wall preventing it from "winging", and abducts and upwardly rotates the scapula. Patients with injury to this nerve will have their scapulae protruding on their back like a wing. The axillary nerve supplies the deltoid and teres minor muscles. The deltoid abducts, flexes, and extends and the teres minor laterally rotates the arm. The spinal accessory nerve is responsible for supplying the trapezius and sternocleidomastoid muscles. The trapezius elevates and upwardly rotates the scapula while the sternocleidomastoid flexes and pulls the chin upward to the opposite side. The dorsal scapular nerve supplies the rhomboid major and minor muscles and are responsible for retraction of the scapula. The thoracodorsal nerve supplies the latissimus dorsi muscle, which adducts, medially rotates, and extends the arm.

Fourth Order Question

7 A 35-year-old man is admitted to the emergency department after a severe car crash. The emergency medicine physician examines the patient and observes what is shown in Figure 1-1. Which of the following functions will the patient most likely be unable to perform during physical examination?

- ☐ **A.** Lateral rotation of the shoulder joint
- ☐ **B.** Abduction of the shoulder joint from 0 to 90 degrees
- ☐ **C.** Flexion of the shoulder joint
- ☐ **D.** Extension of the shoulder joint
- ☐ **E.** Abduction of the shoulder joint above 90 degrees

Explanation

E: In this image, the patient has a winged scapula. This occurs as a result of damage to the long thoracic nerve, which innervates the serratus anterior muscle. The functions of this muscle are protraction of the scapula and superior rotation of the glenoid fossa. The supraspinatus abducts the arm for about the first 12 degrees, and then the deltoid abducts the arm to about 90 degrees. Elevating the arm further requires rotation of the scapula (including superior rotation of the glenoid fossa) that is normally done by the serratus anterior.

MAIN QUESTIONS

1 A 55-year-old man with severe coughing is admitted to the hospital. Radiologic examination is consistent with tuberculosis of the right lung, with extension to the thoracic vertebral bodies of T6 and T7, producing a "gibbus deformity." Which of the following conditions is most likely also to be confirmed by radiologic examination?

- ☐ **A.** Hyperlordosis
- ☐ **B.** Hyperkyphosis
- ☐ **C.** Scoliosis
- ☐ **D.** Spina bifida
- ☐ **E.** Osteoarthritis

2 A 68-year-old man is admitted to the hospital due to severe back pain. Radiologic examination reveals severe osteoporosis of the vertebral column, with compression fractures to vertebrae L4 and L5. Which of the following parts of the vertebrae are most likely to be fractured in this patient?

- ☐ **A.** Spinous process
- ☐ **B.** Vertebral bodies
- ☐ **C.** Transverse process
- ☐ **D.** Superior articular process
- ☐ **E.** Intervertebral disc

3 A 45-year-old man is admitted to the hospital because of severe pain in the back and lower limb. Radiologic examination reveals spinal canal stenosis syndrome. Which of the following conditions is most likely to be confirmed by a magnetic resonance imaging (MRI) examination?

- ☐ **A.** Hypertrophy of supraspinous ligament
- ☐ **B.** Hypertrophy of interspinous ligament
- ☐ **C.** Hypertrophy of ligamentum flavum
- ☐ **D.** Hypertrophy of anterior longitudinal ligament
- ☐ **E.** Hypertrophy of nuchal ligament

4 A 35-year-old man is admitted to the hospital after a severe car crash. Radiologic examination reveals an injury to the dorsal surface of the neck and a fracture of the medial border of the right scapula. During physical examination, the patient presents with the scapula retracted laterally on the affected side. Which of the following nerves has most likely been injured on that side?

- ☐ **A.** Axillary
- ☐ **B.** Long thoracic
- ☐ **C.** Dorsal scapular
- ☐ **D.** Greater occipital
- ☐ **E.** Suprascapular

5 A 64-year-old man arrived at the clinic with a painful rash and skin eruptions that are localized entirely on one side of his body, closely following the dermatome level of the spinal nerve C7. The patient was diagnosed with the a herpes zoster virus infection known as "shingles." In what structure has the virus most likely proliferated to cause the patient's current condition?

- ☐ **A.** The sympathetic chain
- ☐ **B.** The dorsal root ganglion of the C7 spinal nerve
- ☐ **C.** The lateral horn of the C7 spinal cord segment
- ☐ **D.** The posterior cutaneous branch of the dorsal primary ramus of C7
- ☐ **E.** The ventral horn of the C7 spinal cord segment

6 A 45-year-old woman states that she has experienced moderate pain for 2 years over her left lower back; pain that radiates to her left lower limb. She states that after lifting a case of soft drinks, the pain suddenly became intense. She was admitted to the emergency department. Radiologic examination revealed intervertebral disc herniation between vertebral levels L4 and L5. Which of the following nerves was most likely affected by the disc herniation?

- ☐ **A.** L1
- ☐ **B.** L2
- ☐ **C.** L3
- ☐ **D.** L4
- ☐ **E.** L5

7 A 3-year-old boy is brought by his mother to the emergency department with severe headache, high fever, malaise, and confusion. Radiologic and physical examinations reveal that the patient suffers from meningitis. A lumbar puncture is ordered to confirm the diagnosis. Which vertebral level is the most appropriate location for the lumbar puncture?

- ☐ **A.** T12 to L1
- ☐ **B.** L1 to L2
- ☐ **C.** L2 to L3
- ☐ **D.** L4 to L5
- ☐ **E.** L5 to S1

8 When a lumbar puncture is performed to sample cerebrospinal fluid, which of the following external landmarks is the most reliable to determine the position of the L4 vertebral spine?

- ☐ **A.** The inferior angles of the scapulae
- ☐ **B.** The highest points of the iliac crests
- ☐ **C.** The lowest pair of ribs bilaterally
- ☐ **D.** The sacral hiatus
- ☐ **E.** The posterior inferior iliac spines

9 A 39-year-old man presents with severe neck pain after a whiplash injury, sustained when his car was struck from behind. Radiologic studies reveal trauma to the ligament lying on the anterior surface of the cervical vertebral bodies. Which ligament is most likely disrupted?

- ☐ **A.** Anterior longitudinal ligament
- ☐ **B.** Ligamentum flavum
- ☐ **C.** Nuchal ligament
- ☐ **D.** Posterior longitudinal ligament
- ☐ **E.** Transverse cervical ligament

10 A 65-year-old man complains of severe back pain and the inability to move his left lower limb. Radiologic studies demonstrate compression of nerve elements at the intervertebral foramen between vertebrae L5 and S1. Which structure is most likely responsible for this space-occupying lesion?

- ☐ **A.** Anulus fibrosus
- ☐ **B.** Nucleus pulposus
- ☐ **C.** Posterior longitudinal ligament
- ☐ **D.** Anterior longitudinal ligament
- ☐ **E.** Ligamentum flavum

11 A 27-year-old man is admitted to the emergency department after a car crash. Physical examination reveals weakness during medial rotation and adduction of the humerus. Which of the following nerves was most probably injured?

- ☐ **A.** Thoracodorsal
- ☐ **B.** Axillary
- ☐ **C.** Dorsal scapular
- ☐ **D.** Spinal accessory
- ☐ **E.** Radial

12 A 39-year-old woman complains of an inability to reach the top of her head to brush her hair with her right hand. History reveals that she had undergone a mastectomy procedure of her right breast 2 months earlier. Physical examination demonstrates winging of her right scapula. Which nerves were most likely damaged during surgery?

- ☐ **A.** Axillary
- ☐ **B.** Spinal accessory
- ☐ **C.** Long thoracic
- ☐ **D.** Dorsal scapular
- ☐ **E.** Thoracodorsal

13 A 19-year-old man is brought to the emergency department after dislocating his shoulder while playing football. Following treatment of the dislocation, he cannot initiate abduction of his arm. An MRI of the affected shoulder shows a torn muscle. Which muscle was most likely damaged by the injury?

- ☐ **A.** Coracobrachialis
- ☐ **B.** Long head of the triceps brachii
- ☐ **C.** Pectoralis minor
- ☐ **D.** Supraspinatus
- ☐ **E.** Teres major

14 A 1-year-old girl is brought to the clinic for a routine checkup. The child appears normal except for a dimpling of the skin in the midline of the lumbar region with a tuft of hair growing over the dimple. What is this relatively common condition that results from incomplete embryologic development?

- ☐ **A.** Meningomyelocele
- ☐ **B.** Meningocele
- ☐ **C.** Spina bifida occulta
- ☐ **D.** Spina bifida cystica
- ☐ **E.** Rachischisis

15 A young resident complains of an itch on his back that appears to be caused by an insect bite. Which nerve fibers carry the sensation of a mosquito bite on the back, just lateral to the spinous process of the T4 vertebra?

- ☐ **A.** Somatic afferent
- ☐ **B.** Somatic efferent
- ☐ **C.** Visceral afferent
- ☐ **D.** Visceral efferent
- ☐ **E.** Somatic efferent and visceral afferent

16 A 15-year-old woman was suspected of having meningitis. To obtain a sample of cerebrospinal fluid by spinal tap in the lumbar region (lumbar puncture), the tip of the needle must be placed in which of the following locations?

- ☐ **A.** In the epidural space
- ☐ **B.** Between anterior and posterior longitudinal ligaments
- ☐ **C.** Superficial to the ligamentum flavum
- ☐ **D.** Between arachnoid mater and dura mater
- ☐ **E.** In the subarachnoid space

17 A 19-year-old man is diagnosed with a herniated disc but he has no symptoms of spinal cord injury. In the event of intervertebral disc herniation in the cervical region, which of the following ligaments is in an anatomic position to protect the spinal cord from direct compression?

- ▢ **A.** Supraspinous
- ▢ **B.** Posterior longitudinal
- ▢ **C.** Anterior longitudinal
- ▢ **D.** Ligamentum flavum
- ▢ **E.** Nuchal ligament

18 In spinal anesthesia, the needle is often inserted between the spinous processes of the L4 and L5 vertebrae to ensure that the spinal cord is not injured. This level is safe because in the adult the spinal cord usually terminates at the disc between which of the following vertebral levels?

- ▢ **A.** T11 and T12
- ▢ **B.** T12 and L1
- ▢ **C.** L1 and L2
- ▢ **D.** L2 and L3
- ▢ **E.** L3 and L4

19 A 22-year-old woman is diagnosed with Raynaud's disease. In such a case, the patient suffers chronic vasospasm in response to cold. This can lead to arterial constriction and painful ischemia, especially in the fingers or toes. Relief from the symptoms in the hands would require surgical division of which of the following neural elements?

- ▢ **A.** Lower cervical and upper thoracic sympathetic fibers
- ▢ **B.** Lower cervical and upper thoracic ventral roots
- ▢ **C.** Lower cervical and upper thoracic dorsal roots
- ▢ **D.** Lower cervical and upper thoracic spinal nerves
- ▢ **E.** Bilateral spinal accessory nerves

20 A 69-year-old woman visits her physician due to severe neck pain. Radiologic studies reveal bony growths (osteophytes) in the intervertebral foramen between vertebrae C2 and C3. Which of the following muscles would be most likely affected by this condition?

- ▢ **A.** Rhomboideus major
- ▢ **B.** Serratus anterior
- ▢ **C.** Supraspinatus
- ▢ **D.** Diaphragm
- ▢ **E.** Latissimus dorsi

21 A 42-year-old woman is diagnosed with stenosis of the cervical vertebral canal. A laminectomy of two vertebrae is performed. Which of the following ligaments will most likely also be removed?

- ▢ **A.** Anterior longitudinal
- ▢ **B.** Denticulate
- ▢ **C.** Ligamentum flavum
- ▢ **D.** Nuchal
- ▢ **E.** Cruciate

22 A 28-year-old pregnant woman is admitted to the obstetrics department for delivery. In the final stages of labor, a caudal anesthetic is administered via the sacral hiatus. Into which of the following spaces in the sacral canal is the anesthetic placed?

- ▢ **A.** Vertebral canal
- ▢ **B.** Vertebral venous plexus
- ▢ **C.** Epidural space
- ▢ **D.** Subarachnoid space
- ▢ **E.** Subdural space

23 A 12-year-old child was brought to the emergency department by his parents because he has been suffering from a very high fever and severe stiffness in his back. The initial diagnosis is meningitis. The attending physician orders a lumbar puncture to confirm the diagnosis. Upon microscopic examination of the cerebrospinal fluid, hematopoietic cells are seen. Which of the following ligaments was most likely penetrated by the needle?

- ▢ **A.** Supraspinous
- ▢ **B.** Denticulate
- ▢ **C.** Anterior longitudinal
- ▢ **D.** Posterior longitudinal
- ▢ **E.** Nuchal ligament

24 A 25-year-old male racing car driver is admitted to the emergency department after a severe car crash. Radiologic studies reveal damage to the tip of the transverse process of the third cervical vertebra, with a significantly large pulsating hematoma. What artery is the most likely to have been damaged?

- ▢ **A.** Anterior spinal artery
- ▢ **B.** Vertebral artery
- ▢ **C.** Ascending cervical artery
- ▢ **D.** Deep cervical artery
- ▢ **E.** Posterior spinal arteries

25 A 79-year-old man, a retired military veteran, presents to the outpatient clinic with an abnormal curvature of the vertebral column. He complains that it has become increasingly painful to walk around town. Upon physical examination, he has an abnormally increased convexity to his thoracic curvature resulting from osteoporosis. Which of the following is the most likely clinical condition of this patient's spine?

- ☐ **A.** Scoliosis
- ☐ **B.** Hyperkyphosis
- ☐ **C.** Spinal stenosis
- ☐ **D.** Lordosis
- ☐ **E.** Herniated disc

26 A 42-year-old woman complains of pain and stiffness in her neck. She was injured sliding into second base headfirst during her company's softball game. Radiographs reveal no fractures of her spine. However, upon physical examination, her right shoulder is drooping and she has difficulty in elevating that shoulder. If you ordered an MRI, it would most likely reveal soft tissue damage involving which of the following nerves?

- ☐ **A.** Thoracodorsal nerve
- ☐ **B.** Spinal accessory nerve
- ☐ **C.** Dorsal scapular nerve
- ☐ **D.** Greater occipital nerve
- ☐ **E.** Axillary nerve

27 A 53-year-old man was in a head-on vehicle collision that resulted in compression of his spinal cord by the dens (odontoid process) of the axis, with resulting quadriplegia. Which of the following ligaments was most probably torn?

- ☐ **A.** Anterior longitudinal ligament
- ☐ **B.** Transverse ligament of the atlas
- ☐ **C.** Ligamentum flavum
- ☐ **D.** Supraspinous ligament
- ☐ **E.** Nuchal ligament

28 An 18-year-old woman passenger injured in a rollover car crash was rushed to the emergency department. After the patient is stabilized, she undergoes physical examination. She demonstrates considerable weakness in her ability to flex her neck, associated with injury to CN XI. Which of the following muscles is most probably affected by nerve trauma?

- ☐ **A.** Iliocostalis thoracis
- ☐ **B.** Sternocleidomastoid
- ☐ **C.** Rhomboid major
- ☐ **D.** Rhomboid minor
- ☐ **E.** Teres major

29 A 23-year-old man was killed in a high-speed motor vehicle collision after racing his friend on a local highway. When the medical examiner arrives at the scene, it is determined that the most likely cause of death was a spinal cord injury. Upon confirmation by autopsy, the medical examiner officially reports that the patient's cause of death was a fracture of the pedicles of the axis (C2). Breaking of which of the following ligaments would be most likely implicated in this fatal injury?

- ☐ **A.** Ligamentum flavum
- ☐ **B.** Nuchal ligament
- ☐ **C.** Cruciform ligament
- ☐ **D.** Posterior longitudinal ligament
- ☐ **E.** Supraspinous ligament

30 A 65-year-old man is injured when a vehicle traveling at a high rate of speed hits his car from behind. Radiologic examination reveals that two of his articular processes are now locked together, a condition known as "jumped facets." In which region of the spine is this injury most likely to occur?

- ☐ **A.** Cervical
- ☐ **B.** Thoracic
- ☐ **C.** Lumbar
- ☐ **D.** Lumbosacral
- ☐ **E.** Sacral

31 Following a car crash, a 47-year-old woman complains of severe headache and back pain. Radiologic examination reveals bleeding of the internal vertebral venous plexus (of Batson), resulting in a large hematoma. In what space has the blood most likely accumulated?

- ☐ **A.** Subarachnoid space
- ☐ **B.** Subdural space
- ☐ **C.** Central canal
- ☐ **D.** Epidural space
- ☐ **E.** Lumbar cistern

32 A 32-year-old man, an elite athlete, was lifting heavy weights during an intense training session. The athlete felt severe pain radiating to the posterior aspect of his right thigh and leg. The patient was taken to the hospital where MRI revealed a ruptured L4/L5 intervertebral disc. Which nerve is most probably affected?

- ☐ **A.** L3
- ☐ **B.** L4
- ☐ **C.** L2
- ☐ **D.** L5
- ☐ **E.** S1

33 A 24-year-old patient suffered a lower back strain after a severe fall while skiing. MRI studies reveal injury to the muscles responsible for extending and laterally bending the trunk. What arteries provide blood supply for these muscles?

- ☐ **A.** Subscapular
- ☐ **B.** Thoracodorsal
- ☐ **C.** Anterior intercostal
- ☐ **D.** Suprascapular
- ☐ **E.** Posterior intercostal

34 A 22-year-old male soccer player is forced to leave the game following a head-to-head collision with another player. He is admitted to the hospital, and radiologic examination reveals slight dislocation of the atlantoaxial joint. As a result, he experiences decreased range of motion at that joint. What movement of the head would most likely be severely affected?

- ☐ **A.** Rotation
- ☐ **B.** Flexion
- ☐ **C.** Abduction
- ☐ **D.** Extension
- ☐ **E.** Adduction

35 A 42-year-old man is struck in the back, rupturing the internal vertebral venous plexus (of Batson). Radiologic studies reveal a hematoma causing compression of the spinal cord. When aspirating the excess blood, the physician performing the procedure should stop the needle just before puncturing which of the following structures?

- ☐ **A.** Spinal cord
- ☐ **B.** Pia mater
- ☐ **C.** Arachnoid mater
- ☐ **D.** Dura mater
- ☐ **E.** Ligamentum flavum

36 A 35-year-old man pedestrian is crossing a busy intersection and is hit by a truck. He is admitted to the emergency department, and a CT scan reveals a dislocation of the fourth thoracic vertebra. Which of the following costal structures is most likely also involved in the injury?

- ☐ **A.** Head of the fourth rib
- ☐ **B.** Neck of the fourth rib
- ☐ **C.** Head of the third rib
- ☐ **D.** Tubercle of the third rib
- ☐ **E.** Head of the fifth rib

37 A 20-year-old male hiker suffers a deep puncture wound during a fall. Physical examination reveals a lesion between the trapezius and latissimus dorsi muscles on the right lateral side of his back. Upon admission to the hospital, physical examination reveals weak adduction and medial rotation of his arm. Which of the following muscles is most probably injured?

- ☐ **A.** Teres minor
- ☐ **B.** Triceps brachii
- ☐ **C.** Supraspinatus
- ☐ **D.** Infraspinatus
- ☐ **E.** Teres major

38 A 22-year-old man is thrown through a plate glass wall in a fight. Radiologic examination reveals that the lateral border of his right scapula is shattered. He is admitted to the emergency department, and physical examination reveals difficulty laterally rotating his arm. Which of the following muscles is most probably injured?

- ☐ **A.** Teres major
- ☐ **B.** Infraspinatus
- ☐ **C.** Latissimus dorsi
- ☐ **D.** Trapezius
- ☐ **E.** Supraspinatus

39 A 24-year-old woman presents with severe headache, photophobia, and stiffness of her back. Physical examination reveals positive signs for meningitis. The attending physician decides to perform a lumbar puncture to determine if a pathogen is in the cerebrospinal fluid (CSF). What is the last structure the needle will penetrate before reaching the lumbar cistern?

- ☐ **A.** Arachnoid mater
- ☐ **B.** Dura mater
- ☐ **C.** Pia mater
- ☐ **D.** Ligamentum flavum
- ☐ **E.** Posterior longitudinal ligament

40 A 19-year-old presents at the emergency department with high fever, severe headache, nausea, and stiff neck that have persisted for 3 days. The attending physician suspects meningitis and obtains a sample of CSF using a lumbar puncture. From which of the following spaces was the CSF collected?

- ☐ **A.** Epidural space
- ☐ **B.** Subdural space
- ☐ **C.** Subarachnoid space
- ☐ **D.** Pretracheal space
- ☐ **E.** Central canal of the spinal cord

41 A 38-year-old man is admitted to the emergency department after a car collision. During physical examination several lacerations to the back are discovered. Pain from lacerations or irritations of the skin of the back is conveyed to the central nervous system by which of the following?

- ☐ **A.** Dorsal primary rami
- ☐ **B.** Communicating rami
- ☐ **C.** Ventral primary rami
- ☐ **D.** Ventral roots
- ☐ **E.** Intercostal nerves

42 A 66-year-old woman had been diagnosed with a tumor on her spine. She has started to retain urine and is experiencing rectal incontinence. Both of these symptoms are signs of conus medullaris syndrome. At which of the following vertebral levels is the tumor probably located?

- ☐ **A.** L3/L4
- ☐ **B.** L3
- ☐ **C.** L4
- ☐ **D.** T12 to L2
- ☐ **E.** T11

43 Examination of a 3-day-old male infant reveals protrusion of his spinal cord and meninges from a defect in the lower back. Which of the following describes this congenital anomaly?

- ☐ **A.** Avulsion of meninges
- ☐ **B.** Meningitis
- ☐ **C.** Spina bifida occulta
- ☐ **D.** Spina bifida with myelomeningocele
- ☐ **E.** Spina bifida with meningocele

44 A 32-year-old mother complains of serious pain in the coccygeal area some days after giving birth. To determine whether the coccyx is involved, a local anesthetic is first injected in the region of the coccyx and then dynamic MRI studies are performed. Physical examination reveals pain with palpation to the region of the coccyx. The local anesthetic is used to interrupt which of the following nerve pathways?

- ☐ **A.** Visceral afferents
- ☐ **B.** Somatic efferent
- ☐ **C.** Somatic afferent
- ☐ **D.** Sympathetic preganglionic
- ☐ **E.** Parasympathetic preganglionic

45 During a routine physical examination, a 65-year-old man is tested for ease and flexibility of the movements of his lumbar region. Which of the following movements is most characteristic of the intervertebral joints in the lumbar region?

- ☐ **A.** Circumduction
- ☐ **B.** Lateral flexion
- ☐ **C.** Abduction
- ☐ **D.** Adduction
- ☐ **E.** Inversion

46 A 72-year-old man with cancer of the prostate gland presents with loss of consciousness and seizures. A CT scan is performed and a brain tumor is diagnosed. The tumor spread to the brain from the pelvis via the internal vertebral venous plexus (of Batson). What feature of the plexus allows this to happen?

- ☐ **A.** The internal venous plexus contains the longest veins in the body.
- ☐ **B.** The internal venous plexus has valves that ensure one-way movement of blood.
- ☐ **C.** The internal venous plexus is located in the subarachnoid space.
- ☐ **D.** The internal venous plexus is, in general, valveless.
- ☐ **E.** The internal venous plexus is located in the subdural space.

47 A 26-year-old man painting his house slipped and fell from the ladder, landing on the pavement below. After initial examination in the emergency department, the patient is sent to the radiology department. Radiographs reveal that the portion of his left scapula that forms the tip, or point, of the shoulder has been fractured. Which part of the bone was fractured?

- ☐ **A.** Coracoid process
- ☐ **B.** Superior angle of the scapula
- ☐ **C.** Glenoid
- ☐ **D.** Spine of the scapula
- ☐ **E.** Acromion

48 A 43-year-old male construction worker survived a fall from a two-story building but lost all sensation in his lower limbs and was admitted to the hospital for examination and treatment. Radiologic studies revealed that he crushed his spinal cord at vertebral level C6. Which of the following muscles will most likely be paralyzed?

- ☐ **A.** Sternocleidomastoid
- ☐ **B.** Trapezius
- ☐ **C.** Diaphragm
- ☐ **D.** Latissimus dorsi
- ☐ **E.** Deltoid

49 A maternal serum sample with high alpha-fetoprotein alerted the obstetrician to a possible neural tube defect. Ultrasound diagnosis revealed a myelomeningocele protruding from the back of the child. Which of the following is the most likely diagnosis of this congenital anomaly?

- ☐ **A.** Cranium bifida
- ☐ **B.** Spina bifida occulta
- ☐ **C.** Spina bifida cystica
- ☐ **D.** Hemothorax
- ☐ **E.** Caudal regression syndrome

50 A 7-year-old girl who is somewhat obese is brought to the emergency department because of a soft lump above the buttocks. Upon physical examination you note the lump is located just superior to the iliac crest unilaterally on the left side. The protrusion is deep to the skin and pliable to the touch. Which of the following is the most probable diagnosis?

- ☐ **A.** Tumor of the external abdominal oblique muscle
- ☐ **B.** Herniation at the lumbar triangle (of Petit)
- ☐ **C.** Indirect inguinal hernia
- ☐ **D.** Direct inguinal hernia
- ☐ **E.** Femoral hernia

51 A 54-year-old woman is admitted to the emergency department due to increasing back pain over the preceding year. MRI reveals that her intervertebral discs have been compressed. It is common for the discs to decrease in size in people older than 40, and this can result in spinal stenosis and disc herniation. At which locations are the spinal nerves most likely to be compressed?

- ☐ **A.** Between the denticulate ligaments
- ☐ **B.** As they pass through the vertebral foramen
- ☐ **C.** Between the superior and inferior articular facets
- ☐ **D.** Between inferior and superior vertebral notches
- ☐ **E.** Between the superior and inferior intercostovertebral joints

52 A 37-year-old pregnant woman is given a caudal epidural block to alleviate pain during vaginal delivery. Caudal epidural blocks involve injection of local anesthetic into the sacral canal. Which of the following landmarks is most commonly used for the caudal epidural block?

- ☐ **A.** Anterior sacral foramina
- ☐ **B.** Posterior sacral foramina
- ☐ **C.** Cornua of the sacral hiatus
- ☐ **D.** Intervertebral foramina
- ☐ **E.** Median sacral crest

53 A 34-year-old pregnant woman in the maternity ward was experiencing considerable pain during labor. Her obstetrician decided to perform a caudal epidural block. What are the most important bony landmarks used for the administration of such anesthesia?

- ☐ **A.** Ischial tuberosities
- ☐ **B.** Ischial spines
- ☐ **C.** Posterior superior iliac spines
- ☐ **D.** Sacral cornua
- ☐ **E.** Coccyx

54 A 22-year-old man is brought into the emergency department following a brawl in a tavern. He has severe pain radiating across his back and down his left upper limb. He supports his left upper limb with his right hand, holding it close to his body. Any attempt to move the left upper limb greatly increases the pain. A radiograph is ordered and reveals an unusual sagittal fracture through the spine of the left scapula. The fracture extends superiorly toward the suprascapular notch. Which nerve is most likely affected?

- ☐ **A.** Suprascapular nerve
- ☐ **B.** Thoracodorsal nerve
- ☐ **C.** Axillary nerve
- ☐ **D.** Subscapular nerve
- ☐ **E.** Suprascapular nerve and thoracodorsal nerve

55 A 5-year-old boy is admitted to the hospital because of pain in the upper back. Radiologic examination reveals abnormal fusion of the C5 and C6 vertebrae and a high-riding scapula. Which of the following is the most likely diagnosis?

- ☐ **A.** Lordosis
- ☐ **B.** Kyphosis
- ☐ **C.** Scoliosis
- ☐ **D.** Spina bifida
- ☐ **E.** Klippel-Feil syndrome

56 A 53-year-old man is admitted to the emergency department due to severe back pain. MRI examination reveals anterior dislocation of the body of the L5 vertebra upon the sacrum. Which of the following is the most likely diagnosis?

- ☐ **A.** Spondylolysis
- ☐ **B.** Spondylolisthesis
- ☐ **C.** Herniation of intervertebral disc
- ☐ **D.** Lordosis
- ☐ **E.** Scoliosis

57 A male newborn infant is brought to the clinic by his mother and diagnosed with a congenital malformation. MRI studies reveal that the cerebellum and medulla oblongata are protruding inferiorly through the foramen magnum into the vertebral canal. What is this clinical condition called?

- ☐ **A.** Meningocele
- ☐ **B.** Klippel-Feil syndrome
- ☐ **C.** Chiari II malformation
- ☐ **D.** Hydrocephalus
- ☐ **E.** Tethered cord syndrome

58 A 62-year-old woman is admitted to the hospital because of her severe back pain. Radiologic examination reveals that the L4 vertebral body has slipped anteriorly, with fracture of the zygapophysial joint (Fig. 1-2). What is the proper name of this condition?

- ☐ **A.** Spondylolysis and spondylolisthesis
- ☐ **B.** Spondylolisthesis
- ☐ **C.** Crush vertebral fracture
- ☐ **D.** Intervertebral disc herniation
- ☐ **E.** Klippel-Feil syndrome

59 A 40-year-old woman survived a car crash in which her neck was hyperextended when her vehicle was struck from behind. At the emergency department, a plain radiograph of her cervical spine revealed a fracture of the odontoid process (dens). Which of the following was also most likely injured?

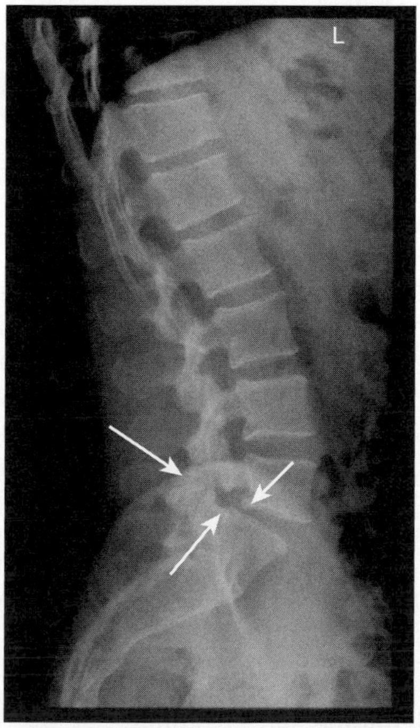

Fig. 1-2

- ☐ **A.** Anterior arch of the atlas
- ☐ **B.** Posterior tubercle of the atlas
- ☐ **C.** Atlanto-occipital joint
- ☐ **D.** Inferior articular process of the axis
- ☐ **E.** Anterior tubercle of the atlas

60 A 34-year-old woman is admitted to the emergency department after a car crash. Radiologic examination reveals a whiplash injury in addition to hyperextension of her cervical spine. Which of the following ligaments will most likely be injured?

- ☐ **A.** Ligamentum flavum
- ☐ **B.** Anterior longitudinal ligament
- ☐ **C.** Posterior longitudinal ligament
- ☐ **D.** Anulus fibrosus
- ☐ **E.** Interspinous ligament

61 A 23-year-old college student is admitted to the emergency department after jumping from a 50-foot high waterfall. The MRI of his back reveals a lateral shift of the spinal cord to the left. Which of the following structures has most likely been torn to cause the deviation?

- ☐ **A.** Posterior longitudinal ligament
- ☐ **B.** Tentorium cerebelli
- ☐ **C.** Denticulate ligaments
- ☐ **D.** Ligamentum flavum
- ☐ **E.** Nuchal ligament

62 A 6-year-old boy is admitted to the hospital with coughing and dyspnea. During taking of the history, he complains that it feels like there is glass in his lungs. Auscultation reveals abnormal lung sounds. The abnormal lung sounds are heard most clearly during inhalation with the scapulae protracted. Which of the following form the borders of a triangular space where one should place the stethoscope in order to best hear the lung sounds?

- ☐ **A.** Latissimus dorsi, trapezius, medial border of scapula
- ☐ **B.** Deltoid, levator scapulae, trapezius
- ☐ **C.** Latissimus dorsi, external abdominal oblique, iliac crest
- ☐ **D.** Quadratus lumborum, internal abdominal oblique, inferior border of the twelfth rib
- ☐ **E.** Rectus abdominis, inguinal ligament, inferior epigastric vessels

63 A 45-year-old woman is admitted to the outpatient clinic for shoulder pain. During physical examination she presents with weakened shoulder movements.

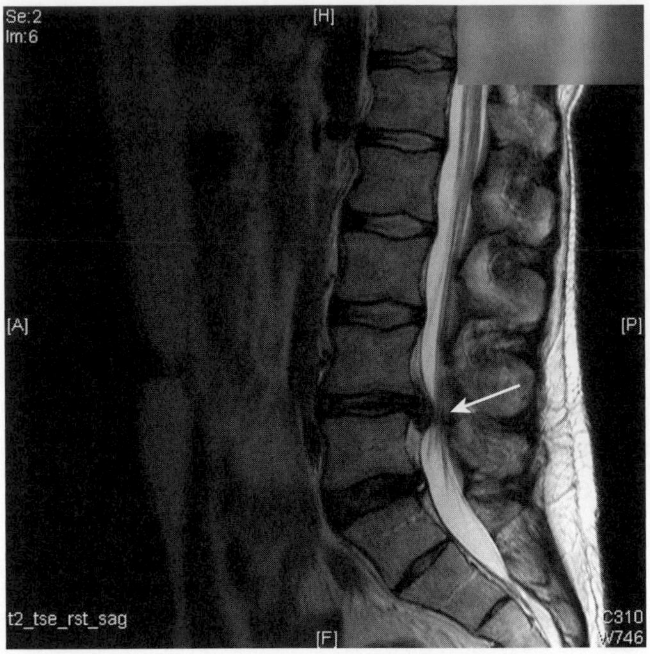

Fig. 1-3

Radiologic examination reveals signs of quadrangular space syndrome, causing weakened shoulder movements. Which of the following nerves is most likely affected?

- ▢ **A.** Suprascapular
- ▢ **B.** Subscapular
- ▢ **C.** Axillary
- ▢ **D.** Radial
- ▢ **E.** Ulnar

64 A 29-year-old female elite athlete was lifting heavy weights during an intense training session. The athlete felt severe pain radiate suddenly to the posterior aspect of her right thigh and leg. The patient was taken to the hospital where an MRI was performed (Fig. 1-3). Which nerve was most probably affected?

- ▢ **A.** L3
- ▢ **B.** L4
- ▢ **C.** L2
- ▢ **D.** L5
- ▢ **E.** S1

65 A 58-year-old man in the intensive care ward exhibited little voluntary control of urinary or fecal activity following repair of an abdominal aortic aneurysm. In addition, physical examination revealed widespread paralysis of his lower limbs. These functions were essentially normal prior to admission to the hospital. The most likely cause of this patient's problems is which of the following?

- ▢ **A.** Injury to the left vertebral artery
- ▢ **B.** Injury of the great radicular artery (of Adamkiewicz)
- ▢ **C.** Ligation of the posterior spinal artery
- ▢ **D.** Transection of the conal segment of the spinal cord
- ▢ **E.** Division of the thoracic sympathetic chain

66 A 23-year-old woman is admitted to the hospital due to back pain. Radiologic examination reveals that she suffers from a clinical condition affecting her vertebral column. Her history reveals that she suffered from polio and has a muscular dystrophy. Which of the following conditions of the vertebral column will most likely be present in this patient?

- ▢ **A.** Hyperlordosis
- ▢ **B.** Hyperkyphosis
- ▢ **C.** Scoliosis
- ▢ **D.** Spina bifida
- ▢ **E.** Osteoarthritis

67 A 26-year-old competitive football player has been complaining of pain, weakness, numbness, and tingling for the past 2 months in his upper limb. Imaging studies reveal a cervical disc herniation compressing the nerve roots and a portion of the spinal cord. An anterior cervical discectomy and fusion (ACDF) surgery is performed. The intervertebral disc is examined upon removal and the anulus fibrosus and nucleus pulposus are severely damaged posterolaterally. What type of cartilage most likely gives the tensile strength of the intervertebral disc?

- ▢ **A.** Hyaline
- ▢ **B.** Elastic
- ▢ **C.** Fibrous
- ▢ **D.** Epiphysial
- ▢ **E.** Elastic and fibrous

68 A 26-year-old competitive football player has been complaining of pain, weakness, numbness, and tingling for the past 2 months in his upper limb. Imaging studies reveal a cervical disc herniation compressing the nerve roots and a portion of the spinal cord. An ACDF surgery is performed. The intervertebral disc is examined upon removal and the nucleus and anulus and nucleus pulposus are severely damaged posterolaterally. What is the embryologic origin of the anulus fibrosus and nucleus pulposus, respectively?

- ▢ **A.** Notochord and neural crest cells
- ▢ **B.** Neural crest cells and ectoderm
- ▢ **C.** Sclerotome and myotome

- ☐ **D.** Mesenchymal cells from sclerotome and neural crest cells
- ☐ **E.** Mesenchymal cells from sclerotome and notochord

69 A 55-year-old woman has suffered from a middle ear infection for the past month. She recently developed right-sided miosis, partial ptosis, anhydrosis, and redness of the conjunctiva. Biopsy examination of which of the following structures would show the cell bodies of neurons affected by this disease?

- ☐ **A.** Anterior gray horn of the spinal cord
- ☐ **B.** Lateral gray horn of the spinal cord
- ☐ **C.** Posterior gray horn of the spinal cord
- ☐ **D.** Spinal ganglia
- ☐ **E.** Lateral column of spinal cord white matter

70 A 62-year-old man is admitted to the emergency department after a severe car crash resulting in a whiplash injury. MRI examination reveals several hairline vertebral fractures in the cervical region impinging the dorsal primary rami of the same levels. Two months after the injury the patient recovered well, however, there is still some weakness in the function of a muscle. Which of the following muscles is most likely affected?

- ☐ **A.** Rhomboid major
- ☐ **B.** Levator scapulae
- ☐ **C.** Rhomboid minor
- ☐ **D.** Semispinalis capitis
- ☐ **E.** Latissimus dorsi

71 A 22-year-old man has suffered from headaches and some muscle weakness to his upper muscles of the back for the last 6 months. An MRI shows a large tumor compressing the suboccipital and greater occipital nerves. Which of the following muscles will most likely still be functioning normally?

- ☐ **A.** Rectus capitis posterior major and minor
- ☐ **B.** Semispinalis capitis
- ☐ **C.** Splenius capitis
- ☐ **D.** Obliquus capitis superior
- ☐ **E.** Obliquus capitis inferior and lateral

72 A 36-year-old man was found guilty of first-degree murder and sentenced to death by judicial hanging. The radiological image below shows the vertebra that is fractured as a result of the hanging. The mechanism of injury resulting in death is forcible hyperextension resulting in a fracture of which of the following structures?

- ☐ **A.** Odontoid process
- ☐ **B.** Transverse process
- ☐ **C.** Lateral mass
- ☐ **D.** Pedicle (pars articularis)
- ☐ **E.** Spinous process

73 A 72-year-old woman presented to her primary care physician after sustaining a fall in her bathroom. Her vital signs were normal and routine blood work was obtained for analysis. As part of her work up, a radiograph of her vertebral column was performed and revealed a wedge fracture at the fourth thoracic vertebra and thin cortical bone showing signs of osteoporotic changes. What will be the most likely type of abnormal spinal curvature in such a patient?

- ☐ **A.** Hyperkyphosis
- ☐ **B.** Scoliosis
- ☐ **C.** Hyperlordosis
- ☐ **D.** Normal
- ☐ **E.** Primary

74 A 65-year-old woman who has been otherwise well presents to her physician with complaints of a group of painful blisters over her back in the distribution of the T9 dermatome. She noticed that a few days prior to the eruption of the blisters she experienced an intense burning sensation over her skin. She was diagnosed with herpes zoster (shingles). Where are the neural cell bodies located that are responsible for the pain sensation?

- ☐ **A.** Dorsal horn
- ☐ **B.** Lateral horn
- ☐ **C.** Dorsal root ganglia
- ☐ **D.** Sympathetic chain ganglia
- ☐ **E.** White rami communicans

75 A 53-year-old man was in a head-on collision resulting in the dens crushing the spinal cord. Which ligament was most likely torn for the dens to crush the spinal cord?

- ☐ **A.** Anterior and posterior longitudinal ligaments
- ☐ **B.** Transverse ligament of the atlas
- ☐ **C.** Interspinous ligament
- ☐ **D.** Supraspinous ligament
- ☐ **E.** Nuchal ligament

76 A 16-year-old girl is sent for a presports physical examination prior to the beginning of her school year. She has no medical complaints or any clinical past history. On physical examination, the physician notices one shoulder is higher than the other. The student is then asked to bend forward at the waist to touch her toes. This maneuver results in a posterior bulging of the ribs on the right side. Which one of the following is most likely diagnosis?

- ▢ **A.** Kyphosis
- ▢ **B.** Spondylosis
- ▢ **C.** Lordosis
- ▢ **D.** Spondylolisthesis
- ▢ **E.** Scoliosis

77 A 60-year-old man has been feeling sharp pains over his left lower chest and back for several days. A rash of red erupted vesicles is seen at the left border of the sternum just at the level of the xiphoid process. Antiviral treatment is given for herpes zoster. Which of the following locations will contain the neural cell bodies responsible for the painful sensation?

- ▢ **A.** Ventral horn of T6 spinal cord segment
- ▢ **B.** Lateral horn of T6 spinal cord segment
- ▢ **C.** Dorsal root ganglion of T4 spinal nerve
- ▢ **D.** Dorsal root ganglion of T6 spinal nerve
- ▢ **E.** Dorsal root ganglion of T10 spinal nerve

78 A 70-year-old man with prostate cancer is experiencing sharp shooting pains radiating from his neck into the upper limb. An MRI of his spine demonstrates a small metastatic mass in the cervical region extending into the left intervertebral foramen between C6 and C7. The intervertebral discs appear normal. Which neural structure is most likely being compressed by the metastatic mass to account for the pain?

- ▢ **A.** C8 spinal nerve
- ▢ **B.** Dorsal horn of C6 spinal cord segment
- ▢ **C.** C6 spinal nerve
- ▢ **D.** Dorsal horn of C7 spinal nerve
- ▢ **E.** C7 spinal nerve

79 A 3-day-old girl develops a fever. She is irritable and not feeding. As part of the workup for fever of unknown origin, a lumbar puncture is performed. This puncture must be done below the spinal cord which usually ends at which vertebral level in a patient of this age?

- ▢ **A.** L1
- ▢ **B.** S1
- ▢ **C.** L3
- ▢ **D.** S3
- ▢ **E.** L5

80 During a surgical procedure to debride an abscess involving the erector spinae muscle at vertebral level T8, the nerve branch supplying the skin and this muscle is unavoidably severed. What are the anatomical locations of the cell bodies of the nerve fibers normally found in this branch?

- ▢ **A.** Ventral horn and dorsal horn
- ▢ **B.** Ventral horn, dorsal horn, and lateral horn
- ▢ **C.** Ventral horn, dorsal root ganglion, and lateral horn
- ▢ **D.** Ventral horn, dorsal root ganglion, and sympathetic paravertebral ganglion
- ▢ **E.** Ventral horn, dorsal horn, and dorsal root ganglion

81 While waiting in his car at a stop sign, a 28-year-old man was rear-ended by a van, resulting in neck hyperextension. He was admitted to the emergency department and a whiplash injury was diagnosed. The next day his neck was stiff and painful. Which structure was most likely damaged to cause the pain?

- ▢ **A.** Anterior longitudinal ligament
- ▢ **B.** Posterior longitudinal ligament
- ▢ **C.** Ligamentum flavum
- ▢ **D.** Intervertebral disc
- ▢ **E.** Supraspinous ligament

82 A 38-year-old man who is a professional golfer complains of chronic lower back pain with radiating pain to the heel. The pain is so debilitating that he now has trouble ambulating. MRI of the lower back reveals severe narrowing of an intervertebral foramen (IVF), which has caused compression of the exiting nerve root. Surgery is required to correct the problem. During surgery the neurosurgeon carefully accesses the IVF using a lateral approach and shaves bone off the superior margin (roof) of the IVF to decompress the exiting nerve root. Which of the following vertebral bony features is the neurosurgeon most likely shaving off?

- ▢ **A.** Superior articular process
- ▢ **B.** Lamina
- ▢ **C.** Inferior articular process
- ▢ **D.** Pedicle
- ▢ **E.** Spinous process

83 The following statement was found in the radiology report of a magnetic resonance imaging scan of the cervical spine: "An acute posterolateral herniation of the most superiorly located intervertebral disc is located within the corresponding intervertebral foramen and compressing the exiting nerve." Which of the following nerves was the radiologist most likely referring to in the report?

- ▢ **A.** C1
- ▢ **B.** C2

- ▢ **C.** C3
- ▢ **D.** C4
- ▢ **E.** C5

84 A 14-year-old girl accidentally flipped her bicycle off a curb, fell, and landed on her face. Although she was wearing a helmet, she landed in such a way that her neck was forced into hyperextension. Which of the following ligaments of the cervical spine was stretched to the greatest degree during her injury?

- ▢ **A.** Posterior longitudinal ligament
- ▢ **B.** Ligamentum nuchae
- ▢ **C.** Ligamenta flava
- ▢ **D.** Supraspinous ligament
- ▢ **E.** Anterior longitudinal ligament

85 An orthopedic surgeon was teaching two residents during a workshop. For the purpose of learning, one resident acted as the patient and the other as the clinician. The surgeon asked the resident-clinician to use a marker and draw a horizontal line connecting the highest points of the iliac crests on the skin of the resident-patient. The surgeon then asked the resident-clinician to palpate the midline area on the skin where the subarachnoid space terminates inferiorly. Which of the following most likely represents the area on the skin where the resident-physician palpated?

- ▢ **A.** Three spinous processes superior to the horizontal line
- ▢ **B.** Two spinous processes inferior to the horizontal line
- ▢ **C.** Three spinous processes inferior to the horizontal line
- ▢ **D.** Two spinous processes superior to the horizontal line
- ▢ **E.** The spinous process bisected by the horizontal line

86 An MRI scan of the thoracic spine of a 68-year-old man with acute midback pain revealed a large tumor arising from the anterior median fissure of the spinal cord at the level of the T3 vertebra. The artery compressed by the tumor is most likely formed superiorly by direct branches from which of the following arteries?

- ▢ **A.** Ascending cervical
- ▢ **B.** Segmental medullary
- ▢ **C.** Vertebral
- ▢ **D.** Segmental spinal
- ▢ **E.** Posterior spinal

87 Radiographs of a 12-year-old girl with midback pain reveal a hemivertebra of the lower thoracic spine. Which additional finding would most likely be demonstrated on the radiographs?

- ▢ **A.** Osteoporosis
- ▢ **B.** Scoliosis
- ▢ **C.** Hyperlordosis
- ▢ **D.** Spondylolisthesis
- ▢ **E.** Sacralization

88 In a report of a radiograph of the cervical spine the radiologist wrote the following: "Severe narrowing of the C7-T1 intervertebral foramen (IVF) on the left." Which nerve was most likely compressed as a result of this finding?

- ▢ **A.** C6
- ▢ **B.** C7
- ▢ **C.** C8
- ▢ **E.** T1

89 A mother brought her 15-month-old previously healthy child to the pediatrician and nervously told the physician that her child now had "a curvature in her low back." The mother stated that this curvature was not present previously and that she noticed it when the child started standing and walking. The physician examined the child and then reassured the mother that the spinal curvature was normal. Which curvature did the mother most likely observe?

- ▢ **A.** Thoracic kyphosis
- ▢ **B.** Cervical lordosis
- ▢ **C.** Lumbar lordosis
- ▢ **D.** Cervical kyphosis
- ▢ **E.** Thoracic lordosis

90 During a gross anatomy laboratory session, a professor demonstrates a large back muscle that inserts onto the floor of the intertubercular sulcus of the humerus. Which of the following structures is most likely the vertebral origin of the muscle that the professor is demonstrating?

- ▢ **A.** Spinous processes of T7 to L5
- ▢ **B.** Spinous processes of C7 to T12
- ▢ **C.** Transverse processes of C1 to C4
- ▢ **D.** Spinous processes of T2 to T5
- ▢ **E.** Spinous processes of C7 and T1

91 A drug that preferentially destroys sclerotomes during embryogenesis would most likely result in underdevelopment of which of the following structures?

- ☐ **A.** Nucleus pulposus of intervertebral disc
- ☐ **B.** Vertebral bodies
- ☐ **C.** Dorsal root ganglion
- ☐ **D.** Spinal cord
- ☐ **E.** Anulus fibrosus of intervertebral disc

92 Which of the following muscles is most likely located immediately deep to the semispinalis muscles, pass from a lateral point of origin in a superomedial direction to attach to spinous processes, and cross between 2 and 4 vertebrae?

- ☐ **A.** Multifidus
- ☐ **B.** Rotatores
- ☐ **C.** Longissimus
- ☐ **D.** Iliocostalis
- ☐ **E.** Spinalis

93 A 32-year-old construction worker falls from a scaffold and is brought to the emergency department with severe lower back pain. Radiographs of the lumbar spine reveal bilateral pars interarticularis fractures of the L5 vertebra. Which of the following radiographic views would most likely reveal these fractures?

- ☐ **A.** Anteroposterior
- ☐ **B.** Lateral
- ☐ **C.** Posteroanterior
- ☐ **D.** Oblique
- ☐ **E.** Anteroposterior open mouth

94 A radiology report of a cervical spine MRI scan contains the following statement: "A small 1-cm tumor is located within a muscle on the lateral border of the right suboccipital triangle." The muscle to which the radiologist is most likely referring inserts on which of the following bony features?

- ☐ **A.** Transverse process of atlas
- ☐ **B.** Lateral portion of occipital bone below inferior nuchal line
- ☐ **C.** Occipital bone between superior and inferior nuchal lines
- ☐ **D.** Medial portion of occipital bone below inferior nuchal line
- ☐ **E.** Posterior tubercle of atlas

95 Radiographs of the lumbar spine of a 68-year-old woman with lower back pain were taken and in the radiology report the following was written: "The anteroposterior view demonstrates marked bilateral enlargement of the transverse processes of a single vertebra. The length and width of both transverse processes of this single vertebra are enlarged and the inferior aspects of these bony features appear to be articulating with the bone immediately below it, so much so that the single vertebra appears to have morphologic characteristics similar to the bone immediately below it." The single vertebra referred to by the radiologist in the report is most likely which of the following?

- ☐ **A.** L1 vertebra
- ☐ **B.** L4 vertebra
- ☐ **C.** S2 vertebra
- ☐ **D.** S1 vertebra
- ☐ **E.** L5 vertebra

96 A 45-year-old man was injured in a motor vehicle crash and brought to the emergency department. Radiographs of the upper cervical spine revealed a type III dens fracture demonstrated by a horizontal radiolucent line on the superior half of the posterior aspect of the C2 vertebral body. Which of the following ligaments most likely has direct attachment to the bony area where the fracture was located?

- ☐ **A.** Apical ligament of dens
- ☐ **B.** Superior longitudinal band of cruciform ligament
- ☐ **C.** Transverse ligament of atlas
- ☐ **D.** Inferior longitudinal band of cruciform ligament
- ☐ **E.** Ligamenta flava

97 A 35-year-old man underwent a laminectomy of the T8 to T9 vertebrae. During the surgery, the neurosurgeon observed that the posterior roots were compressed at that level due to a space-occupying lesion. Which of the following arteries was most likely directly compressed by the lesion?

- ☐ **A.** Radicular
- ☐ **B.** Segmental spinal
- ☐ **C.** Segmental medullary
- ☐ **D.** Anterior spinal
- ☐ **E.** Posterior spinal

98 An 8-year-old girl was brought to a pediatrician for a routine physical examination. The figure associated with this question is a photograph of the child (Fig. 1-4). Which of the following best describes the embryologic basis for this child's condition?

- ☐ **A.** Underdevelopment of the secondary ossification center in the vertebral arch
- ☐ **B.** Underdevelopment of the primary ossification center in the spinous process

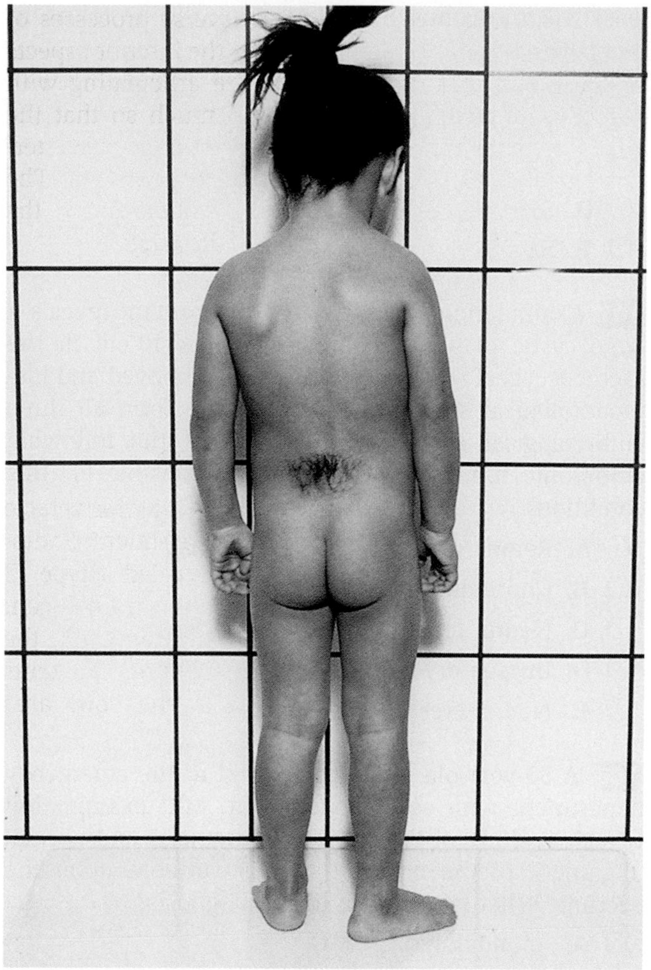

Fig. 1-4

- ▢ **C.** Underdevelopment of the primary ossification center in the vertebral body
- ▢ **D.** Underdevelopment of the secondary ossification center in the vertebral body
- ▢ **E.** Underdevelopment of the primary ossification center in the vertebral arch

99 The following statement is written in the radiology report of an MRI scan of the cervical spine: "A large osteophyte is emanating from the posterolateral area of the vertebral body of the vertebra immediately above the C3 nerve root and is severely compressing the C3 nerve root." The osteophyte is most likely emanating from which of the following vertebrae?

- ▢ **A.** C2
- ▢ **B.** C3
- ▢ **C.** C4
- ▢ **D.** C5
- ▢ **E.** C1

100 A 38-year-old woman has been in labor for 14 hours and has agreed to have an epidural anesthetic injection for pain control. Which of the following structures is most likely to be the last penetrated by the needle before it reaches the epidural space?

- ▢ **A.** Supraspinous ligament
- ▢ **B.** Interspinous ligament
- ▢ **C.** Anterior longitudinal ligament
- ▢ **D.** Posterior longitudinal ligament
- ▢ **E.** Ligamenta flava

101 A 48-year-old man underwent suboccipital surgery whereby the surgeon made a midline incision through the ligamentum nuchae that began 1-cm inferior to the external occipital protuberance and ended at the level of the C2 vertebra. The surgeon then placed self-retaining retractors into the incision to forcibly separate the tissue so that an adequate surgical field existed for the duration of the surgery which lasted for 3 hours. During recovery, the patient complained of severe occipital pain and was diagnosed with postsurgical occipital neuralgia. Which of the following nerves was most likely directly stretched by the retractors during the surgery and resulted in this patient's post-surgical pain?

- ▢ **A.** Third occipital
- ▢ **B.** Suboccipital
- ▢ **C.** Greater occipital
- ▢ **D.** Lesser occipital
- ▢ **E.** Spinal accessory

102 A 7-year-old boy is undergoing a surgery to remove a tumor from his spinal cord. During surgery of the spinal cord, which of the following structures is used as a landmark to identify anterior rootlets from posterior rootlets?

- ▢ **A.** Denticulate ligament
- ▢ **B.** Filum terminale
- ▢ **C.** Conus medullaris
- ▢ **D.** Posterior longitudinal ligament
- ▢ **E.** Ligamenta flava

103 A 45-year-old male driver involved in a motor vehicle crash was taken to the emergency department and MRI revealed a complete tear of the right alar ligament. None of the other ligaments of the upper cervical spine were torn. Upon physical examination, which of the following cervical spine movements will be most likely increased as a result of the tear?

- ▢ **A.** Flexion
- ▢ **B.** Extension
- ▢ **C.** Lateral flexion

- ☐ **D.** Rotation
- ☐ **E.** Abduction

104 A 25-year-old male bodybuilder complains of difficulty moving his right shoulder for the past 2 weeks. Upon physical examination, the muscles of the left upper back and shoulder were notably larger than the right side. There was a notable decrease of muscle power on his right sided upper back and shoulder muscles when he was asked to pull the shoulder blades toward the middle of his back against resistance. Nerve conduction examination confirmed neurapraxia of the nerves supplying the rhomboid major and minor muscles. In which of the following functions will the bodybuilder most likely also demonstrate weakness?

- ☐ **A.** Abduction of the right arm above the horizontal level and protraction of the scapula
- ☐ **B.** Medial rotation and adduction of the right arm
- ☐ **C.** Extensions, adduction, and medial rotation of the right arm
- ☐ **D.** Elevation of the scapula and inferior rotation of the right shoulder
- ☐ **E.** Abduction of the right arm from 0 to 15 degrees

105 A 38-year-old woman with a history of carcinoma of the left breast and who had had a lumpectomy 2 years previously, presents to her surgeon with complaints of a hard mass in the left breast. On ultrasound examination, a 3 cm × 4 cm hard mass is discovered in the upper outer quadrant extending in the axillary tail (of Spence). A radical mastectomy is performed successfully and the tumor is removed. Three weeks postoperatively the patient complains of difficulty raising her left arm above her head. Which of the following is most likely expected to be found during physical examination?

- ☐ **A.** Protraction of the both scapulae
- ☐ **B.** Protrusion of the medial border of the left scapula when hands are pushed against the wall
- ☐ **C.** Weak abduction of the left upper limb in the 15 to 90 degree range
- ☐ **D.** Weak retraction of the scapula
- ☐ **E.** Weak adduction of the humerus

106 A 2-month-old infant is admitted to the emergency department with symptoms of meningitis. A lumbar puncture is performed in order to examine the CSF to confirm the diagnosis. The needle is inserted into the lumbar cistern (dural sac). At which vertebral level will the conus medullaris typically be found in this patient?

- ☐ **A.** L3
- ☐ **B.** L4
- ☐ **C.** L5
- ☐ **D.** S1
- ☐ **E.** S2

107 Examination of a 3-day-old male infant reveals a large cystic of approximately 15 cm × 10 cm in the sacrococcygeal region. The mass was removed and histopathological studies identified tissue from all three embryological germ layers. Which of the following embryonic tissues is most likely responsible for this condition?

- ☐ **A.** Remnants of the primitive streak
- ☐ **B.** Chorionic villi
- ☐ **C.** Neural folds
- ☐ **D.** Intraembryonic coelom
- ☐ **E.** Neural crest

108 A 53-year-old man is admitted to the emergency department with severe back pain. MRI examination reveals fracture of the pars interarticularis and normal alignment of the body of the L5 vertebra upon the sacrum. What is the most likely diagnosis?

- ☐ **A.** Spondylolysis
- ☐ **B.** Spondylolisthesis
- ☐ **C.** Herniation of intervertebral disc
- ☐ **D.** Lordosis
- ☐ **E.** Scoliosis

109 A 22-year-old pregnant woman underwent epidural anesthesia in anticipation of labor. After delivery she developed back pain and right lower extremity weakness. Imaging revealed a hematoma in the epidural space resulting in compression of the nerve that exits at the level of L2 to L3. Which of the following vessels is most likely responsible for the hematoma?

- ☐ **A.** Internal vertebral plexus
- ☐ **B.** Great radicular artery (of Adamkiewicz)
- ☐ **C.** Anterior spinal artery
- ☐ **D.** Posterior spinal artery
- ☐ **E.** External vertebral plexus

110 Idling at a stoplight in his vintage car without headrests, a 71-year-old-man's car is struck from behind by a truck. The man is brought to the emergency department suffering from a severe hyperextension neck injury due to the crash. The T2-weighted MRI shows a rupture of the anterior anulus fibrosus of the C4 to C5 intervertebral disc and a prevertebral hematoma which compromised his airway and required intubation. Which of the following ligaments is most likely disrupted in this injury?

- ☐ **A.** Anterior longitudinal ligament
- ☐ **B.** Posterior longitudinal ligament
- ☐ **C.** Ligamentum flavum
- ☐ **D.** Interspinous ligament
- ☐ **E.** Intertransverse ligament

111 An anesthesiologist administers epidural anesthetic immediately lateral to the spinous processes of vertebrae L3 and L4 of a pregnant woman in labor. During this procedure, what would be the last ligament perforated by the needle in order to access the epidural space?

- ☐ **A.** Ligamentum flavum
- ☐ **B.** Anterior longitudinal ligament
- ☐ **C.** Posterior longitudinal ligament
- ☐ **D.** Interspinous ligament
- ☐ **E.** Intertransverse ligament

112 A 38-year-old man presents to the emergency department with complaints of lower back pain during the past 5 days. Examination revealed tenderness of the spine over the L5 vertebra with an obvious "step-off" defect at that level. There was some weakness of the limbs. An MRI examination revealed an anterior displacement of the L5 vertebral body and narrowing of the vertebral canal. This pathology will most likely be associated with which of the following?

- ☐ **A.** Compression of the spinal cord and bilateral lower limb weakness
- ☐ **B.** Compression of the spinal cord and unilateral lower limb weakness
- ☐ **C.** Compression of the spinal nerve roots and L5 with unilateral lower limb weakness
- ☐ **D.** Compression of the cauda equina and bilateral lower limb weakness
- ☐ **E.** Compression of the cauda equina and low back pain only

113 A 62-year-old man visits his physician for his annual medical check-up. During physical examination it is noted that the patient has noticeable pulsations on palpation of the lower abdomen. Ultrasound examination reveals a large abdominal aortic aneurysm. The patient is operated on and during the repair his aorta is temporarily clamped. Which of the following arterial anastomoses will most likely prevent ischemia of the spinal cord if the blood pressure drops dangerously low?

- ☐ **A.** Segmental arteries from the vertebral, intercostals, superficial epigastric, lumbar, and medial sacral arteries
- ☐ **B.** Segmental arteries from the vertebral, intercostal, lumbar, spinal anterior, and posterior and lateral sacral arteries
- ☐ **C.** Anterior and posterior spinal arteries
- ☐ **D.** Radicular arteries of the vertebral, lumbar, intercostal, lateral sacral arteries, and artery of Adamkiewicz
- ☐ **E.** Segmental arteries from vertebral and intercostals

114 A 22-year-old woman is diagnosed with the presence of a chondroma at her index finger. Which of the following structures are sharing the same embryologic with the tumor?

- ☐ **A.** Denticulate ligament
- ☐ **B.** Dentate ligament
- ☐ **C.** Nucleus pulposus
- ☐ **D.** Apical ligament of the atlas
- ☐ **E.** Alar ligament

115 A 40-year-old woman survived a car crash in which her neck was hyperextended when her vehicle was struck from behind. At the emergency department a plain radiograph of her cervical spine is shown below (Fig. 1-5). Which of the following was also most likely injured?

- ☐ **A.** Anterior arch of the atlas
- ☐ **B.** Posterior tubercle of the atlas
- ☐ **C.** Atlanto-occipital joint
- ☐ **D.** Inferior articular process of the axis
- ☐ **E.** Anterior tubercle of the atlas

116 A 32-year-old man was lifting heavy weights during an intense training session. He felt severe pain radiating to the posterior aspect of his right thigh and leg. He was taken to hospital where an MRI scan (see Fig. 1-3) revealed a ruptured intervertebral disc. Which of the following nerves was most likely affected?

- ☐ **A.** L2
- ☐ **B.** L3
- ☐ **C.** L4
- ☐ **D.** L5
- ☐ **E.** S1

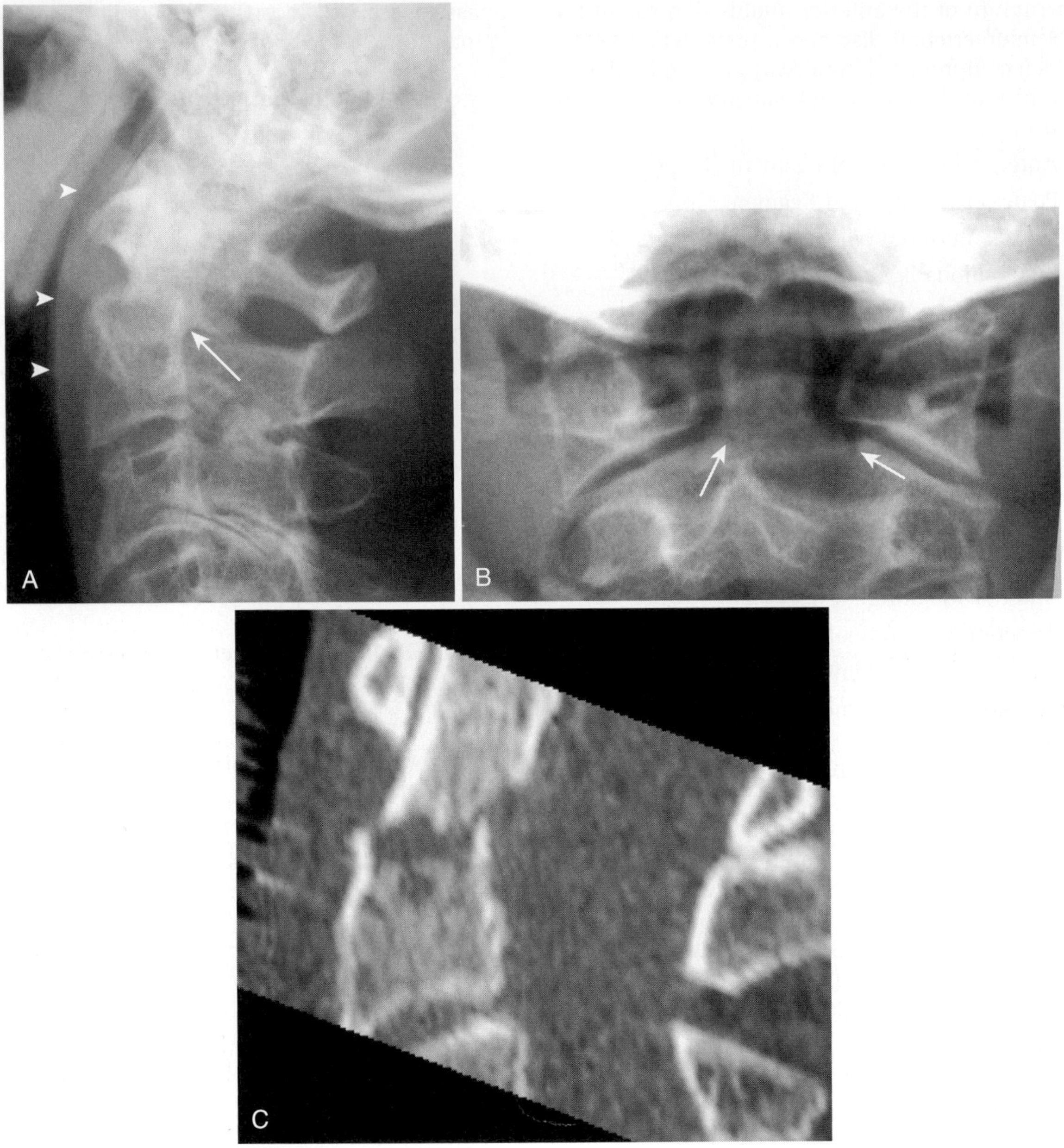

Fig. 1-5

ANSWERS

1 B. Hyperkyphosis is characterized by a "hunchback" due to an abnormal increase in curvature of the thoracic region of the vertebral column. Hyperlordosis, or "swayback," is an increase in lumbar curvature of the spine. Lordosis can be physiologic, such as seen in a pregnant woman. Scoliosis is a lateral curvature of the spine with rotation of the vertebrae. Spina bifida is a neural tube defect characterized by failure of closure of the vertebral arch. Osteoarthritis is a degenerative disorder that affects the articular cartilage of joints and is not specifically related to the thoracic region of the spine.

GAS 76; N 153; McM 97

2 B. A crush fracture is characterized by compression of the entire vertebral body. The wedge fracture is similar in that it affects the vertebral bodies, but it involves small fractures around the perimeter of the vertebral body. Both of these fractures cause reductions in overall height. Fracture of the spinal, transverse, or superior articular processes can be due to an oblique, transverse, or comminuted fracture.

Intervertebral discs are associated with disc herniation, not compression fractures.
GAS 82; N 153-154; McM 88, 107

3 C. The ligamentum flavum connects the laminae of two adjacent vertebrae and forms the posterior wall of the vertebral canal. It is the only answer choice that is in direct contact with the vertebral foramen. Therefore, hypertrophy of only the ligamentum flavum would present as spinal canal stenosis. The supraspinous and interspinous ligaments connect spinous processes. The anterior longitudinal ligament connects the anterior portion of the vertebral bodies and intervertebral discs. Finally, the nuchal ligament is a thickened extension of the supraspinous ligament above the level of C7.
GAS 84; N 159; McM 99

4 C. The dorsal scapular nerve (from the ventral ramus of C5) is responsible for innervating rhomboids major and minor. The rhomboids are responsible for retraction of the scapula. Therefore, if this nerve is damaged, individuals present with a laterally displaced scapula. In this case, the levator scapulae remains functional due to additional innervation provided by C3 to C4 spinal nerves. The axillary nerve innervates the deltoid and teres minor muscles. The deltoid muscle abducts the humerus, and the teres minor laterally rotates the humerus. The long thoracic nerve innervates the serratus anterior, which functions to protract and upwardly rotate the scapula. The greater occipital nerve is mainly sensory but also contributes to the innervation of the semispinalis capitis. In addition, the greater occipital nerve can be involved in occipital neuralgias. The suprascapular nerve innervates the supraspinatus and infraspinatus muscles. The supraspinatus abducts the humerus, and the infraspinatus muscles laterally rotate the humerus. Injury to any of these other nerves would not present with a laterally retracted scapula.
GAS 90; N 174; McM 133

5 B. Herpes zoster is a viral disease that remains latent in the dorsal root ganglia of the sensory nerves and when the virus becomes active presents as a painful skin lesion. It is associated only with sensory nerve fibers and has no motor involvement. The only answer choice that is solely responsible for sensory innervation is the dorsal root ganglion.
GAS 109; N 161-162; McM 95

6 E. Disc herniation in the lumbar region between L4 and L5 affects the L5 spinal nerve roots. Even though the L4 spinal nerve root lies directly between the L4 and L5 vertebrae, it exits from the spinal canal superior to the intervertebral disc, whereas the L5 spinal nerve root lies directly posterior to the disc.
GAS 79; N 161; McM 97

7 D. A lumbar puncture is performed by taking a sample of CSF from the lumbar cistern (the subarachnoid space below the spinal cord) between vertebrae L4 and L5 or sometimes between L3 and L4. It is done in this region because the spinal cord typically ends at the level of L1 to L2 and the dural sac ends at the level of S2. Therefore, it is the safest place to do the procedure because it lies between these areas and the risk of injuring the spinal cord is minimized. (Remember in children the cord ends more caudally.)
GAS 116; N 160-161; McM 97

8 B. The highest points of the iliac crests are used as a landmark for locating the position of L4 to L5 for a lumbar puncture; they are identified and traced medially toward the vertebral column (Tuffier's line). The inferior angles of the scapulae lie at vertebral level T7; the lowest ribs lead one to T12; the sacral hiatus is located lower at the distal portion of the sacrum; the posterior inferior iliac spines lie below S2.
GAS 106, 114-116; N 160-161; McM 97

9 A. The anterior longitudinal ligament lies anterior to the vertebral bodies along the vertebral column. The ligamentum flavum connects the laminae of two adjacent vertebrae. The nuchal ligament is a continuation of the supraspinous ligament above C7, which connects spinous processes. The posterior longitudinal ligament lies on the posterior margin of the vertebral bodies. The transverse cervical (cardinal) ligament is associated with the pelvic region of the body and not the spinal column (*GAS* Figs. 2-31 and 2-34).
GAS 80; N 159; McM 98

10 B. Compression of nerves at the intervertebral foramen indicates a disc herniation. A disc herniation is characterized by protrusion of the nucleus pulposus through the anulus fibrosus posterolaterally into the spinal canal or intervertebral foramen. In general, the ligaments may be affected by the herniation but are not responsible for the compression of the spinal nerve roots.
GAS 79; N 158; McM 99

11 A. The thoracodorsal nerve innervates the latissimus dorsi, one of major muscles that adduct and medially rotate the humerus. The axillary nerve

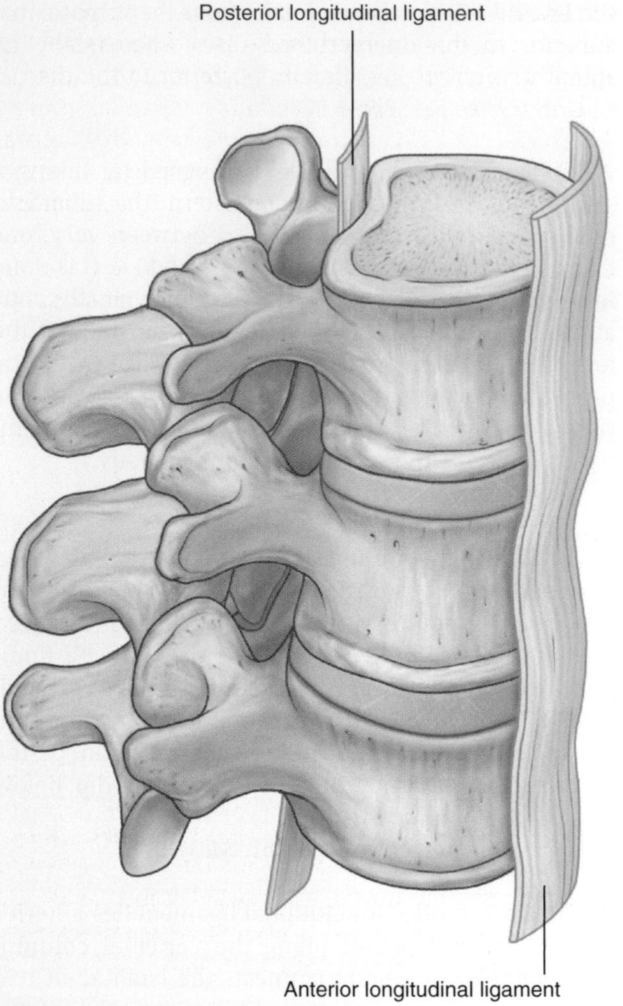

GAS Fig. 2-31

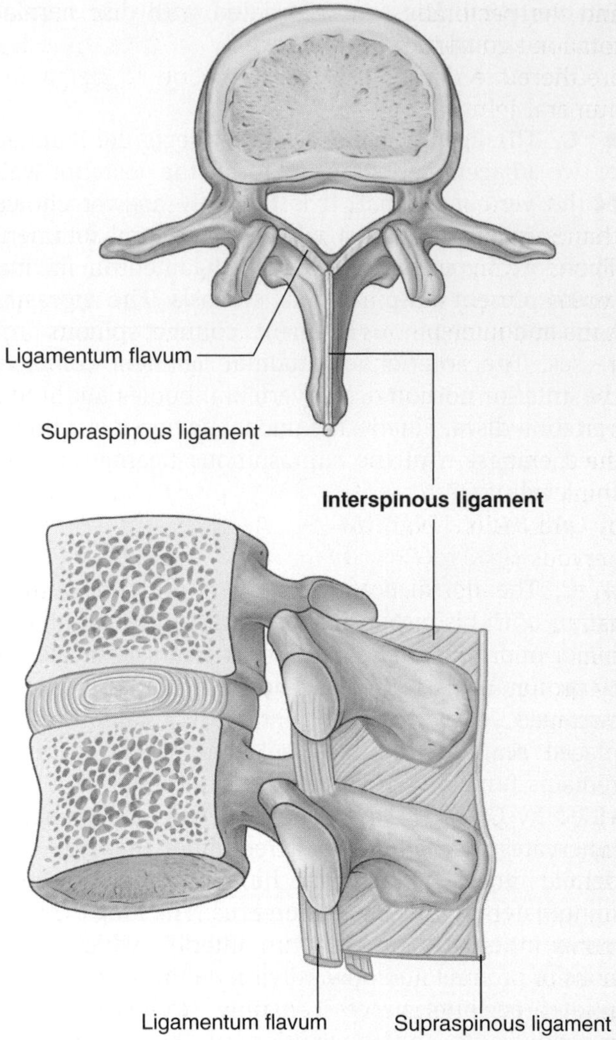

GAS Fig. 2-34

supplies the deltoid muscle, the dorsal scapular nerve supplies the rhomboids and levator scapulae muscles, and the spinal accessory nerve innervates the trapezius. None of these nerves medially rotates or adducts the humerus. The radial nerve is responsible for the innervation on the posterior aspect of the arm and forearm. The medial and lateral pectoral nerves and the lower subscapular nerve supply the other medial rotators of the humerus.

GAS 87, 99; N 174; McM 101

12 **C.** The long thoracic nerve innervates the serratus anterior, which is responsible for elevation and protraction of the scapula beyond the horizontal level while maintaining its position against the thoracic wall. Along with the thoracodorsal nerve, the long thoracic nerve runs superficially along the thoracic wall and is subject to injury during a mastectomy procedure. The axillary nerve, the spinal accessory nerve, and the thoracodorsal nerve supply the deltoid muscle, trapezius muscle, and latissimus dorsi muscles, respectively. The dorsal scapular nerve is responsible for innervation of the rhomboids and levator scapulae. Aside from the long thoracic and thoracodorsal nerves, the remaining nerves do not course along the lateral thoracic wall.

GAS 726; N 180, 413; McM 140

13 **D.** The rotator cuff muscles are common sites of damage during shoulder injuries. These muscles include the supraspinatus, infraspinatus, teres minor, and subscapularis (SITS). Initiation of abduction of the humerus (the first 15 degrees) is performed by the supraspinatus, followed by the deltoid from 15 to 90 degrees. Above the horizontal, the scapula is rotated by the trapezius and serratus anterior muscles, causing the glenoid fossa to turn superiorly and allowing the humerus to move above 90 degrees. The teres major and the pectoralis major are responsible for medial rotation and adduction of the humerus. These muscles are therefore not involved in abduction at the glenohumeral joint.

GAS 711-712, 717; N 134-135; McM 411, 413

14 C. Spina bifida is a developmental condition resulting from incomplete fusion of the vertebral arches within the lumbar region. Spina bifida occulta commonly presents asymptomatically with midline, lumbar, cutaneous stigmata such as a tuft of hair and a small dimple. More severe forms (spina bifida cystica) are categorized into three types: Spina bifida cystica with meningocele presents with protrusion of the meninges through the unfused vertebral arches; spina bifida with myelomeningocele is characterized by protrusion both of the meninges and central nervous system (CNS) tissues and is often associated with neurologic deficits; and rachischisis, also known as spina bifida cystica with myeloschisis, results from a failure of neural folds to fuse and is characterized by protrusion of the spinal cord or spinal nerves and meninges.

GAS 74; N 14, 160; McM 77, 88

15 A. Somatic afferents are responsible for conveying pain, pressure, touch, temperature, and proprioception to the CNS. Afferent fibers carry only sensory stimuli, whereas efferent fibers convey motor information. Visceral innervation is associated with the autonomic nervous system. Visceral afferents generally carry information regarding the physiologic changes of the internal viscera whereas visceral efferents deliver autonomic motor function to three types of tissue: smooth muscle, cardiac muscle, and glandular epithelium.

GAS 32-35; N 174; McM 211

16 E. CSF is found within the subarachnoid space and is continuous with the ventricles of the brain (CSF flows from the ventricles to the subarachnoid space). The epidural space, positioned between the dura mater and periosteum, contains fat and the internal vertebral venous plexus (of Batson). The subdural space, between the arachnoid mater and dura mater, exists only as a potential space and does not contain cerebrospinal fluid. The anterior and posterior longitudinal ligaments traverse the length of the vertebral bodies.

GAS 106, 114-116; N 166; McM 97

17 B. The posterior longitudinal ligament is the only ligament spanning the posterior aspect of the vertebral bodies and intervertebral discs. With intervertebral disc herniation, the nucleus pulposus of the intervertebral disc protrudes posterolaterally. The anterior longitudinal ligament traverses the anterior side of the vertebral bodies and thus would not protect the spinal cord from direct compression. The supraspinous and ligamentum flavum ligaments connect the spinous processes and the laminae of adjacent vertebrae, respectively. The nuchal ligament is a continuation of the supraspinous ligaments near the C7 vertebrae and runs to the occipital protuberance.

GAS 80-81; N 159; McM 94

18 C. This is the location of the conus medullaris, a tapered conical projection of the spinal cord at its inferior termination. Although the conus medullaris rests at the level of L1 and L2 in adults, it is often situated at L3 in newborns. The cauda equina and filum terminale extend beyond the conus medullaris.

GAS 99, 100; N 161; McM 97

19 A. The sympathetic division of the autonomic nervous system is primarily responsible for vasoconstriction. Separation of ventral or dorsal roots would lead to undesired consequences, such as a loss of motor or sensory activity. Similarly, surgical division of spinal nerves would also have unwanted consequences, but such are not related to the increased arterial constriction and the painful ischemia in the digits. Division of selected sympathetic chain ganglia, however, would decrease the sympathetic outflow to the upper limbs.

GAS 38-39; N 163; McM 94-95

20 D. The diaphragm is innervated by the phrenic nerve, which arises from C3 to C5. The rhomboid, serratus anterior, supraspinatus, and latissimus dorsi are innervated by the ventral rami of the brachial plexus (C5 to T1).

GAS 161-162; N 161; McM 194

21 C. The anterior longitudinal ligament runs along the anterior-most aspect of the vertebral column from C1 to the sacrum and would therefore be unaffected by a laminectomy. Denticulate ligaments extend laterally from the pia mater to the arachnoid mater along the length of the spinal cord. The ligamentum flavum is one of the two ligaments found in the vertebral canal and is adherent to the anterior aspect of the vertebral arches and often greatly thickened in spinal pathology. It is thus simultaneously removed upon excision of the lamina. The nuchal ligament is a thick longitudinal extension continuing from the supraspinous ligament at the level of C7 to the external

occipital protuberance (inion). The cruciate ligament is an incorrect answer because it is located anterior to the spinal cord, and thus would not be involved in laminectomy.
GAS 80; N 159; McM 98

22 C. The vertebral canal is the longitudinal canal that extends through the vertebrae, containing the meninges, spinal cord, and associated ligaments. The internal vertebral venous plexus is the mostly valveless network of veins extending longitudinally along the vertebral canal. Neither of these answer choices describes a specific space. The spinal epidural space is found superficially to the dura mater. It is a fat-filled space extending from C1 to the sacrum. The subarachnoid space is a true space containing CSF. It is found within the CNS and extends to the level of S2. The subdural space is a potential space between the dura and the arachnoid mater. Normally, these two layers are fused due to the pressure of CSF in the subarachnoid space.
GAS 103-110; N 166; McM 94, 96

23 A. Lumbar puncture is generally performed at the level of L4 or L5. The supraspinous ligament extends between spinous processes on the dorsal aspect of the vertebrae. The needle will bypass this structure. The denticulate ligaments are not correct because they terminate with the conus medullaris at the level of L2 and are located laterally. The anterior longitudinal ligament extends along the most anterior aspect of the vertebral bodies and can be reached only ventrally. The posterior longitudinal ligament is present at the correct vertebral level but will be punctured only if the procedure is performed incorrectly as in this case, where hematopoietic cells were aspirated from the vertebral body anterior to the ligament. The nuchal ligament extends cranially from the supraspinous ligament in the lower cervical region to the skull.
GAS 103-110; N 159; McM 94, 96

24 B. The anterior spinal artery is located anteriorly along the spinal cord and is not directly associated with the vertebrae. The vertebral arteries run through the transverse foramina of cervical vertebrae C6 through C1 and are therefore most closely associated with injury to the transverse processes. The ascending cervical artery is usually a very small branch from the thyrocervical trunk of the subclavian artery, running on the anterior aspect of the vertebrae. The deep cervical artery arises from the costocervical trunk and is also a very small artery and courses along the posterior aspect of the cervical vertebrae. The posterior spinal arteries are adherent to the posterior aspect of the spinal cord.
GAS 100; N 167; McM 94-95

25 B. Scoliosis is defined as a lateral deviation of the spinal column to either side. Hyperkyphosis is an increased primary curvature of the spinal column. This curvature is associated with thoracic and sacral regions and is most likely this patient's clinical condition. Spinal stenosis is a narrowing of the vertebral canal and is not directly associated with a displacement of the spinal column. Hyperlordosis is the increased secondary curvature affecting the cervical and lumbar regions. A herniated disc is a rupture of the anulus fibrosus of the intervertebral disc, commonly causing a posterolateral displacement of the nucleus pulposus into the vertebral canal.
GAS 75; N 153; McM 87

26 B. The thoracodorsal nerve innervates the latissimus dorsi, which has no direct action on the shoulder girdle. The spinal accessory nerve is the eleventh cranial nerve (CN XI) and innervates both the trapezius and sternocleidomastoid muscles. The loss of CN XI results in drooping of the shoulder due to paralysis of the trapezius. In addition to the clinical findings of the MRI, one can test the innervation of this nerve by asking the patient to shrug his or her shoulders against resistance (testing the trapezius), as well as turning his or her head against resistance (testing the sternocleidomastoid). The dorsal scapular nerve usually innervates the levator scapulae muscle and the rhomboid muscles. The greater occipital nerve is primarily a sensory nerve innervating the posterolateral aspect of the scalp. The axillary nerve is a branch of the brachial plexus and innervates the deltoid and teres minor muscles. It is not involved in shoulder elevation.
GAS 87, 99; N 171; McM 101

27 B. The anterior longitudinal ligament runs on the anterior aspect of the vertebrae and is not affected. The transverse ligament of the atlas anchors the dens laterally to prevent posterior displacement of the dens. This ligament has been torn in this injury. The ligamentum flavum is found on the posterior aspect of the vertebral canal and does not contact the anteriorly placed dens. The supraspinous ligament is located along the spinous processes of the vertebrae. The nuchal ligament is a longitudinal extension of the supraspinous ligament above the level of C7.
GAS 80; N 159; McM 97

28 B. The iliocostalis thoracis muscle is found in the deep back and functions to maintain posture. It is not associated with neck flexion. The sternocleidomastoid muscle is innervated by CN XI and functions in contralateral rotation (unilateral contraction) and flexion (bilateral contraction) of the neck. Rhomboid major and minor are both innervated by the dorsal scapular nerve and serve to adduct the scapulae. Teres major is innervated by the lower subscapular nerve and serves to medially rotate and adduct the humerus.

GA 93-97; N 171; McM 101

29 **C.** The pedicles are bony structures connecting the vertebral arches to the vertebral body. The ligamentum flavum runs on the posterior aspect of the vertebral canal and is more closely associated with the laminae than to the pedicles of the vertebrae. The nuchal ligament is a longitudinal extension of the supraspinous ligament from C7 to the occiput, both running on the most posterior aspect of the vertebrae along the spinous processes. The cruciform (also called cruciate or transverse ligament of the atlas) ligament is a stabilizing ligament found at the skull base and C1/C2. It attaches to the pedicles and helps stabilize the dens. The posterior longitudinal ligament extends the length of the anterior aspect of the vertebral canal and is anterior to the pedicles.

GAS 68-69; N 23; McM 85

30 **A.** Spondylolysis is the anterior displacement of one or more vertebrae. This is most commonly seen with the cervical vertebrae because of their small size and structure and the oblique angle of the articular facets. Lumbar vertebrae are somewhat susceptible to this problem because of the pressures at lower levels of the spine and the sagittal angles of the articular facets. It is much less common in the thoracic vertebrae due to the stabilizing factor of the ribs. It is not seen in the sacral vertebrae because they are fused together.

GAS 82-83; N 153; McM 86

31 **D.** The internal vertebral plexus (of Batson) surrounds the dura mater in the spinal epidural space; hence the bleeding would cause the hematoma in that space. The subarachnoid space, containing the CSF, is located between pia and arachnoid mater. A subarachnoid hemorrhage would most likely result from a ruptured intercerebral aneurysm. A subdural hematoma would result most likely from a venous bleed from a torn cerebral vein as it enters the superior sagittal venous sinus within the skull. The central canal is located within the gray matter of the spinal cord. The lumbar cistern is an enlargement of the subarachnoid space between the conus medullaris of the spinal cord and the caudal end of the subarachnoid space.

GAS 102; N 169; McM 108

32 **D.** In the lumbar region spinal nerves exit the vertebral column below their named vertebrae. In an L4, L5 intervertebral disc herniation, the L5 spinal nerve would be affected as it descends between L4, L5 vertebrae to exit below the L5 level. L2, L3, and L4 spinal nerves have already exited above the level of herniation; therefore, they would not be affected by this herniation. An "L6" spinal nerve normally does not exist. (The National Board of Medical Examiners does not allow "made up" structures, but in cases of lumbarization of S1, some people recognize an L6 nerve.)

GAS 79, 108; N 161; McM 97

33 **E.** Posterior intercostal arteries supply the deep back muscles, which are responsible for extending and laterally bending the trunk. The subscapular artery supplies the subscapularis muscle, the thoracodorsal artery supplies the latissimus dorsi, the anterior intercostal supplies the upper nine intercostal spaces, and the suprascapular artery supplies the supraspinatus and infraspinatus muscles. These muscles are not responsible for extension and lateral flexion of the trunk.

GAS 100-101; N 168; McM 102

34 **A.** The atlantoaxial joint is a synovial joint responsible for rotation of the head, not flexion, abduction, extension, or adduction. The atlanto-occipital joint is primarily involved in flexion and extension of the head on the neck.

GAS 71; N 19; McM 85

35 **D.** The internal vertebral plexus (of Batson) lies external to the dura mater in the epidural space. To aspirate excess blood, the physician must pass the needle through the ligamentum flavum to reach the epidural space wherein the blood would accumulate. The spinal cord, pia mater, and arachnoid mater are located deep to the epidural space.

GAS 102; N 169; McM 97

36 **E.** The T4 thoracic vertebra articulates with the head of the fifth rib. The head of the rib has two facets. The rib articulates with the superior facet on the body of its own vertebra (the fourth rib articulates with the superior facet T4 vertebra) and with the inferior facet on the body of the vertebra above (the fourth rib articulates with the inferior facet of T3 vertebra). Taking the T4 vertebra into consideration, the superior facet of this vertebra articulates with the head of the fourth rib and the inferior facet articulates with the head of the fifth rib. The head of the fourth rib has two points of articulation (a joint with the vertebral body and a costotransverse joint) on T4, so when it is injured it moves as a unit, whereas the fifth rib has only one articulation with T4.

GAS 124; N 183; McM 174

37 E. The teres major is responsible for adduction and medial rotation of the humerus, the teres minor is responsible for lateral rotation of the humerus, the triceps brachii is responsible for extension of the forearm, the supraspinatus is responsible for the first 0 to 15 degrees of abduction, and the infraspinatus is a lateral rotator.

GAS 717; N 171; McM 103

38 B. The infraspinatus is responsible for lateral rotation of the humerus (along with the teres minor, not a choice here). The teres major is responsible for adduction and medial rotation of the humerus. The latissimus dorsi is responsible for adduction, extension, and medial rotation of the humerus. The trapezius is an elevator of the scapula and rotates the scapula during abduction of the humerus above the horizontal plane. The supraspinatus is responsible for the first 0 to 15 degrees of abduction.

GAS 717; N 171; McM 102

39 A. When a lumbar puncture is performed, the needle must penetrate the ligamentum flavum, the dura mater, and finally the arachnoid mater to reach the subarachnoid space where the CSF is located. The lumbar cistern is a continuation of the subarachnoid space below the conus medullaris. The pia mater is adherent to the spinal cord, and the posterior longitudinal ligament is attached to the posterior aspect of the vertebral bodies.

GAS 106, 114-116; N 161; McM 97

40 C. The subarachnoid space, containing the CSF, is located between the pia and the arachnoid mater. Neither the epidural space, the subdural space, nor the pretracheal space contains CSF. Although the central canal, contained within the substance of the spinal cord, does contain CSF, extraction of CSF from this space would result in spinal cord injury. CSF circulates within the subarachnoid space and can be aspirated only from that location. The subdural space is only a potential space between the dura and arachnoid mater. The epidural space contains the epidural fat and Batson's venous plexus and is the site to inject an anesthetic for epidural anesthesia. CSF is not located in the pretracheal space.

GAS 106; N 166; McM 97

41 A. General somatic afferent fibers are conveyed from the skin of the back via the dorsal primary rami. Communicating rami contain general visceral efferent (sympathetic) fibers and general visceral afferent fibers of the autonomic nervous system. Ventral primary rami convey mixed spinal nerves to/from all other parts of the body excluding the back, and parts of the head innervated by cranial nerves. The ventral roots contain only efferent (motor) fibers. Intercostal nerves are the ventral rami of T1 to T11. The ventral ramus of T12 is the subcostal nerve.

GAS 32-48; N 177; McM 98

42 D. The conus medullaris is usually located at the L1 to L2 vertebral level; therefore, any choice that contains that region is the correct answer. L3 to L4 is a common location to perform lumbar puncture, but it is caudal to the apex of the conus medullaris. L3 and L4 are caudal to the conus medullaris. T11 is superior to the conus medullaris.

GAS 99-110; N 161, 163, 164; McM 97

43 D. Because the meninges and spinal cord are included in the protrusion, the patient's condition is a classic presentation of spina bifida with myelomeningocele. If the protrusion contains only meninges but no CNS tissue, it is known as spina bifida with meningocele. Meningitis is an inflammation of the meninges caused by bacteria, viral, or numerous other irritants (e.g., blood). It does not cause deformation of the vertebrae or result in protrusion of spinal cord contents. Spina bifida occulta is a normally asymptomatic condition in which the vertebral laminae fail to fuse completely during embryologic development. A tuft of hair is commonly seen growing over the affected region (usually lumbar in position).

GAS 74; N 160; McM 97

44 C. Somatic afferent fibers convey localized pain, typically from the body wall and limbs. Visceral afferents convey autonomic nervous system sensory information. Pain from these fibers will present as dull and diffuse. Somatic efferent fibers convey motor information to skeletal muscle. Sympathetic preganglionic fibers are visceral efferent fibers and do not contain sensory information. Parasympathetic preganglionic fibers are also visceral efferents and do not contain sensory information.

GAS 32-48; N 174; McM 97

45 **B.** Lateral flexion is the best answer because other movements of the lumbar portion of the vertebral column are very limited due to the orientation of the articular facets.
GAS 64-73; N 155; McM 97

46 **D.** Batson's venous plexus, in general, is a valveless network of veins located in the epidural space of the vertebral canal. The lack of valves can provide a route for the metastasis of cancer (e.g., from prostate or breast to brain) because the flow of blood is bidirectional due to local pressures. The length of Batson's plexus is irrelevant to the question. B is incorrect because Batson's plexus, in general, does not have valves or one-way movement of blood. Batson's plexus is located within the epidural space, not the subarachnoid or subdural spaces.
GAS 102; N 169; McM 88

47 **E.** The acromion (the highest point of the shoulder) is the part of the scapula that forms the "point" of the shoulder. The coracoid process is located more medially. The superior angle of the scapula is located near the midline of the back. The glenoid of the scapula articulates with the head of the humerus to form the glenohumeral joint. The spine of the scapula is located posteriorly and separates supraspinous and infraspinous fossae.
GAS 702-711; N 183; McM 110

48 **D.** All of the spinal nerves from C6 and below will be affected. The trapezius and sternocleidomastoid muscles will be intact because they are innervated by the spinal accessory nerve. The deltoid will be affected because its nerve motor supply is from the axillary nerve derived from C5 and C6. The diaphragm will work properly as its motor nerve supply is derived from the phrenic nerve (C3 to C5).
GAS 89; N 171; McM 102

49 **C.** Spina bifida cystica refers to spina bifida with a meningocele or myelomeningocele and is the correct answer. Cranium bifida could present with meningocele in the skull, but it would not be located in the lower back. Spina bifida occulta is a defect in the formation of the vertebral arches and does not usually present with meningocele. Hemothorax refers to blood accumulation in the pleural space surrounding the lungs. Caudal regression syndrome presents with loss or deformation of the distal part of the spine and/or spinal cord and is not related to a meningocele or myelomeningocele, in general.
GAS 74; N 160; McM 97

50 **B.** The lumbar triangle (of Petit) is bordered medially by the latissimus dorsi, laterally by the external abdominal oblique, and inferiorly by the iliac crest. The floor of Petit's triangle is formed by the internal abdominal oblique, and this is a possible site of herniation. An indirect inguinal hernia is located in the inguinal canal of the anterior abdominal wall. A direct inguinal hernia is located in Hesselbach's triangle of the anterior abdominal wall. A femoral hernia occurs below the inguinal ligament. Answer A is not the best answer because this lump is described as soft and pliable, which would not likely indicate a tumor, as tumors tend to be hard masses.
GAS 84-89; N 171; McM 101

51 **D.** This question tests anatomic knowledge relating to typical vertebra and the spinal cord. Intervertebral disc herniations occur when the nucleus pulposus of the intervertebral disc protrudes through the anulus fibrosus into the intervertebral foramen or vertebral canal. The most common protrusion is posterolaterally, where the anulus fibrosus is not reinforced by the posterior longitudinal ligament. The inferior and superior vertebral notches frame the intervertebral foramen, so this is the most likely location of compression. The denticulate ligaments are lateral extensions of pia mater that anchor to the dura mater, and help maintain the spinal cord in position within the subarachnoid space. The vertebral foramen is the canal through which the spinal cord passes; while this may also be a place of compression, it is not the most likely site of herniation. Articular facets are the locations where vertebral bodies articulate with each other. Intercostovertebral joints are locations where vertebral bodies articulate with ribs.
GAS 99-110; N 166; McM 98

52 **C.** Caudal anesthesia is used to block the spinal nerves that carry sensation from the perineum. This procedure is commonly used by anesthesiologists to relieve pain during labor and childbirth. Administration of local anesthetic to the epidural space is via the sacral hiatus, which opens between the sacral cornua. The anterior sacral foramina are located on the pelvic surface of the sacrum and are not palpable from a dorsal approach. The posterior sacral foramina and intervertebral foramina are the openings through which sacral nerves exit and are not palpable landmarks. The median sacral crest is cranial to the injection site.
GAS 106-110; N 152; McM 90

53 **D.** The sacral cornua lie on either side of the sacral hiatus, from which one can gain access to the sacral canal. This is the best landmark for administration of anesthesia. The ischial tuberosities are more commonly used as landmarks for a pudendal nerve block. The ischial spines are only palpated intravaginally. The posterior superior iliac spines, though palpable, are not proximal enough for an epidural block within the sacral canal. The coccyx is not part of the sacral canal.

GAS 106-110; N 152; McM 90

54 A. The suprascapular nerve passes through the suprascapular notch, deep to the superior transverse scapular ligament. This nerve is most likely affected in a fracture of the scapula as described in the question. The thoracodorsal nerve runs behind the axillary artery and lies superficial to the subscapularis muscle and would therefore be protected. The axillary nerve passes posteriorly through the quadrangular space, which is distal to the suprascapular notch. The subscapular nerve originates from the posterior cord of the brachial plexus, which is distal to the site of fracture.

GAS 717-718; N413; McM 111

55 E. Klippel-Feil syndrome is a congenital defect in which there is a reduction, or extensive fusion of one or more cervical vertebrae. It often manifests as a short, stiff neck with limited motion. Hyperlordosis is an abnormal increase in lumbar curvature. Hyperkyphosis ("hunchback") is an abnormal increase in thoracic curvature. Scoliosis is a lateral curvature of the spine. Spina bifida can present with deformities in the lumbar region.

GAS 76; N 153; McM 83

56 B. Spondylolisthesis is an anterior vertebral displacement created by an irregularity in the anterior margin of the vertebral column such that L5 and the overlying L4 (and sometimes L3) protrude forward rather than being restrained by S1. Spondylolysis is a condition in which the region between the superior and inferior articular facets (on the posterior arch of the L5 vertebra) is damaged or missing, which is not the case in this example. Herniation is a protrusion of the nucleus pulposus through the anulus fibrosus, and this is not associated with vertebral dislocation. Hyperlordosis and scoliosis are excessive curvatures that do not involve dislocations.

GAS 82-83; N 153; McM 83

57 C. Chiari II malformation results from herniation of the medulla and cerebellum into the foramen magnum. Meningocele is a small defect in the cranium in which only the meninges herniate. Klippel-Feil syndrome results from an abnormal number of cervical vertebral bodies. Hydrocephalus results from an overproduction of cerebrospinal fluid, obstruction of its flow, or interference with CSF absorption. Tethered cord syndrome is a congenital anomaly often caused by a defective closure of the neural tube. This syndrome is characterized by a low conus medullaris and a thickened filum terminale.

N 107; McM 51

58 A. Spondylolisthesis is an anterior displacement created by an irregularity in the anterior margin of the vertebral column such that L5 and the overlying L4 (and sometimes L3) protrude forward. Spondylolysis is a condition in which the region between the superior and inferior articular facets (on the posterior arch of the L5 vertebra) is damaged or missing, which is not the case in this example. Compression vertebral fracture is a collapse of vertebral bodies as a result of trauma. Intervertebral disc herniations occur when the nucleus pulposus protrudes through the anulus fibrosus into the intervertebral foramen or vertebral canal. The most common protrusion is posterolaterally, where the anulus fibrosus is not reinforced by the posterior longitudinal ligament. Klippel-Feil syndrome results from an abnormal number of cervical vertebral bodies.

GAS 82-83; N 166; McM 83

59 A. The odontoid process, or the dens, projects superiorly from the body of the axis and articulates with the anterior arch of the atlas. The posterior and anterior tubercles of the atlas are bony eminences on the outer surface. The inferior articular facet is where the axis articulates with the C3 vertebra (*GAS* Fig. 2-21).

GAS 69-70; N 19; McM 85

60 B. The anterior longitudinal ligament is a strong fibrous band that covers and connects the anterolateral aspect of the vertebrae and intervertebral discs; it maintains stability and prevents hyperextension. It can be torn by cervical hyperextension. The ligamentum flavum helps maintain upright posture by connecting the laminae of two adjacent vertebrae. The posterior longitudinal ligament runs within the vertebral canal supporting the posterior aspect of the vertebrae and prevents hyperflexion. The anulus fibrosus is the outer fibrous part of an intervertebral disc. The interspinous ligament connects adjacent spinous processes.

GAS 80; N 159; McM 94

61 C. The denticulate ligaments are lateral extensions of pia mater that attach to the dura mater

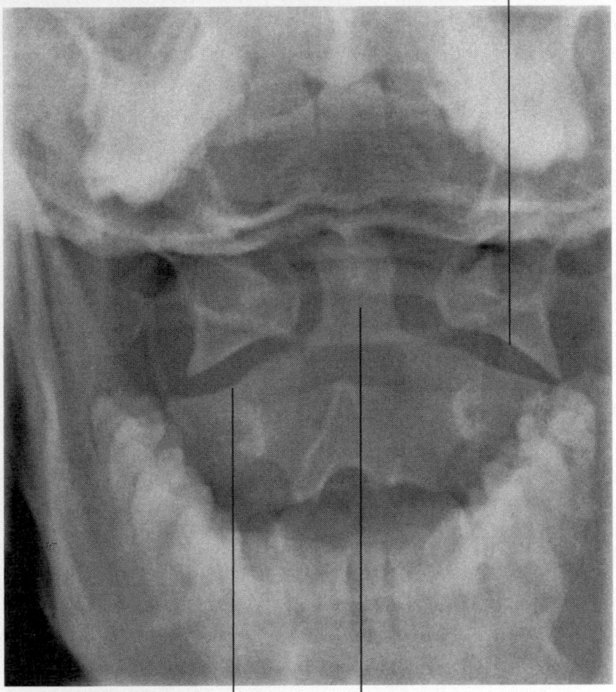

GAS Fig. 2-21

between the dorsal and ventral roots of the spinal nerves. These ligaments function to keep the spinal cord in the midline position. The posterior longitudinal ligament supports the posterior aspect of the vertebrae within the vertebral canal. The tentorium cerebelli is a layer of dura mater that supports the occipital lobes of the cerebral hemispheres and covers the cerebellum. The ligamentum flavum helps maintain upright posture by connecting the laminae of two adjacent vertebrae. The nuchal ligament is a thickening of the supraspinous ligaments extending from the C7 vertebra to the external occipital protuberance.

GAS 99-110; N 165; McM 94-96

62 A. The region bounded by the upper border of the latissimus dorsi, the lateral border of the trapezius, and the medial border of the scapula is known as the triangle of auscultation. Lung sounds can be heard most clearly from this location because minimal tissue intervenes between the skin of the back and the lungs. The deltoid, levator scapulae, and trapezius do not form the borders of the so-called "triangle of auscultation." The latissimus dorsi, external abdominal oblique, and iliac crest form the border of Petit's inferior lumbar triangle. The quadratus lumborum, internal abdominal oblique, and inferior border of the twelfth rib form the border of the Grynfeltt's superior lumbar triangle. The rectus abdominis, inguinal ligament, and inferior epigastric vessels form the border of the inguinal triangle (of Hesselbach).

GAS 84-89; N 409; McM 131

63 C. The weakness in shoulder movement results from denervation of the teres minor and deltoid by the axillary nerve, which passes through the quadrangular space. Quadrangular space syndrome occurs when there is hypertrophy of the muscles that border the quadrangular space or fibrosis of portions of the muscles that are in contact with the nerve.

GAS 718; N 413; McM 102

64 D. In this MRI a posterolateral herniation between L4/L5 exists. In the lumbar region, spinal nerves exit the vertebral column below their named vertebrae. In an L4/L5 intervertebral disc herniation, the L5 spinal nerve would be affected as it descends between L4/L5 vertebrae to exit below the L5 level.

GAS GAS 79; N 161; McM 97

65 B. The (great radicular) artery of Adamkiewicz is important for blood supply to anterior and posterior spinal arteries. The location of this artery should be noted during surgery because damage to it can result in dire consequences, including paraplegia (loss of all sensation and voluntary movement inferior and at the level of the injury). Injury to the left vertebral artery would not be likely due its superior location to the surgical site. Ligation of the posterior spinal artery would not occur because of its protected location inside the vertebral canal. Transection of the conus medullaris of the spinal cord would not occur as this structure is located at L1, L2 levels and is, again, protected inside the vertebral canal. Division of the thoracic sympathetic chain would not be likely as the symptoms described include limb paralysis, which would not be a consequence of sympathetic disruption (*GAS* Fig. 2-49A).

GAS 100-101; N 167

66 C. Scoliosis can be a secondary condition in such disorders as muscular dystrophy and polio in which abnormal muscle does not keep the normal alignment of the vertebral column and results in a lateral curvature. Hyperlordosis is increased secondary curvature of the lumbar region. It can be caused by stress on the lower back and is quite common during late pregnancy. Hyperkyphosis is increased primary curvature of the thoracic regions and produces a hunchback deformity. It can be secondary to tuberculosis, producing a "gibbus deformity," which results in angulated kyphosis at the lesion site. Spina

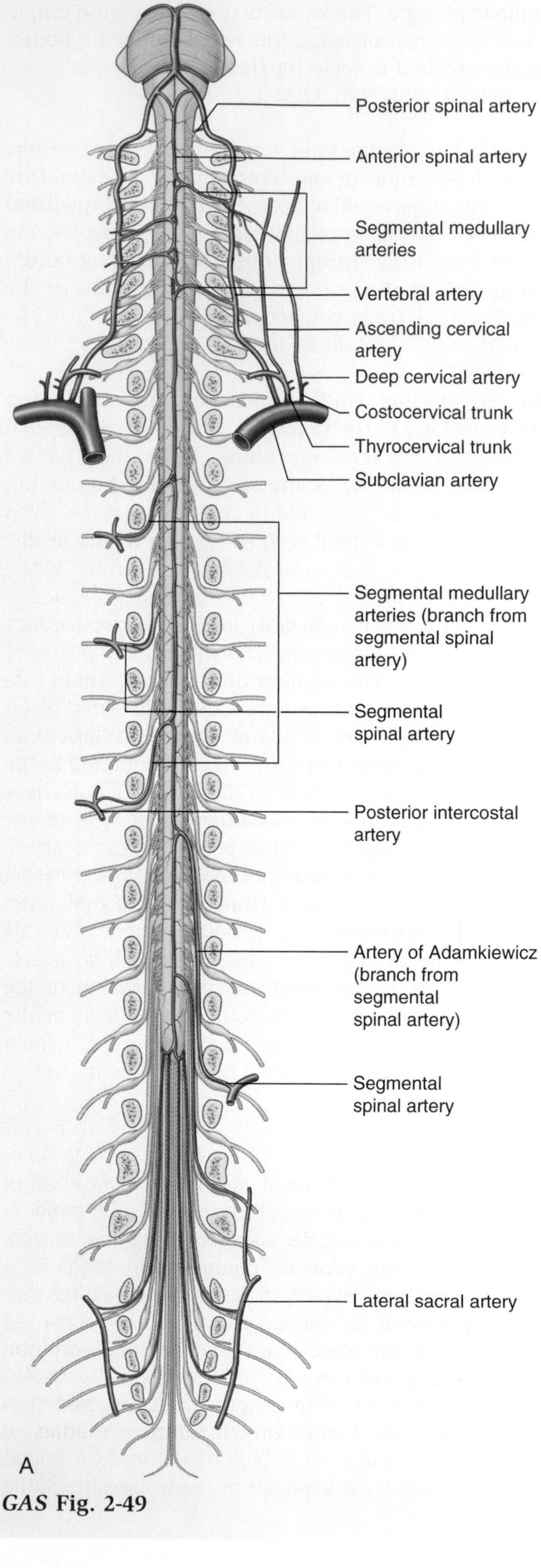

GAS **Fig. 2-49**

bifida is a congenital defect and would not present as a result of muscular dystrophy or polio. Osteoarthritis most commonly presents with age from normal "wear and tear." It is highly unlikely in a 23-year-old woman.

GAS 75; N 153; McM 83

67 C. The intervertebral disc consists of an outer anulus fibrosus and inner nucleus pulposus. The tensile strength comes from the anulus fibrosus, which limits rotation between vertebrae. Hyaline cartilage is found in the joint capsule and epiphysial plate. Elastic cartilage is found in, for example, the epiglottis.

GAS 78; N 155; McM 99

68 A. Notochord remnant forms the gelatinous nucleus pulposus and the surrounding mesenchyme which is derived from the adjacent sclerotome forms the concentric fibrous anulus fibrosus. There is no direct neural crest or ectoderm involvement.

GAS 78; N 155; McM 99

69 B. Horner's syndrome is characterized by, among other things, constricted pupils, sunken eyes, partially drooping eyelid (ptosis), and dryness of the skin on the face. It is caused by problems in sympathetic autonomic pathways such as damage to the lateral horn. Horner's syndrome is a result of disruption to the sympathetic nerves whose cell bodies are located in the lateral gray horn of the spinal cord. The anterior gray horn has cell bodies for somatic efferent fibers whereas the posterior gray serves as a location for the axons of sensory fibers whose cell bodies are located in the spinal ganglion. There are no cell bodies located in the white matter of the spinal cord.

McM 98

70 D. Semispinalis capitis is the only muscle among the choices that is supplied by the dorsal rami. All of the other muscles are supplied by the ventral rami. The rhomboid major and minor are innervated by the ventral primary rami of the dorsal scapular nerve. The levator scapulae is innervated by branches of C4 and C5, as well as from branches of dorsal scapular nerve. The latissimus dorsi is innervated by thoracodorsal nerve.

GAS 95; N 172; McM 103

71 C. The splenius capitis is supplied by the dorsal rami. The obliquus capitis muscles are innervated by branches of the suboccipital nerve which also supplies the rectus capitus posterior major and minor. The greater occipital nerve supplies the semispinalis capitis.

GAS 95; N 172; McM 105

72 **D.** Following judicial hanging the pedicles of C2 are fractured and the cruciform ligament is torn which results in the upper spinomedullary junction being crushed by the odontoid process, killing the victim. The odontoid process is typically not fractured in such cases. The C1 vertebra is not necessarily involved so there may be no lateral mass involvement. Similarly, there is no transverse or spinous process involvement.

GAS 64-71; N 23; McM 85

73 **A.** The thoracic vertebrae contribute to the primary curvature and wedge fracture here from osteoporosis, infection or trauma leads to kyphosis. Hyperlordosis occurs when the above changes occur in the lumbar region. Scoliosis is an abnormal lateral curvature of the vertebrae, which also involves rotation of the vertebrae on one another.

GAS 64-71; N 153; McM 81

74 **C.** Somatic afferent fibers convey localized pain, typically from the body wall and limbs and the cell bodies are found in the dorsal root ganglia. The dorsal horn is found at all spinal cord levels and is comprised of sensory nuclei that receive and process incoming somatosensory information. The lateral horn comprises autonomic neurons innervating visceral and pelvic organs. The sympathetic chain ganglia deliver the sympathetic information to the body. White rami communicans carry preganglionic sympathetic fibers and are called *white* because the fibers it contains are myelinated.

GAS 31-48; N 177; McM 96

75 **B.** The transverse ligament of the atlas anchors the dens laterally to prevent posterior displacement of the dens, which has been torn in this injury. The anterior longitudinal ligament runs on the anterior aspect of the vertebrae and is not affected. The ligamentum flavum is found on the posterior aspect of the vertebral canal and does not contact the anteriorly placed dens. The supraspinous ligament is located along the spinous processes of the vertebrae. The nuchal ligament is a longitudinal extension of the supraspinous and interspinous ligaments above the level of C7.

GAS 71-72; N 23; McM 85

76 **E.** Scoliosis is defined as a lateral deviation of the spinal column to either side and is often associated with a "rib-hump" as seen on examination when bending forward to touch the toes. Hyperkyphosis is an increased primary curvature of the spinal column. This curvature is associated with thoracic and sacral regions and is most likely this patient's clinical condition. Hyperlordosis is the increased secondary curvature affecting the cervical and lumbar regions.

GAS 75; N 153; McM 83

77 **D.** Cells from a specific somite develop into the dermis of the skin in a precise location, somatic sensory fibers originally associated with that somite enter the posterior region of the spinal nerve. The somatic sensory (afferent) fibers convey localized pain, typically from the body wall and limbs and the cell bodies are found in the dorsal root ganglia. The lateral horn comprises autonomic neurons innervating visceral and pelvic organs. The lateral horn comprises autonomic neurons innervating visceral and pelvic organs. The anterior horn contains motor neurons that supply muscles of the body wall and the limbs.

GAS 32-48; N 162; McM 96

78 **E.** In the cervical region, spinal nerves exit the vertebral column above their named vertebrae. From the thoracic region and below the spinal nerves exit the vertebral column below their named vertebrae.

GAS 107-110; N 161; McM 94

79 **C.** Lumbar puncture is generally performed at the level of L4, L5. The spinal cord ends at the level of L1/L2 in adults and at the level of L2/L3 in newborns.

GAS 103-104, 106; N 161; McM 97

80 **D.** The erector spinae muscle is supplied by the dorsal rami, which carry motor, sensory, and autonomic fibers. The cell bodies of the motor part are found in the anterior horn, while the cell bodies of the sensory fibers are found in the dorsal root ganglia. The cell bodies of the sympathetic fibers are found in the paravertebral ganglia.

GAS 23-48, 92-99; N 177; McM 103

81 **A.** The anterior longitudinal ligament is a strong fibrous band that covers and connects the anterolateral aspect of the vertebrae and intervertebral discs; it maintains stability and prevents hyperextension. It can be torn by cervical hyperextension. The ligamentum flavum helps maintain upright posture by connecting the laminae of two adjacent vertebrae. The posterior longitudinal ligament runs within the vertebral canal supporting the posterior aspect of the vertebrae and prevents hyperflexion. The anulus fibrosus is the outer fibrous part of an intervertebral disc. The interspinous ligament connects adjacent spinous processes.

GAS 80-83; N 159; McM 94

82 D. The boundaries of an intervertebral foramen (clockwise) include the following: the superior margin (roof) is formed by the inferior vertebral notch of the vertebra above, the anterior margin by the intervertebral disc between the vertebral bodies of the adjacent vertebrae, the inferior margin (floor) by the superior vertebral notch of the vertebra below, and the posterior margin by the zygapophysial (facet) joint of the adjacent vertebrae. Each pedicle contains superior and inferior vertebral notches.

GAS 66-72; N 158; McM 98

83 C. The most superiorly positioned intervertebral disc is between the C2 to C3 vertebrae. In the cervical region the spinal nerves exit superior to their corresponding vertebrae and take a somewhat horizontal path. The C3 nerve therefore exits through the C2 to C3 intervertebral foramen and would be affected by a posterolateral disc herniation at this level. The C1 nerve exists between the C1 vertebra and the occipital bone of the cranium and would not be affected. The C2 nerve passes superior to the second vertebra and would not be affected by a herniated disc between C2 and C3. C4 and C5 both exit superior to their corresponding vertebrae which is below the level of the herniated disc and will therefore not be affected.

GAS 79, 108; N 161; McM 94

84 E. Ligaments serve to restrict movement. The anterior longitudinal ligament courses downward on the anterior surface of the vertebral bodies attaching to the intervertebral discs along its way. It is stretches from the base of the skull inferiorly to the anterior surface of the sacrum. The anterior longitudinal ligament is the most anteriorly positioned ligament of the vertebral column and limits its extension. The posterior longitudinal ligament travels on the posterior surface of the vertebral bodies attaching to the intervertebral discs along the way. This ligament serves to prevent excessive flexion of the vertebral column and extends from C2 to the sacrum. The supraspinous ligament attaches the tips of the spinous processes to each other from C7 to the sacrum. Superiorly the ligament broadens becoming more distinct and triangular and is termed the ligamentum nuchae. Ligamentum nuchae limits excessive flexion of the cervical spine and serves as an attachment for muscles. Ligamentum flava attach the internal surfaces of adjacent lamina to each other and prevent them from pulling apart during flexion.

GAS 80-81; N 159; McM 94

85 C. A horizontal line that connects the highest points of the iliac crests typically bisects the spinous process of the L4 vertebra or L4-L5 interspace (Tuffier's line). The lumbar cistern, which represents the subarachnoid space, terminates at the level corresponding to the S2 spinous process. Three spinous processes inferiorly from the drawn line between the iliac crests would correspond to S2 spinous processes. Two and three spinous processes above the drawn line would be at the vertebral level L2 and L1, respectively, which would correspond to the approximate location where the spinal cord ends and therefore the pia mater.

GAS 99; N 166; McM 100

86 C. The anterior spinal artery lies in the anterior median fissure and would likely be compressed by the tumor. This artery is formed superiorly by the union of two branches that directly arise from the vertebral arteries. Ascending cervical artery is not found within the vertebral canal and does not contribute to the blood supply of the spinal cord. The segmental spinal arteries follow the spinal nerves and provide the segmental medullary vessels which run along the dorsal and ventral roots to supply the lateral aspect of the spinal cord. There are two posterior spinal arteries, each are located in the posterolateral sulcus on the posterior aspect and have only small branches to the direct area.

GAS 100-101; N 167; McM 94

87 B. Hemivertebra is a condition where part of one or more vertebrae does not develop. This causes an abnormal lateral bending of the spinal column known as scoliosis, which may also include rotational deformities. Osteoporosis is a condition where bones become gradually less dense and may cause fractures even in minor traumas. Hyperlordosis is characterized by an increase in the anterior curvature of the lumbar or cervical spines. It is a result of an increase in thickness anterior, or a decrease in thickness posterior, on the vertebral bodies. Spondylolisthesis is an anterior displacement of a portion of the vertebra consequent to a fracture of the pars interarticularis (spondylolysis). Sacralization is when the fifth lumbar vertebra fuses to the sacrum.

GAS 74-77; N 153; McM 83

88 C. There are seven (7) cervical vertebrae and eight (8) cervical spinal nerves. Nerves C1 to C7 exit superior to their corresponding vertebrae, whereas nerve C8 exits inferiorly to the C7 vertebra. The nerves of the thoracic and subsequent regions all exit inferior to their corresponding vertebrae.

GAS 99-100, 108; N 158; McM 94

89 **C.** When a child is born only one curvature is present in the vertebral column, the primary curvature, which is concave anteriorly and termed kyphosis. During postnatal development two additional curvatures form, secondary curvatures, which are convex anteriorly and termed lordosis. The first forms in response to the child lifting its head and is in the cervical spine, the second forms once the child is sitting and completes once the child starts to walk. Thoracic kyphosis is the normal curvature with which we are born and cervical lordosis is associated with the neck and develops much earlier on. Cervical kyphosis and thoracic lordosis would both be considered abnormal curvatures in a child of this age.
GAS 54; N 153; McM 83

90 **A.** The muscle that was demonstrated by the professor was the latissimus dorsi, which attaches to the spinous processes of vertebrae T7 to L5 and the floor of the intertubercular sulcus. None of the other options describes attachments sites for muscles attaching to the upper limb.
GAS 84-90; N 171; McM 102

91 **B.** Sclerotomes are the derivatives of somites that develop into bone and if eliminated will result in underdevelopment of the vertebrae. The nucleus pulposus is a remnant of the notochord. The dorsal root ganglion is formed by neural crest cells that migrate during development. The neural tube is the precursor for the spinal cord and the anulus fibrosus develops from the sclerotome component of the somite.
GAS 67; N 153; McM 83

92 **A.** Multifidus is a deep muscle, which attaches from the transverse processes to the spinous processes usually crossing four to six segments. Longissimus, iliocostalis, and spinalis are not deep to semispinalis but are superficial. The rotators typically attach between the spinous processes or lamina of vertebrae and the transverse processes of the vertebra one or two segments below.
GAS 92, 98; N 173; McM 103

93 **D.** The oblique radiographic view is ideal to show the pars interarticularis. In this projection a "Scottie dog" can be seen; the neck of the dog is the pars interarticularis, where the fracture may be seen. In the lateral view, the pedicles are superimposed on the pars interarticularis and so it cannot be easily seen. In the anteroposterior and posteroanterior views, the vertebral bodies make it difficult to see the pars interarticularis. The anteroposterior open mouth is a radiographic view of the upper cervical region.
GAS 83; N 153; McM 107

94 **A.** The muscle that forms the lateral border of the suboccipital triangle is the obliquus capitis superior. This muscle originates from the transverse process of the atlas and inserts untoon the occipital bone between superior and inferior nuchal lines. The muscle that inserts at the transverse process of the atlas is the obliquus capitis inferior which forms the inferior border of the suboccipital triangle. The rectus capitis posterior major inserts on the lateral portion of occipital bone below the inferior nuchal line and the rectus capitis posterior minor inserts on the medial portion of occipital bone below the inferior nuchal line. These muscles form the medial border of the triangle. The rectus capitis posterior minor originates from the posterior tubercle of the atlas.
GAS 97-98; N 175; McM 104

95 **E.** Sacralization is a process where the L5 vertebra completely or incompletely fuses with the sacrum. This vertebra adapts the characteristics of the sacrum with an increase in the length and width of both transverse processes.
GAS 76; N 157; McM 91

96 **D.** The inferior longitudinal band of the cruciform ligament runs inferiorly from the transverse ligament of the atlas and attaches to the posterosuperior aspect of the vertebral body of the axis (C2). The transverse ligament of the atlas spans the distance between the medial aspects of the lateral masses, holding the dens in place. The superior longitudinal band of the cruciform ligament runs from the transverse cervical ligament superiorly to attach to the occiput. The apical ligament runs from the tip of the dens to the anterior margin of the foramen magnum. The ligamentum flavum is located in the vertebral canal and connects the laminae of adjacent vertebrae.
GAS 71-72; N 23; McM 85

97 **A.** The radicular arteries are branches of the segmental spinal arteries. They occur at every vertebral level and follow and provide blood supply to the anterior and posterior roots. A space occupying lesion that compresses the posterior roots will also compress the arteries that supply them. The segmental spinal arteries are feeder arteries that reinforce the blood supply to the spinal cord and arise from the vertebral and deep cervical arteries in the neck, the posterior intercostals in the thorax, and the lumbar arteries in the abdomen. The anterior and posterior spinal arteries arise from the vertebral artery and supply the spinal cord directly. The segmental medullary arteries are also branches of the segmental spinal arteries that anastomose directly with the anterior and posterior spinal arteries.

GAS 100-101; N 168; McM 96

98 E. The patient in the figure above has spina bifida occulta. This is a developmental condition resulting from incomplete ossification and failure of fusion of the vertebral arches. Three primary ossification centers should be present in the fetus by the eighth week: one in the centrum (to form the vertebral body) and one in each half of the vertebral arch. Five secondary ossification centers develop in the vertebrae after puberty: one at the tip of the spinous processes, the tips of the transverse processes, and on the inferior and superior rims of the vertebral body.

GAS 74; N 160; McM 93

99 A. In the cervical region, the spinal nerve exits in the intervertebral foramen above the correspondingly named vertebrae. Therefore, the C3 spinal nerve exits above the C3 vertebrae and lies directly below the C2 vertebrae.

GAS 106-109; N 161; McM 94

100 E. The ligamentum flavum lies within the vertebral canal on the anterior aspect of the vertebral arches connecting the lamina of adjacent vertebrae. Puncturing this ligament allows the needle to enter into the epidural/extradural space for the injection of the anesthetic. Although the posterior longitudinal ligament lies within the spinal canal, it will not be punctured during the procedure. The supraspinous ligament connects and passes along the tips of the vertebral spinous processes. The interspinous ligament lies between adjacent spinous processes. The anterior longitudinal ligament connects the anterior aspect of the vertebral body. These ligaments do not lie within the vertebral canal.

GAS 80-84; N 159; McM 97

101 A. The third occipital nerve is the medial branch of the dorsal ramus of C3. It pierces the trapezius muscle medially in the neck below the external occipital protuberance and supplies the skin of the nuchal region. The greater occipital and lesser occipital nerves lie lateral to the midline and are less likely to be affected in this patient. The suboccipital nerve lies within and supplies the muscles of the suboccipital triangle. The spinal accessory nerve supplies the trapezius and sternocleidomastoid muscles and has no cutaneous supply in the neck (*GAS* Fig. 2-46).

GAS 98; N 174; McM 104

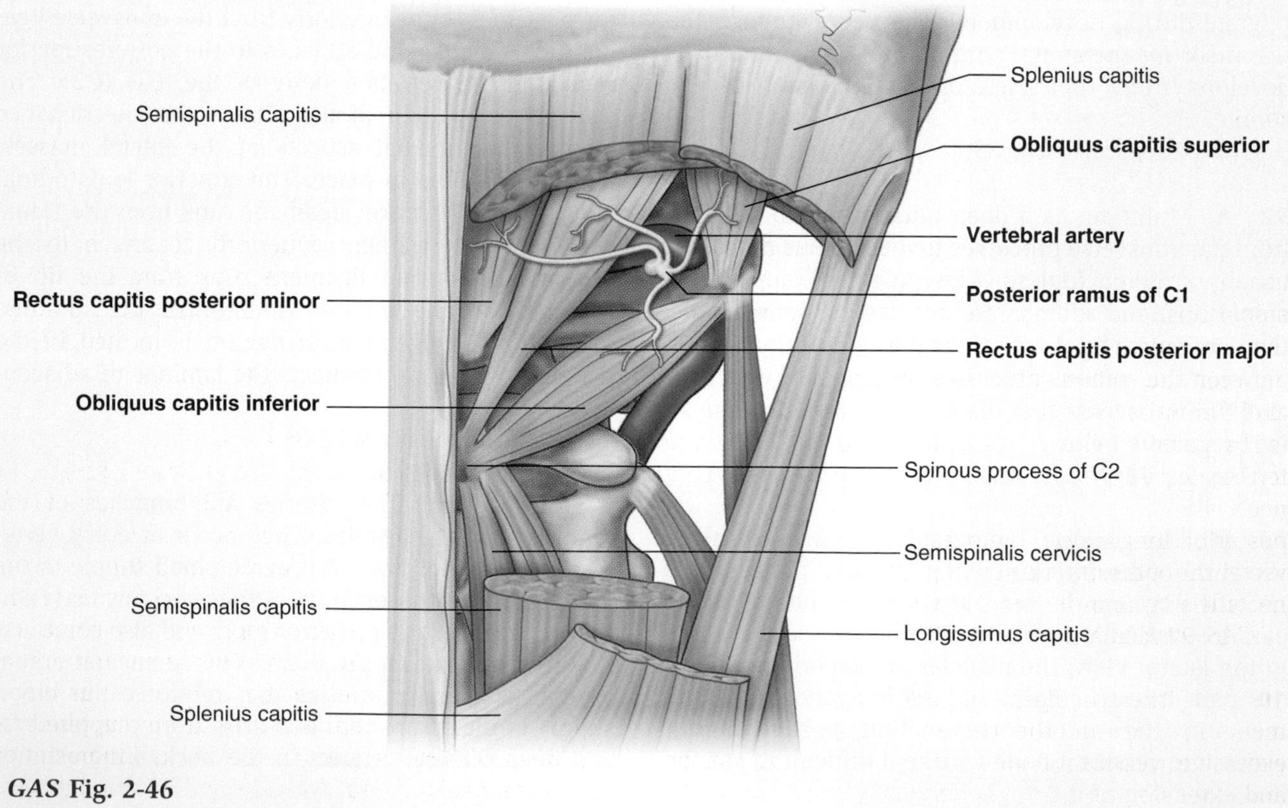

***GAS* Fig. 2-46**

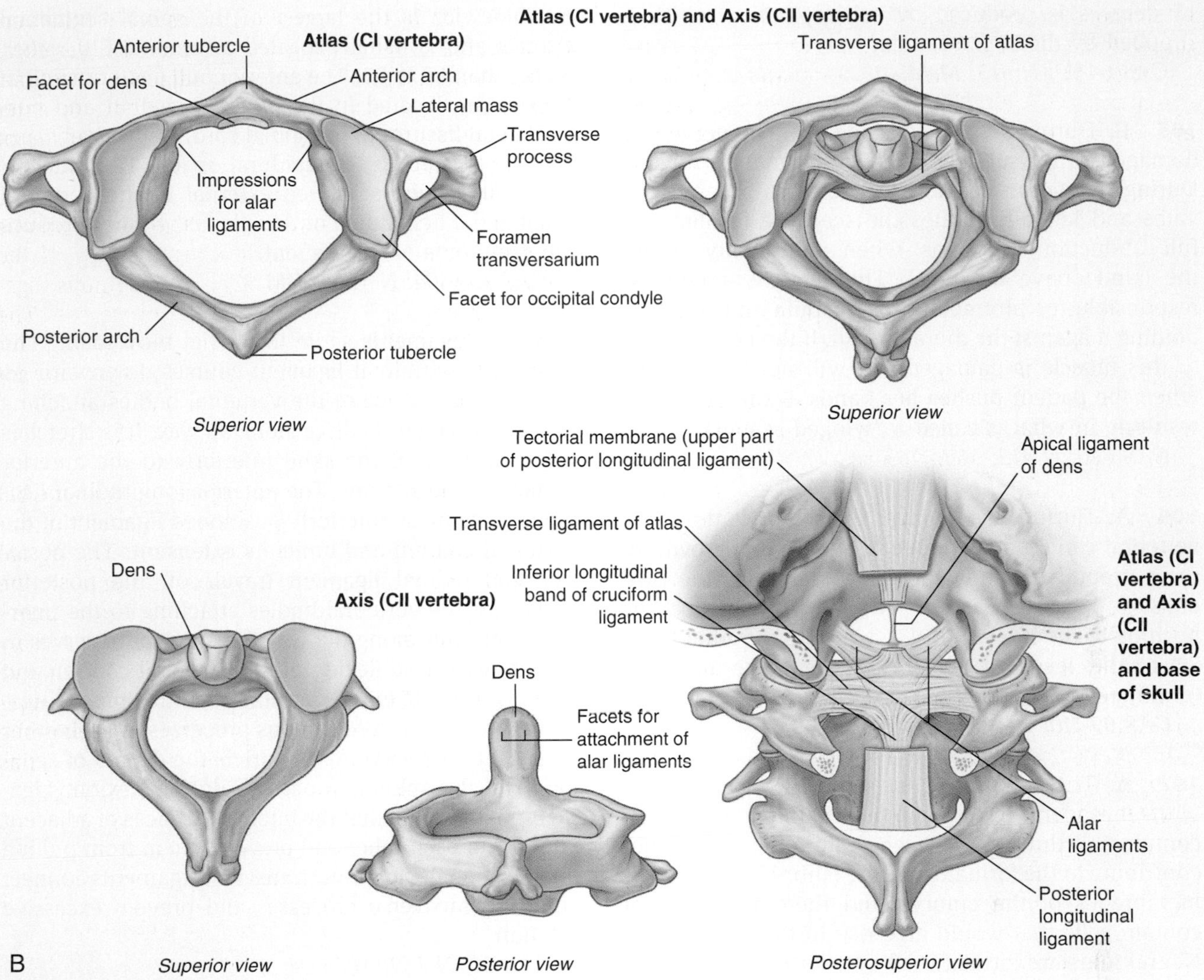

GAS **Fig. 2-20**

102 A. The denticulate ligament is a sheet of pia mater running longitudinally on either side of the spinal cord, connecting it to the dura mater. Medially, the denticulate ligament lies between the origin of the anterior and posterior rootlets serving as a landmark to differentiate between them. The conus medullaris is the terminal end of the spinal cord and the filum terminale is an extension of the pia mater that connects the conus medullaris to the dural sac. The posterior longitudinal ligament lies posterior to the vertebral bodies, while the ligamentum flavum connects the lamina of adjacent vertebrae.

GAS 99-104; N 165; McM 96

103 D. The alar ligament connects the dens to the medial surface of the occipital condyles. It limits excessive rotation of the atlanto-axial joints. Flexion and extension of the upper cervical spine occur at the atlanto-occipital joints and the zygapophysial joints. Lateral flexion (abduction) as a combination movement at the uncovertebral joints (of Luschka). These are not limited by the alar ligament (*GAS* Fig. 2-20B).

GAS 71-72; N 23; McM 85

104 D. The rhomboid major and minor are supplied by the dorsal scapular nerve which also supplies the levator scapulae. The function of levator scapulae is elevation and inferior rotation of the scapulae. Abduction of the arm above 90 degrees and protraction of the scapula are possible due to the action of serratus anterior, which is supplied by the long thoracic nerve. Medial rotation and adduction of the arm is performed mainly by the pectoralis major and latissimus dorsi, which also extends the arm. These are supplied by the medial and lateral pectoral nerves and thoracodorsal, respectively. Abduction of the arm through 0 to

15 degrees is produced by supraspinatus, which is supplied by the suprascapular nerve.

GAS 84-90; N 413; McM 102

105 B. During surgery the long thoracic nerve was damaged which supplies the serratus anterior muscle. During abduction of the arm, serratus anterior elevates and laterally rotates the scapulae to allow for full abduction, such as when the ability to lift the hand above the head. The serratus anterior is responsible for protracting the scapula and therefore holding it against the thoracic wall. If the nerve supply to this muscle is damaged this will not be achieved when the patient pushes her hands against the wall, resulting in what is called a "winged scapula".

GAS 726; N 413; McM 103

106 A. During development the spinal cord fills the vertebral canal entirely. Due to differential growth of the vertebral column and the spinal cord, the cord ends at L3 in an infant. It gradually changes its position to the level of L1/L2, which is the adult level. S2 is the level at which the dural sac normally terminates.

GAS 99-110; N 161; McM 97

107 A. The primitive streak aids in the development of the mesoderm resulting in the trilaminar disc which contains all three germ layers. Chorionic villi do not contribute to the formation of the embryo itself but the membranes of the embryo and therefore does not contain cells that would give rise to the germ layers. Neural folds are formed from ectoderm and gives rise to neural crest cells. The intraembryonic coelom forms the embryonic cavities and is therefore a space.

N 153

108 A. A fracture of the pars interarticularis is termed spondylolysis. Spondylolisthesis is when the anterior portion of the vertebra is displaced after fracture of the pars interarticularis. A herniated disc is when the nucleus pulposus protrudes through the anulus fibrosus. Lordosis is the normal curvature of the cervical and lumbar spine. Scoliosis is an abnormal lateral curvature of the spine which usually also has a degree of rotation of the vertebrae.

GAS 83; N 153; McM 88

109 A. An epidural anesthetic procedure is performed in the epidural space which contains fat and the internal vertebral (Batson's) plexus. A hematoma in this region would cause compression on the spinal nerves and possibly the cord resulting in severe pain and deficits. The great anterior medullary artery of Adamkiewicz is the largest of the spinal segmental arteries and is usually located at around T10, much higher than L2 to L3. The anterior and posterior spinal arteries are located in the anterior median and posterolateral fissures of the spinal cord, respectively, and are not located in the epidural space. The external vertebral plexus is located external to the vertebral canal and a hematoma of this plexus will not produce the symptoms of this patient.

GAS 100-104; N 166; McM 97

110 A. Ligaments serve to restrict movement. The anterior longitudinal ligament courses downward on the anterior surface of the vertebral bodies attaching to the intervertebral discs along its way. It is stretches from the base of the skull inferiorly to the anterior surface of the sacrum. The anterior longitudinal ligament is the most anteriorly positioned ligament of the vertebral column and limits its extension. The posterior longitudinal ligament travels on the posterior surface of the vertebral bodies attaching to the intervertebral discs along the way. This ligament serves to prevent excessive flexion of the vertebral column and extends from C2 to the sacrum. The interspinous ligaments attach adjacent spinous processes to each other from C2 to the sacrum, it restricts the degree of separation of the spinous processes during flexion. Ligamentum flava attaches the internal surfaces of adjacent laminae to each other and prevents them from pulling apart during flexion. Intertransverse ligaments connect adjacent transverse processes and prevent excessive rotation.

GAS 80; N 159; McM 94

111 A. The order of structures pierced during an epidural procedure is skin, subcutaneous tissue, muscle, supraspinous ligament, interspinous ligament, and ligamentum flavum (there is often a midline gap in the ligamentum flavum). The anterior longitudinal ligament is anterior to the vertebral body and cannot be reached by this approach. The posterior longitudinal ligament is posterior to the vertebral body and can also not be reached by this procedure. The intertransverse ligaments are too lateral and may not be perforated by this technique.

GAS 100-104, 115-116; N 166; McM 97

112 D. The spinal cord ends at the level between the L1/L2 vertebra but the spinal nerves continue as the caudal equina below this level. As a result, narrowing of the canal at the level of L5 will impact on all of the nerves resulting in bilateral lower limb weakness.

GAS 99-104; N 161; McM 97

113 **B.** The anterior and posterior spinal arteries do not provide sufficient blood supply to the spinal cord below cervical levels and will receive additional supply segmentally along its course from multiple sources. The largest of these vessels are usually termed the artery of Adamkiewicz and arises at the lower thoracic or upper lumbar region.

GAS 100-104; N 167; McM 94

114 **D.** A chondroma is typically a benign tumor of cartilaginous origin, which is encapsulated. It has the same origin as the apical ligament of the atlas which is considered as a rudimentary intervertebral fibrocartilage derived from the notochord.

GAS 99-104; N 155; McM 99

115 **A.** The odontoid process, or the dens, projects superiorly from the body of the axis and articulates with the anterior arch of the atlas. The posterior and anterior tubercles of the atlas are bony eminences on the outer surface. The inferior articular facet is where the axis joins to the C3 vertebra. **A,** Lateral radiograph shows that this patient has only mild prevertebral swelling, which is centered at the odontoid (see *arrowheads* in Fig. 1-5, p. 20). The odontoid is displaced posteriorly relative to the C2 body *(arrow)* and is angled posteriorly. These findings indicate a fracture. **B,** The fracture is extremely subtle on the open-mouth odontoid radiograph *(arrows)*. C, Sagittal CT reconstruction shows the fracture.

GAS 68-73; N 19; McM 85

116 **D.** The herniated disc is between vertebrae L4 and L5. In the lumbar region spinal nerves exit below their corresponding vertebrae in which case the L4 nerve would pass superior to the herniation. As the L5 nerve crosses the intervertebral disc to exit below the fifth lumbar vertebra it will be compressed by the herniation. Compression of nerves L2, L3, and S1 would produce symptoms different to those seen in this patient.

GAS 79; N 161; McM 99

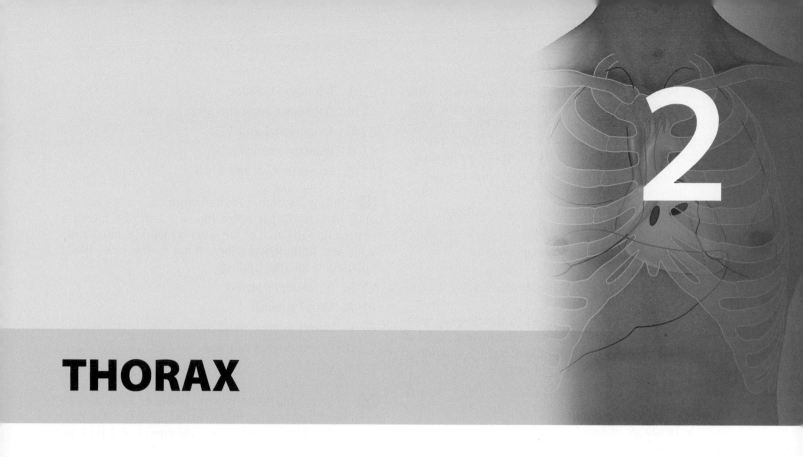

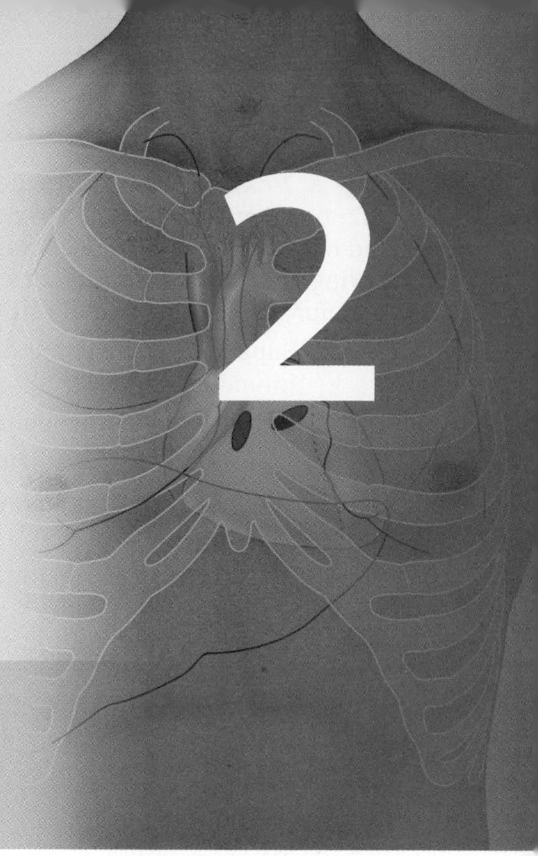

2 THORAX

QUESTIONS

1 A 2-day-old newborn is diagnosed with transposition of the great arteries. Which structure is primarily responsible for the division of the truncus arteriosus into the great arteries?

- ▢ **A.** Septum secundum
- ▢ **B.** Septum primum
- ▢ **C.** Bulbar septum
- ▢ **D.** Aorticopulmonary septum
- ▢ **E.** Endocardial cushions

2 A 32-year-old woman in her third trimester of pregnancy is undergoing a routine ultrasound examination. The examination of the fetus reveals enlarged and echogenic lungs, an inverted diaphragm, and fetal ascites. Which condition is best characterized by these signs?

- ▢ **A.** Laryngeal atresia
- ▢ **B.** Tracheal atresia
- ▢ **C.** Polyhydramnios
- ▢ **D.** Lung hypoplasia
- ▢ **E.** Oligohydramnios

3 A 2-year-old child is seen in the pediatric cardiology unit for a congenital heart condition. Which of the following conditions occurs most often?

- ▢ **A.** Membranous ventricular septal defect (VSD)
- ▢ **B.** Tetralogy of Fallot
- ▢ **C.** Muscular VSD
- ▢ **D.** Ostium secundum defect
- ▢ **E.** Ostium primum defect

4 A 2-day-old infant is diagnosed with transposition of the great arteries. If this condition were to be left untreated for more than 4 months, it would be fatal. Which of the following structures must remain patent so that the infant can survive until surgical correction of the malformation?

- ▢ **A.** Ductus arteriosus
- ▢ **B.** Umbilical arteries
- ▢ **C.** Umbilical vein
- ▢ **D.** Coarctation of the aorta
- ▢ **E.** Pulmonary artery stenosis

5 A 2-day-old newborn female is diagnosed with pulmonary artery stenosis, overriding of the aorta, VSD, and hypertrophy of the right ventricle. Which condition is best characterized by these signs?

- ▢ **A.** Tetralogy of Fallot
- ▢ **B.** Atrial septal defect
- ▢ **C.** Transposition of the great vessels
- ▢ **D.** Pulmonary atresia
- ▢ **E.** VSD

6 A 2-day-old newborn female is diagnosed with pulmonary artery stenosis, overriding of the aorta, VSD, and hypertrophy of the right ventricle. Which of the following embryologic mechanisms is most likely responsible for the development of this cluster of anomalies?

- ☐ **A.** Superior malalignment of the subpulmonary infundibulum
- ☐ **B.** Defect in the aorticopulmonary septum
- ☐ **C.** Endocardial cushion defect
- ☐ **D.** Total anomalous pulmonary venous connections
- ☐ **E.** Atrioventricular canal malformation

7 A 5-year-old boy is admitted to the hospital with severe dyspnea. During physical examination, a loud systolic murmur and a wide, fixed, split S_2 sound is noted. What is the most likely diagnosis?

- ☐ **A.** VSD
- ☐ **B.** Atrial septal defect
- ☐ **C.** Tetralogy of Fallot
- ☐ **D.** Transposition of the great arteries
- ☐ **E.** Aortic stenosis

8 A 3-month-old infant is diagnosed with Down syndrome (trisomy 21). A routine cardiovascular examination reveals that the infant suffers from arrhythmias. What other cardiac conditions are most likely to occur with Down syndrome?

- ☐ **A.** Tetralogy of Fallot
- ☐ **B.** Transposition of the great arteries
- ☐ **C.** Atrial septal and VSDs
- ☐ **D.** Truncus arteriosus
- ☐ **E.** Coarctation of the aorta

9 A 3-month-old infant is diagnosed with a deletion at the 22q11 chromosome. A routine cardiovascular examination reveals severe congenital cardiac malformation. Which of the following malformations will most likely be associated with 22q11 syndrome?

- ☐ **A.** Tetralogy of Fallot and truncus arteriosus
- ☐ **B.** Transposition of the great arteries
- ☐ **C.** Atrial septal and VSDs
- ☐ **D.** Coarctation of the aorta
- ☐ **E.** Aortic atresia

10 A 28-year-old woman in her third trimester of pregnancy with a complaint of dizziness for several days is admitted to the hospital. Physical examination reveals that she has diabetes mellitus. Which of the following cardiac malformations is most likely to affect the fetus when the mother has this disease?

- ☐ **A.** Tetralogy of Fallot
- ☐ **B.** Transposition of the great arteries
- ☐ **C.** Atrial septal and VSDs
- ☐ **D.** Truncus arteriosus
- ☐ **E.** Coarctation of the aorta

11 During cardiac catheterization of a 6-year-old child, the radiologist notes that the contrast medium released into the arch of the aorta is visible immediately in the left pulmonary artery. What is the most likely explanation for this finding?

- ☐ **A.** Atrial septal defect
- ☐ **B.** Mitral stenosis
- ☐ **C.** Patent ductus arteriosus
- ☐ **D.** Patent ductus venosus
- ☐ **E.** VSD

12 A 3-year-old male patient presents with a clinically significant atrial septal defect (ASD). The ASD usually results from incomplete closure of which of the following structures?

- ☐ **A.** Foramen ovale
- ☐ **B.** Ligamentum arteriosum
- ☐ **C.** Ductus arteriosus
- ☐ **D.** Sinus venarum
- ☐ **E.** Coronary sinus

13 A premature infant has progressive difficulty in breathing and is diagnosed with respiratory distress syndrome. Which cells are deficient in synthesizing surfactant in this syndrome?

- ☐ **A.** Alveolar capillary endothelial
- ☐ **B.** Bronchial mucous
- ☐ **C.** Bronchial respiratory epithelium
- ☐ **D.** Type I alveolar
- ☐ **E.** Type II alveolar

14 A newborn baby is diagnosed with eventration of the diaphragm. In this condition, half of the diaphragm ascends into the thorax during inspiration, while the other half contracts normally. What is the cause of this condition?

- ☐ **A.** Absence of a pleuropericardial fold
- ☐ **B.** Absence of musculature in one half of the diaphragm
- ☐ **C.** Failure of migration of diaphragm
- ☐ **D.** Failure of the septum transversum to develop
- ☐ **E.** Absence of a pleuroperitoneal fold

15 A 35-year-old man is admitted to the emergency department because of a severe nosebleed (epistaxis) and a headache that had become worse during the weekend. On physical examination, his upper body appears much better developed than his lower body, a loud midsystolic murmur is present on his anterior chest wall and back, his lower extremities are cold, and femoral pulses are absent. Which of the following embryologic structure(s) has been most likely affected to produce such symptoms?

- ☐ **A.** Bulbus cordis
- ☐ **B.** Ductus arteriosus
- ☐ **C.** Third, fourth, and sixth pharyngeal arches
- ☐ **D.** Right and left horns of sinus venosus
- ☐ **E.** Right cardinal vein

16 After a 2-day-old newborn male swallows milk he becomes cyanotic. After 3 days, he develops aspiration pneumonia. A tracheoesophageal fistula is suspected. Failure of development has occurred most specifically in which of the following structures?

- ☐ **A.** Esophagus
- ☐ **B.** Trachea
- ☐ **C.** Tongue
- ☐ **D.** Tracheoesophageal septum
- ☐ **E.** Pharynx

17 After a 2-day-old newborn male swallows milk he becomes cyanotic. After 3 days he develops pneumonia. A tracheoesophageal fistula is suspected. Which of the following conditions is most likely to be associated with a tracheoesophageal fistula?

- ☐ **A.** Oligohydramnios
- ☐ **B.** Rubella
- ☐ **C.** Polyhydramnios
- ☐ **D.** Thalidomide exposure
- ☐ **E.** Toxoplasmosis

18 A 2-day-old newborn male develops mild cyanosis. An ultrasound examination reveals a patent ductus arteriosus (PDA). Which of the following infections will most likely lead to this congenital anomaly?

- ☐ **A.** Toxoplasmosis
- ☐ **B.** Rubella
- ☐ **C.** Cytomegalovirus
- ☐ **D.** Varicella virus
- ☐ **E.** Treponema pallidum

19 A 5-year-old boy has frequent episodes of fatigability and dyspnea. An ultrasound examination reveals an ASD, located at the opening of the superior vena cava. Which of the following types of ASDs are characteristic for this description?

- ☐ **A.** Ostium secundum
- ☐ **B.** Ostium primum
- ☐ **C.** Atrioventricular canal
- ☐ **D.** Common atrium
- ☐ **E.** Sinus venosus

20 A 3-day-old newborn was born with ectopia cordis. Despite the efforts of doctors at the pediatric intensive care unit, the infant died from cardiac failure and hypoxemia. Which of the following embryologic events is most likely responsible for the development of such conditions?

- ☐ **A.** Faulty development of the sternum and pericardium, secondary to incomplete fusion of the lateral folds
- ☐ **B.** Interruption of third pharyngeal arch development
- ☐ **C.** Interruption of fourth pharyngeal arch development
- ☐ **D.** Interruption of fifth pharyngeal arch development
- ☐ **E.** Faulty development of sinus venosus

21 A 2-day-old newborn male is admitted to the pediatric intensive care unit with cyanosis and tachypnea. Cardiac ultrasound (echocardiography) and magnetic resonance imaging (MRI) examinations reveal totally anomalous pulmonary connections. Which of the following embryologic events is responsible for this malformation?

- ☐ **A.** Abnormal septation of the sinus venosus
- ☐ **B.** Abnormal development of the septum secundum
- ☐ **C.** Abnormal development of the left sinus horn
- ☐ **D.** Abnormal development of the coronary sinus
- ☐ **E.** Abnormal development of common cardinal vein

22 A 3-day-old newborn has difficulties breathing. A computed tomography (CT) scan of his chest and abdomen reveals the absence of the central tendon of the diaphragm. Which of the following structures failed to develop normally?

- ☐ **A.** Pleuroperitoneal folds
- ☐ **B.** Pleuropericardial folds
- ☐ **C.** Septum transversum
- ☐ **D.** Cervical myotomes
- ☐ **E.** Dorsal mesentery of the esophagus

23 A 30-year-old man is diagnosed with a blockage of arterial flow in the proximal part of the thoracic aorta. Brachial arterial pressure is markedly increased, femoral artery pressure is decreased, and the femoral pulses are delayed. The patient shows no external signs of inflammation. Which of the following structures failed to develop normally?

- ☐ **A.** Second aortic arch
- ☐ **B.** Third aortic arch
- ☐ **C.** Fourth aortic arch
- ☐ **D.** Fifth aortic arch
- ☐ **E.** Ductus venosus

24 A 1-year-old child was admitted to the pediatric clinic due to severe dyspnea. An electrocardiogram (ECG) reveals cardiac arrhythmia and right ventricular hypertrophy. An angiogram reveals a PDA. From which of the following embryologic arterial structures does the PDA take origin?

- ☐ **A.** Left sixth aortic arch
- ☐ **B.** Right sixth aortic arch
- ☐ **C.** Left fifth aortic arch
- ☐ **D.** Right sixth aortic arch
- ☐ **E.** Left fourth aortic arch

25 A 4-year-old girl is admitted to the hospital with high fever. *Staphylococcus aureus* is isolated from her blood cultures and antibiotic therapy is initiated. A loud, harsh murmur is heard on auscultation. A chest radiograph shows prominent pulmonary arteries. Echocardiography shows all the valves to be normal. Which congenital heart disease most likely explains these findings?

- ☐ **A.** Atrial septal defect
- ☐ **B.** Tetralogy of Fallot
- ☐ **C.** Coarctation of the aorta
- ☐ **D.** Patent ductus arteriosus
- ☐ **E.** Aortic atresia

26 A 3-day-old infant is admitted to the cardiology unit with severe cyanosis. During echocardiographic examination a right-to-left shunt is identified. Which of the following conditions will most likely produce this type of shunt?

- ☐ **A.** Interatrial septal defect
- ☐ **B.** Interventricular septal defect
- ☐ **C.** Patent ductus arteriosus
- ☐ **D.** Corrected transposition of the great arteries
- ☐ **E.** Common truncus arteriosus

27 A 4-day-old infant is admitted to the pulmonary unit suffering from dyspnea and cyanosis. Radiologic examination revealed a left hypoplastic lung and herniation of the abdominal intestines into the left thoracic cavity. Which of the following embryologic structures most likely failed to develop properly?

- ☐ **A.** Septum transversum
- ☐ **B.** Pleuroperitoneal membrane
- ☐ **C.** Tracheoesophageal septum
- ☐ **D.** Laryngotracheal groove
- ☐ **E.** Foregut

28 A 3-month-old infant is diagnosed with a VSD at the area of the subpulmonary infundibulum. Which of the following structures must be avoided carefully by the surgeon when the sutures are placed at the site of the defect?

- ☐ **A.** Right bundle branch
- ☐ **B.** Right coronary artery
- ☐ **C.** Tricuspid valve
- ☐ **D.** Left anterior descending coronary artery
- ☐ **E.** Aortic valve

29 A 2-day-old infant is diagnosed with incomplete division of the foregut into respiratory and digestive portions. Which is the most common congenital condition characteristic of this description?

- ☐ **A.** Esophageal atresia
- ☐ **B.** Esophageal achalasia
- ☐ **C.** Tracheoesophageal fistula
- ☐ **D.** Congenital diaphragmatic hernia
- ☐ **E.** Esophageal fistula

30 An unconscious 2-month-old infant is admitted to the emergency department after an automobile collision. An emergency tracheostomy is performed. Which of the following structures is most commonly at high risk of injury during this procedure?

- ☐ **A.** Left brachiocephalic vein
- ☐ **B.** Left common carotid artery
- ☐ **C.** Vagus nerve
- ☐ **D.** Phrenic nerve
- ☐ **E.** Thoracic duct

31 A 45-year-old woman is admitted to the hospital with difficulty breathing. Radiologic examination reveals a tumor invading the lung surface anterior to the hilum. Which nerve is most likely compressed by the tumor to result in dyspnea?

☐ **A.** Phrenic
☐ **B.** Vagus
☐ **C.** Intercostal
☐ **D.** Recurrent laryngeal
☐ **E.** Cardiopulmonary

32 A 62-year-old male patient expresses concern that his voice has changed over the preceding months. Imaging reveals a growth located within the aortic arch, adjacent to the left pulmonary artery. Which neural structure is most likely being compressed to cause the changes in the patient's voice?

☐ **A.** Left phrenic nerve
☐ **B.** Esophageal plexus
☐ **C.** Left recurrent laryngeal nerve
☐ **D.** Left vagus nerve
☐ **E.** Left sympathetic trunk

33 A 39-year-old woman visits the outpatient clinic and complains of inability to reach a pantry shelf just above her head. History reveals that 2 months ago she underwent a mastectomy procedure and she did not have this complaint prior to the surgery. Which nerve was most likely damaged during surgery to result in the patient's complaint?

☐ **A.** Axillary
☐ **B.** Spinal accessory
☐ **C.** Long thoracic
☐ **D.** Radial
☐ **E.** Thoracodorsal

34 A 41-year-old woman is admitted to the emergency department with a complaint of severe, sharp, but poorly localized pain on the chest wall. Radiologic examination gives evidence of pleural effusion. What is the location of the neuronal cell bodies responsible for the nerve fibers that carry this pain to the central nervous system (CNS)?

☐ **A.** Dorsal root ganglia
☐ **B.** Sympathetic chain ganglia
☐ **C.** Dorsal horn of the spinal cord
☐ **D.** Lateral horn of the spinal cord
☐ **E.** Ventral horn of the spinal cord

35 A 23-year-old man is admitted to the emergency department after an automobile collision. Physical examination reveals tachycardia. What is the location of the preganglionic neural cell bodies involved in increasing the heart rate?

☐ **A.** Deep cardiac plexus
☐ **B.** Dorsal motor nucleus of vagus
☐ **C.** Lateral horn T5 to T9
☐ **D.** Lateral horn T1 to T4
☐ **E.** Inferior cervical ganglia

36 A 55-year-old man is admitted to the emergency department with a diagnosis of possible myocardial infarction. Which nerves carry pain fibers from the heart to the CNS?

☐ **A.** Vagus
☐ **B.** Greater thoracic splanchnic
☐ **C.** Least thoracic splanchnic
☐ **D.** Cardiopulmonary (thoracic visceral)
☐ **E.** T5 to T9 ventral rami

37 A 17-year-old girl is admitted to the hospital with severe dyspnea. Physical examination reveals that the patient is suffering from an asthma attack, with associated bronchospasm. Which of the following nerves is responsible for the innervation of the bronchial smooth muscle cells?

☐ **A.** Greater thoracic splanchnic
☐ **B.** Phrenic
☐ **C.** Vagus
☐ **D.** Intercostal
☐ **E.** Lesser thoracic splanchnic

38 A 42-year-old woman is admitted to the hospital with an inability to speak. The patient's personal history reveals that she has experienced hoarseness for the past month. A chest radiograph reveals a mass at the aortopulmonary window. Which of the following nerves is most likely compressed?

☐ **A.** Vagus
☐ **B.** Phrenic
☐ **C.** Left recurrent laryngeal
☐ **D.** Right recurrent laryngeal
☐ **E.** Greater thoracic splanchnic

39 Following the diagnosis of breast cancer, a 42-year-old woman underwent a total mastectomy, including excision of the axillary tail (of Spence). Postoperatively, the patient complains of dysesthesia in the inner aspect of the arm and axilla. Which of the following nerves was most likely injured during the procedure?

☐ **A.** Ulnar
☐ **B.** Long thoracic
☐ **C.** Intercostobrachial
☐ **D.** Lateral cutaneous nerve of T4
☐ **E.** Axillary nerve

40 A 39-year-old man is admitted to the hospital with a complaint of severe retrosternal pain that radiates to the left shoulder. The pain is relieved by leaning forward. Auscultation reveals a pericardial friction rub, leading to a diagnosis of pericarditis. Which of the following nerves is responsible for the radiating pain to the shoulder?

- ☐ **A.** Intercostobrachial
- ☐ **B.** Phrenic
- ☐ **C.** Long thoracic
- ☐ **D.** Greater thoracic splanchnic
- ☐ **E.** Cardiopulmonary

41 A 72-year-old man is admitted to the hospital with complaints of severe chest pain radiating to his left arm. ECG examination provides evidence of significant myocardial infarction of the posterior wall of the left ventricle. Which of the following nerves is responsible for the radiation of pain to the arm during myocardial infarction?

- ☐ **A.** Phrenic
- ☐ **B.** Vagus
- ☐ **C.** Intercostobrachial
- ☐ **D.** Greater splanchnic
- ☐ **E.** Suprascapular

42 A 43-year-old male hunter is admitted to the emergency department after falling over a barbed wire fence, as a result of which he suffered several deep lacerations along the left midaxillary line. When the patient is examined in the outpatient clinic several days later, numbness and anhydrosis are observed anterior to the area of the cuts. Which structures were most likely damaged to result in these signs?

- ☐ **A.** Dorsal roots
- ☐ **B.** Ventral roots
- ☐ **C.** Cutaneous branches of dorsal rami
- ☐ **D.** Cutaneous branches of ventral rami
- ☐ **E.** Rami communicans

43 A 62-year-old patient is admitted to the hospital with a complaint of suddenly occurring, tearing pain radiating to his back. A CT examination reveals that the patient has an aortic aneurysm. An urgent placement of an endovascular stent-graft is performed. Which of the following nerves are most likely responsible for the tearing sensation radiating to his back?

- ☐ **A.** Somatic afferent
- ☐ **B.** Thoracic visceral afferent
- ☐ **C.** Sympathetic postganglionics
- ☐ **D.** Sympathetic preganglionics
- ☐ **E.** Parasympathetic afferent

44 A 22-year-old woman had undergone elective breast enhancement, with the insertion of 250-ml saline bags bilaterally. This resulted, unfortunately, in loss of sensation bilaterally in the nipples and areolae and some reduction of sensation of the skin from the areolae laterally to the midaxillary lines. Which of the following nerves were most likely subject to iatrogenic injury?

- ☐ **A.** Anterior cutaneous branches of second and third intercostal nerves
- ☐ **B.** Anterior and lateral cutaneous branches of the fourth intercostal nerves
- ☐ **C.** Lateral pectoral nerves
- ☐ **D.** Cutaneous branches of the second thoracic spinal nerves (intercostobrachial nerves)
- ☐ **E.** Lateral cutaneous branches of the second and third intercostal nerves

45 A 32-year-old woman is admitted to the emergency department with dyspnea, dysphagia, hoarseness, and severe anxiety. Her medical history reveals that she has lived on a liquid diet for some months and has lost more than 30 lb. Over the past several weeks, she has had bloody sputum during attacks of coughing. Fluoroscopy and a barium swallow reveal a 4-cm mass associated with a bronchus and associated compression of the esophagus. Which of the following nerves is most likely to be affected?

- ☐ **A.** Right recurrent laryngeal nerve
- ☐ **B.** Left vagus nerve, posterior to the hilum of the lung
- ☐ **C.** Left recurrent laryngeal nerve
- ☐ **D.** Greater splanchnic nerve
- ☐ **E.** Phrenic nerve

46 A 35-year-old man is admitted to the hospital with pain on swallowing. Imaging reveals a dilated left atrium. Which structure is most likely being compressed by the expansion of the left atrium to result in the patient's symptoms?

- ☐ **A.** Esophagus
- ☐ **B.** Root of the lung
- ☐ **C.** Trachea
- ☐ **D.** Superior vena cava
- ☐ **E.** Inferior vena cava

47 A 69-year-old woman with advanced stage of laryngeal cancer has a tracheostomy and needs to be tube fed. A nasogastric tube is inserted. What is the last site at which resistance would be expected as the tube passes from the nose to the stomach?

- ▢ **A.** Pharyngoesophageal junction
- ▢ **B.** Level of the superior thoracic aperture
- ▢ **C.** Posterior to the aortic arch
- ▢ **D.** Posterior to the left main bronchus
- ▢ **E.** Esophageal hiatus of the diaphragm

48 A 59-year-old man is admitted to the hospital with severe chest pain. During examination a slight rhythmic pulsation on the chest wall at the left fifth intercostal space is noted in the midclavicular line. What part of the heart is responsible for this pulsation?

- ▢ **A.** Right atrium
- ▢ **B.** Left atrium
- ▢ **C.** Aortic arch
- ▢ **D.** Apex of the heart
- ▢ **E.** Mitral valve

49 A 42-year-old man was admitted to the hospital after a head-on vehicular collision in which he received severe blunt trauma to his sternum from the steering wheel. What part of the heart would be most likely to be injured by the impact?

- ▢ **A.** Right ventricle
- ▢ **B.** Apex of left ventricle
- ▢ **C.** Left ventricle
- ▢ **D.** Right atrium
- ▢ **E.** Anterior margin of the left atrium

50 A 54-year-old man is admitted to the hospital with dyspnea. Physical examination and echocardiographic studies reveal severe mitral valve prolapse. Auscultation of this valve is best performed at which location?

- ▢ **A.** Left fifth intercostal space, just below the nipple
- ▢ **B.** Right lower part of the body of the sternum
- ▢ **C.** Right second intercostal space near the lateral border of the sternum
- ▢ **D.** Directly over the middle of the manubrium
- ▢ **E.** Left second intercostal space near the lateral border of the sternum

51 A 48-year-old male patient is admitted with chronic angina. Coronary angiography reveals nearly total blockage of the circumflex artery near its origin from the left coronary artery. When this artery is exposed to perform a bypass procedure, what accompanying vein must be protected from injury?

- ▢ **A.** Middle cardiac
- ▢ **B.** Great cardiac
- ▢ **C.** Small cardiac
- ▢ **D.** Anterior cardiac
- ▢ **E.** Posterior cardiac

52 A 55-year-old patient is to undergo a coronary bypass operation. The artery of primary concern is the vessel that supplies much of the left ventricle and the right and left bundle branches of the cardiac conduction system. Which artery is the surgeon most concerned with?

- ▢ **A.** Right marginal
- ▢ **B.** Anterior interventricular
- ▢ **C.** Circumflex
- ▢ **D.** Artery to the sinu-atrial (SA) node
- ▢ **E.** Posterior interventricular

53 A 58-year-old male patient presents himself to the emergency department with severe angina. Upon cardiac catheterization, it is found that he has a significant occlusion in his right coronary artery, just distal to the right sinus of the aortic valve. His collateral cardiac circulation is minimal. Assuming the patient is right coronary dominant, which of the following arteries would be most likely to still have normal blood flow?

- ▢ **A.** Right (acute) marginal artery
- ▢ **B.** Atrioventricular nodal artery
- ▢ **C.** Posterior interventricular artery
- ▢ **D.** SA nodal artery
- ▢ **E.** Anterior interventricular artery

54 A 55-year-old man is admitted to the emergency department with severe chest pain. Coronary angiography reveals that the patient's right coronary artery is free of pathology. The left coronary artery is found to be 70% to 80% occluded at three points proximal to its bifurcation into the circumflex and left anterior descending arteries. Having a left dominant coronary circulation, and without surgery, what is the most likely explanation for a poor prognosis for recovery of this patient to a normally active life?

- ▢ **A.** All the branches of the coronary artery are end arteries, precluding the chance that anastomotic connections will occur.
- ▢ **B.** It is probable that the anterior and posterior papillary muscles of the tricuspid valve have been damaged.
- ▢ **C.** The blood supply of the SA node is inadequate.
- ▢ **D.** The development of effective collateral circulation between anterior and posterior interventricular arteries will not be possible.

- ▢ **E.** The blood supply of the atrioventricular (AV) node will be inadequate.

55 A 35-year-old woman is admitted to the hospital with dyspnea. During physical examination her S_1 heart sound is very loud. Which of the following valves is most likely defective?

- ▢ **A.** Mitral valve
- ▢ **B.** Aortic
- ▢ **C.** Pulmonary
- ▢ **D.** Aortic and pulmonary
- ▢ **E.** Tricuspid

56 A 72-year-old man is admitted to the hospital with severe chest pain. ECG examination provides evidence of severe myocardial infarction of the lower part of the muscular interventricular septum. The function of which of the following valves will be most severely affected?

- ▢ **A.** Pulmonary
- ▢ **B.** Aortic
- ▢ **C.** Tricuspid
- ▢ **D.** Mitral
- ▢ **E.** Eustachian

57 A 35-year-old woman is admitted to the hospital with a complaint of shortness of breath. During physical examination it is noted that there is wide splitting in her S_2 heart sound. ECG reveals a right bundle branch block. Which of the following valves is most likely defective?

- ▢ **A.** Mitral valve
- ▢ **B.** Pulmonary
- ▢ **C.** Aortic and mitral
- ▢ **D.** Tricuspid
- ▢ **E.** Tricuspid and aortic

58 A 3-month-old infant is diagnosed with a membranous VSD. A cardiac operation is performed, and the septal defect is patched inferior to the noncoronary cusp of the aorta. Two days postoperatively, the infant develops severe arrhythmias affecting both ventricles. Which part of the conduction tissue was most likely injured during the procedure?

- ▢ **A.** Right bundle branch
- ▢ **B.** Left bundle branch
- ▢ **C.** Bundle of His
- ▢ **D.** Posterior internodal pathway
- ▢ **E.** Atrioventricular node

59 A 62-year-old man was admitted to the hospital with intense left chest pain. ECG and echocardiography reveal myocardial infarction and pulmonary valve regurgitation. Emergency coronary angiography is performed and provides evidence that the artery supplying the upper portion of the anterior right ventricular free wall is occluded. Which of the following arteries is most likely to be occluded?

- ▢ **A.** Circumflex
- ▢ **B.** Anterior interventricular artery
- ▢ **C.** Posterior interventricular artery
- ▢ **D.** Artery of the conus
- ▢ **E.** Acute marginal branch of the right coronary artery

60 A 3-month-old male infant died unexpectedly in his sleep. The pathologist examined the histologic slides of tissue samples taken from the heart of the infant and observed that a portion of the conduction tissue that penetrates the right fibrous trigone had become necrotic. As a result, a fatal arrhythmia probably developed, leading to the death of the infant. Which of the following parts of the conduction tissue was most likely interrupted?

- ▢ **A.** Right bundle branch
- ▢ **B.** The bundle of Bachmann
- ▢ **C.** The left bundle branch
- ▢ **D.** The atrioventricular bundle of His
- ▢ **E.** The posterior internodal pathway

61 A 42-year-old woman is admitted to the hospital after blunt trauma to her sternum by the steering wheel during a car crash. Ultrasound examination reveals a cardiac tamponade. ECG data indicate that the heart has been severely injured. Which of the following cardiac structures will most likely be injured?

- ▢ **A.** Right ventricle
- ▢ **B.** Obtuse margin of the left ventricle
- ▢ **C.** Right atrium
- ▢ **D.** Left atrium
- ▢ **E.** Apex of the left ventricle

62 A 69-year-old man is admitted to the hospital with intense left chest pain. ECG reveals hypokinetic ventricular septal muscle, myocardial infarction in the anterior two thirds of the interventricular septum and left anterior ventricular wall. The patient's ECG also exhibited left bundle branch block. Which of the following arteries is most likely occluded?

- ▢ **A.** Circumflex
- ▢ **B.** Proximal right coronary

- ▢ **C.** Proximal left coronary
- ▢ **D.** Proximal left anterior interventricular artery
- ▢ **E.** Posterior interventricular artery

63 A 49-year-old woman is admitted to the hospital complaining of severe, crushing, retrosternal pain during the preceding hour. An ECG reveals that she is suffering from acute myocardial infarction in the posterior aspect of her left ventricle and posteromedial papillary muscle. A coronary angiogram is performed and the patient is found to have left dominant coronary circulation. Which of the following arteries is the most likely to be occluded?

- ▢ **A.** Artery of the conus
- ▢ **B.** Right coronary artery
- ▢ **C.** Circumflex
- ▢ **D.** Right acute marginal
- ▢ **E.** Left diagonal

64 A 75-year-old man is scheduled for his routine annual medical examination. During echocardiographic examination a large, mobile structure resembling a thrombus is identified in the right atrium near the opening of the inferior vena cava. After careful examination the doctor identifies the large mobile structure as a normal component of the heart. Which of the following structures could most likely resemble a thrombus in this location?

- ▢ **A.** Tricuspid valve
- ▢ **B.** Eustachian valve
- ▢ **C.** Thebesian valve
- ▢ **D.** Septum primum
- ▢ **E.** Fossa ovalis

65 A 4-year-old boy is operated on for a correction of a small, muscular interventricular septal defect. To access the right side of the interventricular septum, a wide incision is first made in the anterior surface of the right atrium. Instruments are then inserted through the tricuspid valve to correct the VSD. Which of the following structures is the most crucial to protect during the opening of the right atrium?

- ▢ **A.** Crista terminalis
- ▢ **B.** Pectinate muscles
- ▢ **C.** Tricuspid valve
- ▢ **D.** Eustachian valve
- ▢ **E.** Coronary sinus

66 A 52-year-old patient is admitted to the hospital with severe chest pain. ECG and radiologic examinations provide evidence of a significant myocardial infarction and cardiac tamponade. An emergency pericardiocentesis is performed. At which of the following locations will the needle best be inserted to relieve the tamponade?

- ▢ **A.** Right seventh intercostal space in the midaxillary line
- ▢ **B.** Left fifth intercostal space in the midclavicular line
- ▢ **C.** Right third intercostal space, 1 inch lateral to the sternum
- ▢ **D.** Left sixth intercostal space, ½ inch lateral to the sternum
- ▢ **E.** Triangle of auscultation

67 A 55-year-old man is brought to the emergency department after his motorcycle collided with an automobile. He is hypotensive, his pulse is irregular, and he shows other signs of substantial blood loss. MRI and CT scan evaluations reveal profuse abdominal bleeding. A decision is made to enter the chest so that the descending thoracic aorta can be clamped to minimize blood loss and to preserve cerebral blood flow. After surgical entrance into the thorax, the fibrous pericardium is elevated with forceps and punctured. A midline, longitudinal incision of the pericardium would best be made to prevent injury to which of the following structures?

- ▢ **A.** Auricular appendage of the left atrium
- ▢ **B.** Coronary sinus
- ▢ **C.** Left anterior descending artery
- ▢ **D.** Left phrenic nerve
- ▢ **E.** Left sympathetic trunk

68 During cardiac surgery of a 45-year-old man, the cardiac surgeon can place her fingers in the transverse pericardial sinus, if necessary. This allows the surgeon to easily place a vascular clamp upon which of the following vessels?

- ▢ **A.** Right and left pulmonary veins
- ▢ **B.** Superior and inferior vena cava
- ▢ **C.** Right and left coronary arteries
- ▢ **D.** Pulmonary trunk and ascending aorta
- ▢ **E.** Pulmonary trunk and superior vena cava

69 A 48-year-old male patient is scheduled to have a coronary arterial bypass because of chronic angina. Coronary arteriography reveals nearly total blockage of the posterior descending interventricular artery. In exposing this artery to perform the bypass procedure, which accompanying vessel is most susceptible to injury?

- ▢ **A.** Middle cardiac vein
- ▢ **B.** Great cardiac vein

- ▢ **C.** Small cardiac vein
- ▢ **D.** Anterior cardiac vein
- ▢ **E.** Coronary sinus

70 A 54-year-old man is admitted to the hospital with severe chest pain. ECG examination reveals a myocardial infarction. If the posterior interventricular branch in the patient arises from the right coronary artery, which part of the myocardium will most likely have its blood supply reduced if the circumflex branch of the left coronary artery becomes occluded from an atherosclerotic plaque?

- ▢ **A.** Anterior part of the interventricular septum
- ▢ **B.** Diaphragmatic surface of the right ventricle
- ▢ **C.** Infundibulum
- ▢ **D.** Lateral wall of the left ventricle
- ▢ **E.** Posterior part of the interventricular septum

71 A 70-year-old man with a history of two previous myocardial infarctions is admitted to the hospital with severe chest pain. ECG reveals a new myocardial infarction and ventricular arrhythmia. Coronary angiography reveals that the right coronary artery is blocked just distal to the origin of the right marginal artery in a right coronary dominant circulation. Which of the following structures would most likely be affected after such a blockade?

- ▢ **A.** Right atrium
- ▢ **B.** SA node
- ▢ **C.** AV node
- ▢ **D.** Lateral wall of the left ventricle
- ▢ **E.** Anterior interventricular septum

72 A 43-year-old woman is diagnosed with mitral valve stenosis. During physical examination the first heart sound is abnormally loud. Which of the following heart valves are responsible for the production of the first heart sound?

- ▢ **A.** Aortic and mitral
- ▢ **B.** Aortic and tricuspid
- ▢ **C.** Tricuspid and mitral
- ▢ **D.** Mitral and pulmonary
- ▢ **E.** Tricuspid and pulmonary

73 A 75-year-old woman is admitted to the hospital with anginal pain. ECG reveals myocardial infarction and a right bundle branch block. During physical examination the patient has a loud second heart sound. Which of the following heart valves are responsible for the production of the second heart sound?

- ▢ **A.** Aortic and pulmonary
- ▢ **B.** Aortic and tricuspid
- ▢ **C.** Tricuspid and mitral
- ▢ **D.** Mitral and pulmonary
- ▢ **E.** Tricuspid and pulmonary

74 Ten days after a surgical procedure to correct her cardiac malformation, a 3-month-old infant died unexpectedly in her sleep. After an autopsy, the pathologist reported as follows: "A significant portion of the conduction tissue was found to be necrotic. The area of the necrotic tissue was located inferior to the central fibrous body, membranous septum, and septal leaflet of the tricuspid valve. Further examination revealed infarction of the surrounding tissue. The rest of the heart was unremarkable." Which of the following arteries was most likely occluded?

- ▢ **A.** Artery of the conus
- ▢ **B.** SA node artery
- ▢ **C.** AV node artery
- ▢ **D.** First septal perforator of the anterior interventricular artery
- ▢ **E.** All of the above

75 A 55-year-old man is undergoing an aortic valve replacement. During the procedure the heart is connected to the heart lung machine. As the surgeon explores the oblique pericardial sinus, which of the following is not directly palpable with the tips of the fingers?

- ▢ **A.** Inferior vena cava
- ▢ **B.** Superior vena cava
- ▢ **C.** Posterior wall of the left atrium
- ▢ **D.** Inferior right pulmonary vein
- ▢ **E.** Right atrium

76 A 42-year-old woman is admitted urgently to the emergency department after suffering a penetrating wound to her chest from an ice pick during a violent domestic dispute. Physical and ultrasound examinations reveal that the patient has cardiac tamponade. Which of the following will most likely be found during physical examination?

- ▢ **A.** There will be a visible or palpable decrease in the dimensions of the external jugular and internal jugular vein
- ▢ **B.** There will be gradual enlargement of the ventricles in diastole
- ▢ **C.** The difference between systolic and diastolic arterial pressures will increase significantly
- ▢ **D.** There will be diminished heart sounds
- ▢ **E.** The pulses in the internal carotid arteries will become increasingly distinct, as detected behind the angles of the mandible

77 During surgical repair of a congenital cardiac anomaly in a 15-year-old boy with a right dominant coronary arterial system, the surgeon accidentally injured a vessel that usually supplies part of the conduction system. This results in intermittent periods of atrioventricular block and severe arrhythmia. The injured artery was most likely a direct branch of which of the following arteries?

- ☐ **A.** Distal anterior interventricular artery
- ☐ **B.** Circumflex artery
- ☐ **C.** Left coronary artery
- ☐ **D.** Marginal artery
- ☐ **E.** Right coronary artery

78 A 42-year-old woman is admitted to the hospital with dyspnea. Imaging reveals severe mitral valve regurgitation. Which of the following structures prevents regurgitation of the mitral valve cusps into the left atrium during systole?

- ☐ **A.** Crista terminalis
- ☐ **B.** Crista supraventricularis
- ☐ **C.** Pectinate muscles
- ☐ **D.** Chordae tendineae
- ☐ **E.** Trabeculae carneae

79 A 58-year-old woman with cardiac arrhythmia has undergone a procedure to implant a pacemaker. The electrical conducting leads for the pacemaker must be passed into the heart from the pacemaker. Which of the following is the correct order of structures for passage of the leads into the right ventricle?

- ☐ **A.** Brachiocephalic vein, superior vena cava, mitral valve, right ventricle
- ☐ **B.** Superior vena cava, right atrium, mitral valve, right ventricle
- ☐ **C.** Superior vena cava, right atrium, tricuspid valve, right ventricle
- ☐ **D.** Brachiocephalic vein, superior vena cava, right atrium, tricuspid valve, right ventricle
- ☐ **E.** Brachiocephalic vein, superior vena cava, right atrium, mitral valve, right ventricle

80 A 68-year-old man patient in the cardiology ward complains at each mealtime of difficulty in swallowing (dysphagia). Radiologic studies reveal significant cardiac hypertrophy. A barium swallow, followed by radiologic examination of the thorax, reveals esophageal constriction directly posterior to the heart. Which of the following is the most likely cause of the patient's dysphagia?

- ☐ **A.** Mitral valve stenosis
- ☐ **B.** Pulmonary valve stenosis
- ☐ **C.** Regurgitation of the aorta
- ☐ **D.** Occlusion of the anterior interventricular artery
- ☐ **E.** Occlusion of the posterior interventricular artery

81 A 35-year-old woman is admitted to the emergency department because of cardiac arrhythmia. ECG examination reveals that the patient suffers from atrial fibrillation. Where is the mass of specialized conducting tissue that initiates the cardiac cycle located?

- ☐ **A.** At the junction of the coronary sinus and the right atrium
- ☐ **B.** At the junction of the inferior vena cava and the right atrium
- ☐ **C.** At the junction of the superior vena cava and the right atrium
- ☐ **D.** Between the left and right atria
- ☐ **E.** In the interventricular septum

82 A 45-year-old woman is admitted to the hospital with swelling (edema) of the lower limbs. Ultrasound examination reveals an incompetent tricuspid valve. Into which area will regurgitation of blood occur in this patient?

- ☐ **A.** Pulmonary trunk
- ☐ **B.** Left atrium
- ☐ **C.** Ascending aorta
- ☐ **D.** Right atrium
- ☐ **E.** Left ventricle

83 A 34-year-old man with a complaint of sharp, localized pain over the thoracic wall is diagnosed with pleural effusion. Through which intercostal space along the midaxillary line is it most appropriate to insert a chest tube to drain the effusion fluid?

- ☐ **A.** Fourth
- ☐ **B.** Sixth
- ☐ **C.** Eighth
- ☐ **D.** Tenth
- ☐ **E.** Twelfth

84 A 51-year-old man is admitted to the hospital with severe dyspnea. Radiologic examination reveals a tension pneumothorax. Adequate local anesthesia of the chest wall prior to insertion of a chest tube is necessary for pain control. Of the following layers, which is the deepest that must be infiltrated with the local anesthetic to achieve adequate anesthesia?

- ☐ **A.** Endothoracic fascia
- ☐ **B.** Intercostal muscles

- ▢ **C.** Parietal pleura
- ▢ **D.** Subcutaneous fat
- ▢ **E.** Visceral pleura

85 A 5-year-old boy had been playing with a small toy car. Soon after, he put a wheel from one of the cars in his mouth and began choking and coughing. Where in the tracheobronchial tree is the most common site for a foreign object to lodge?

- ▢ **A.** The right primary bronchus
- ▢ **B.** The left primary bronchus
- ▢ **C.** The carina of the trachea
- ▢ **D.** The beginning of the trachea
- ▢ **E.** The left tertiary bronchus

86 A 3-year-old child is admitted to the emergency department with a particularly severe attack of asthma. Which of the following is the most important factor in increasing the intrathoracic capacity in inspiration?

- ▢ **A.** "Pump handle movement" of the ribs—thereby increasing anterior-posterior dimensions of the thorax
- ▢ **B.** "Bucket handle movement" of the ribs—increasing the transverse diameter of the thorax
- ▢ **C.** Straightening of the forward curvature of the thoracic spine, thereby increasing the vertical dimensions of the thoracic cavity
- ▢ **D.** Descent of the diaphragm, with protrusion of the abdominal wall, thereby increasing vertical dimensions of the thoracic cavity
- ▢ **E.** Orientation and flexibility of the ribs in the baby, thus allowing expansion in all directions

87 A 54-year-old woman is admitted to the hospital with a stab wound of the thoracic wall in the area of the right fourth costal cartilage. Which of the following pulmonary structures is present at this site?

- ▢ **A.** The horizontal fissure of the left lung
- ▢ **B.** The horizontal fissure of the right lung
- ▢ **C.** The oblique fissure of the left lung
- ▢ **D.** The apex of the right lung
- ▢ **E.** The root of the left lung

88 A 55-year-old woman visited her doctor because of a painful lump in her right breast and a bloody discharge from her right nipple. Radiologic studies and physical examination reveal unilateral inversion of the nipple, and a tumor in the right upper quadrant of the breast is suspected. In addition, there is an orange-peel appearance of the skin *(peau d'orange)* in the vicinity of the areola. Which of the following best explains the inversion of her nipple?

- ▢ **A.** Retention of the fetal and infantile state of the nipple
- ▢ **B.** Intraductal cancerous tumor
- ▢ **C.** Retraction of the suspensory ligaments of the breast by cancer
- ▢ **D.** Obstruction of the cutaneous lymphatics, with edema of the skin
- ▢ **E.** Inflammation of the epithelial lining of the nipple and underlying hypodermis

89 A 58-year-old woman is admitted to the emergency department with severe dyspnea. Bronchoscopy reveals that the carina is distorted and widened. Enlargement of which group of lymph nodes is most likely responsible for altering the carina?

- ▢ **A.** Pulmonary
- ▢ **B.** Bronchopulmonary
- ▢ **C.** Inferior tracheobronchial
- ▢ **D.** Superior tracheobronchial
- ▢ **E.** Paratracheal

90 A 72-year-old patient vomited and then aspirated some of the vomitus while under anesthesia. On bronchoscopic examination, partially digested food is observed blocking the origin of the right superior lobar bronchus. Which of the following groups of bronchopulmonary segments will be affected by this obstruction?

- ▢ **A.** Superior, medial, lateral, medial basal
- ▢ **B.** Apical, anterior, posterior
- ▢ **C.** Posterior, anterior, superior, lateral
- ▢ **D.** Apical, lateral, medial, lateral basal
- ▢ **E.** Anterior, superior, medial, lateral

91 A 35-year-old woman is admitted to a surgical ward with a palpable mass in her right breast and swollen lymph nodes in the ipsilateral axilla. Radiologic studies and biopsy reveal carcinoma of the breast. Which group of axillary lymph nodes is the first to receive lymph drainage from the secretory tissue of the breast and therefore most likely to contain metastasized tumor cells?

- ▢ **A.** Lateral
- ▢ **B.** Central
- ▢ **C.** Apical
- ▢ **D.** Anterior (pectoral)
- ▢ **E.** Posterior (subscapular)

92 An 18-year-old man is admitted to the emergency department because of a significant nose bleed and a headache that has worsened over several days. He also complains of fatigue. Upon examination it is noted that brachial artery pressure is markedly increased, femoral pressure is decreased, and the femoral pulses are delayed. The patient shows no external signs of inflammation. Which of the following is the most likely diagnosis?

- ▢ **A.** Coarctation of the aorta
- ▢ **B.** Cor pulmonale
- ▢ **C.** Dissecting aneurysm of the right common iliac artery
- ▢ **D.** Obstruction of the superior vena cava
- ▢ **E.** Pulmonary embolism

93 A 22-year-old man is diagnosed with signs of reduced aortic flow. Upon examination it is noted that brachial artery pressure is markedly increased, femoral pressure is decreased, and the femoral pulses are delayed. The patient shows no external signs of inflammation. Which of the following conditions will most likely be observed in a radiologic examination?

- ▢ **A.** Flail chest
- ▢ **B.** Pneumothorax
- ▢ **C.** Hydrothorax
- ▢ **D.** Notching of the ribs
- ▢ **E.** Mediastinal shift

94 A patient who has undergone a radical mastectomy with extensive axillary dissection exhibits winging of the scapula when she pushes against resistance on an immovable object, such as a wall. Injury of which of the following nerves would result in this condition?

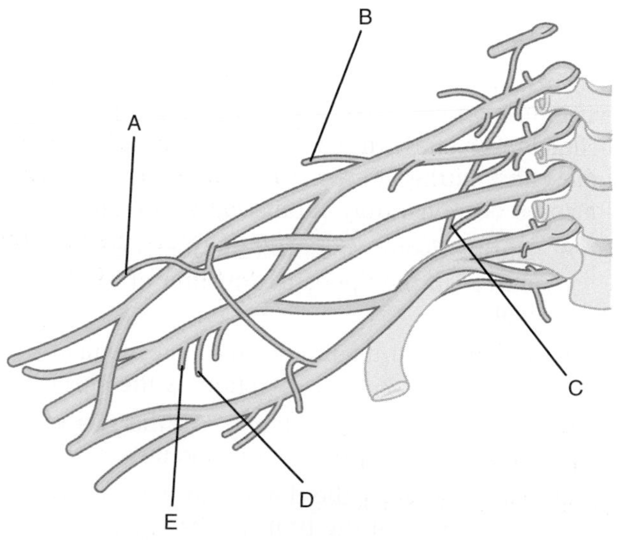

- ▢ **A.** A
- ▢ **B.** B
- ▢ **C.** C
- ▢ **D.** D
- ▢ **E.** E

95 A 22-year-old woman sustained a chest injury upon impact with the steering wheel during a car crash. Upon admission of the patient to the hospital, physical examination revealed profuse swelling, inflammation, and deformation of the chest wall. A radiograph revealed an uncommon fracture of the sternum at the manubriosternal joint. Which of the following ribs would be most likely to also be involved in such an injury?

- ▢ **A.** First
- ▢ **B.** Second
- ▢ **C.** Third
- ▢ **D.** Fourth
- ▢ **E.** Fifth

96 A 47-year-old man is admitted to the emergency department, due to severe dysphagia. Edema of the left upper limb is apparent upon physical examination. A barium sulfate swallow imaging procedure reveals esophageal dilation, with severe inflammation, due to constriction at the esophageal hiatus from a large lipoma. What is the most likely cause of the severe edema of the left upper limb?

- ▢ **A.** Thoracic aorta constriction
- ▢ **B.** Thoracic duct blockage
- ▢ **C.** Superior vena cava occlusion
- ▢ **D.** Aortic aneurysm
- ▢ **E.** Femoral artery disease

97 In coronary bypass graft surgery of a 49-year-old woman, the internal thoracic artery is used as the coronary artery bypass graft. The anterior intercostal arteries in intercostal spaces three to six are ligated. Which of the following arteries will be expected to supply these intercostal spaces?

- ▢ **A.** Musculophrenic
- ▢ **B.** Superior epigastric
- ▢ **C.** Posterior intercostal
- ▢ **D.** Lateral thoracic
- ▢ **E.** Thoracodorsal

98 A 10-year-old boy is admitted to the hospital with retrosternal discomfort. A CT scan reveals a midline tumor of the thymus gland. Which of the following veins would most likely be compressed by the tumor?

- ▢ **A.** Right internal jugular
- ▢ **B.** Left internal jugular
- ▢ **C.** Right brachiocephalic
- ▢ **D.** Left brachiocephalic
- ▢ **E.** Right subclavian

99 A 25-year-old man is admitted to the emergency department with a bullet wound in the neck just above the middle of the right clavicle and first rib. Radiologic examination reveals collapse of the right lung and a tension pneumothorax. Injury to which of the following respiratory structures resulted in the pneumothorax?

- ▢ **A.** Costal pleura
- ▢ **B.** Cupula
- ▢ **C.** Right mainstem bronchus
- ▢ **D.** Right upper lobe bronchus
- ▢ **E.** Mediastinal parietal pleura

100 A 51-year-old woman with a history of brain tumor and associated severe oropharyngeal dysphagia develops right lower lobe pneumonia after an episode of vomiting. Which of the following is the best reason that this type of aspiration pneumonia most commonly affects the right lower lung lobe?

- ▢ **A.** Pulmonary vascular resistance is higher in the right lung than the left lung
- ▢ **B.** The right main bronchus is straighter than the left main bronchus
- ▢ **C.** The right main bronchus is narrower than the main bronchus
- ▢ **D.** The right main bronchus is longer than the left main bronchus
- ▢ **E.** The right lower lung lobe has poorer venous drainage than the other lobes

101 A 41-year-old man is admitted to the emergency department with complaints of shortness of breath, dizziness, and sharp chest pain. The large arrow in his chest radiograph indicates the region of pathology (Fig. 2-1). What is this structure?

- ▢ **A.** Superior vena cava
- ▢ **B.** Right ventricle
- ▢ **C.** Left ventricle
- ▢ **D.** Arch of the aorta
- ▢ **E.** Pulmonary artery

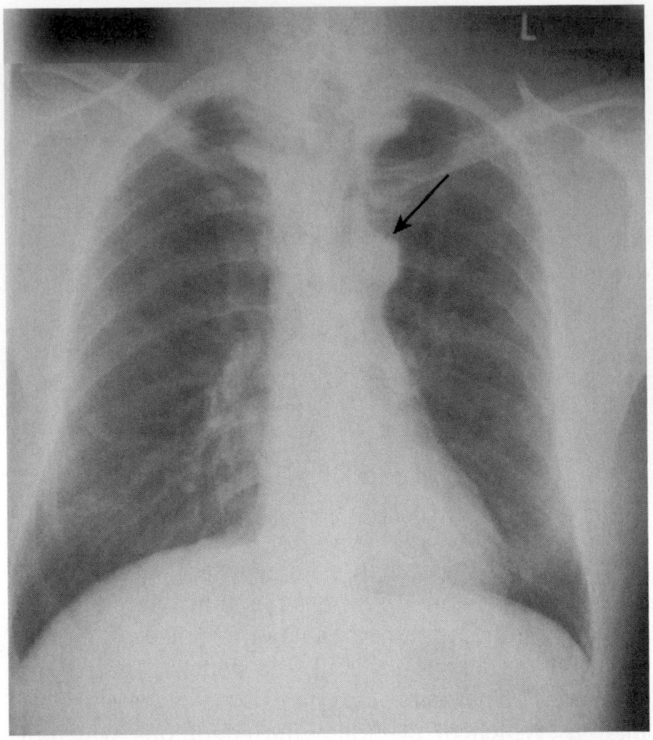

Fig. 2-1

102 A 42-year-old woman is seen by her family physician because she has a painful lump in her right breast and a bloody discharge from her right nipple. Upon physical examination it is noted that there is unilateral inversion of the right nipple and a hard, woody texture of the skin over a mass of tissue in the right upper quadrant of the breast. Which of the following conditions is most frequently characterized by these symptoms?

- ▢ **A.** *Peau d'orange*
- ▢ **B.** Cancer *en cuirasse*
- ▢ **C.** Intraductal cancerous tumor
- ▢ **D.** Obstruction of the lymphatics draining the skin of the breast, with edema of the skin
- ▢ **E.** Inflammation of the epithelial lining of the nipple and underlying hypodermis

103 A 25-year-old woman is admitted to the hospital after an automobile crash. Radiologic examination reveals four broken ribs in the left thoracic wall, producing a flail chest observable on physical examination. Which of the following conditions is most likely to also be observed during physical examination?

- ▢ **A.** During deep inspiration the flail segment moves in the opposite direction of the chest wall
- ▢ **B.** During deep inspiration the flail segment moves in the same direction as the chest wall
- ▢ **C.** "Pump handle movements" of the ribs will not be affected by the rib fractures
- ▢ **D.** The descent of the diaphragm will be affected on the side of the broken ribs

☐ **E.** The descent of the diaphragm will be affected on the side of the broken ribs and also on the opposite side

104 A 33-year-old man is admitted to the hospital with severe traumatic injuries. His blood pressure is 89/39 mm Hg, and a central venous line is placed. Which of the following injuries is most likely to occur when a subclavian central venous line procedure is performed?

☐ **A.** Penetration of the subclavian artery

☐ **B.** Injury of the phrenic nerve

☐ **C.** Penetration of the superior vena cava

☐ **D.** Penetration of the left common carotid artery

☐ **E.** Impalement of the vagus nerve

105 A 39-year-old man is admitted to the hospital with odynophagia. A barium swallow reveals an esophageal constriction at the level of the diaphragm. A CT scan and a biopsy further indicate the presence of an esophageal cancer. Which of the following lymph nodes will most likely be affected first?

☐ **A.** Posterior mediastinal and left gastric

☐ **B.** Bronchopulmonary

☐ **C.** Tracheobronchial

☐ **D.** Inferior tracheobronchial

☐ **E.** Superior tracheobronchial

106 A 42-year-old man is admitted to the hospital with retrosternal pain. Endoscopy and biopsy examinations of the trachea reveal a malignant growth at the right main bronchus. Which of the following lymph nodes will most likely be the first infiltrated by cancerous cells from the malignancy?

☐ **A.** Inferior tracheobronchial

☐ **B.** Paratracheal

☐ **C.** Bronchomediastinal trunk

☐ **D.** Bronchopulmonary

☐ **E.** Thoracic duct

107 A 60-year-old man is admitted to the hospital with severe abdominal pain. A CT scan reveals a dissecting aneurysm of the thoracic aorta. While in the hospital, the patient's aneurysm ruptures and he is transferred urgently to the operating theater. Postoperatively, the patient suffers from paraplegia. Which of the following arteries was most likely injured during the operation to result in the paralysis?

☐ **A.** Right coronary artery

☐ **B.** Left common carotid

☐ **C.** Right subclavian

☐ **D.** Great radicular (of Adamkiewicz)

☐ **E.** Esophageal

108 A 47-year-old woman is admitted to the hospital with pain in her neck. During physical examination it is observed that the thyroid gland is enlarged and is displacing the trachea. A biopsy reveals a benign tumor. A CT scan examination reveals tracheal deviation to the left. Which of the following structures will most likely be compressed as a result of the deviation?

☐ **A.** Left brachiocephalic vein

☐ **B.** Left internal jugular vein

☐ **C.** Left subclavian artery

☐ **D.** Vagus nerve

☐ **E.** Phrenic nerve

109 A 33-year-old man is admitted to the hospital after a multiple car collision. His blood pressure is 89/39 mm Hg, and a central venous line is placed. Which of the following structures is used as a landmark to verify that the the tip of the catheter of the central venous line is in the correct place?

☐ **A.** Carina

☐ **B.** Subclavian artery

☐ **C.** Superior vena cava

☐ **D.** Left atrium

☐ **E.** Right atrium

110 A 42-year-old man is diagnosed with liver and pancreatic disease as a result of alcoholism. During physical examination it is noted that he has abnormal enlargement of his mammary glands, as a secondary result of his disease process. Which of the following clinical conditions will most likely describe this case?

☐ **A.** Polythelia

☐ **B.** Supernumerary breast

☐ **C.** Polymastia

☐ **D.** Gynecomastia

☐ **E.** Amastia

111 A 21-year-old woman gymnast is admitted to the hospital with severe dyspnea after a fall from the uneven parallel bars. Radiologic examination reveals that her right lung is collapsed and the left lung is compressed by the great volume of air in her right pleural cavity. During physical examination she has no signs of external injuries. Which of the following conditions will most likely describe this case?

☐ **A.** Flail chest with paradoxical respiration

☐ **B.** Emphysema

- ☐ **C.** Hemothorax
- ☐ **D.** Chylothorax
- ☐ **E.** Tension pneumothorax

112 A 34-year-old man unconscious patient is admitted to the hospital. His blood pressure is 85/45 mm Hg. A central venous line is placed. During subsequent radiologic examination, a chylothorax is detected. Which of the following structures was most likely accidentally damaged during the placement of the central venous line?

- ☐ **A.** Left external jugular vein
- ☐ **B.** Site of origin of the left brachiocephalic vein
- ☐ **C.** Right subclavian vein
- ☐ **D.** Proximal part of right brachiocephalic vein
- ☐ **E.** Right external jugular vein

113 A 28-year-old woman in the third trimester of pregnancy has experienced severe dizziness for several days and is admitted to the hospital. During physical examination her blood pressure is normal when standing or sitting. When the patient is supine, her blood pressure drops to 90/50 mm Hg. What is the most likely explanation for these findings?

- ☐ **A.** Compression of the inferior vena cava
- ☐ **B.** Compression of the superior vena cava
- ☐ **C.** Compression of the aorta
- ☐ **D.** Compression of the common carotid artery
- ☐ **E.** Compression of the internal jugular veins

114 A 17-year-old girl is admitted to the hospital with dyspnea and fever. Radiologic examination reveals lobar pneumonia in one of the lobes of her right lung. During auscultation at the level of the sixth intercostal space at the midaxillary line, rales (or crackles) are heard and dull sounds are produced during percussion. Which of the following lobes is most likely to be involved by pneumonia?

- ☐ **A.** Upper lobe of the right lung
- ☐ **B.** Middle lobe of the right lung
- ☐ **C.** Lower lobe of the right lung
- ☐ **D.** Lower lobes of the right and left lungs
- ☐ **E.** Upper lobes of the right and left lungs

115 A 35-year-old man is admitted to the hospital with severe chest pain, dyspnea, tachycardia, cough, and fever. Radiologic examination reveals significant pericardial effusion. When pericardiocentesis is performed, the needle is inserted up from the infrasternal angle. The needle passes too deeply, piercing the visceral pericardium and entering the heart. Which of the following chambers would be the first to be penetrated by the needle?

- ☐ **A.** Right ventricle
- ☐ **B.** Left ventricle
- ☐ **C.** Right atrium
- ☐ **D.** Left atrium
- ☐ **E.** The left cardiac apex

116 A 45-year-old man is admitted to the hospital with severe chest pain radiating to his left arm and left upper jaw. An emergency ECG reveals an acute myocardial infarction of the posterior left ventricular wall. Which of the following spinal cord segments would most likely receive the sensations of pain in this case?

- ☐ **A.** T1, T2, T3
- ☐ **B.** T1, T2, T3, T4
- ☐ **C.** T1, T2
- ☐ **D.** T4, T5, T6
- ☐ **E.** T5, T6, T7

117 A 55-year-old woman is admitted to the hospital with cough and severe dyspnea. Radiologic examination reveals that the patient suffers from emphysema. Upon physical examination the patient shows only "bucket handle movements" during deep inspiration. Which of the following movements of the thoracic wall is characteristic for this type of breathing?

- ☐ **A.** Increase of the transverse diameter of the thorax
- ☐ **B.** Increase of the anteroposterior diameter of the thorax
- ☐ **C.** Increase of the vertical dimension of the thorax
- ☐ **D.** Decrease of the anteroposterior diameter of the thorax
- ☐ **E.** Decrease of the transverse diameter of the thorax

118 A 15-year-old male is admitted to the hospital with cough and severe dyspnea. Physical examination reveals expiratory wheezes, and a diagnosis is made of acute asthma. The expiratory wheezes are characteristic signs of bronchospasm of the smooth muscle of the bronchial airways. Which of the following nerves could be blocked to result in relaxation of the smooth muscle?

- ☐ **A.** Phrenic
- ☐ **B.** Intercostal
- ☐ **C.** Vagus
- ☐ **D.** T1 to T4 sympathetic fibers
- ☐ **E.** Recurrent laryngeal nerve

119 A 34-year-old man with a complaint of sharp, localized pain over the thoracic wall is diagnosed with pleural effusion. A chest tube is inserted to drain the effusion through an intercostal space. At which of the following locations is the chest tube most likely to be inserted?

- ▢ **A.** Superior to the upper border of the rib
- ▢ **B.** Inferior to the lower border of the rib
- ▢ **C.** At the middle of the intercostal space
- ▢ **D.** Between the internal and external intercostal muscles
- ▢ **E.** Between the intercostal muscles and the posterior intercostal membrane

120 A 42-year-old woman is admitted to the emergency department after a fall from the balcony of her apartment. During physical examination there is an absence of heart sounds, reduced systolic pressure, reduced cardiac output, and engorged jugular veins. Which condition is most likely characterized by these signs?

- ▢ **A.** Hemothorax
- ▢ **B.** Cardiac tamponade
- ▢ **C.** Hemopneumothorax
- ▢ **D.** Pneumothorax
- ▢ **E.** Deep vein thrombosis

121 A 35-year-old woman is admitted to the hospital with a complaint of shortness of breath. During physical examination it is noted that there is wide splitting in her S_2 heart sound. Which of the following valve(s) is/are responsible for production of the S_2 heart sound?

- ▢ **A.** Mitral valve
- ▢ **B.** Pulmonary and aortic
- ▢ **C.** Aortic and mitral
- ▢ **D.** Tricuspid
- ▢ **E.** Tricuspid and aortic

122 A 35-year-old woman is admitted to the hospital with dyspnea. During physical examination her S_1 heart sound is very loud. Which of the following valve(s) is/are responsible for production of the S_1 heart sound?

- ▢ **A.** Mitral valve
- ▢ **B.** Pulmonary and aortic
- ▢ **C.** Aortic and mitral
- ▢ **D.** Tricuspid
- ▢ **E.** Tricuspid and mitral

123 A 57-year-old man is admitted to the emergency department after he was struck by a truck while crossing a busy street. Radiologic examination reveals flail chest. During physical examination, the patient complains of severe pain during inspiration and expiration. Which of the following nerves is most likely responsible for the sensation of pain during respiration?

- ▢ **A.** Phrenic
- ▢ **B.** Vagus
- ▢ **C.** Cardiopulmonary
- ▢ **D.** Intercostal
- ▢ **E.** Thoracic splanchnic

124 A 62-year-old woman is admitted to the hospital with severe dyspnea and also complains of pain over her left shoulder. A radiologic examination reveals an aneurysm of the aortic arch. Which of the following nerves is most likely affected by the aneurysm?

- ▢ **A.** Phrenic
- ▢ **B.** Vagus
- ▢ **C.** Cardiopulmonary
- ▢ **D.** Intercostal
- ▢ **E.** Thoracic splanchnic

125 A 62-year-old woman accountant is admitted to the emergency department with severe chest pains that radiate to her left arm. ECG reveals that the patient suffers from an acute myocardial infarction. Coronary angiography is performed and a stent is placed at the proximal portion of the anterior interventricular artery (left anterior descending). Because of the low ejection fraction of the right and left ventricles, a cardiac pacemaker is also placed in the heart. The function of which of the following structures is essentially replaced by the insertion of a pacemaker?

- ▢ **A.** AV node
- ▢ **B.** SA node
- ▢ **C.** Purkinje fibers
- ▢ **D.** Bundle of His
- ▢ **E.** Bundle of Kent

126 A 22-year-old marathon runner is admitted to the emergency department with severe dyspnea. Physical examination reveals that the patient is experiencing an acute asthma attack, and a bronchodilating drug is administered. Which of the following elements of the nervous system must be inhibited by the drug to achieve relaxation of the smooth muscle of the tracheobronchial tree?

- ▢ **A.** Postganglionic sympathetic fibers
- ▢ **B.** Preganglionic sympathetic fibers
- ▢ **C.** Postganglionic parasympathetic fibers
- ▢ **D.** Visceral afferent fibers
- ▢ **E.** Somatic efferent fibers

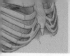

127 Radiologic examination of a 3-day-old infant who was cyanotic gives evidence of abnormalities within the heart. Blood tests reveal abnormally high levels of TGF-β factor *Nodal*. Which of the following conditions is most likely to be associated with these findings?

- ☐ **A.** Dextrocardia
- ☐ **B.** Ectopia cordis
- ☐ **C.** Transposition of the great arteries
- ☐ **D.** Unequal division of the truncus arteriosus
- ☐ **E.** Coarctation of the aorta

128 A 35-year-old woman who was brought into the emergency department for a drug overdose requires insertion of a nasogastric tube and administration of activated charcoal. What are the three sites in the esophagus where one should anticipate resistance due to compression on the organ?

- ☐ **A.** At the aortic arch, the cricopharyngeal constriction, and the diaphragmatic constriction
- ☐ **B.** The cardiac constriction, the cricoid cartilage constriction, and the thoracic duct
- ☐ **C.** The pulmonary constriction, cricothyroid constriction, and the azygos vein arch
- ☐ **D.** The cardiac constriction, the azygos vein arch, and the pulmonary trunk
- ☐ **E.** The cricopharyngeal constriction, cricothyroid constriction, and thymus gland

129 A 29-year-old patient complains of severe pain radiating across her back and chest. Upon clinical examination you observe a rash characteristic of herpes zoster infection passing from her upper left back and across her left nipple. Which of the following spinal nerve roots sheds the active virus?

- ☐ **A.** Dorsal root of T3
- ☐ **B.** Ventral root of T3
- ☐ **C.** Dorsal root of T4
- ☐ **D.** Ventral root of T4
- ☐ **E.** Dorsal root of T5

130 A 3-year-old man who fell from a tree complains of severe pain over the right side of his chest because of a rib fracture at the midaxillary line. He is admitted to the hospital due to his difficulty breathing. Radiologic and physical examinations reveal atelectasis, resulting from the accumulation of blood in his pleural space and resulting hemothorax. What is the most likely the source of bleeding to cause the hemothorax?

- ☐ **A.** Left common carotid artery
- ☐ **B.** Intercostal vessels
- ☐ **C.** Pulmonary arteries
- ☐ **D.** Pulmonary veins
- ☐ **E.** Internal thoracic artery

131 A 45-year-old woman is admitted to the hospital with severe dyspnea. Radiologic examination confirms the presence of a Pancoast tumor (Fig. 2-2). Physical examination reveals that the patient has miosis of the pupil, partial ptosis of the eyelid, and anhydrosis of the face. Which of the following structures has most likely been injured?

- ☐ **A.** Sympathetic chain
- ☐ **B.** Vagus nerve
- ☐ **C.** Phrenic nerve

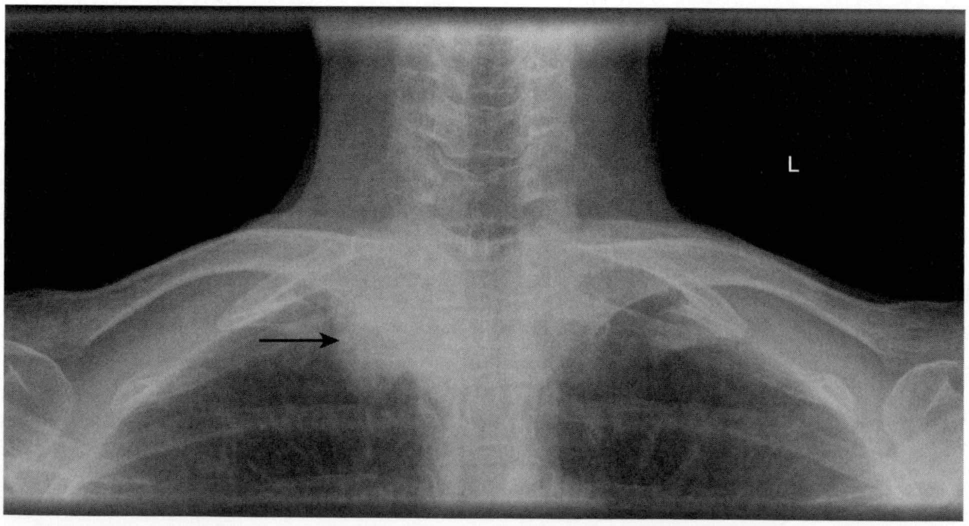

 Fig. 2-2

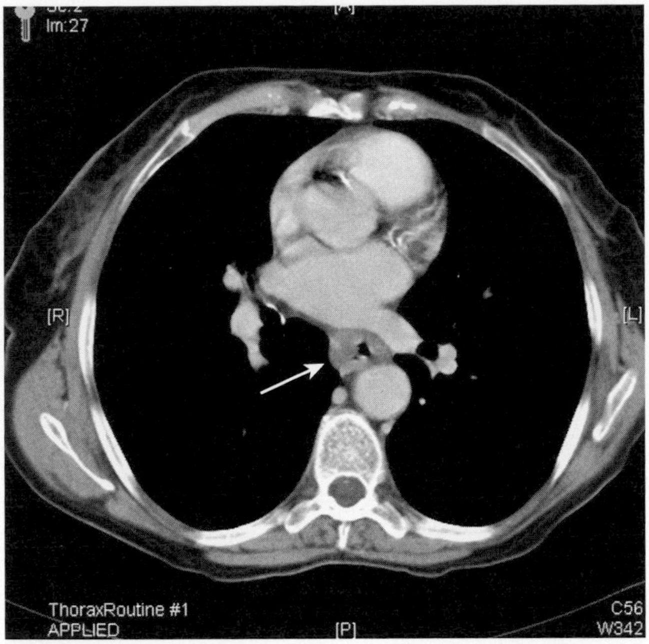

Fig. 2-3

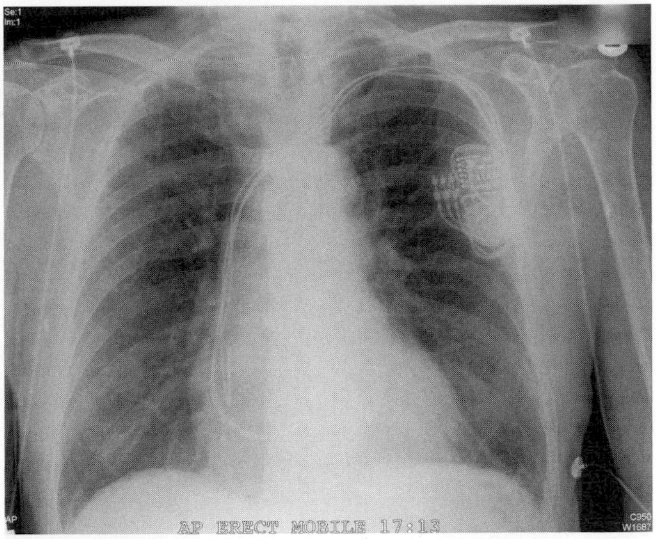

Fig. 2-4

- ▢ **D.** Arch of aorta
- ▢ **E.** Cardiopulmonary plexus

132 A 35-year-old male bartender is admitted to the hospital due to severe dysphagia. A CT scan (Fig. 2-3) reveals carcinoma of the middle segment of the esophagus. Which of the following structures will most likely be affected if the carcinoma increases greatly in size?

- ▢ **A.** Inferior vena cava
- ▢ **B.** Left atrium
- ▢ **C.** Pulmonary artery
- ▢ **D.** Left ventricle
- ▢ **E.** Vertebral body

133 A 62-year-old male internist is admitted to the emergency department with a complaint of severe chest pain. Physical examination reveals acute myocardial infarction. After the patient is stabilized, angiography is performed and the ejection fraction of the left ventricle is reduced to 30% of normal values. A cardiac pacemaker is placed to prevent fatal arrhythmias (Fig. 2-4). What is the location of the tip of the pacemaker?

- ▢ **A.** Right atrium
- ▢ **B.** Left atrium
- ▢ **C.** Right ventricle
- ▢ **D.** Left ventricle
- ▢ **E.** Superior vena cava

134 Postoperative examination of a 68-year-old man who underwent mitral valve replacement demonstrates

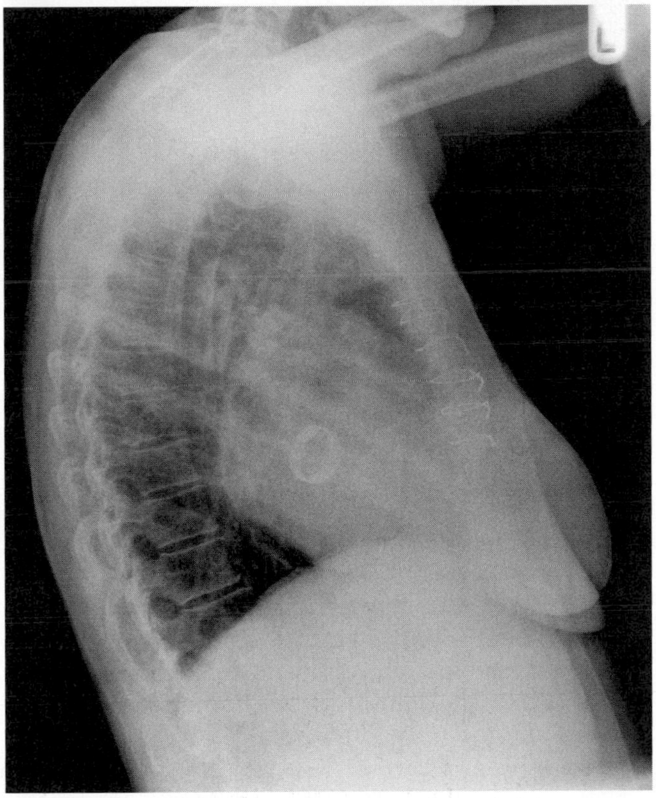

Fig. 2-5

significant cardiac hypertrophy (Fig. 2-5). Which of the following structures would be most likely compressed?

- ▢ **A.** Esophagus
- ▢ **B.** Pulmonary trunk
- ▢ **C.** Superior vena cava
- ▢ **D.** Trachea
- ▢ **E.** Inferior vena cava

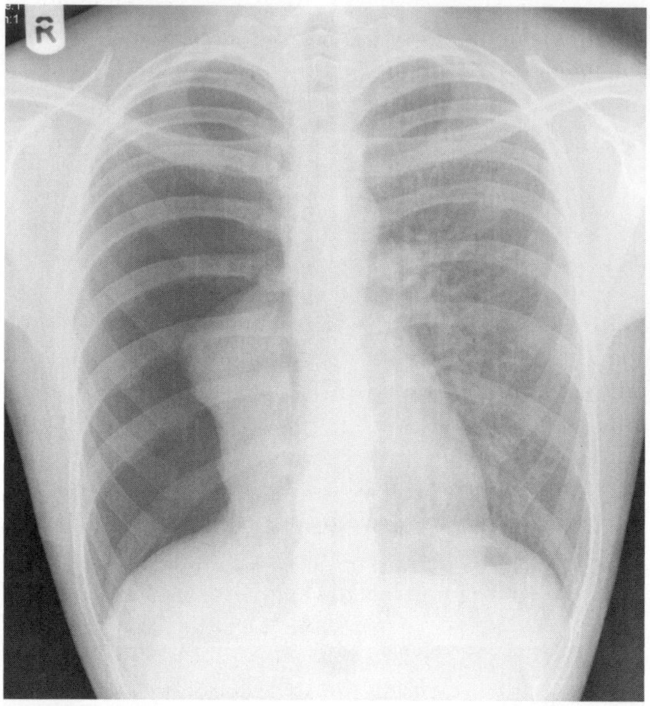

Fig. 2-6

135 A 29-year-old man is admitted to the hospital with great difficulty breathing after an automobile accident. Radiologic examination (Fig. 2-6) reveals no fractured bones or mediastinal shift. During physical examination he has no signs of external injuries, but the dyspnea becomes progressively worse. Which of the following conditions would best describe this case?

- A. Flail chest with paradoxical respiration
- B. Emphysema
- C. Hemothorax
- D. Spontaneous pneumothorax
- E. Tension pneumothorax

136 A 56-year-old male swimming coach is admitted to the hospital with dyspnea, cough, and high fever. A radiologic examination reveals lobar pneumonia (Fig. 2-7). Which of the following lobes of the lung is affected as shown in the image?

- A. Right upper
- B. Right middle
- C. Right lower
- D. Right upper, middle, and lower
- E. Right upper and lower

137 Having fallen while jogging, a 62-year-old man is admitted to the emergency department with severe chest pain. Physical examination reveals acute myocardial infarction. After the patient is stabilized, angiography is performed and one of the major coronary arteries is found to be occluded (Fig. 2-8). Which of

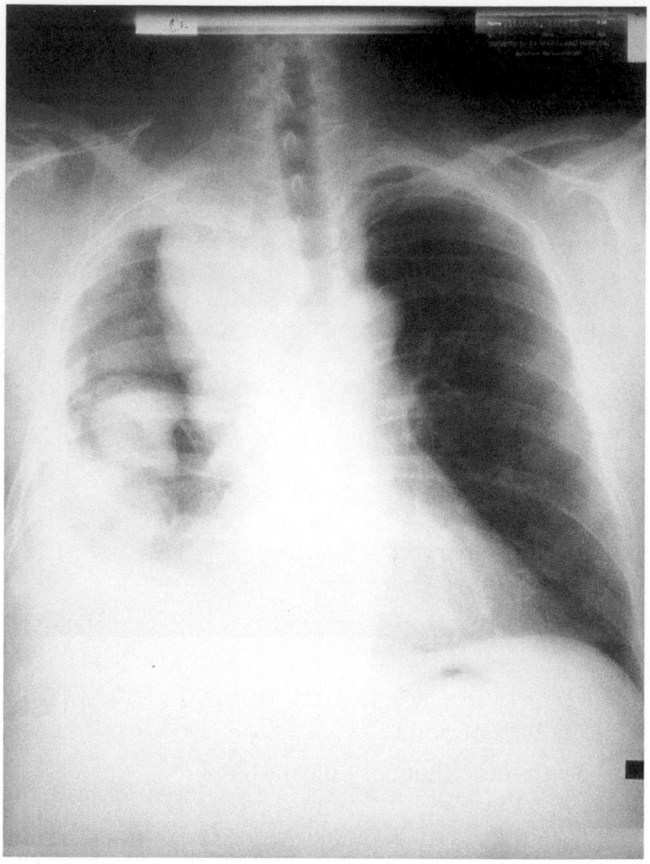

Fig. 2-7

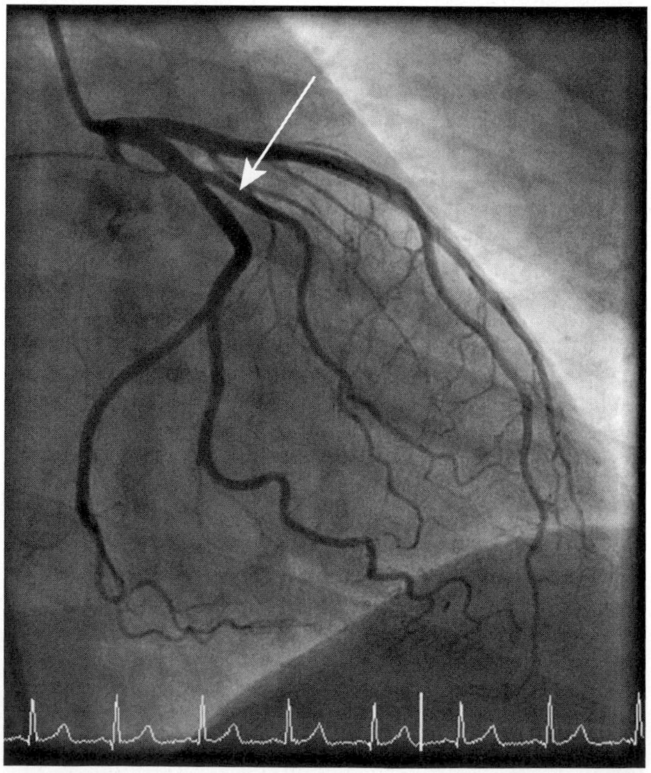

Fig. 2-8

the following arteries is most obviously blocked by atherosclerotic plaque or clot?

- ▢ **A.** Right coronary
- ▢ **B.** Left anterior interventricular
- ▢ **C.** Posterior interventricular
- ▢ **D.** Diagonal
- ▢ **E.** Circumflex

138 A 47-year-old woman patient's right breast exhibited *peau d'orange* characteristics. This condition is primarily a result of which of the following occurrences?

- ▢ **A.** Blockage of cutaneous lymphatic vessels
- ▢ **B.** Shortening of the suspensory ligaments by cancer in the axillary tail of the breast
- ▢ **C.** Contraction of the retinacula cutis of the areola and nipple
- ▢ **D.** Invasion of the pectoralis major by metastatic cancer
- ▢ **E.** Ipsilateral (same side) inversion of the nipple from cancer of the duct system of the breast

139 A 27-year-old male billiards player received a small-caliber bullet wound to the chest in the region of the third intercostal space, several centimeters to the left of the sternum. The patient is admitted to the emergency department and a preliminary notation of "Beck's triad" is entered on the patient's chart. Which of the following are features of this triad?

- ▢ **A.** There was injury to the left pulmonary artery, left primary bronchus, and esophagus
- ▢ **B.** The patient has bleeding into the pleural cavity, a collapsed lung, and mediastinal shift to the right side of the thorax
- ▢ **C.** The patient has a small, quiet heart; decreased pulse pressure; and increased central venous pressure
- ▢ **D.** The young man is suffering from marked diastolic emptying, dyspnea, and dilation of the aortic arch
- ▢ **E.** The left lung has collapsed, there is paradoxical respiration, and there is a mediastinal shift of the heart and trachea to the left

140 A 34-year-old patient had been diagnosed earlier in the week with Guillain-Barré syndrome. He is now in extreme respiratory distress. His thoracic wall contracts and relaxes violently, but there is little movement of the abdominal wall. The degenerative disease has obviously affected the muscle that is most responsible for increasing the vertical dimensions of the thoracic cavity (and pleural cavities). Which of the following is the most likely cause of his disease?

- ▢ **A.** Paralysis of his intercostal muscles and loss of the "bucket handle movement" of his ribs
- ▢ **B.** Generalized intercostal nerve paralysis that resulted in loss of the "pump handle movement" of his ribs
- ▢ **C.** Paralysis of his medial and lateral pectoral nerves, interrupting the function of his pectoralis major muscles, an important accessory muscle of respiration
- ▢ **D.** Paralysis of his sternocleidomastoid muscles
- ▢ **E.** Degeneration of the myelin of his phrenic nerves

141 Two days after the patient's breathing had become assisted by mechanical ventilation, a patient with Guillain-Barré syndrome began experiencing severe cardiac arrhythmia, with perilously slow cardiac contractions, resulting in reduced cardiac output. This most likely resulted from interruption of the contractile stimulus carried by which of the following?

- ▢ **A.** Left vagus nerve
- ▢ **B.** Right phrenic nerve
- ▢ **C.** Preganglionic sympathetic fibers in upper thoracic spinal nerves
- ▢ **D.** Cardiac pain fibers carried by upper thoracic spinal nerves
- ▢ **E.** Ventral horn neurons of spinal cord levels T1 to T4

142 During transesophageal echocardiography (TEE), an ultrasound transducer is placed through the nose or mouth to lie directly behind the heart. The closer a structure is to the transducer, the better the ultrasound image that can be obtained. In TEE, which heart valve can be best visualized?

- ▢ **A.** Tricuspid
- ▢ **B.** Pulmonary
- ▢ **C.** Mitral
- ▢ **D.** Aortic
- ▢ **E.** Valve of the inferior vena cava

143 A 65-year-old alcoholic man is admitted to the emergency department because of severe dehydration due to continuous vomiting for the past 2 days. The patient was placed on fluid replacement and he recovers well. His chest radiograph reveals a mild pneumomediastinum. The presence of which of the following anatomic structures is a radiologic landmark for the diagnosis of pneumomediastinum?

- ▢ **A.** Left superior intercostal vein
- ▢ **B.** Vagus nerve
- ▢ **C.** Superior vena cava
- ▢ **D.** Pulmonary vein
- ▢ **E.** Aortic arch

144 A neonate was born at 34 weeks of gestation and was admitted for pneumonitis. A CT scan examination reveals that the upper segment of the esophagus ends blindly and the presence of an abnormal communication between the trachea and the lower segment of esophagus. Which of the following clinical condition is commonly seen in association with this congenital anomaly?

- ▢ **A.** Polyhydramnios
- ▢ **B.** Oligodramnios
- ▢ **C.** Anhydramnios
- ▢ **D.** Hydatidiform mole
- ▢ **E.** Choriocarcinomas

145 A 55-year-old woman is admitted to the hospital with cough and severe dyspnea. Radiologic examination reveals that the patient suffers from emphysema. Upon physical examination the patient shows only "bucket-handle" movements during deep inspiration. Which movements of the thoracic wall are characteristic of this type of breathing?

- ▢ **A.** Increase of the transverse diameter of the thorax
- ▢ **B.** Increases of the anteroposterior diameter of the thorax
- ▢ **C.** Increase of the vertical dimension of the thorax
- ▢ **D.** Decrease of the anteroposterior diameter of the thorax
- ▢ **E.** Decrease of the transverse diameter of the thorax

146 A 34-year-old man with a complaint of sharp, localized pain over the thoracic wall is diagnosed with pleural effusion. A chest tube is inserted to drain the effusion through an intercostal space. Where should the chest tube be inserted?

- ▢ **A.** Just superior to the upper border of the rib
- ▢ **B.** Just inferior to the lower border of the rib
- ▢ **C.** At the middle of the intercostal space
- ▢ **D.** Between the internal and external intercostal muscles
- ▢ **E.** Between the intercostal muscles and the posterior intercostal membrane

147 A 30-year-old man is admitted to the emergency department because of a significant nose bleed and a headache that has worsened over several days. He also complains of fatigue. Upon examination it is noted that brachial artery pressure is markedly increased, femoral pressure is decreased, and the femoral pulses are delayed. The patient shows no external signs of inflammation. Which of the following is the most likely embryologic defect of this condition?

- ▢ **A.** Fourth pharyngeal arch
- ▢ **B.** Third pharyngeal arch
- ▢ **C.** Left dorsal aorta
- ▢ **D.** Left fifth pharyngeal arch
- ▢ **E.** Sixth pharyngeal arch

148 A 3-day-old newborn is admitted to the surgical unit with severe dyspnea and cyanosis. On physical examination the patient appears to have a flat abdomen. Imaging reveals a left side pneumothorax and pockets of air in the left hemithorax. Which of the following conditions is the most likely diagnosis?

- ▢ **A.** Congenital diaphragmatic hernia
- ▢ **B.** Laryngeal atresia
- ▢ **C.** Emphysema
- ▢ **D.** Respiratory distress syndrome
- ▢ **E.** Tracheoesophageal fistula

149 A 55-year-old man is admitted to the hospital with complaints of severe chest pain radiating to his left arm and increased sweating over his chest. ECG examination provides evidence of a myocardial infarction of the posterior wall of the left ventricle. Which nerve fibers are most likely responsible for the increased sweating?

- ▢ **A.** Preganglionic parasympathetics
- ▢ **B.** Postganglionic sympathetics in the cardiopulmonary nerve
- ▢ **C.** Thoracic visceral afferents
- ▢ **D.** Postganglionic sympathetic fibers from T1 to T4
- ▢ **E.** Postganglionic sympathetic fibers from superior, middle, and inferior cervical ganglia

150 A 35-year-old woman patient has a hard tumor about 1 cm in diameter slightly above, and lateral, to her right areola. A specific dye was injected into the tissue around the tumor which was taken up by the lymph vessels, draining the area. An incision was made to expose the lymphatic vessels which were then visible to the naked eye. The vessels were traced to surgically expose the lymph nodes receiving the lymph from the tumor. Which nodes will most likely first receive lymph from the tumor?

- ▢ **A.** Anterior axillary (pectoral)
- ▢ **B.** Lateral axillary
- ▢ **C.** Parasternal
- ▢ **D.** Central axillary
- ▢ **E.** Apical (infraclavicular)

151 A 51-year-old woman visited her physician complaining of dyspnea. Examination revealed edema of the lower limbs and a systolic murmur was heard in the left second intercostal space. Which of the following valve abnormalities is she most likely suffering from?

- ▢ **A.** Regurgitation through aortic valve
- ▢ **B.** Regurgitation through pulmonary valve
- ▢ **C.** Stenosis of aortic valve
- ▢ **D.** Regurgitation through mitral valve
- ▢ **E.** Stenosis of pulmonary valve

152 A 58-year-old man was brought to the emergency department complaining of breathlessness and chest pains radiating out into his left arm. A diagnosis of angina pectoris was made resulting from ischemia of the myocardium. Sublingual nitroglycerine relieved the condition by causing vasodilation and improving blood flow to the heart. Which of the following nerves referred the pain to the arm?

- ▢ **A.** Vagus
- ▢ **B.** Intercostals
- ▢ **C.** Phrenic
- ▢ **D.** Intercostobrachial
- ▢ **E.** Cardiopulmonary

153 A 41-year-old woman is examined in the outpatient surgical clinic for a lump in her right breast. Physical examination reveals dimpling of skin of the breast over the mass. A CT scan of the breast reveals a 3-cm mass at the right upper quadrant of her right breast with multiple calcifications. The dimpling of the breast is most likely caused by invasion of the tumor into which of the following structure(s)?

- ▢ **A.** Lactiferous ducts
- ▢ **B.** Mammary and apical lymph nodes
- ▢ **C.** Suspensory ligaments
- ▢ **D.** Deltopectoral fascia
- ▢ **E.** Medial and lateral pectoral nerves

154 A 65-year-old woman is admitted to the emergency department with severe chest pain. Laboratory examination reveals that the patient has suffered a myocardial infarction. Cardiac catheterization is performed and the portion of the heart immediately behind the sternum is found to be infarcted. Which artery is most likely occluded?

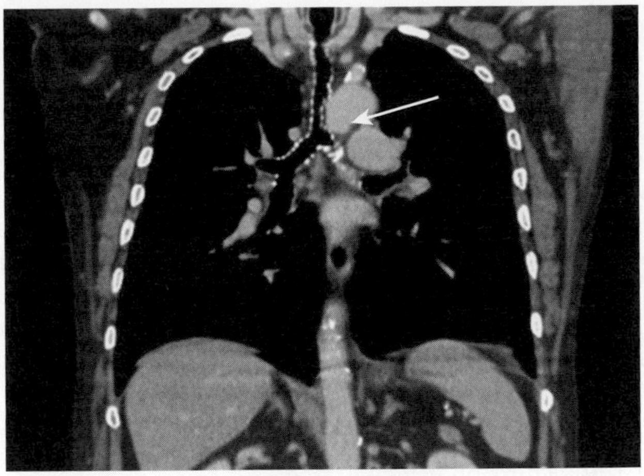

Fig. 2-9

- ▢ **A.** Circumflex
- ▢ **B.** Anterior interventricular
- ▢ **C.** Posterior interventricular
- ▢ **D.** Left marginal
- ▢ **E.** Right coronary

155 A 42-year-old woman is admitted to the emergency department with severe dysphagia. A CT scan (Fig. 2-9) reveals a small aortic aneurysm. Which of the following nerves will most likely be compressed if the aortic aneurysm continues to grow?

- ▢ **A.** Vagus
- ▢ **B.** Phrenic
- ▢ **C.** Left recurrent laryngeal
- ▢ **D.** Right recurrent laryngeal
- ▢ **E.** Greater thoracic splanchnics

156 A 59-year-old man is admitted to the hospital with a severe inferior myocardial infarction. The patient was brought to the catheterization lab for an emergency catheterization of his coronary arteries. During passage of the catheter from his right radial artery it is noted that the patient has a right subclavian artery passing posteriorly to the esophagus and thus requires a longer catheter. Which of the following structures failed to regress in this condition?

- ▢ **A.** Right dorsal aorta distal to the seventh intersegmental artery
- ▢ **B.** Left dorsal aorta distal to the seventh intersegmental artery
- ▢ **C.** Right dorsal aorta proximal to the seventh intersegmental artery

- ▢ **D.** Fifth arch artery
- ▢ **E.** Ventral part of the first arch artery

157 A 25-year-old man is admitted to the hospital with severe headache, cold feet and legs, and pain in his legs when he runs a short distance. During physical examination, femoral pulses are much weaker than radial pulses. Three-dimensional CT scan angiography reveals a coarctation of the aorta proximal to the left subclavian artery. The condition that creates these symptoms is a result of a failure of normal development of which structure?

- ▢ **A.** Fourth pharyngeal arch
- ▢ **B.** Third pharyngeal arch
- ▢ **C.** Left dorsal aorta
- ▢ **D.** Left fifth pharyngeal arch
- ▢ **E.** Sixth pharyngeal arch

158 A newborn girl is diagnosed with tricuspid valve atresia. An ultrasonographic examination reveals a widely patent oval foramen, VSD, hypoplastic right ventricle, and hypertrophied left ventricle. The patent foramen ovale most likely reflects a developmental failure of which of the following structures?

- ▢ **A.** Endocardial cushions
- ▢ **B.** Foramen primum
- ▢ **C.** Septum secundum
- ▢ **D.** Truncus arteriosus
- ▢ **E.** Bulbus cordis

159 A 25-year-old woman is admitted to hospital with dyspnea. Radiologic examination reveals a tumor invading the lung surface just anterior to the hilum. Which nerve is being compressed by the tumor?

- ▢ **A.** Phrenic
- ▢ **B.** Vagus
- ▢ **C.** Intercostal
- ▢ **D.** Recurrent laryngeal
- ▢ **E.** Cardiopulmonary

160 A 60-year-old woman with a history of severe rheumatic heart disease is in the clinic for a routine follow-up. Her cardiac symptoms have been relatively stable since valve replacement surgery 2 years ago, but she has developed some new symptoms over the past few months. A chest radiograph reveals sternotomy wires, prosthetic aortic and mitral valves, and a greatly enlarged left atrium. Which symptom could most likely develop as a direct result of her left atrial enlargement?

- ▢ **A.** Nausea and vomiting
- ▢ **B.** Pain and tenderness over thoracic vertebral spinous processes
- ▢ **C.** Difficulty swallowing
- ▢ **D.** Epigastric pain after eating fatty foods
- ▢ **E.** Increased coughing

161 A 59-year-old man is admitted to emergency department with severe chest pain. During examination a slight rhythmic pulsation on the chest wall at the left fifth intercostal space is noted. What causes this pulsation?

- ▢ **A.** Right atrium
- ▢ **B.** Left atrium
- ▢ **C.** Aortic arch
- ▢ **D.** Apex of the heart
- ▢ **E.** Mitral valve

162 A 48-year-old man is admitted to the emergency department with chronic angina. Coronary angiography reveals nearly total blockage of the anterior interventricular artery just after it arises from the left coronary. In exposing this artery for a bypass procedure, which accompanying vein must be protected from injury?

- ▢ **A.** Middle cardiac
- ▢ **B.** Great cardiac
- ▢ **C.** Small cardiac
- ▢ **D.** Anterior cardiac
- ▢ **E.** Posterior cardiac

163 A 25-year-old man is brought to the emergency department because of a 1-week history of fever and cough productive of purulent sputum. His temperature is 38.9° C (102° F), pulse is 110/min, respirations are 24/min, and blood pressure is 110/70 mm Hg. Crackles, decreased breath sounds, and decreased fremitus are present in the right lower lobe. A chest x-ray shows a pleural effusion over the lower third of the thorax on the right in the midclavicular line. A thoracocentesis is scheduled. Which intercostal space in the midclavicular line in this patient would be most appropriate for insertion of the needle during this procedure?

- ▢ **A.** Fifth
- ▢ **B.** Seventh
- ▢ **C.** Ninth
- ▢ **D.** Eighth
- ▢ **E.** Eleventh

164 When inserting a nasogastric tube, which is the most distal site in, or in relation to, the esophagus that might offer resistance to the tube as it passes to the stomach?

- ☐ **A.** Posterior to the left atrium
- ☐ **B.** Level of the superior thoracic aperture
- ☐ **C.** Posterior to the aortic arch
- ☐ **D.** Posterior to the left main bronchus
- ☐ **E.** Esophageal hiatus of the diaphragm

165 A 55-year-old woman is to undergo a coronary bypass operation. The artery of primary concern is the vessel that arises from the circumflex artery in a left dominant heart. Which artery is this?

- ☐ **A.** Right marginal
- ☐ **B.** Anterior interventricular
- ☐ **C.** Left marginal
- ☐ **D.** Artery to the SA node
- ☐ **E.** Posterior interventricular

166 A 35-year-old woman is admitted to emergency department with dyspnea. Examination reveals a systolic (S1) murmur, suggestive of regurgitation of the tricuspid valve. What is the best site to auscultate this valve?

- ☐ **A.** Fourth intercostal space at left border of sternum
- ☐ **B.** Fifth intercostal space at left midclavicular line
- ☐ **C.** Fifth intercostal space at right border of sternum
- ☐ **D.** Third intercostal space at right border of sternum
- ☐ **E.** Second intercostal space at right border of sternum

167 A 42-year-old woman is admitted to the emergency department after a fall from the balcony of her apartment. During physical examination there is an absence of heart sounds, reduced systolic pressure, and engorged jugular veins. The condition that was created can be alleviated with which of the following procedures?

- ☐ **A.** Chest tube insertion superior to the rib
- ☐ **B.** Central venous line
- ☐ **C.** Nasogastric tube
- ☐ **D.** Thoracocentesis
- ☐ **E.** Pericardiocentesis

168 A 55-year-old man is admitted to the hospital with reduced heart rate and cardiac output. Which nerve fibers may have been damaged to cause these symptoms?

- ☐ **A.** Preganglionic parasympathetics from the vagus nerve in the cardiac plexus
- ☐ **B.** Somatic efferents in the phrenic nerve
- ☐ **C.** Visceral afferents in the cardiopulmonary nerve
- ☐ **D.** Preganglionic sympathetics from T1 to T4 lateral horn
- ☐ **E.** T1 to T4 ventral horn neurons

169 During a dissection of the posterior mediastinum, a medical student identifies a vessel that lies on the anterior surface of the vertebral bodies between the thoracic aorta on the left and the azygos vein on the right. In a living human being, this vessel would most likely contain which of the following?

- ☐ **A.** Lymph
- ☐ **B.** Deoxygenated blood
- ☐ **C.** Saliva
- ☐ **D.** Urine
- ☐ **E.** Oxygenated blood

170 Diagnostic imaging of a 10-year-old boy revealed a single but large tumor in a structure located in the most anterior part of the superior mediastinum immediately posterior to the manubrium. This structure is most likely derived from which of the following pharyngeal pouches?

- ☐ **A.** First
- ☐ **B.** Second
- ☐ **C.** Third
- ☐ **D.** Fourth
- ☐ **E.** Fifth

171 A 25-year-old woman was brought to the emergency department after suffering a gunshot wound to the back. During physical examination, she was found to be in cardiopulmonary distress. Vital signs: P 110 beats/min, BP 90/50, RR 32/min. The entry wound of a bullet was noted on the left thoracic area of her back. The left thorax was notably larger than the right with decreased breath sounds on auscultation and hyperresonance to percussion of the left chest. A tracheal tug to the right side was noted. She was assessed as having a tension pneumothorax and the physician prepared to perform an emergency decompression of the left thorax. Between which layers will the needle have to be placed to relieve the pneumothorax?

- ☐ **A.** Between the visceral and parietal layers of the pericardium
- ☐ **B.** Between the serous and fibrous layers of the pericardium

- ☐ **C.** Between the mediastinal pleura and fibrous pericardium
- ☐ **D.** Between the parietal and visceral layers of the pleura
- ☐ **E.** Between the endothoracic fascia and parietal pleura

172 A 38-year-old woman delivered a live male infant at 37 weeks by elective cesarean section. Ultrasound at 16 weeks' gestation showed that the fetal heart was located outside the chest cavity but the mother opted against termination of the pregnancy. On examination, the infant was pink, he was in no cardiopulmonary distress, and vital signs were normal. A pulsatile mass 5 cm × 6 cm was seen outside the skin in the midline of the thorax. A chest radiograph revealed a "split" in the sternum. The infant was diagnosed with ectopia cordis. What was the most likely embryological cause of this defect?

- ☐ **A.** Failed fusion of pleuropericardial folds at the midline
- ☐ **B.** Failed fusion of the septum transversum with pleuropericardial folds
- ☐ **C.** Failed fusion of lateral body wall folds in the midline
- ☐ **D.** Failed fusion of pleuroperitoneal at the midline
- ☐ **E.** Failed fusion of pericardial coelom and peritoneal coelom

173 A 42-year-old woman delivered a male infant at term. On examination of the infant, vital signs were normal. Although he moved all limbs equally, there was generalized decreased muscle tone. His face was broad and flat with oblique eye fissures, flattened nose bridge, and protruding tongue from a small jaw. Auscultation of the chest revealed a systolic ejection murmur. Cardiac ultrasound showed a defect in the wall separating the right from left atria. The patient was diagnosed with trisomy 21 with an ASD. What is the most likely cause of the defect in this patient?

- ☐ **A.** Failed fusion of septum primum with the atrioventricular septum
- ☐ **B.** Failed fusion of septum primum with septum secundum
- ☐ **C.** Excess resorption of the cranial part of the septum primum
- ☐ **D.** Short septum secundum
- ☐ **E.** Incomplete resorption of the sinus venosus into the right atrium

174 A 6.5 pound female infant was born to a 32-year-old woman by cesarean section. There was no cyanosis but a pansystolic murmur was auscultated. Cardiac ultrasound showed a small jet of blood directly between left and right ventricles during systole, through a defect in the cranial part of the interventricular septum. The infant was admitted to the Neonatal Intensive Care Unit and discharged on day 2. Which of the following is the most likely cause of the cardiac defect discovered in this patient?

- ☐ **A.** There is uneven partitioning of the bulbus cordis
- ☐ **B.** It causes a right to left shunt of blood at birth
- ☐ **C.** It is a cause of cyanosis at birth
- ☐ **D.** Failed fusion of the interventricular septum and endocardial cushions
- ☐ **E.** Failed closure of the septum primum and septum secundum at birth

175 A 30-year-old woman delivered a 6-lb female infant at term via spontaneous vaginal delivery. The infant was noted to have an elevated respiratory rate and was admitted to the neonatal intensive care unit. She developed a fever day later with no resolution of the tachypnea. A chest radiograph showed bilateral basal hazy opacification and a right-sided cardiac shadow. A whole-body CT scan was ordered which showed normal orientation of the other viscera. What is the most likely cause of this infant's cardiac condition?

- ☐ **A.** Posterior and superior growth of the primordial atrium
- ☐ **B.** Anterior and inferior growth of the primordial ventricle
- ☐ **C.** Anterior and inferior growth of the bulbus cordis
- ☐ **D.** Growth of primordial heart tube to the left
- ☐ **E.** Growth of the primordial heart tube to the right

176 A 54-year-old man was admitted to hospital for elective esophageal surgery. He had been diagnosed with Barrett's esophagus and opted for surgery that would excise the distal part of the esophagus. Postoperatively, he complained of gradually increasing chest discomfort. Vital signs: P 90 beats/min, BP 160/90, RR 20/min. Auscultation revealed normal heart and breath sounds. A chest radiograph showed hazy opacity of the mediastinum. A CT image of the chest showed a collection in the posterior mediastinum. Which of the following structures is most likely damaged in this patient?

- ☐ **A.** Thoracic duct
- ☐ **B.** Esophagus
- ☐ **C.** Descending aorta

- D. Azygos vein
- E. Bronchial lymphatics

177 A 3-day-old male infant is admitted to the cardiology unit with cyanosis. During echocardiographic examination a right-to-left shunt is identified. Which condition is most likely to produce this type of shunt at birth?

- A. Atrial septal defect
- B. VSD
- C. Patent ductus arteriosus
- D. Persistent truncus arteriosus with VSD
- E. Tetralogy of Fallot

178 During cardiac catheterization of a 4-year-old girl, the radiologist notes that the contrast medium released into the arch of the aorta is visible immediately in both pulmonary arteries. What is the most likely explanation for this finding?

- A. Aortic atresia
- B. Tetralogy of Fallot
- C. Patent (persistent) ductus arteriosus
- D. Patent ductus venosus
- E. VSD

179 A 4-day-old female infant was admitted to the pulmonary unit suffering from dyspnea and cyanosis. Radiographic examination revealed herniation of bowel into the left thoracic cavity and a hypoplastic left lung. Which embryologic structure probably failed to develop and resulted in the herniation?

- A. Septum transversum
- B. Pleuroperitoneal membrane
- C. Tracheoesophageal septum
- D. Laryngotracheal groove
- E. Ventral mesogastrium

180 A 30-year-old man is admitted emergency department following involvement in a domestic dispute with a jilted lover. The man reported that he was stabbed in his right anterior chest wall with a sharp instrument. Initial assessment revealed a man in acute respiratory distress. Physical examination showed a puncture wound in the third right intercostal space at the midclavicular line and distended neck veins. There was a hyperresonance on percussion and absent breath sounds on right hemithorax. A radiograph revealed a deviated trachea to the left. Which one of the following is the most likely diagnosis?

- A. Right tension pneumothorax
- B. Right simple pneumothorax
- C. Right simple pneumothorax and cardiac tamponade
- D. Right tension pneumothorax and cardiac tamponade
- E. Cardiac tamponade

181 A 35-year-old man was involved in a hit and run accident. A chest radiograph reveals broken ribs 5 to 7. On physical examination there are lacerations and radiography shows no evidence of punctured pleura. Several hours later the patient appears cyanotic. What is the most likely cause of the new cyanosis?

- A. Hemothorax
- B. Flail chest
- C. Paralysis of the diaphragm
- D. Tension pneumothorax
- E. Spontaneous pneumothorax

182 A 55-year-old man is admitted to the emergency department because of chills followed by a painful dry cough and fever for the past 3 days. The patient complains of painful breathing and upon auscultation, a pleural rub is heard when the patient breathes. A radiograph shows signs of pleurisy. The physician decides to administer lidocaine (a local anesthetic agent) to which of the following nerves?

- A. Intercostal nerves
- B. Phrenic nerve
- C. Vagus nerve
- D. Cardiopulmonary
- E. Recurrent laryngeal nerve

183 A 3-week-old prematurely born male neonate with respiratory distress is found to have a systolic murmur crossing the S_2 heart sound. The murmur is accompanied by a thrill, is best heard below the left clavicle, and radiates over the chest. On a chest radiograph, the cardiac silhouette is enlarged and pulmonary vascular markings are increased. Echocardiography reveals a congenital defect. A video-assisted thoracoscopic procedure is considered for correction of the underlying defect. Which of the following structures is the most common site of injury?

- A. Left vagus nerve
- B. Right vagus nerve
- C. Left phrenic nerve
- D. Right phrenic nerve
- E. Left recurrent laryngeal nerve

184 A 27-year-old man is stabbed in the chest during a bar fight and is taken to the emergency department.

He is conscious with tachypnea, hypotension, and pleuritic chest pain. On physical examination there is jugular venous distension, right-sided hyper resonance to percussion, and decreased breath sounds over the right lung. A radiograph of the chest shows decreased vascular markings on the right side and a tracheal deviation to the left. Which of the following is the most likely diagnosis?

- ☐ **A.** Spontaneous pneumothorax
- ☐ **B.** Tension pneumothorax
- ☐ **C.** Cardiac tamponade
- ☐ **D.** Lung contusion
- ☐ **E.** Pneumonia

185 A 72-year-old patient is admitted to the emergency department with tight, burning substernal chest pain. An ECG reveals a myocardial infarction of the cardiac muscle forming the diaphragmatic surface of the heart. Which of the following coronary arteries is most likely occluded in this patient?

- ☐ **A.** Left anterior descending coronary artery
- ☐ **B.** Left circumflex coronary artery
- ☐ **C.** Left main coronary artery
- ☐ **D.** Right coronary artery
- ☐ **E.** Acute marginal branches

186 A newborn boy is examined due to his cyanosis. On radiographic examination his right ventricle is enlarged and his heart shows a characteristic boot shape. Which of the following embryological events most likely underlies this condition?

- ☐ **A.** Abnormal neural crest cell migration
- ☐ **B.** Endocardial cushion defect
- ☐ **C.** Aortic arch constriction
- ☐ **D.** Pulmonary hypertension
- ☐ **E.** Abnormal primitive heart tube looping

187 A 70-year-old man is admitted to the emergency department for evaluation of his fever, chills, and chest pain. Physical examination reveals a holosystolic murmur that radiates toward the axilla. Blood cultures are ordered and he undergoes TEE. The ultrasound transducer is placed in the midesophagus facing posteriorly. Which of the following structures will be immediately posterior to the transducer?

- ☐ **A.** Left atrium
- ☐ **B.** Pulmonary veins
- ☐ **C.** Right atrium
- ☐ **D.** Right ventricle
- ☐ **E.** Aorta

188 A 52-year-old man with a long history of alcoholic cirrhosis complained of severe dysphagia and retrosternal "burning" pain. During esophagoscopy, the endoscopist advanced the endoscope until its tip reached the esophageal hiatus of the diaphragm. Which of the following vertebral levels did the tip of the endoscope most likely end?

- ☐ **A.** T7
- ☐ **B.** T8
- ☐ **C.** T10
- ☐ **D.** T11
- ☐ **E.** T12

189 A famous crocodile hunter was snorkeling among giant stingrays when the tail (barb) of one of the stingrays suddenly pierced his chest. The tip of the barb pierced the right ventricle and the man instinctively removed it in the water. When he was brought onto the boat, there were muffled heart sounds, reduced cardiac output, and engorged jugular veins. Which of the following is the most likely diagnosis?

- ☐ **A.** Pneumothorax
- ☐ **B.** Deep vein thrombosis
- ☐ **C.** Cardiac tamponade
- ☐ **D.** Pulmonary embolism
- ☐ **E.** Hemothorax

190 During a routine physical examination of a healthy 38-year-old man, the physician auscultates the heart by placing a stethoscope on the anterior surface of the patient's chest between the left second and third costal cartilages. Which of the following heart valves is the physician most likely auscultating?

- ☐ **A.** Pulmonary
- ☐ **B.** Aortic
- ☐ **C.** Mitral
- ☐ **D.** Tricuspid
- ☐ **E.** Bicuspid

191 Chest radiographs were taken of a 70-year-old woman who complained of a cough of 3 weeks' duration but was able to ambulate. While reading the films with a medical student, the radiologist asked the student to identify the sternal angle (of Louis). Which of the following radiographic views would best demonstrate this landmark?

- ☐ **A.** Anteroposterior
- ☐ **B.** Posteroanterior
- ☐ **C.** Lateral
- ☐ **D.** Apical lordotic
- ☐ **E.** Axial

192 A 50-year-old man was involved in a motor vehicle crash and was rushed to the emergency department where a chest tube was placed to drain fluid. The following anatomic structures comprise the wall of the thorax.

1. Internal intercostal muscle
2. Skin
3. Innermost intercostal muscle
4. Parietal pleura
5. External intercostal muscle
6. Visceral pleura

Which of the following best represents the order of structures traversed by the tube during the procedure?

- ▢ **A.** 4-6-5-1-3-2
- ▢ **B.** 2-5-1-3-6-4
- ▢ **C.** 2-3-1-5-6-4
- ▢ **D.** 2-1-3-5-4-6
- ▢ **E.** 2-5-1-3-4-6

ANSWERS

1 D. The aorticopulmonary septum functions to divide the truncus arteriosus and bulbus cordis into the aorta and pulmonary trunk. The septum secundum forms an incomplete separation between the two atria. The septum primum divides the atrium into right and left halves. The bulbar septum is derived from the bulbus cordis and will give rise to the interventricular septum inferior to the aorticopulmonary septum, eventually fusing with it. The endocardial cushions play a role in the division of the AV canal into right and left halves, by causing the AV cushions to approach each other.
GAS 203; N 209; McM 185, 191

2 A. Laryngeal atresia (congenital high airway obstruction syndrome) is a rare obstruction of the upper fetal airway. Distal to the site of the atresia, the airways dilate, lungs enlarge and become echogenic, the diaphragm flattens or inverts, and fetal ascites and/or hydrops develop. Tracheal atresia is a rare obstruction of the trachea, commonly found with a tracheoesophageal fistula, probably resulting from the unequal division of foregut into esophagus and trachea. Polyhydramnios is an excess of amniotic fluid, often associated with esophageal atresia or tracheoesophageal fistula. Lung hypoplasia is reduced lung volume, often seen in infants with a congenital diaphragmatic hernia. Oligohydramnios, or a decrease in amniotic fluid, is associated with stunted lung development and pulmonary hypoplasia.
GAS 172-178; N 230; McM 200, 201, 204

3 A. VSDs account for 25% of congenital heart defects. The most common of these are defects in the membranous portion of the interventricular septum (membranous VSDs).
GAS 203; N 209; McM 185, 191

4 A. In a case of transposition of the great arteries, oxygenated blood travels from the left ventricle into the pulmonary trunk, where it will eventually reach the lungs. In contrast, the aorta would be carrying deoxygenated blood into the systemic circulation. A PDA acts as a shunt between the aorta and pulmonary trunk, allowing oxygenated and deoxygenated blood to mix and therefore allowing some oxygenated blood to reach the tissues. None of the other answer choices would be correct for this problem; with these structures remaining patent, the body would still not receive sufficient oxygenated blood for survival to be possible.
GAS 203; N 226; McM 195

5 A. Tetralogy of Fallot is characterized by four cardiac defects: pulmonary stenosis, VSD, overriding aorta, and these in turn lead to right ventricular hypertrophy. An ASD is characterized by the communication between the two atria. In a case of transposition of the great vessels, the aorta arises from the right ventricle and the pulmonary trunk arises from the left ventricle.
GAS 203; N 221; McM 188, 189

6 A. Superior malalignment of the subpulmonary infundibulum causes stenosis of the pulmonary trunk. This leads to the four symptoms mentioned and is known as *tetralogy of Fallot*. A defect in formation of the aorticopulmonary septum is characteristic of transposition of the great arteries. An endocardial cushion defect is associated with membranous VSDs.
GAS 192-193, 203; N 221; McM 188, 189

7 B. The murmur at S_2 localizes the defect at an atrioventricular valve. An ASD causes a diastolic murmur in the tricuspid valve, whereas a VSD would cause a pansystolic murmur. Transposition of the great arteries and aortic stenosis will cause a murmur

at S_1, and tetralogy of Fallot does not cause a murmur at S_1 or S_2.
GAS 203; N 217, 218; McM 189

8 C. Down syndrome (more properly called "trisomy 21") is associated with cardiovascular abnormalities such as arrhythmias and atrial and VSDs. It is also characterized by mental retardation, brachycephaly, flat nasal bridge, upward slant of the palpebral fissure, protruding tongue, simian crease, and clinodactyly of the fifth digit.
GAS 203; N 217, 218; McM 188

9 A. Tetralogy of Fallot and truncus arteriosus are associated with DiGeorge syndrome (22q11). Transposition of the great arteries is associated with maternal diabetes. ASDs and VSDs are present in individuals with Down syndrome. Coarctation of the aorta is related to Turner syndrome. Marfan syndrome is present in individuals with aortic atresia.
GAS 203; N 211; McM 188

10 B. Transposition of the great arteries is associated with maternal diabetes. Tetralogy of Fallot and truncus arteriosus are associated with DiGeorge syndrome (22q11). ASDs and VSDs are present in individuals with Down syndrome. Coarctation of the aorta is related to Turner syndrome. Marfan syndrome is present in individuals with aortic atresia.
GAS 197, 203; N 211; McM 185, 191

11 C. The ductus arteriosus is an embryologic structure that acts as a communication between the pulmonary trunk and the aorta. If it remains patent, the injected contrast medium would flow from the aorta through this communication and into the pulmonary artery. An ASD is a communication between the atria. Mitral stenosis is a narrowing of the AV valve between the left atrium and left ventricle. The ductus venosus transports blood from the left umbilical vein to the inferior vena cava, bypassing the liver. A VSD is a communication between the ventricles.
GAS 203; N 211; McM 195

12 A. An ASD is a communication between the right and left atria. In the formation of the partition between the two atria, the opening in the foramen secundum, also known as the foramen ovale, typically closes at birth. If it remains patent, an ASD will result. The rest of the structures are not associated with ASDs.
GAS 203; N 217-218; McM 187

13 E. Type II alveolar cells are the only cells that produce surfactant.
GAS 167-174; N 193; McM 200

14 B. An absence of musculature in one half of the diaphragm causes it to protrude into the thoracic cavity forming a pouch into which the abdominal viscera protrude. Pleuropericardial folds are responsible for separating the pericardial cavity from the pleural cavity. Typically, the diaphragm migrates to its position with the fibrous pericardium. The septum transversum is the primordial central tendon of the diaphragm that separates the heart from the liver. The pleuroperitoneal folds form the pleuroperitoneal membranes that separate the pleural cavity from the peritoneal cavity. Absence of any of these would not have anything to do with eventration of the diaphragm.
GAS 262; N 191; McM 184

15 C. The anomalies present in this individual are all caused by a coarctation of the aorta. The portion of the aortic arch that is constricted arises from the third, fourth, and sixth pharyngeal arches. The bulbus cordis becomes part of the ventricular system. The ductus arteriosus becomes the ligamentum arteriosum.
GAS 217; N 209; McM 195

16 D. The tracheoesophageal septum is a primordial structure that separates the trachea from the esophagus. If this structure fails to develop, a tracheoesophageal fistula will result, in which event the two structures will not separate completely. When the infant attempts to swallow milk, it spills into the esophageal pouch and is regurgitated. The child becomes cyanotic because an insufficient amount of oxygen is reaching the lungs as a result of the malformed trachea.
GAS 218; N 230; McM 197

17 C. Polyhydramnios is an excess of amniotic fluid, often associated with esophageal atresia or a tracheoesophageal fistula. This abnormality affects fetal ability to swallow the normal amount of amniotic fluid; therefore, excess fluid remains in the amniotic sac. None of the other factors listed has an association with this type of fistula.
GAS 336; N 231; McM 197

18 B. Congenital heart defects are common problems that can be caused by teratogens, such as the rubella virus, or single-gene factors, or chromosomal abnormalities.
GAS 203; N 211; McM 195

19 E. Sinus venosus ASDs occur close to the entry of the superior vena cava in the superior portion of the interatrial septum. Ostium secundum ASDs are located near the fossa ovale and encompass both septum primum and septum secundum defects. An ostium primum defect is a less common form of ASD and is associated with endocardial cushion defects because the septum primum fails to fuse with the endocardial cushions, resulting in a patent foramen primum. An AV canal defect is not a clinically significant type of ASD. A common atrium is an uncommon type of ASD in which the interatrial septum is absent (Figs. 2-10 and 2-11).

GAS 191-193, 203; N 217, 218; McM 187

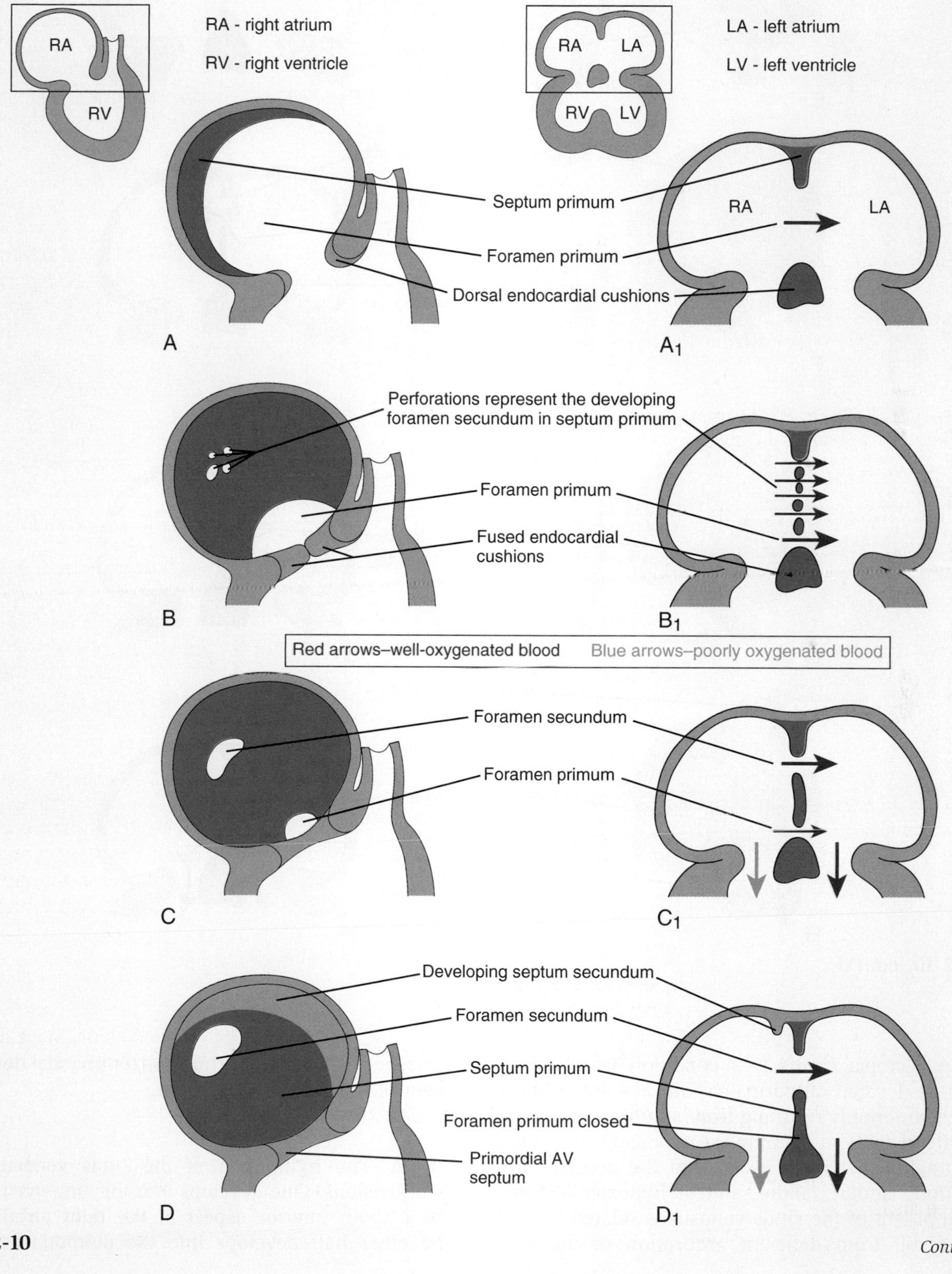

Fig. 2-10

Continued

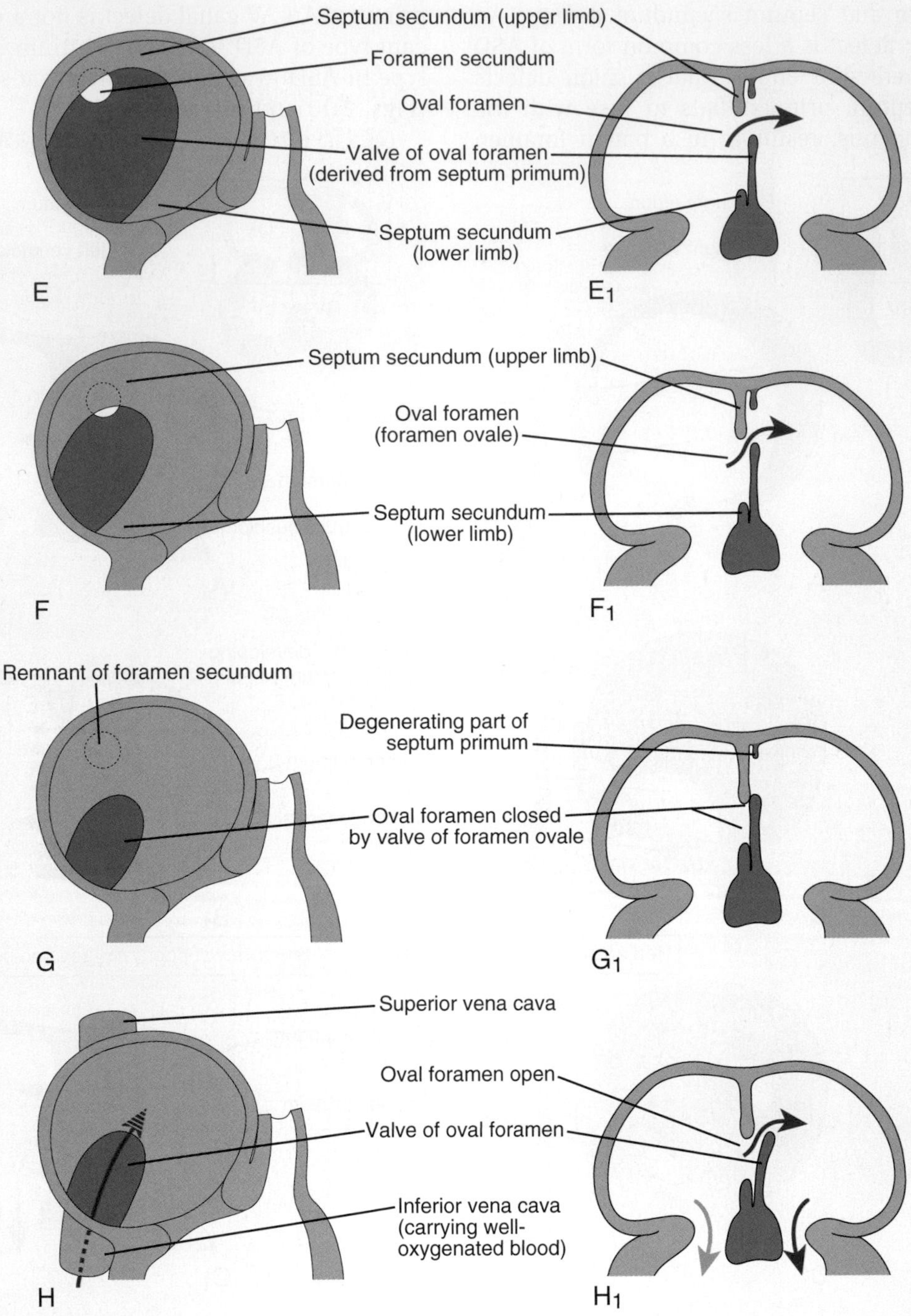

Fig. 2-10, cont'd

20 A. Ectopia cordis is a condition in which the heart is located abnormally, outside the thoracic cavity, commonly resulting from a failure of fusion of the lateral folds in forming the thoracic wall. This is incompatible with life because of the occurrence of infection, cardiac failure, and/or hypoxemia. Faulty development of the sinus venosus is related to ASDs that result from deficient absorption of the sinus venosus into the right atrium and/or unusual development of the septum secundum.

GAS 191-193; N 209; McM 184

21 A. The right horn of the sinus venosus has two divisions: One develops into the sinus venarum, the smooth interior aspect of the right atrial wall; the other half develops into the pulmonary veins.

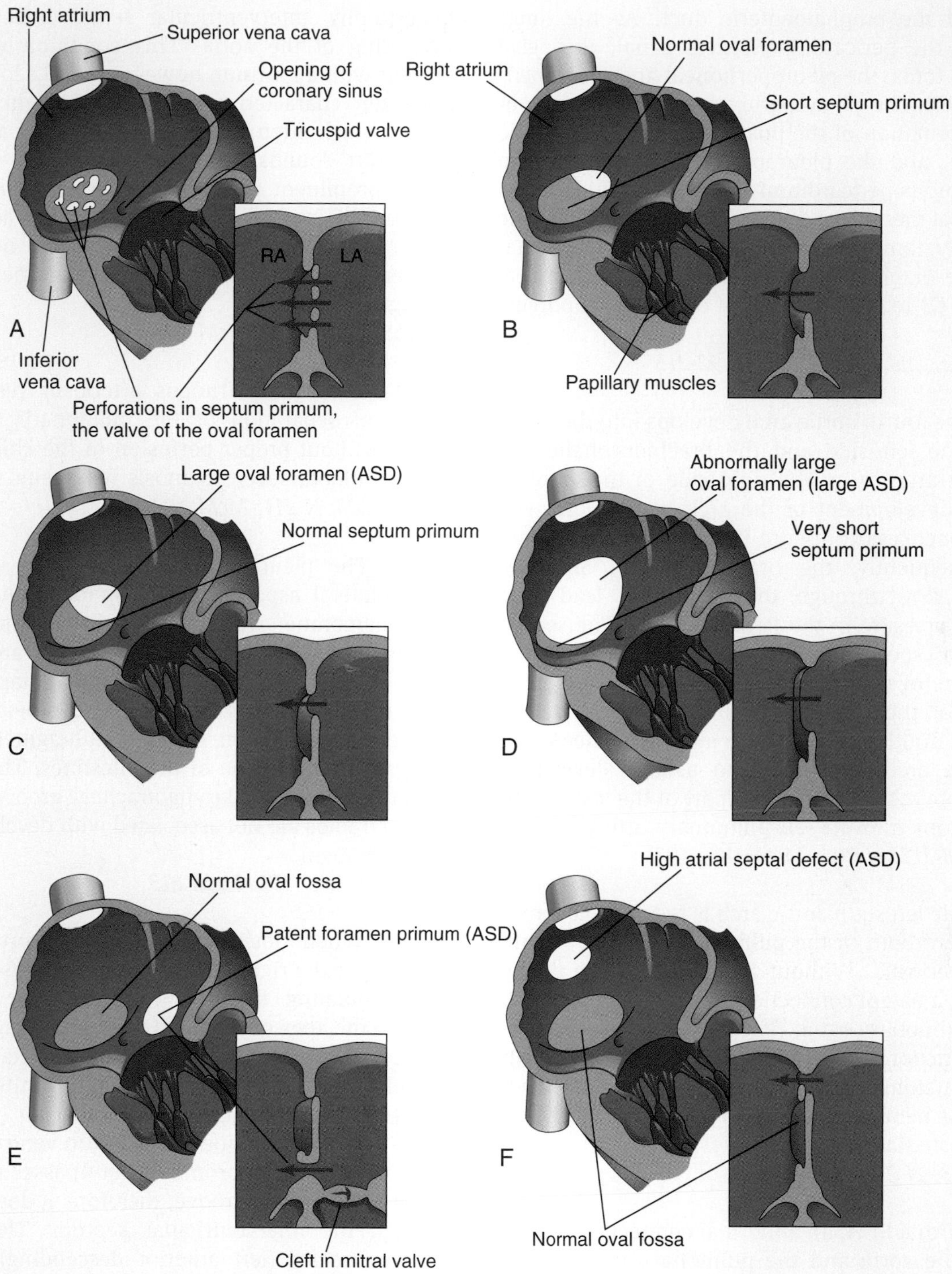

Fig. 2-11

Abnormal septation of the sinus venosus can lead to inappropriate pulmonary connections. Abnormal development of the left sinus horn would present with abnormalities in the coronary sinus, whereas incorrect development of the septum secundum can result in an ASD but would not be involved with anomalous pulmonary veins. The left sinusal horn develops into the coronary sinus, and the right sinusal horn is incorporated into the right atrial wall.

GAS 191-193, 203; N 211; McM 191-193

22 C. The septum transversum is a thickened layer of mesoderm that gives origin to the central tendon of the diaphragm. It is situated between the thoracic cavity and the omphaloenteric duct. As the lungs grow into the pericardioperitoneal canal, they give rise to two folds: the pleuroperitoneal and pleuropericardial folds. The pleuroperitoneal folds are responsible for formation of the posterolateral aspect of the diaphragm, and the pleuropericardial folds develop into the fibrous pericardium. The crura provide origin of the dorsal mesentery of the esophagus, whereas the cervical myotomes are responsible for the musculature of the diaphragm. (Note that these are cervical myotomes C3 to C5, the levels of origin of the phrenic nerve.)

GAS 262, 203; N 192; McM 192-213

23 C. The fourth aortic arch develops into the aortic arch on the left side and the brachiocephalic and subclavian arteries on the right side of the embryo. Improper development of the arch of the aorta will cause an increased pressure in the subclavian artery and, subsequently, the brachial artery. Similarly, decreased flow through the aorta will lead to a decreased pressure in the femoral artery. The second aortic arch, specifically the dorsal aspect, develops into aspects of the small stapedial artery. The proximal part of the third aortic arch gives rise to the common carotid arteries, which supply the head. The fifth aortic arch is said not to usually develop in human embryos. The proximal part of the sixth aortic arch develops into the left pulmonary artery.

GAS 213-215; N 204; McM 185, 193

24 A. The left sixth aortic arch is responsible for the development both of the pulmonary arteries and the ductus arteriosus. Without regression of the ductus arteriosus, a patent connection remains between aorta and the pulmonary trunk. The ductus arteriosus often reaches functional closure within 24 hours after birth, whereas anatomic closure and subsequent formation of the ligamentum arteriosum often occur by the twelfth postnatal week.

GAS 203; N 211; McM 195

25 D. With a PDA, an abnormal connection persists between the aorta and the pulmonary trunk. Blood leaving the left ventricle of the heart and into the aorta is reshunted back into the left pulmonary artery. This is responsible for the murmur heard during auscultation of the heart. The diversion of blood to the pulmonary arteries causes increased atrial pressure, leading to enlarged, and therefore noticeable, pulmonary arteries on the chest radiograph. The tetralogy of Fallot often presents with a right-to-left shunt of blood flow through the ventricles. It is also associated with pulmonary artery stenosis, right ventricular hypertrophy, interventricular septal defect, and an overriding of the aorta. This condition would not present with a murmur, however. Atrial septal defects are often characterized by a left-to-right shunt of blood, which often presents with dyspnea and abnormal heart sounds. A chest radiograph would not reveal prominent pulmonary arteries in such cases. Both aortic atresia and coarctation of the aorta result in a narrowing of the aorta but would not lead to noticeable prominent pulmonary arteries on the radiograph.

GAS 203; N 211; McM 195

26 E. A common truncus arteriosus results from failure of separation of the pulmonary trunk and aorta. Without proper perfusion of the child by oxygenated blood, severe cyanosis will result.

GAS 203; N 211; McM 193, 195

27 B. The pleuroperitoneal membrane forms the posterolateral aspect of the diaphragm. A defect in this membrane would allow for communication between the upper left abdominal cavity and thoracic cavity and could result in a congenital diaphragmatic hernia. The septum transversum provides origin to the central tendon of the diaphragm but is not involved in herniation of the intestines. The tracheoesophageal septum, laryngotracheal groove, and oligohydramnios are not associated with development of the diaphragm.

GAS 262; N 191; McM 213

28 A. When closing a VSD, it is important not to suture over the right bundle branch because it carries the stimulating impulse from the atrioventricular node to the apex of the heart through the right bundle of His. Following the course of the right bundle branch on the interventricular septum, the impulses travel along the septomarginal trabecula (moderator band) and Purkinje fibers, leading to ventricular contraction. The right coronary artery passes dorsally in the atrioventricular groove; therefore, it does not pass through the interventricular septum. The anterior interventricular (left anterior descending) coronary artery is superficial to the IV septum on the anterior surface of the heart. The tricuspid valve and aortic valve are not directly associated with the interventricular septum.

GAS 192, 203; N 217; McM 187, 188

29 A. Esophageal atresia is often the result of an incomplete division of the tracheoesophageal septum, thus causing an absence of, or blind ending of, the esophagus. Though similar to an esophageal atresia,

a tracheoesophageal fistula is an atypical connection between the trachea and the esophagus.
GAS 172-174; N 230; McM 197

30 A. In a tracheotomy, an incision is made at the level of the sixth cervical vertebra, near the cricoid cartilage. The left brachiocephalic vein passes across the trachea immediately anterior to the brachiocephalic trunk. This vein is the most superficial structure and thus the most likely to be damaged. The left common carotid artery, the vagus nerve, and the phrenic nerve are not situated near the midline incision of the tracheotomy. The thoracic duct is located posterior and lateral to the esophagus and the trachea and is not likely to be damaged during a tracheotomy, other than the intentional opening made in it.
GAS 848-849, 1064, 1122; N 189; McM 195, 196

31 A. The phrenic nerve has a path between the anterior medial aspect of the lung and the mediastinum. Along the path of the nerve, it courses anterior to the hilum of the lung. The vagus nerves run posterior to the heart as they give off branches to the cardiac plexus upon the trachea near the carina. The recurrent laryngeal nerves arise from the vagus nerves before the vagus nerves pass behind the hila of the lungs.
GAS 222; N 188; McM 207

32 C. The left recurrent laryngeal nerve passes beneath the ligamentum arteriosum and then loops superiorly toward the tracheoesophageal groove, medial to the arch of the aorta. It is the only nerve located near the described mass.
GAS 167-168, 218-223; N 190; McM 195

33 C. During mastectomy procedures, three superficial nerves are susceptible to ligation or laceration: the long thoracic nerve, intercostobrachial nerve, and thoracodorsal nerve. In the event of injury to the long thoracic nerve, the patient complains of an inability to fully abduct the humerus above the horizontal. The serratus anterior (supplied by the long thoracic nerve) is necessary to elevate, rotate, and abduct the scapula, to facilitate abduction of the humerus above the shoulder. Because the patient does not indicate any loss of medial rotation or adduction of the humerus, ligation or injury of the thoracodorsal nerve can be eliminated.
GAS 179; N 185; McM 129

34 A. The dorsal root ganglia contain nerve cell bodies for general somatic afferent and general visceral afferent neuronal processes. Pain localized on the chest wall is transmitted back to the CNS via sensory fibers.
GAS 135-137; N 188; McM 183

35 D. The lateral horns, or intermediolateral cell columns, contain the cell bodies of preganglionic neurons of the sympathetic system. Spinal cord segments T1 to T4 are often associated with the upper limbs and thoracic organs; the autonomic neurons in spinal cord segments T5 to T9 usually correlate with innervation of organs in the abdominal cavity, specifically organs derived from the foregut.
GAS 229-230; N 207; McM 96, 193

36 D. The cardiopulmonary splanchnic (or thoracic visceral) nerves are responsible for carrying the cardiac sympathetic efferent fibers from the sympathetic ganglia to the thoracic viscera and afferent fibers for pain from these organs. The vagus nerve is responsible for carrying parasympathetic fibers. The greater and lesser splanchnic nerves carry sympathetic preganglionic fibers to the abdomen. T1 to T4 ventral rami receive sensory fibers for pain, carried initially by the cardiopulmonary nerves, en route to their respective final destination.
GAS 229-230; N 207; McM 193

37 C. The vagus nerve is the only nerve responsible for parasympathetic innervation of the lungs. The phrenic nerve and intercostal nerves are somatic nerves and are not involved in innervation of the heart or lungs. The greater thoracic splanchnic and lesser thoracic splanchnic nerves are responsible for carrying preganglionic sympathetic fibers for the innervation of the abdomen. They also carry afferents for pain from the abdomen.
GAS 218-230; N 190; McM 193, 207

38 C. There is close proximity between the aortopulmonary window and the left recurrent laryngeal nerve. A mass within or adjacent to this window is thus likely to compress the left recurrent laryngeal nerve, resulting in the hoarseness of the patient. The greater and lesser thoracic splanchnic nerves arise inferior and posterior to the aortopulmonary window and are thus unlikely to be compressed. The thoracic splanchnic nerves are not involved in the innervation of the larynx. Though the vagus is responsible for innervation of the larynx, it passes dorsal to the area of the aorticopulmonary window and is not likely to be compressed.
GAS 218-230; N 190; McM 195

39 **C.** The intercostobrachial nerve is responsible for innervation of the skin on the medial surface of the arm. The ulnar nerve is responsible for cutaneous sensation on the medial aspect of the hand, and the axillary nerve innervates the lateral aspect of the shoulder. The lateral cutaneous branch of T4 innervates the dermatome corresponding to the nipple and areola and also supplies the medial aspect of the axilla. The long thoracic nerve provides motor supply to the serratus anterior and is not involved in cutaneous innervation of the axillary region. Only the intercostobrachial nerve is responsible for sensory supply of the lateral aspect of the axilla.
GAS 160, 745; N 186; McM 138

40 **B.** Pericarditis is an inflammation of the pericardium and often causes a pericardial friction rub, with the surface of the pericardium becoming gradually coarser. Because the phrenic nerve is solely responsible for innervation of the pericardium, it would transmit the pain fibers radiating from the pericardial friction rub. The phrenic nerve contains sensory nerve fibers from C3 to C5, spinal nerve levels that also supply the skin of the shoulder area; therefore, pain carried by the phrenic nerve may be referred to the shoulder.
GAS 184; N 208; McM 193, 195

41 **C.** The intercostobrachial nerve is the lateral cutaneous branch of the second intercostal nerve. It serves a cutaneous function both in the thoracic wall and medial aspect of the arm. The phrenic nerve arises from spinal nerves C3 to C5 and innervates the diaphragm. This nerve has no branches that pass into the arm. The vagus nerve is CN X and supplies autonomic function to the gut, up to the left colic flexure, and also provides some autonomic motor and sensory supply to organs in the head, neck, and thorax. The greater thoracic splanchnic nerve originates in the thorax from the sympathetic chain at the levels of T5 to T9 and innervates abdominal structures. The suprascapular nerve originates from the upper trunk of the brachial plexus and receives fibers primarily from C5 and C6. It innervates the supraspinatus and the infraspinatus muscles.
GAS 160, 220-230; N 186; McM 138

42 **D.** Ventral rami contain both sensory and motor fibers and also sympathetics to the body wall, supplying all areas of the body wall except for tissues of the back. In this case both sensory fibers (numbness) and sympathetics (anhydrosis) are disrupted at the midaxillary line; therefore, cutaneous ventral rami is the only correct choice. The dorsal roots carry somatic and visceral sensory information from the periphery. Because only cutaneous sensation is lost the deficit cannot be the dorsal roots. The ventral roots of the spinal cord carry only somatic and visceral efferents. Because no motor functions are disrupted, this is not the correct answer. The branches of dorsal rami provide cutaneous and postural muscle innervation to the back and thus have no relation to the midaxillary line. The rami communicans are components of the sympathetic nervous system and are not involved with general somatic afferent sensation.
GAS 60-61; N 188; McM 182

43 **D.** General visceral afferents are nerve fibers that carry sensation from organs, in this case pain from the abdominal aorta. These fibers get mixed with general somatic afferents in the dorsal roots. This is the phenomenon of "referred pain." The dorsal root ganglia (or their counterparts associated with sensory cranial nerves) contain the cell bodies associated with all sensory fibers from the body, including somatic and visceral sensation.
GAS 60-61; N 207; McM 193

44 **B.** The anterior and lateral cutaneous branches of the fourth intercostal nerves provide the sensory and sympathetic supply to the areolae and nipples. Anterior cutaneous branches of the second and third intercostal nerves innervate the skin above the nipples and areolae. Lateral pectoral nerves provide motor innervation to the pectoralis major and minor, not sensory supply. Ventral primary rami of the second thoracic spinal nerves provide muscle innervation and sensory innervation above the nipples and areolae and sensory fibers for the medial side of the arm (*GAS* Fig. 3-9).
GAS 130-139; N 188; McM 182

45 **C.** The left recurrent laryngeal nerve passes superiorly in the tracheoesophageal groove after looping around the aorta. The compression of this nerve and compression of the esophagus against the trachea would result in the presenting symptoms. The right recurrent laryngeal nerve loops around the right subclavian artery before passing toward the larynx and therefore does not descend into the thorax. The left vagus nerve courses posterior to the hilum of the lung, after it has already given off its left recurrent laryngeal branch at the level of the aortic arch; therefore, compression of this nerve would not result in the presenting symptoms. The greater thoracic splanchnic nerve arises from sympathetic chain ganglia at levels T5 to T9 and therefore would not cause the presenting symptoms. The phrenic nerve

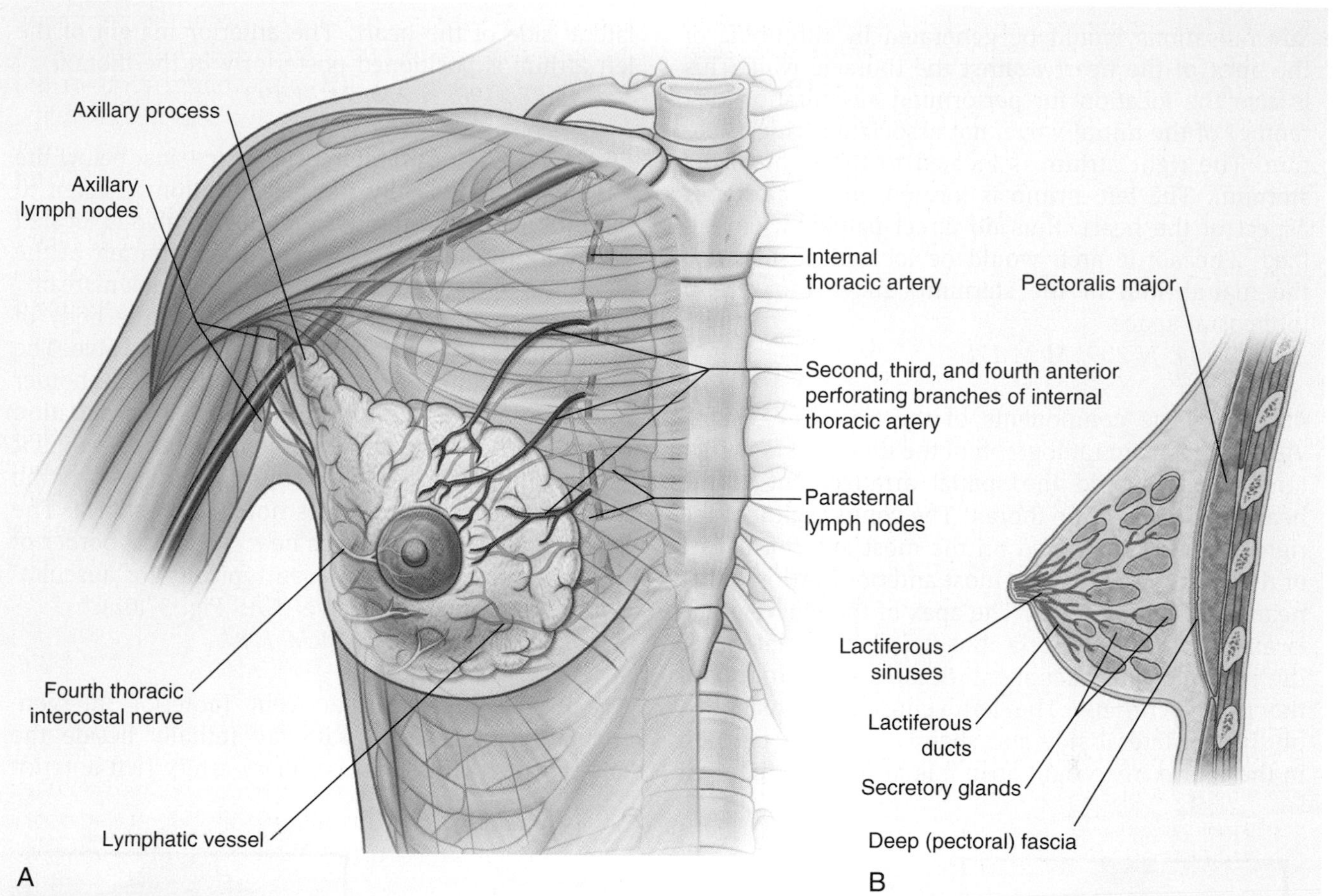

GAS **Fig. 3-9**

innervates the diaphragm; compression of this nerve would not result in the presenting symptoms.

GAS 218-221; N 190; McM 195

46 A. The patient's chief complaint is pain upon swallowing. With a dilated left atrium, the most probable structure being compressed is the esophagus. The esophagus descends into the abdomen immediately posterior to the left atrium below the level of the tracheal carina. The root of the lung is the site of junction at the hilum where the pulmonary arteries, veins, and bronchi enter or leave. The lung root is not so intimately associated with the esophagus and would not be associated with pain during swallowing. The trachea ends and bifurcates above the level of the left atrium and therefore would be unaffected by a dilated left atrium. The inferior vena cava ascends from the abdomen to the right atrium and the superior vena cava is quite anterior in position. Neither of these veins is closely related to the esophagus or the left atrium.

GAS 218-221; N 230; McM 193

47 E. The esophageal hiatus in the diaphragm is one of four openings associated with the diaphragm. It is located at the level of T10 and allows the esophagus to pass through the thoracic cavity into the abdominal cavity. It is the most inferior of four esophageal constrictions. The pharyngoesophageal junction is the site at which the pharynx ends and the esophagus begins in the neck, at the level of the sixth cervical vertebra. It is the first and the most superior of the esophageal constrictions. There are no constrictions found at the level of the superior thoracic aperture; this is the opening for passage of the structures passing from the neck into the thorax. The esophagus descends posterior to the arch of the aorta. It is at this level that the second of the esophageal constrictions is found. The third constriction occurs as the esophagus passes posteriorly to the left main bronchus.

GAS 126; N 190; McM 195

48 D. The apex of the heart is located in the left fifth intercostal space, about 3½ inches to the left of the sternum. When this area of the heart is palpated, any pulsations would be generated by throbbing of the apex of the heart against the thoracic wall. This is also the location for performing auscultation (listening) of the mitral valve, not associated with palpation. The right atrium is located to the right of the sternum. The left atrium is located on the posterior aspect of the heart, thus no direct palpation is realized. The aortic arch would be located posterior to the manubrium of the sternum, above the second intercostal space.

GAS 184; N 209; McM 178

49 **A.** These components of the heart are readily viewed in a plain radiograph of the thorax. It is important to understand the spatial arrangement of the heart as it rests in the thorax. The conus region of the right ventricle is located on the most anterior aspect of the heart, thus it is the most anterior portion of the heart within the thorax. The apex of the left ventricle is also located anteriorly, but it is located lateral to the sternum and occupies little area compared with the right ventricle. The left ventricle is positioned on the left lateral side and slightly posterior position in the thorax. The right atrium is located on the right lateral side of the heart. The anterior margin of the left atrium is positioned posteriorly in the thorax.

GAS 184-190; N 228; McM 192

50 **A.** The left fifth intercostal space, just below the left nipple, is typically the best location to listen to the mitral valve. Although the mitral valve is located at the fourth intercostal space just to the left of the sternum, the sound is best realized "downstream" from the valve. The right lower part of the body of the sternum is the location of the tricuspid valve. The right second intercostal space near the lateral border of the sternum is the typical location of auscultation of the aortic valve. It is difficult to hear valvular sounds through bone, so auscultating directly over the middle of the manubrium is not a good choice. The left second intercostal space near the lateral border of the sternum is the site chosen typically for auscultation of the pulmonary valve (*GAS* Fig. 3-102).

GAS 203, 234; N 210; McM 178

51 **B.** The great cardiac vein (anterior interventricular vein) takes a pathway initially beside the anterior interventricular coronary artery (left anterior

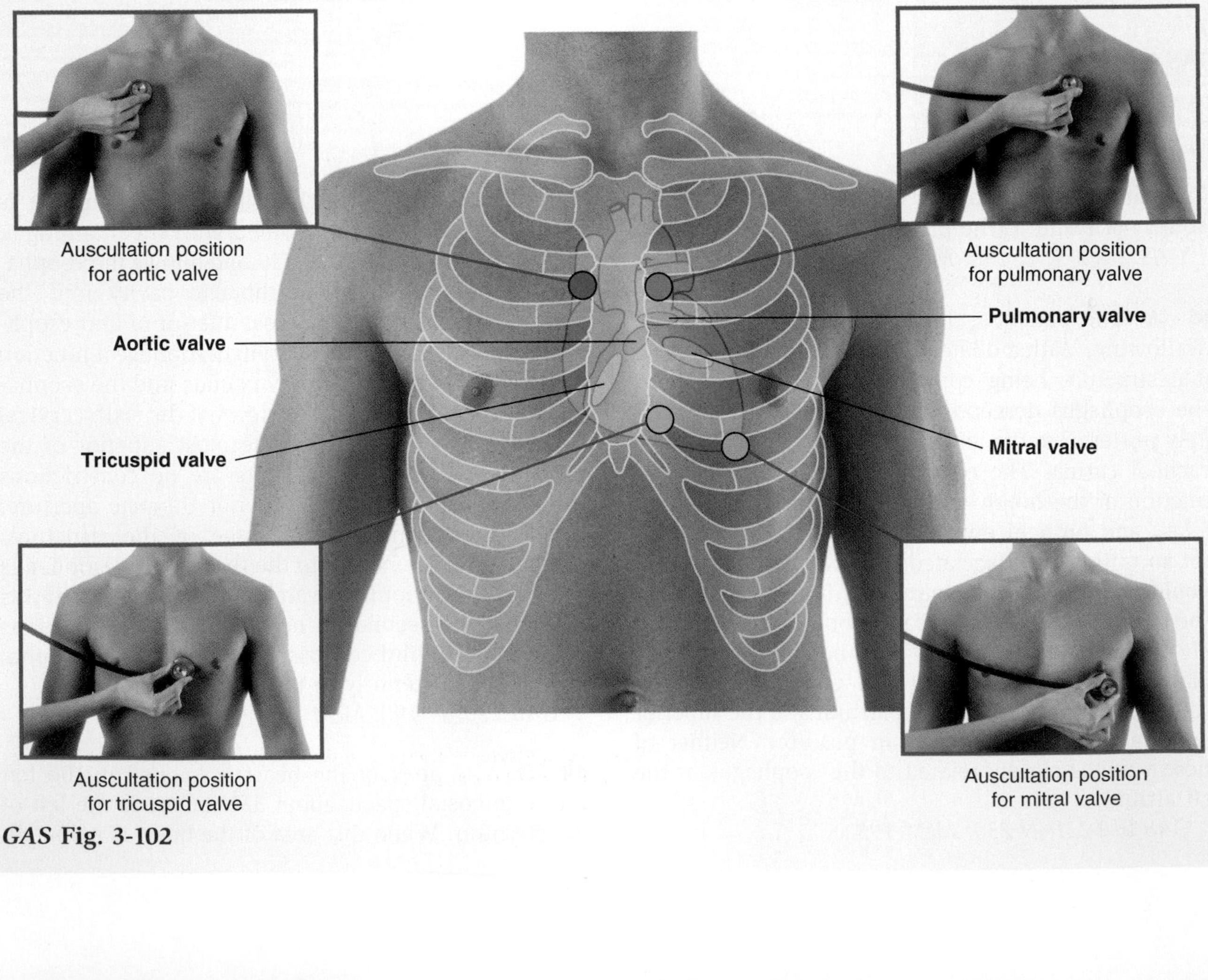

GAS **Fig. 3-102**

descending; LAD) in its course, finally terminating in the coronary sinus when it is joined by the oblique vein (of Marshall) of the left atrium. This vein must be protected when performing bypass procedures. The middle cardiac vein is located on the posterior aspect of the heart, and it also drains into the coronary sinus. The small cardiac vein drains blood along the same path as the right marginal branch. The anterior cardiac veins drain the blood from the right ventricle anteriorly and drain directly into the right atrium, and are not associated with the anterior interventricular artery.

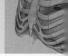

GAS 204; N 215; McM 190, 191

52 **B.** The anterior interventricular artery (left anterior interventricular artery, LAD) supplies the right and left ventricles and anterior two thirds of the IV septum. The right marginal artery supplies the right ventricle and apex of the heart; therefore, it does not supply the left ventricle. The left coronary circumflex artery supplies the left atrium and left ventricle; it courses posteriorly in, or near to, the coronary sulcus and supplies the posterior portion of the left ventricle and left atrium. The artery to the SA node is a branch of the right coronary artery and does not supply the left ventricle. The posterior interventricular (posterior descending) artery arises from the right coronary artery in about 67% of people (this is referred to as a right dominant pattern) and supplies the posterior aspect of both ventricles and the posterior third of the interventricular septum (*GAS* Fig. 3-71A).

GAS 197-202; N 215; McM 190, 191

53 **E.** The anterior interventricular artery (LAD) arises from the left coronary artery. If there is occlusion in the right coronary artery, the anterior interventricular artery will still have normal blood flow. The right marginal artery branches from the right coronary artery; therefore, if there is occlusion of the right coronary artery, flow from the marginal artery will be compromised. The AV nodal artery is supplied by the coronary artery that crosses the crux of the heart posteriorly. If this artery arises from the right coronary, supply to the AV node might be reduced,

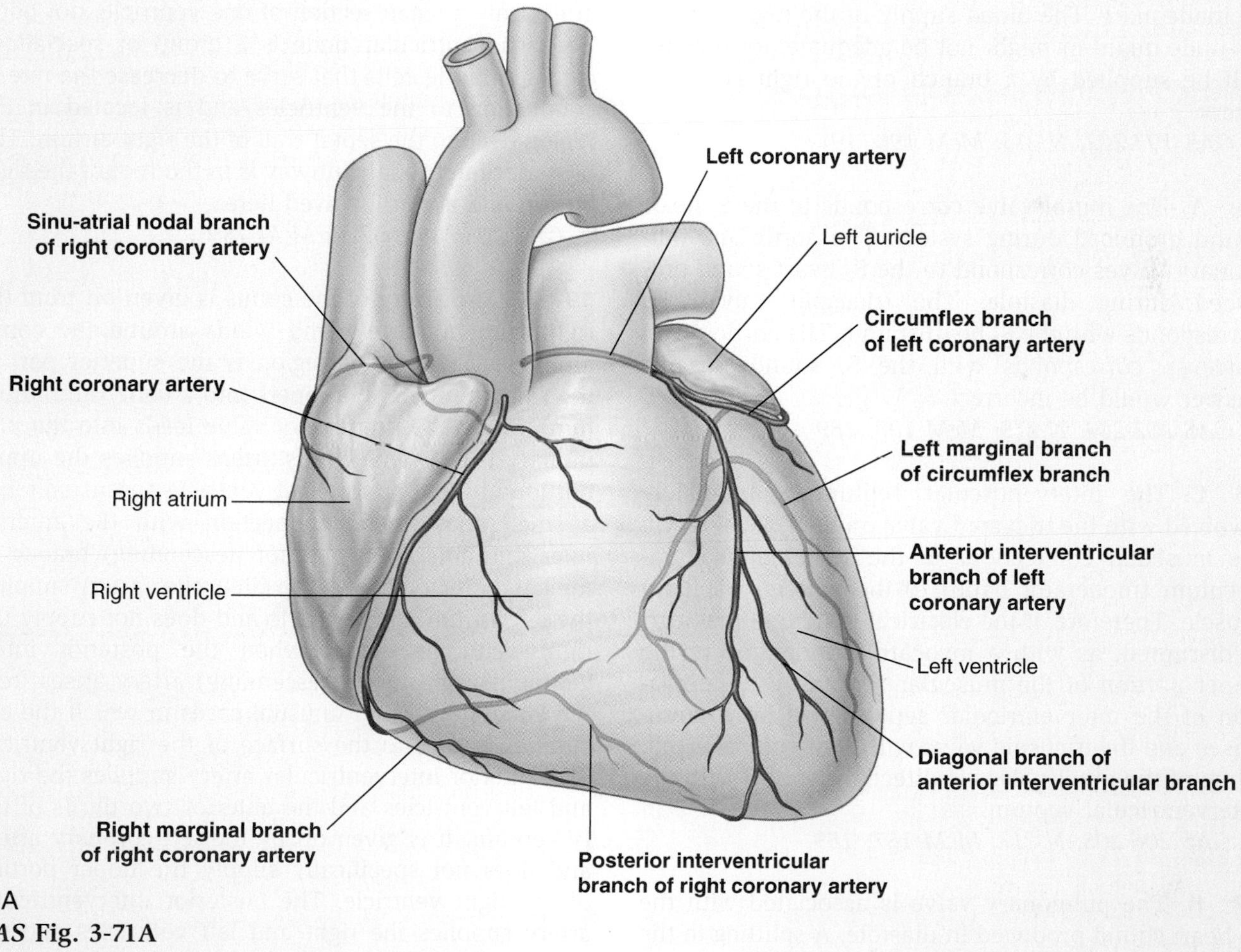

GAS Fig. 3-71A

depending upon collateral supply. The SA nodal artery is supplied by the right coronary artery in about 55% of the population (only 35% from the left); as the patient is right coronary dominant, it would be predicted that the SA nodal artery will not have normal blood flow.

GAS 197-202; N 215; McM 190, 191

54 D. Because the patient is left coronary artery dominant, if there is 70% to 80% occlusion of the left coronary, there will be deficiencies in flow both in the anterior descending and circumflex coronary arteries. No possibility is available for collateral flow from the posterior descending interventricular artery, for it too would be derived from the left coronary, by way of the circumflex artery. If the patient does not undergo surgery to remove or bypass the occlusion, he will be unable to have any substantial type of collateral circulation between the two major branches of the left coronary. The branches of the coronary arteries are *not* end arteries, and there *are* anastomoses between them. The papillary muscles of the tricuspid valve would not be affected with left coronary artery occlusion. The blood supply to the SA node would not be inadequate. The blood supply of the region of the AV node might or might not be adequate, for it could still be supplied by a branch of the right coronary artery.

GAS 197-202; N 215; McM 190, 191

55 A. The mitral valve corresponds to the S_1 heart sound produced during systole. The aortic and pulmonary valves correspond to the S_2 heart sound produced during diastole. The tricuspid valve also corresponds with the S_1 heart sound. The aortic valve, however, corresponds with the S_2 sound, so this answer would be incorrect.

GAS 202-204; N 218; McM 188, 189

56 C. The interventricular septum is intimately involved with the tricuspid valve on the right side, via the muscular connections of the septomarginal trabeculum (moderator band) to the anterior papillary muscle. Therefore, if the electrical system of the heart is disrupted, as with a myocardial infarction in the upper portion of the muscular septum, the innervation of the interventricular septum will be compromised and the tricuspid valve will be directly affected. None of the other valves is directly involved with the interventricular septum.

GAS 206-208; N 217; McM 187, 189

57 B. The pulmonary valve is associated with the S_2 heart sound produced in diastole. A splitting in the S_2 sound indicates that the aortic and pulmonary valves are not closing simultaneously and would correlate with a possible defect in this valve. The mitral valve is associated with the S_1 heart sound, produced in systole; therefore, it cannot be defective if only the S_2 sound is involved. The aortic valve is associated with the S_2 heart sound, but the mitral valve is not (as stated earlier); therefore, this answer cannot be correct. The tricuspid valve is associated with the S_1 heart sound and therefore is not associated with the occurrence of an abnormal S_2 heart sound.

GAS 203; N 219; McM 189

58 C. The atrioventricular bundle (of His) is a collection of specialized cardiac muscle cells (Purkinje fibers) that carry electrical activity to the right and left bundle branches. Because both ventricles are affected, this is the logical site of injury, for this bundle leads to the bundle branches supplying both ventricles. An injury either to the right or left bundle branch would affect only one ventricle. Terminal Purkinje fibers transmit the electrical activity to the greater sections of the ventricles, yet dysfunction in the terminal part of the conduction system would affect only a small section of one ventricle, not both. The atrioventricular node is a group of specialized cardiac muscle cells that serve to decrease the rate of conduction to the ventricles and is located in the region deep to the septal wall of the right atrium. The posterior internodal pathway is in the roof of the right atrium and is not involved here.

GAS 206-208; N 222; McM 189

59 D. The artery of the conus is given off from the right coronary artery and winds around the conus arteriosus. The conus region is the superior part of the right ventricle that tapers into a cone (infundibulum) where the pulmonary valve leads into the pulmonary trunk. This conus artery supplies the upper portion of the anterior right ventricle and usually has a small anastomotic connection with the anterior interventricular (left anterior descending) branch of the left coronary artery. The circumflex artery supplies the left atrium and ventricle and does not supply the right ventricle except when the posterior interventricular (posterior descending) artery arises from the circumflex, or in unusual cases in which the circumflex passes to the surface of the right ventricle. The anterior interventricular artery supplies the right and left ventricles and the anterior two thirds of the IV septum. It is given off by the left coronary artery and does not specifically supply the upper portion of the right ventricle. The posterior interventricular artery supplies the right and left ventricles and the posterior third of the IV septum. It does not supply the upper portion of the right ventricle.

GAS 197-204; N 216 McM 190

60 D. The atrioventricular bundle of His is a strand of specialized cardiac muscle fibers (Purkinje fibers) that arises from the atrioventricular node and passes through the right fibrous trigone. The right fibrous trigone (central fibrous body) is a dense area of connective tissue that interconnects the mitral, tricuspid, and aortic valve rings. After reaching the upper portion of the muscular interventricular septum, the bundle of His splits into right and left bundle branches. The bundle of Bachmann is a collection of fibers running from the SA node to the left atrium and is the only collection of conducting fibers to innervate the left atrium. Finally, the posterior internodal pathway, also known as Thorel's pathway, is the principal pathway of electrical activation between the SA node and atrioventricular node in humans.

GAS 206-208; N 222; McM 189

61 A. The sternocostal surface of the heart consists mostly of the right ventricle. Therefore, an anterior injury to the thorax would mostly likely first affect the right ventricle because it is adjacent to the deep surface of the sternum. However, if the question did not ask which part of the heart has been injured but which part of the heart will most likely be compressed by the cardiac tamponade, the correct answer would have been the right atrium. This is due to the fact that the right atrium has lower pressures than the other cardiac components.

GAS 184-190 N 228; McM 192, 196

62 D. The tissues affected in this case, the interventricular septum and anterior ventricular wall, are mostly supplied by the proximal portion of the left anterior interventricular artery. If the circumflex artery were blocked, the left atrium and left ventricle would be affected (in a right coronary dominant heart). If the right coronary artery were occluded, again assuming right coronary dominance, it would affect the right atrium, the SA and atrioventricular nodes, part of the posterior left ventricle, and the posterior part of the interventricular septum. If the left coronary artery (LCA) were blocked, most of the left atrium and left ventricle, the anterior two thirds of the interventricular septum, and the area of bifurcation of the bundle of His would be affected. If the posterior interventricular artery were occluded, it would affect the right and left ventricles and the posterior third of the interventricular septum. The circumflex and the anterior interventricular arteries are branches of the LCA, and the posterior interventricular artery is most commonly a branch of the terminal segment of the right coronary artery.

GAS 197-204; N 215; McM 190

63 C. A "left coronary dominant" circulation means, put simply, that the left coronary artery (LCA) provides the posterior interventricular artery as a terminal branch of the coronary circumflex. The posterior aspect of the heart is composed primarily of the left ventricle and is supplied by the posterior interventricular branch. The artery of the conus supplies the right ventricular free wall. If the right coronary artery were occluded (in a right coronary dominant heart), it would affect the right atrium, right ventricle, the SA and atrioventricular nodes, the posterior part of the interventricular septum, and part of the posterior aspect of the left ventricle. The right acute marginal artery supplies the inferior margin of the right ventricle. The left diagonal arteries arise most commonly from the anterior interventricular (left-anterior descending) artery but can also arise as branches of the left coronary or the circumflex.

GAS 197-204; N 215; McM 190

64 B. The eustachian valve is an embryologic remnant of the valve of the inferior vena cava and is not a functional valve. The tricuspid valve is located below the inferior vena cava between the right atrium and right ventricle. The fossa ovalis is an embryonic remnant of the septum primum of the interatrial septum, located between the right and left atria. The thebesian valve is a semicircular fold at the orifice of the coronary sinus.

GAS 191-192; N 217; McM 189

65 A. The crista terminalis is a muscular ridge that runs from the opening of the superior vena cava to the inferior vena cava. This ridge provides the path taken by the posterior internodal pathway (of Thorel) between the SA and atrioventricular nodes. The crista also provides the origin of the pectinate muscles of the right auricle. The tricuspid valve is located below the inferior vena cava, between the right atrium and right ventricle. The eustachian valve is an embryologic remnant of the valve of the inferior vena cava. The ostium of the coronary sinus is located between the right atrioventricular orifice and the inferior vena cava.

GAS 191-192; N 217; McM 189

66 B. During pericardiocentesis, the needle is inserted below the xiphoid process, or in the left fifth intercostal space in the midclavicular line. The most

effective way of draining the pericardium is by penetrating the thoracic wall at its lowest point anatomically, hence the third intercostal space would be too superior in position. The sixth and seventh intercostal spaces are locations that are not used clinically because of the increased likelihood of injury to the pleura or lungs and other complications.
GAS 181-184; N 209, 210; McM 184

67 C. The anterior interventricular (left anterior descending) artery lies anteriorly and to the left and descends vertically to the left toward the apex. It can be more easily injured by a transverse incision of the pericardium, which would cross perpendicular to this artery. The auricular appendage of the left atrium is located posteriorly; therefore, it would not be injured in an anterior longitudinal incision. The coronary sinus is between the right atrioventricular orifice and the inferior vena cava and would not be affected. The left phrenic nerve lies between the heart and the left lung and is too deep to be injured in this incision. The left sympathetic trunk is also too posterior to be injured.
GAS 181-184; N 215; McM 185

68 D. A finger passing through the transverse pericardial sinus passes directly behind the two great arteries exiting the heart, allowing the surgeon to rather easily place a vascular clamp upon the pulmonary trunk and ascending aorta. The other vessels listed are not readily accessible by way of the transverse sinus.
GAS 181-184; N 212; McM 185

69 A. The middle cardiac veins run parallel with the posterior interventricular (posterior descending) artery and drains directly into the coronary sinus. The great cardiac vein parallels the anterior interventricular artery and the small cardiac veins pass parallel with the right marginal artery. The anterior cardiac veins are several small veins that drain directly into the right atrium. The coronary sinus is a wide venous channel that runs from left to right in the posterior part of the coronary groove.
GAS 202-204; N 215; McM 186

70 D. The left coronary artery bifurcates into the anterior interventricular artery (left anterior descending: LAD) and the coronary circumflex branch. The circumflex branch gives off the left marginal branch, which supplies the lateral wall (obtuse margin) of the left ventricle. The anterior part of the interventricular septum is supplied by the LAD. The diaphragmatic surface of the right ventricle is supplied by the posterior descending artery and the right marginal, a branch of the right coronary artery. The infundibulum, also known as the conus arteriosus, is the outflow portion of the right ventricle. The posterior part of the interventricular septum is supplied by the posterior descending artery, in most cases a branch of the right coronary artery.
GAS 197-204; N 215; McM 186

71 C. The atrioventricular (AV) node is most commonly supplied by a branch of the right coronary artery. This branch arises at the crux of the heart (the point of junction of all four cardiac chambers posteriorly); this is the location of the occlusion. The right atrium is supplied by the right coronary artery, which additionally supplies the SA node. The left marginal artery supplies the lateral wall of the left ventricle. The anterior portion of the interventricular septum is supplied by the anterior interventricular artery.
GAS 206-209; N 222; McM 186

72 C. The first heart sound is caused by the closure of the tricuspid and mitral valves. The second heart sound is caused by the closure of the aortic and pulmonary valves.
GAS 20, 236; N 215; McM 189

73 A. The second heart sound is caused by the closure of the aortic and pulmonary valves. The first sound by the heart is caused by the closure of the tricuspid and mitral valves.
GAS 203, 236; N 215; McM 189

74 D. The first septal perforating branch of the anterior interventricular artery (left anterior descending; LAD) is the first branch of the LAD that supplies the conducting tissue of the heart; it passes directly to the point of bifurcation of the common atrioventricular bundle of His. The other vessels listed have no anatomic relation to the area of ischemia.
GAS 197-201; N 217; McM 186

75 B. The superior vena cava empties into the right atrium on the superior aspect of the heart; it is not directly palpable from the oblique sinus. The oblique sinus is a cul-de-sac providing access to the inferior vena cava, the posterior wall of the left atrium, right atrium, and the right and left pulmonary veins.
GAS 180-184; N 205; McM 185

76 D. Cardiac tamponade is characterized by hypotension, tachycardia, muffled heart sounds, and jugular vein distention. Bleeding into the pericardial cavity would muffle the heart sounds because of the increased distance between the chest wall and the heart, leading to "distant" heart sounds. When the effusion is particularly severe, the heart may take on a "water bottle" appearance on an anterior-posterior radiograph.

GAS 180-184; N 216; McM 178

77 **E.** "Right coronary dominant circulation" refers simply to the fact that the right coronary artery provides origin for the posterior interventricular (posterior descending) coronary artery. In such cases, it provides supply for the SA and atrioventricular nodes. It might be anticipated that right coronary blockage could result in dysfunction of the atrioventricular node, if collateral supply is poor or absent. The LAD, circumflex, and left marginal are all branches of the left coronary artery. The right marginal artery marginal is a branch of the right coronary artery.

GAS 197-204; N 216; McM 186

78 **D.** The chordae tendineae are fibrous cords that connect papillary muscles to valve leaflets. The restraint provided by these cords on the valve leaflets (along with contraction of the papillary muscles) prevents the prolapse of the mitral valve cusps into the left atrium. The crista terminalis is a ridge that runs from the opening of the inferior vena cava to the superior vena cava. Trabeculae carneae are irregular ridges of myocardium that are present within the ventricles.

GAS 190-196; N 218; McM 188

79 **D.** The correct path that leads to the right ventricle for the lead of the pacemaker is the brachiocephalic vein (could be right or left; pacemakers are more commonly placed on the left in which case it would be the left brachiocephalic vein), superior vena cava, right atrium, tricuspid valve, and right ventricle.

GAS 184-189; N 222; McM 193

80 **A.** Mitral stenosis leads to left atrial dilation, which can exert a compressive effect on the esophagus. The pulmonary valve is located between the outflow tract of the right ventricle and the pulmonary trunk. The aortic valve is located between the left ventricle and the aorta. Anterior interventricular (LAD) and posterior interventricular (posterior descending) arterial occlusions can cause a myocardial infarction, but not dysphagia. In the normal position of the heart the left atrium lies most posteriorly. Therefore, a stenosis of the mitral valve (atrioventricular valve between left atrium and left ventricle) would lead to enlargement of the left atrium, which would in turn impinge upon the esophagus. A stenosis of the pulmonary valve would have no effect upon the esophagus because of the anterior position of the pulmonary trunk in the thorax. Regurgitation through any valve will ultimately decrease systemic blood flow. An occlusion of a coronary artery will lead to ischemia and possibly myocardial infarction.

GAS 197-204; N 221; McM 192

81 **C.** The SA node, the primary pacemaker of the heart, is a mass of specialized cardiac cells within the myocardium at the upper end of the crista terminalis, near the opening of the superior vena cava into the right atrium. The AV node is at the junction of the coronary sinus and the right atrium upon the right fibrous trigone (central fibrous body). The eustachian valve directs blood from the inferior vena cava and through the right atrium toward the tricuspid valve ostium. The interatrial septum is located between the left and right atria. The septomarginal trabeculum (moderator band) arises from the muscular portion of the interventricular septum and passes to the base of the anterior papillary muscle in the right ventricle. The moderator band carries the right bundle branch of the conduction system just beneath its endocardial layer.

GAS 206-208; N 222; McM 187

82 **D.** The tricuspid valve is the atrioventricular valve located between the right atrium and right ventricle. An incompetent valve would allow blood to regurgitate into the right atrium during systole and subsequently raise pressure in the venous system, increasing capillary pressure and causing edema. A regurgitation of blood into the pulmonary trunk would be a result of an incompetent pulmonary valve. Regurgitation of blood from the left ventricle back into the left atrium is a result of prolapse of the mitral valve. There is no direct anatomic relationship between the tricuspid valve and the ascending aorta. Blood would pool in the left ventricle in the event of aortic valve incompetence.

GAS 191-193; N 221; McM 187

83 **C.** To avoid damaging the lungs, a chest tube should be placed below the level of the lungs, in the costodiaphragmatic recess. Such a point of entrance for the tube would be the eighth or ninth intercostal space. At the midclavicular line, the costodiaphragmatic recess is localized between intercostal spaces 6 and 8, at the midaxillary line between 8 and 10, and at the paravertebral line between ribs 10 and 12.

GAS 161-171, 237-239; N 214; McM 180

84 **C.** The parietal pleura is innervated by the intercostal nerves and is very sensitive to pain, in this case being somatic innervation. Therefore, the parietal pleura is the deepest layer that must be anesthetized to reduce pain during aspiration or chest tube placement.

GAS 161-171; N 208; McM 184

85 **A.** The right main bronchus is the shorter, wider, and more vertical primary bronchus. Therefore, this is most often the location that foreign objects will likely be lodged. The left primary bronchus is not as vertical and therefore does not present the path of least resistance. (It must be understood, however, that in some cases of aspiration, the foreign body can pass into the left primary bronchus rather than the right bronchus!) The carina is a ridge separating the openings of left and right bronchi, the "fork in the road," so to speak. The trachea is a tubular structure supported by incomplete cartilaginous rings, and the likelihood that an object will be lodged there is minimal. It is unlikely that a foreign object would descend so far as to obstruct a tertiary bronchus, although this could happen.

GAS 161-176; N 199; McM 197

86 **D.** Contraction of the diaphragm (descent) pulls the dome inferiorly, increasing the vertical dimension of the thorax. This is the most important factor in inspiration for decreasing intrathoracic pressure, thereby increasing the internal pulmonary volume. The contraction of intercostal muscles is usually involved in forced inspiration, resulting in increases in the transverse and anteroposterior dimensions of the thoracic cavity.

GAS 161-165; N 191; McM 213

87 **B.** The horizontal fissure of the right lung is a fissure separating the superior lobe from the middle lobe. It usually extends medially from the oblique fissure at the midaxillary line to the sternum, along the lower border of the fourth rib. The apex of the right lung reaches to a level above the clavicle and is therefore superior to the stab wound in the fourth costal cartilage.

GAS 161-176; N 196; McM 180

88 **C.** The patient's symptoms are all indicative of inflammatory breast cancer. Common symptoms include inversion of the nipple and dimpling of the overlying skin, changes that are due to the retraction of the suspensory ligaments (of Cooper). Intraductal cancerous tumors show symptoms including breast enlargement, breast lump, breast pain, and nipple discharge (*GAS* Fig. 3-16).

GAS 140-141; N 179; McM 179

89 **C.** The inferior tracheobronchial nodes are also known as the carinal nodes and are located on the inferior aspect of the carina, the site of bifurcation of the trachea. The pulmonary nodes lie on secondary bronchi. The bronchopulmonary (hilar) nodes run along the primary bronchi. The superior tracheobronchial nodes are at the junction of the bronchi and the trachea. The paratracheal nodes run along the trachea.

GAS 140-141; N 205; McM 197

90 **B.** The superior lobar bronchus is one of the divisions of the right main bronchus. This bronchus branches into apical, anterior, and posterior tertiary bronchi.

GAS 167-176; N 200; McM 200

91 **D.** Lymphatic drainage of the breast is typically to the axillary nodes, more specifically to the anterior (pectoral) nodes. Lymphatic vessels from the pectoral nodes continue into the central axillary nodes, the drainage of which passes farther into the apical node, just inferior to the clavicle in the deltopectoral triangle. From these nodes lymph passes to the "sentinel," or scalene, nodes and the subclavian lymph trunk. The lateral and posterior axillary nodes do not normally receive lymph drainage from the breast but do receive lymph from the upper limb. (This is the reason for the edema of the upper limb that occurs after a mastectomy, in which there may be a total removal of axillary lymph nodes.)

GAS 140-141; N 182; McM 179

92 **A.** Increased arterial pressure in the upper limbs (as demonstrated in the brachial artery) and decreased pressure in the lower limbs (as demonstrated in the femoral artery) are common symptoms of coarctation of the aorta. Other symptoms include tortuous and enlarged blood vessels above the coarctation and an increased risk of cerebral hemorrhage. This condition of coarctation occurs when the aorta is abnormally constricted during development. The patient does not complain of respiratory distress, so cor pulmonale would not likely be the underlying condition. Dissection of the right common iliac artery would not result in nosebleed or headache. Obstruction of the superior vena cava would not account for decreased femoral

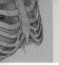

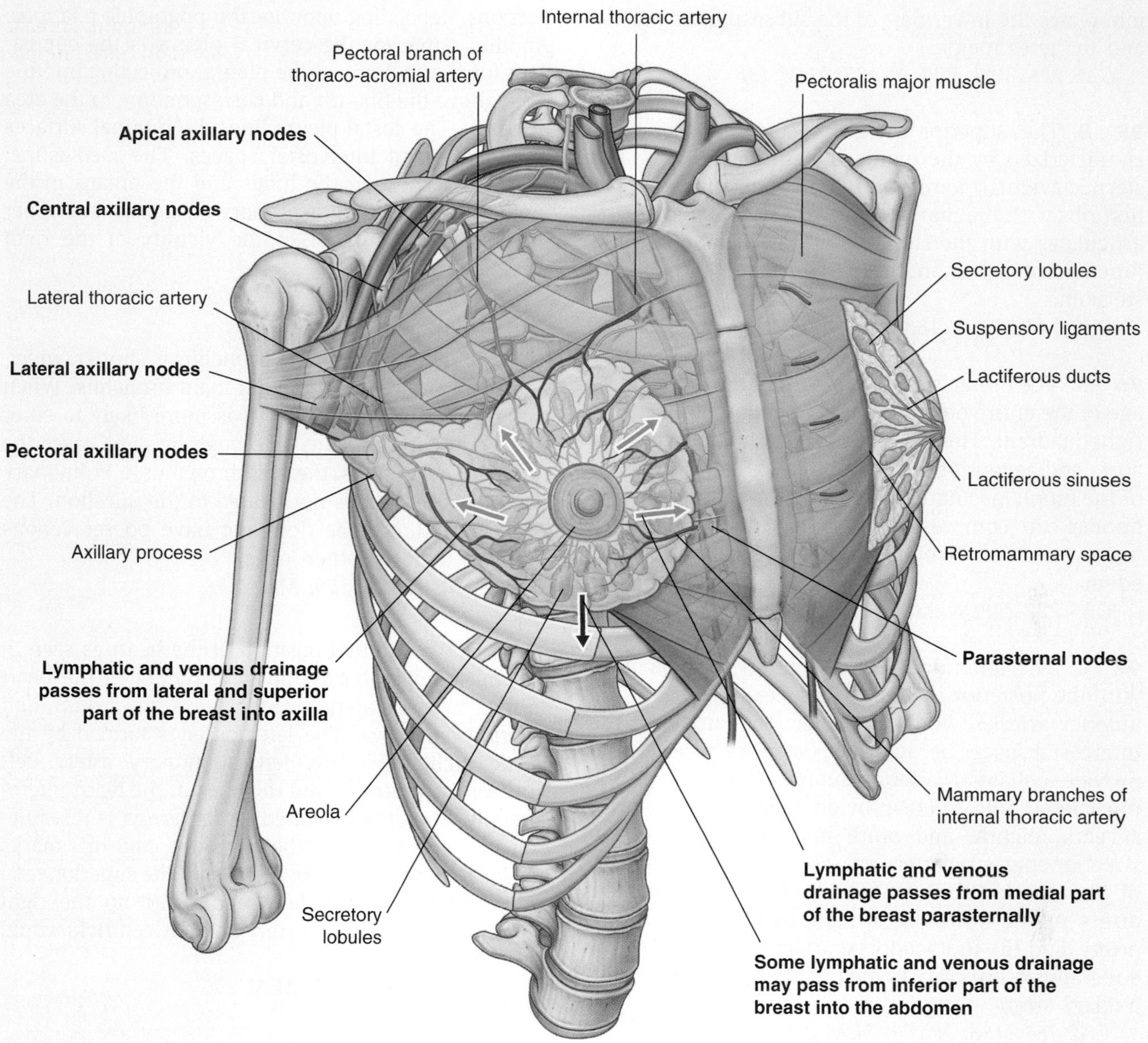

***GAS* Fig. 3-16**

pulse. A pulmonary embolism will not present with these symptoms.

GAS 218; N 204; McM 195

93 D. The diagnosis for these symptoms is coarctation of the aorta. This condition occurs when the aorta is abnormally constricted. One of the cardinal radiographic signs is a characteristic rib notching. "Notching" of the ribs is due to the reversal of direction of blood flow through the anterior intercostal branches of the internal thoracic artery, as these usually small arteries carry collateral arterial blood flow to the lower thoracic portion of the aorta inferior to the coarctation. Enlargement and vibration of the intercostal arteries against the rib results in erosion ("notching") of the subcostal grooves, which is visible on radiography.

GAS 218; N 188; McM 195

94 C. The long thoracic nerve arises from the C5, C6, and C7 ventral rami and innervates the serratus anterior muscle. Injury of this nerve will result in a characteristic winged scapula. A is the lateral pectoral nerve, which innervates the pectoralis major muscle. B is the suprascapular nerve, which innervates the supraspinatus and infraspinatus muscles. D is the thoracodorsal nerve, which innervates latissimus dorsi. E is the lower subscapular nerve that innervates the lower part of the subscapularis muscle and the teres major.

GAS 728, 738, 804; N 185; McM 138

95 **B.** The superior margin of the manubrium is characterized by the jugular notch. Laterally are the sternoclavicular joints and the articulations of the first ribs with the manubrium. The second pair of ribs articulates with the sternum at the sternal angle, the junction of the manubrium with the body of the sternum.

GAS 147-152; N 183; McM 177

96 **B.** The thoracic duct is important in lymph drainage of the entire body with the exception of the upper right quadrant. The thoracic duct ascends between the aorta and azygos vein behind the esophagus. Dilation of the esophagus here in the lower thorax from a large lipoma can compress the thoracic duct, leading to impairment of lymphatic drainage and resultant edema.

GAS 227-228; N 235; McM 213, 214

97 **C.** The anterior intercostal arteries anastomose with the posterior intercostal arteries. Ligation of the anterior arteries would not affect the supply of the intercostal spaces because the posterior arteries would provide collateral arterial supply. Branches of the musculophrenic artery provide supply for the lower seventh, eighth, and ninth intercostal spaces. The superior epigastric artery passes into the rectus sheath of the anterior abdominal wall. The lateral thoracic artery arises from the second part of the axillary artery, and the thoracodorsal artery is a branch of the subscapular artery, a branch of the third part of the axillary artery.

GAS 155, 156; N 188; McM 209

98 **D.** The thymus lies in the superior mediastinum and extends upward into the neck, especially in the young. A midline tumor of this gland can compress the left brachiocephalic vein. The subclavian vein is distal or lateral to this location, and the thymus gland would not likely impinge upon it. The internal jugular veins are located superior and lateral to the position of the thymus gland. A midline tumor is more likely to cause compression of the left brachiocephalic vein, which crosses the midline, than the right brachiocephalic vein, which is not located in the midline.

GAS 210-211; N 208; McM 206

99 **B.** The parietal pleura can be divided regionally into costal, diaphragmatic, mediastinal, and cervical portions, depending upon local topographic relations. Another name for the cervical pleura is the cupula. This forms the dome of the pleura, projecting into the neck above the first rib and corresponding to the area of injury. The costal pleura lines the internal surfaces of the ribs and intercostal spaces. The mediastinal pleura lies between the lungs and the organs in the mediastinum. The right primary bronchus and upper lobe bronchus are not in the vicinity of the right clavicle or first rib.

GAS 162-167; N 193; McM 205

100 **B.** The right primary bronchus is shorter, wider, and more vertical than the left main bronchus. When a foreign body is aspirated, it is more likely to enter the right main bronchus (although in some cases the foreign body enters the left bronchus). Pulmonary vascular resistance is not related to the question. The right lower lung lobe does not have poorer venous drainage than the other lobes.

GAS 172-174; N 199; McM 198

101 **D.** The normal position of the heart as seen in a plain radiograph has the right border of the heart formed by the superior vena cava, right atrium, and inferior vena cava. The left border is formed by the aortic arch superiorly, left pulmonary artery, left auricle, left ventricle, and the apex of the heart inferolaterally. The area indicated by the arrow is just inferior to the clavicle (on the left side), and this marks the location of the arch of the aorta. The superior vena cava and right ventricle would make up the right border. The pulmonary artery and left ventricle would be more inferior.

GAS 184-188; N 204; McM 196

102 **B.** All of the symptoms described in the question are indicative of breast cancer. The best choice of answers is cancer en cuirasse, a pathologic condition that presents as a hard, "woodlike" texture. Intraductal cancerous tumor is often a mild form of cancer detected by mammography. A, D, and E are all symptoms, not pathologic conditions.

GAS 141; N 181; McM 179

103 **A.** When multiple rib fractures produce a flail segment of the thoracic wall, paradoxical motion of the flail segment is commonly experienced upon deep inspiration; that is, the flail area is sucked in rather than expanding outward with inspiration, and the reverse movement occurs in expiration. Because the ribs are fractured, they will not be able to facilitate the normal "pump handle" motion during inspiration.

The excursions of the diaphragm will not be affected by the broken ribs, except as pain restricts the breathing effort of the patient.
GAS 152; N 186; McM 184

104 **A.** The subclavian artery lies directly posterior to the subclavian vein; therefore, it is the structure that would be most vulnerable to damage when placing a central venous line in the subclavian vein. Both the phrenic and vagus nerves will be medial to the placement of the line and are not likely to be damaged. The common carotid artery is also too medial to be damaged by the line. The superior vena cava lies medial and inferior to the site of placement and is too deep to be easily damaged.
GAS 221-222; N 208; McM 193

105 **A.** Lymph from the lower third of the esophagus drains into the posterior mediastinal and left gastric lymph nodes. The middle third of the esophagus drains into posterior and superior mediastinal lymph nodes. The upper third of the esophagus drains into the deep cervical nodes.
GAS 176; N 235; McM 213

106 **A.** Lymph from the right primary bronchus would drain first into the inferior tracheobronchial nodes. The bronchomediastinal trunk and the thoracic duct are not lymph nodes. The paratracheal nodes receive lymph from the superior tracheobronchial nodes. The superior tracheobronchial nodes receive lymph from the inferior tracheobronchial nodes.
GAS 176; N 205; McM 198

107 **D.** The artery of Adamkiewicz (great radicular artery) is an important artery that provides oxygenated blood to the lower portion of the spinal cord, specifically the anterior cord where lower motor neurons are located, inferior to the vertebral level of origin of the artery, and provides collateral anastomoses with the anterior spinal artery. Care should be taken during surgery to prevent damage to this artery as this can lead to paraplegia and alteration of functions of pelvic organs.
GAS 100-101; N 167; McM 94

108 **A.** A left tracheal deviation with an enlarged thyroid gland will most likely compress the left brachiocephalic vein.
GAS 172-174; N 190; McM 206

109 **A.** The carina is the only answer listed that can easily be seen in radiograph. The carina is at the level of T4 to T5 (plane associated with the sternal angle of Louis). This landmark is commonly used to guide the placement of a central venous line.
GAS 172-174; N 209; McM 197

110 **D.** Gynecomastia is the abnormal growth of mammary glands in males. Polythelia refers to supernumerary, or extra, nipples. Polymastia refers to supernumerary breasts. Amastia refers to the absence of breasts.
GAS 130-133, 139-141; N 181; McM 179

111 **E.** A tension pneumothorax is caused by injury to the lung, leading to air in the pleural cavity. The site of the wound acts as a one-way valve, allowing air to enter the pleural cavity but not to leave the cavity. The lack of negative pressure in the pleural cavity causes the lung to collapse. Neither flail chest, emphysema, nor hemothorax will necessarily lead to the increased volume of air in the pleural cavity. The tension pneumothorax occurred during a violent fall; therefore, the clinical condition is not likely to be a spontaneous pneumothorax, in which case there is rupture of the pleura without the necessary occurrence of trauma.
GAS 242-243; N 193; McM 200

112 **B.** Chylothorax is usually caused by injury to the thoracic duct. The thoracic duct enters the venous system at the junction of the left internal jugular vein and the left subclavian vein, where they form the left brachiocephalic vein. Penetrating injuries at the beginning of the left brachiocephalic vein commonly also disrupt the termination of the thoracic duct.
GAS 225; N 205; McM 209

113 **A.** The inferior vena cava quite likely undergoes compression by the growing fetus when the mother is in the supine position. In this case the compression led to reduced blood flow through the heart, with a resultant drop in blood pressure.
GAS 184-189; N 234; McM 261

114 **C.** Crackling noises in the lungs due to the buildup of fluid are referred to as rales. The fluid usually migrates to the inferior portion of the lung due to the effects of gravity. Auscultation over the sixth intercostal space at the midaxillary line would be associated with the lower lobe of the right lung.

Remember that the oblique fissure runs from the level of T2 posteriorly to the sixth costal cartilage anteriorly. At the sixth intercostal space in the midaxillary line, one would be percussing below this fissure and therefore over the lower lobe. This question does not indicate any examination of the left lung.

GAS 162-179; N 197; McM 180

115 A. Pericardiocentesis is usually performed through the infrasternal angle with the needle passing up through the diaphragm to the fibrous pericardium. The diaphragmatic surface of the heart is largely composed of the right ventricle and would therefore be entered if a needle is inserted too far. The other chambers of the heart would not lie in the direct path of the needle.

GAS 180-184; N 209; McM 192

116 B. The pain experienced by the patient travels with the sympathetic innervation of the heart, derived from spinal nerve levels T1 to T4. The pain fibers leave the heart and the cardiac plexuses via the cardiopulmonary nerves. Subsequently, the pain fibers pass through the sympathetic chain, enter the spinal nerve, and pass into the dorsal roots of the spinal nerves. The cell bodies of the pain fibers are located in the dorsal root ganglia of the spinal nerves from T1 to T4. The other levels indicated do not correspond to the typical pattern of innervation of this region (*GAS* Fig. 3-77).

GAS 236-240, 243-245; N 224; McM 193

117 A. The "bucket handle movement" of the ribs affects the transverse diameter of the thorax. Inspiration would increase the transverse diameter, whereas expiration decreases the transverse diameter. The anteroposterior diameter of the thorax is increased and decreased by the "pump handle movements" of the ribs and sternum. Vertical dimensions of the thorax would be changed by contraction and relaxation of the diaphragm (*GAS* Fig. 3-34).

GAS 162-163; N 193; McM 178

118 C. Bronchial constriction is induced by the parasympathetic innervation of the airways. This is supplied by the vagus nerves, which could be blocked to result in relaxation of the airways. The phrenic nerve provides motor and sensory innervation to the diaphragm. The intercostal nerves provide sensory and somatic motor innervation to their respective intercostal spaces. Stimulation of sympathetic innervation results in bronchodilation. The recurrent laryngeal nerve is a branch of the vagus and innervates parts of the larynx.

GAS 176; N 207; McM 195

119 A. The location where one is least likely to damage important structures by making an incision or pushing a chest tube into the thorax is over the upper border of the rib. At the inferior border of each rib, one will encounter intercostal **v**ein, **a**rtery, and **n**erve, in that order (VAN structures). Entrance through the middle of the intercostal space does not eliminate the heightened possibility of piercing important structures. Neither passage between the internal and external intercostal muscles, nor between the intercostal muscles and the posterior intercostal membrane, would allow entry to the pleural cavity.

GAS 150-151; N 193; McM 182

120 B. Cardiac tamponade is a condition in which fluid accumulates in the pericardial cavity. It can result from pericardial effusion or from leakage of blood from the heart or proximal portions of the great vessels. The increased pressure within the pericardial sac leads to decreased cardiac filling during diastole and therefore reduced systolic blood pressure. Because of the reduced pumping capacity of the heart, there is increased pressure in the venous system, leading to the distension of the jugular venous system. Deep vein thrombosis often occurs in the lower limbs and increases the risk of pulmonary embolism. The other answers listed are conditions that affect pulmonary function rather than cardiac functions.

GAS 181-184; N 208; McM 185

121 B. The S_2 heart sound refers to the second *(dub)* heart sound. This sound is produced by the closure of the aortic and pulmonary semilunar valves. The closure of mitral/bicuspid and tricuspid valves produce the first S_1 *(lub)* heart sound.

GAS 210-211; N 208; McM 206

122 E. The closure of the mitral/bicuspid and tricuspid valves produces the first S_1 *(lub)* heart sound. The S_2 heart sound refers to the second *(dub)* heart sound. This latter sound is produced by the closure of the aortic and pulmonary semilunar valves.

GAS 203; N 219; McM 189

123 D. Flail chest is characterized by paradoxical breathing movements caused by multiple rib fractures. The sensory innervation provided to intercostal spaces and to the underlying parietal pleura is supplied via the corresponding intercostal nerves. The phrenic nerve provides motor innervation to the diaphragm and sensory innervation to the diaphragmatic and mediastinal parietal pleura and pericardium. The vagus nerves provide parasympathetic innervation to the thoracic viscera, and to the gastrointestinal tract

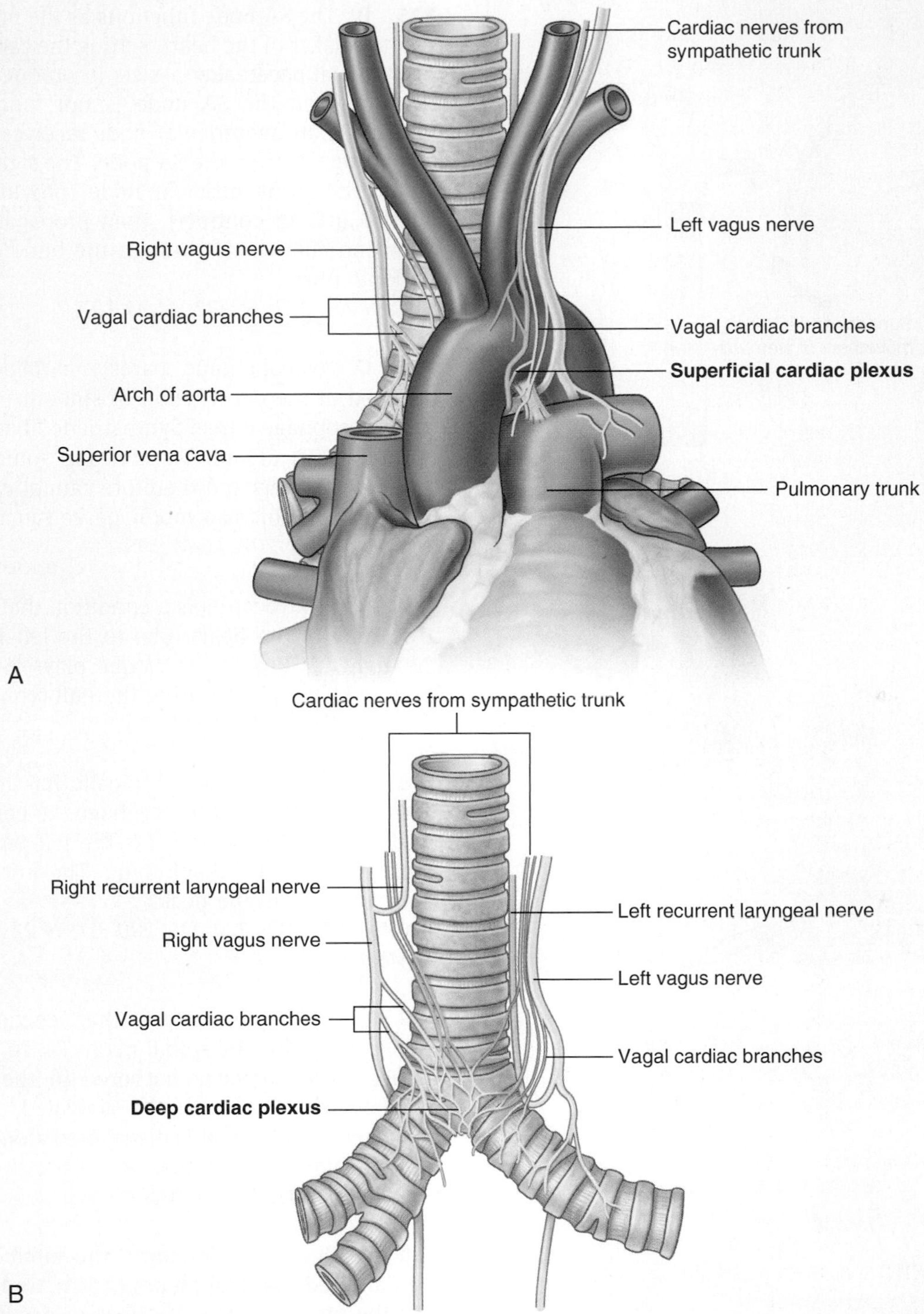

***GAS* Fig. 3-77**

as distal as the left colic flexure. The cardiopulmonary nerves carry sympathetic innervation from T1 to T4 levels to the thoracic organs, and pain fibers from these organs. Thoracic splanchnic nerves carry sympathetic innervation to the abdomen.

GAS 218-219; N 188; McM 182

124 A. An aneurysm of the aortic arch could impinge upon the phrenic nerve, causing referral of pain to the left shoulder. This referral occurs because the root levels of the phrenic nerve are C3 to C5, nerve levels that are also distributed to the skin over the shoulder region. The other choices do not cause

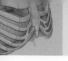

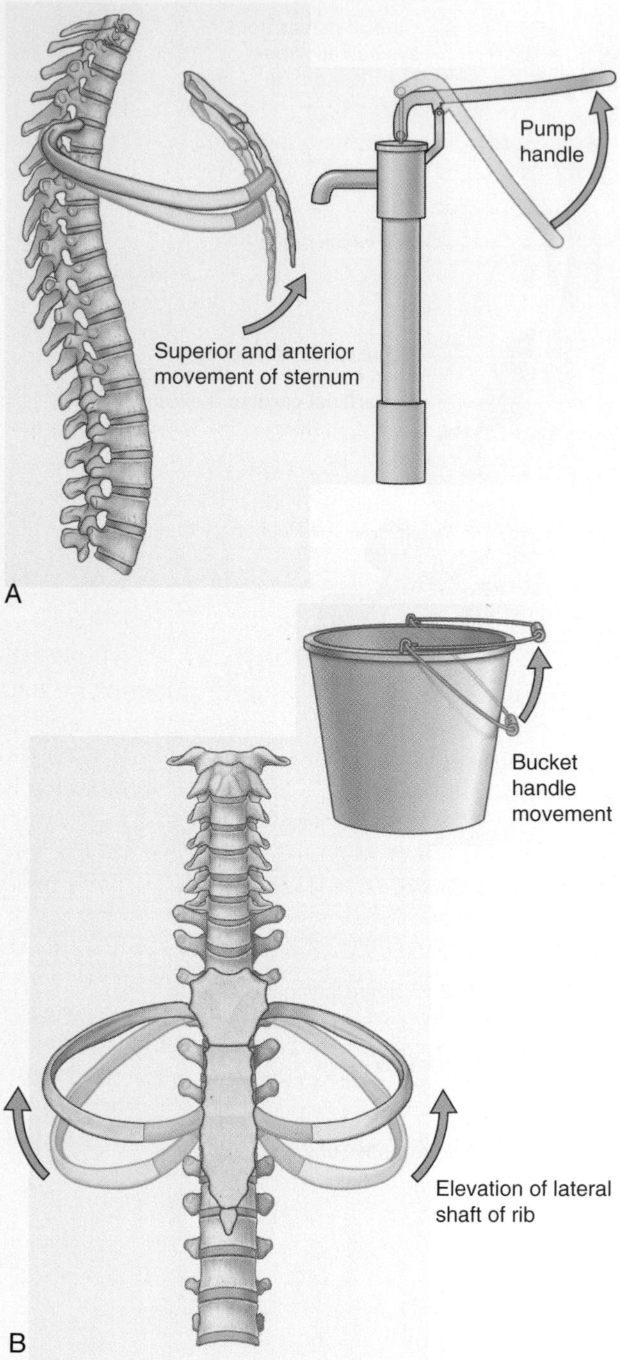

GAS **Fig. 3-34**

referral of pain to the left shoulder. The vagus nerve does not transmit pain sensations except from certain organs in the abdomen and pelvis. The intercostal nerves carry sensory information from the intercostal spaces and parietal pleura, pain that would not be referred to the shoulder. The thoracic splanchnics carry sympathetic innervation to the abdomen.

GAS 217; N 223; McM 195

125 B. The SA node functions as the primary intrinsic pacemaker of the heart, setting the cardiac rhythm. An artificial pacemaker assists in producing a normal rhythm when the SA node is not functioning normally. The atrioventricular node receives the depolarization signals from the SA node. The signal is delayed within the atrioventricular node (providing the time for the atria to contract), then propagated from the atrioventricular node through the bundle of His and Purkinje fibers.

GAS 206-209; N 222; McM 187

126 C. Postganglionic parasympathetic fibers are involved in the constriction of smooth muscle in the tracheoesophageal tree. Sympathetic fibers cause dilation of this structure. Visceral and somatic afferents are sensory fibers and therefore cannot cause dilation of muscle, as this is a motor nerve function.

GAS 176; N 207; McM 195

127 A. Dextrocardia is a condition that results from a bending of the heart tube to the left instead of to the right. TGF-β factor *Nodal* plays a role in the looping of the heart during the embryonic period.

GAS 203; N 226; McM 185

128 A. The esophagus typically has four constrictions. In the thorax the esophagus is compressed by (1) the arch of the aorta, (2) the left principal bronchus, and (3) the diaphragm. The cricopharyngeal constriction is in the neck.

GAS 207, 222, 224-225, 310-311; N 229, 230; McM 214

129 C. The dermatome that encompasses the nipple is supplied by spinal nerve T4. In this case the herpes zoster virus is harbored in the dorsal root ganglion of T4 and can be activated to cause the characteristic rash that is distributed along the dermatome including the nipple.

GAS 139-141; N 162; McM 178

130 B. Due to rib fracture, the intercostal vessels are damaged, parietal pleura is torn, and blood flows into the pleural space. The loss of negative pressure within the pleural cavity results in collapse of the lung. The carotid vessels would not be affected by the described injury. The pulmonary vessels are found within the parenchyma of the lungs and would not be injured due to an external injury such as that described. The internal thoracic artery is well protected by the sternum and is not the cause of this hemothorax.

GAS 148-152; N 230; McM 183

131 A. Miosis, partial ptosis, and anhydrosis are a clinically important constellation of symptoms possibly indicating Horner's syndrome. Horner's syndrome is a lesion of the cervical sympathetic chain and sympathetic chain ganglia and is often a result of a Pancoast tumor, also known as a superior pulmonary sulcus tumor of the apex of the lung. The pupil, eyelid (superior tarsal muscle), and sweat glands are all under sympathetic nervous system control. The arch of the aorta and phrenic nerve are not part of the autonomic nervous system. The vagus nerve does carry parasympathetic fibers to muscles of the trachea, bronchi, digestive tract, and heart but not to any structure in the head and neck (laryngeal supply, and Von Ebner's glands in the tongue). A lesion to the phrenic nerve would result in paralysis of the diaphragm. The cardiopulmonary nerves are splanchnic nerves that are postganglionic and sympathetic. They originate in cervical and upper thoracic ganglia and innervate the thoracic cavity. The cardiopulmonary plexus is the autonomic supply to the heart.

GAS 937-938; N 207; McM 195

132 B. The esophagus lies posterior to the heart. Of the four chambers in the heart, the left atrium lies most posteriorly, just anterior to the esophagus when the heart is in its normal position in the mediastinum. The inferior vena cava runs on the right side within the thoracic cavity and empties its contents into the right atrium. The pulmonary arteries are too anterior to the esophagus to be affected by an esophageal tumor. The left ventricle is too anterior within the mediastinum to be affected by an esophageal tumor. Whereas the esophagus does lie against the vertebral bodies, a growing tumor would affect the esophagus first because it is a smooth muscle structure and therefore the path of least resistance, but this organ can be deviated relatively easily rather than compressed.

GAS 217-219; N 229; McM 193

133 C. Artificial pacemakers are commonly used to treat patients who have weak or failing heart conduction systems. The electrode or "tip" of the pacemaker is threaded through the subclavian vein to the superior vena cava into the right atrium and then the right ventricle where it is used to stimulate the Purkinje fibers to result in ventricular contraction. The right atrium and left atrium do not contain Purkinje fibers and would therefore not be useful in artificially pacing the heart. The left ventricle is more difficult to access. The superior vena cava is not related to cardiac pacing.

GAS 247-248; N 222; McM 188

134 A. Cardiac hypertrophy is a compensatory mechanism of the myocardium in response to increasing demands on the heart due to ischemia, incompetent valves, or hypertension. The increased size of the heart muscle would most likely compress the esophagus, and due to the incompetent mitral valve, a backflow of blood into the left atrium can cause a left atrial dilation. The left atrium lies just anteriorly to the esophagus in the mediastinum. The pulmonary trunk is located superiorly and delivers blood to the lungs, so cardiac hypertrophy would not cause direct compression to this structure. The superior vena cava and inferior vena cava are vessels that deliver blood to the right atrium and are not likely to be compressed in this example of cardiac hypertrophy. The heart is inferior to the trachea.

GAS 217-219; N 230; McM 193

135 E. Tension pneumothorax is a progressive accumulation of air in the pleural cavity that is trapped during inspiration. The resulting increase of pressure diminishes the negative pressure required to maintain an inflated lung, resulting in a collapsed lung as seen on the radiograph. A flail chest is a result of ribs being broken in two or more locations, and no broken ribs are seen on this radiograph. Emphysema is a chronic condition in which elastic tissues and alveoli in the lungs are destroyed, reducing the surface area for gas exchange. Emphysema may result in a secondary spontaneous pneumothorax. A hemothorax is an accumulation of blood in the pleural space. On a radiograph, it is identifiable by a meniscus of fluid. Although spontaneous pneumothorax would present the same way on a radiograph, the patient's history of trauma (car crash) indicates the patient does not have a spontaneous pneumothorax.

GAS 243; N 197; McM 200

136 D. Upper, middle, and lower lobes are affected. The right upper lobe extends from the apex of the lung (above the clavicle) to the fourth rib. The radiograph shows multiple opacities on the right side, eliminating the possibility of it being a left lung pneumonia. Opacity in the right middle lobe extends inferiorly to the sixth rib. In the present case the opacity is inferior to the sixth rib extending to the tenth rib in the midaxillary line affecting the lower lobe of the right lung.

GAS 162-176; N 198; McM 200

137 D. In many people the anterior interventricular branch of the left coronary artery gives rise to a lateral diagonal branch that descends on the anterior surface of the heart. This branch is occluded in the radiograph. The left coronary artery arises from the left aortic sinus of the ascending aorta and passes between the left atrium and the left side of the pulmonary trunk in the coronary groove. The left coronary artery divides into two branches: an anterior interventricular branch (also known as the left anterior descending branch; LAD) and a circumflex branch. The LAD runs along the interventricular groove to the apex of the heart. The right coronary artery arises from the right aortic sinus and runs in the coronary groove. It usually gives off a SA nodal branch; it descends in the coronary groove and gives off a right marginal branch. At the crus of the heart, it gives off an AV nodal branch and a large posterior interventricular branch (in the "right dominant" pattern).

GAS 197-201; N 196; McM 190

138 **A.** Blockage of cutaneous lymphatic vessels results in edema of the skin surrounding the hair follicles, leading to an appearance like an orange peel *(peau d'orange)*. Shortening of the suspensory ligaments leads to dimpling of the overlying skin, not *peau d'orange*. Contraction of retinacula cutis results in retraction and inversion of the nipple and/or areola. Pectoralis major involvement has nothing to do with this condition but can result in fixing the tumor firmly to the chest wall.

GAS 141; N 182; McM 179

139 **C.** The patient is suffering from cardiac tamponade, that is, filling of the pericardial cavity with fluid. The classic signs of this tamponade are referred to as "Beck's triad." This trio, by definition, includes a small heart from compression of the heart by the fluid-filled pericardial sac, and a quiet heart because the tamponade muffles the cardiac sounds; decreased pulse pressure resulting from the reduced difference between systolic and diastolic pressure because the tamponade restricts the ability of the heart to fill in diastole; and increased central venous pressure because venous blood cannot enter the compressed heart.

GAS 181-184; N 208; McM 185

140 **E.** Myelin degeneration of the phrenic nerves, as can occur in Guillain-Barré, results in loss of phrenic nerve function and paralysis of the diaphragm. Diaphragmatic paralysis is predictable with lack of movement of the abdominal wall in respiratory efforts. The ribs are moving "violently" in this case; therefore, intercostal muscles and the pectoral musculature have retained their motor supply.

GAS 212; N 192; McM 213

141 **C.** The loss of myelin from the preganglionic (normally myelinated) sympathetic fibers in T1 to T4 results in interruption in their transmission of electrical stimulating impulses and, therefore, reduction of positive inotropic (force increasing) and chronotropic (rate increasing) stimulation of the heart. Reduction of function of the vagus nerves would not result in slowing cardiac activity; just the opposite would occur. Interruption of phrenic nerve activity has no effect on cardiac rate (as this nerve innervates the diaphragm), nor would the interruption of the thinly myelinated pain fibers from the heart. The ventral horn neurons do not innervate the heart, but rather skeletal muscle; therefore, they would not be directly affected by the disease process affecting the heart.

GAS 208-210; N 207; McM 188

142 **C.** The mitral valve is best visualized by TEE because the transducer within the esophagus is directly posterior to the left atrium. The physical laws that apply to ultrasound imaging dictate that the closer the structure to the transducer, the better the ability to obtain a good image. This question asks which heart valve is most directly related to the posterior aspect of the left atrium, which is the mitral valve.

GAS 184-215; N 219; McM 189

143 **A.** Pneumomediastinum describes the presence of air in the mediastinum and may arise from a wide range of pathological conditions. Despite the well-described imaging of pneumomediastinum, it is sometimes difficult to differentiate from other conditions such as pneumopericardium and medial pneumothorax. The "aortic nipple" is the radiographic term used to describe the lateral nipple-like projection from the aortic knob. The aortic nipple corresponds to the end-on appearance of the left superior intercostal vein coursing around the aortic knob and may be mistaken radiologically for lymphadenopathy or a neoplasm. In cases of pneumomediastinum, it takes on an "inverted aortic nipple" appearance. In this position, the inverted aortic nipple facilitates the radiographic discrimination of pneumomediastinum from similar conditions (*GAS* Fig. 3-88).

GAS 180-183; N 189; McM 212

144 **A.** A tracheoesophageal fistula (TEF) is an abnormal communication between the trachea and esophagus. This is a congenital anomaly that results from incomplete fusion of the tracheoesophageal folds that separate the trachea from the esophagus embryologically. In most cases it is accompanied by esophageal atresia. Polyhydramnios is commonly associated

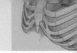

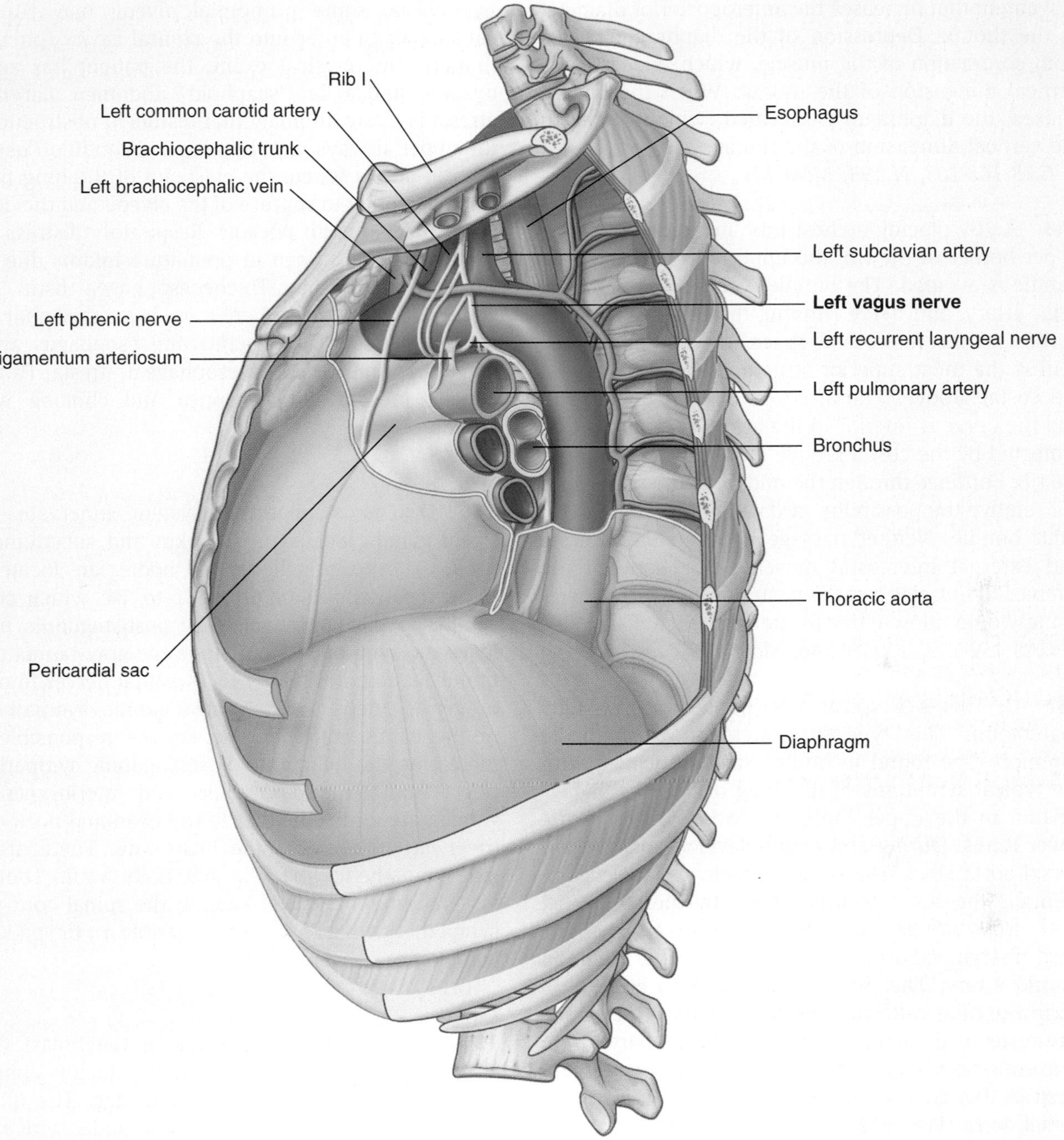

GAS **Fig. 3-88**

with TEF and esophageal atresia, as the amniotic fluid is unable to pass into the stomach and intestines for absorption and collects in the amniotic sac. Oligohydramnios and anhydramnios are associated with genitourinary anomalies. Hydatidiform mole and choriocarcinomas are tumors of the placenta and are not usually associated with polyhydramnios.

GAS 262; N 230; McM 196

145 A. The middles of the shafts of the ribs are lower than the two ends (anterior and posterior). Therefore when the shafts of the ribs are elevated, they move laterally. This "bucket-handle" movement increases the transverse diameter of the thorax. The anterior ends of the ribs are inferior to the posterior ends; therefore when the ribs are elevated, they move the sternum upward and forward in a "pump handle" movement that increases the anteroposterior diameter of the thorax. Depression of the diaphragm results from contraction of the muscle, which increases the vertical dimension of the thorax. When the muscle relaxes, the diaphragm is elevated, which decreases the vertical dimension of the thorax.

GAS 162-163; N 193; McM 177

146 **A.** By placing a chest tube just superior to the upper border of the rib, the important neurovascular bundle is avoided. The bundle consists of intercostal vein, artery, and nerve running through the superior portion of the intercostal space. In each space, the vein is the most superior structure and is highest in the costal groove. The artery is inferior to the vein and the nerve is inferior to the artery and may not be protected by the costal groove on the lower border of the rib. Entrance through the middle of the space does not remove the possibility of damaging the neurovascular bundle. Neither passage between the internal and external intercostal muscles, nor between the intercostal muscles and the posterior intercostal membrane would allow entry to the pleural cavity.

GAS 152-159, 160; N 186; McM 183

147 **C.** This is a typical description of a postductal coarctation. This type of coarctation is the most common type found in adults. It is associated with the typical symptoms of notching of the ribs, hypertension in the upper limb, and weak pulses in the lower limbs. During embryonic development the left dorsal aorta gives rise to the thoracic aorta. Developmentally the aortic arch is formed by the aortic sac, the fourth pharyngeal artery, and the dorsal aorta. The third pharyngeal artery will give rise to the common carotid artery. The fifth pharyngeal arch artery will disappear bilaterally and the sixth will form the ductus arteriosus on the left and part of the pulmonary trunk. Since this case is a postductal coarctation the development of this area of the arch of the aorta is from the dorsal aorta (Fig. 2-12).

GAS 217; N 229; McM 196

148 **A.** Congenital diaphragmatic hernia is a relatively common congenital anomaly. It is most often seen as a posterolateral defect in the diaphragm resulting from the defective formation or fusion of the pleuroperitoneal membranes with the other three embryological parts of the diaphragm. If this defect persists when the intestines return to the stomach from the umbilicus during the tenth week, some of the intestines and abdominal viscera may pass into the thorax. This compresses the developing lungs and results in pulmonary hypoplasia. In cases of severe hypoplasia, some primordial alveoli may rupture, causing air to enter into the pleural cavity (pneumothorax). On physical exam, the patient has severe dyspnea and a flat "scaphoid" abdomen. Laryngeal atresia is a rare anomaly that results in obstruction of the upper airways. Emphysema is a condition usually seen in adults where the elasticity of the lung tissue is lost resulting in rupture of the alveoli and the development of large air pockets. Respiratory distress syndrome is usually seen in premature infants due to a surfactant deficiency. Tracheoesophageal fistula is a congenital condition where there is an abnormal connection between the trachea and esophagus and is usually accompanied by esophageal atresia. Patients usually present with dyspnea and choking when attempting to feed.

GAS 262; N 192; McM 213

149 **D.** The sympathetic system innervates the sweat glands located in the skin and subcutaneous tissue. The postganglionic cell bodies are located in the sympathetic chain from T1 to T4, which corresponds to the chest wall. The postganglionic fibers leave the sympathetic chain via the gray ramus communicans to enter the T1 to T4 spinal nerves in order to get to their target. Postganglionic sympathetics in the cardiopulmonary nerves are responsible for increasing the heart rate. Postganglionic sympathetic fibers from superior, middle, and inferior cervical ganglia are directed either to the head and neck or to the heart to increase the heart rate. There are no parasympathetic fibers in the body wall. Thoracic visceral afferents travel back to the spinal cord with sympathetic fibers but are responsible for the patient's complaint of severe chest pain.

GAS 38-46, 209; N 224; McM 193

150 **A.** The lateral quadrants of the breast drain into the anterior axillary (pectoral), which is approximately 75% of the lymphatic drainage. The medial quadrants drain into the parasternal nodes with some drainage to the parasternal nodes of the opposite breast. There is also a small amount of drainage of the inferior part of the breast into lymph nodes of the anterior abdominal wall. The central and apical axillary nodes receive lymphatic from the pectoral, lateral, and posterior axillary nodes.

GAS 140-141; N 182; McM 179

151 **E.** Pulmonary stenosis of the pulmonary valve results in a systolic murmur that can be auscultated at the left second intercostal space. During systole, blood is forcibly expelled from the ventricles and result in turbulent flow against a narrowed valve.

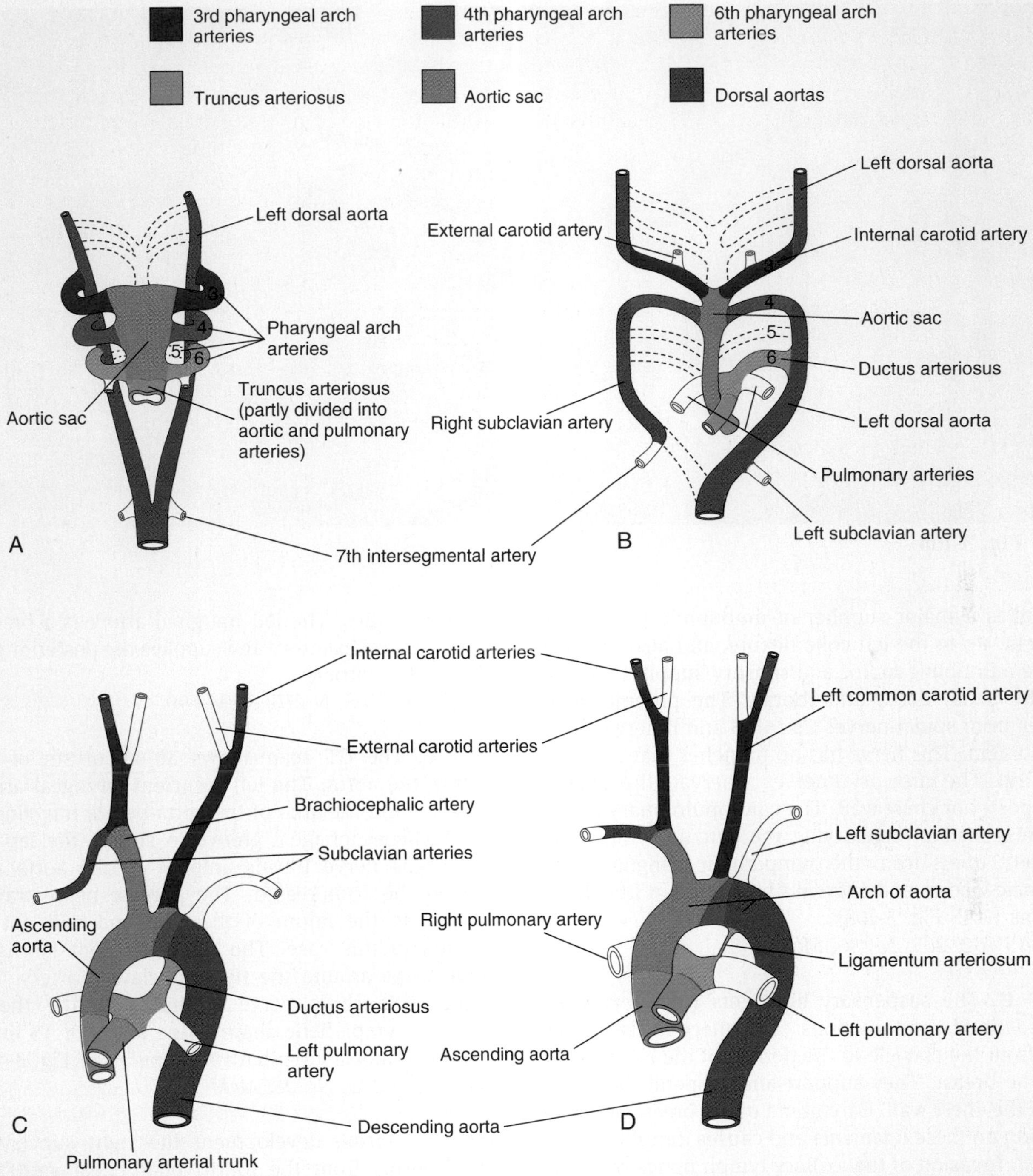

Fig. 2-12

Aortic stenosis also results in a systolic murmur but is auscultated at the right second intercostal space. Regurgitation through the mitral valve results in a systolic murmur that is auscultated at the fourth left intercostal space in the midclavicular line. Pulmonary and aortic valve regurgitation result in diastolic murmurs.

GAS 203-204; N 219; McM 189

152 **D.** The intercostobrachial nerve is the lateral cutaneous branch of the second intercostal nerve and is responsible for the sensation to the medial side of the arm. Ischemia of the myocardium stimulates visceral afferents that travel back to the spinal cord with the sympathetics that innervate the heart. At the level of the spinal cord, this visceral stimulus is interpreted as coming from the body wall. The vagus nerve is CN

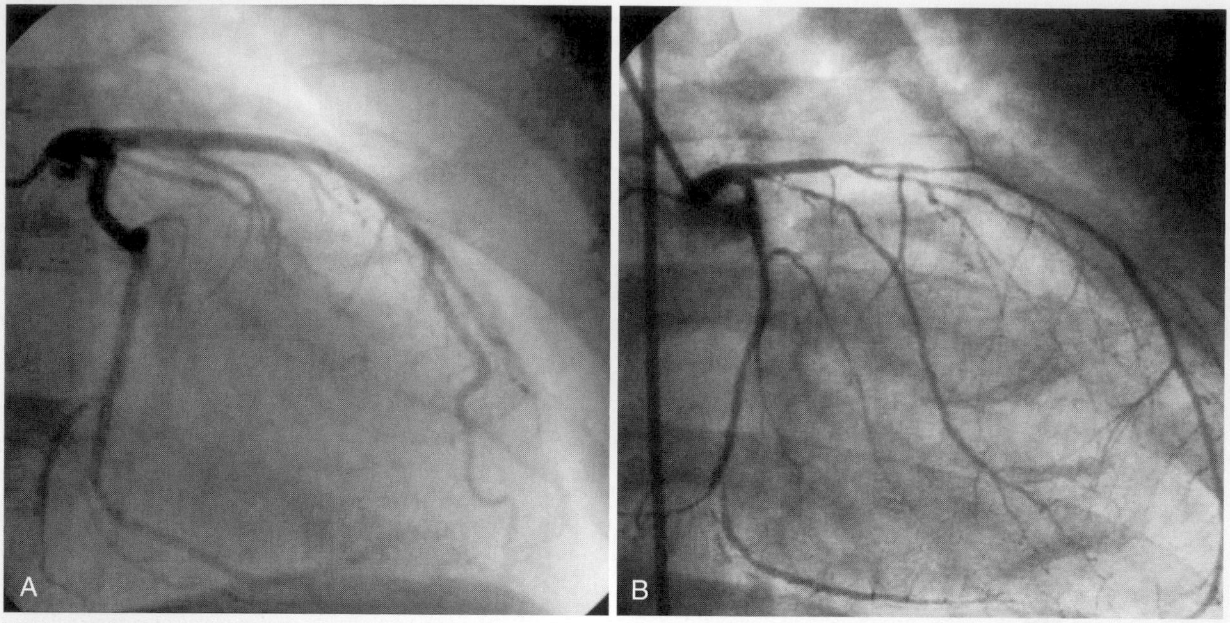

GAS **Fig. 3-108**

X and is a major supplier of autonomic function to the gut, up to the left colic flexure, and also provides some autonomic motor and sensory supply to organs in the head, neck, and thorax. The phrenic nerve arises from spinal nerves C3 to C5 and innervates the diaphragm. This nerve has no branches that pass into the arm. The intercostal nerves innervate the anterior and posterior chest wall. The cardiopulmonary nerves are responsible for carrying the cardiac sympathetic efferent fibers from the sympathetic ganglia to the thoracic viscera and afferent fibers for pain from these organs (*GAS* Fig. 3-108).

GAS 160, 209; N 186; McM 138

153 C. The suspensory ligaments (of Cooper) are well-defined condensations of connective tissue that run from the clavicle to the dermis of the skin overlying the breast. They support and suspend the breast from the chest wall. Carcinoma of the breast produces tension on these ligaments and causes dimpling of the breast. Invasion of the axillary lymph nodes results in stagnation and fibrosis of lymph resulting in the *peau d'orange* appearance of the overlying skin.

GAS 140-141; N 179; McM 179

154 E. The right coronary artery supplies the right ventricle, which lies immediately posterior to the sternum. The circumflex artery supplies the left atrium. The anterior interventricular artery supplies the left ventricle and the anterior two thirds of the interventricular septum. The posterior interventricular artery supplies the posterior third of the interventricular septum. The left marginal artery is a branch of the circumflex artery and supplies the posterior part of the left ventricle.

GAS 197-205; N 216; McM 190

155 C. The CT scan shows an aneurysm of the arch of the aorta. The left recurrent laryngeal artery loops around the arch of the aorta before traveling in the tracheoesophageal groove to supply the larynx. The vagus nerve travels anterior to the aorta and will not be compressed. The phrenic nerve travels anterior to the hilum of the lung and will not be affected in this case. The right recurrent laryngeal nerve loops around the right subclavian artery. The greater splanchnic nerve originates in the thorax from the sympathetic chain at the levels of T5 to T9 and innervates abdominal structures (*GAS* Fig. 3-46).

GAS 221-222; N 228; McM 195

156 A. During development the right subclavian artery forms from the fourth pharyngeal arch and seventh intersegmental arteries. If the fourth pharyngeal arch artery and the right dorsal aorta disappear cranial to the seventh segmental artery the right subclavian artery will be retroesophageal. In this case the right subclavian artery is formed by the right seventh intersegmental artery and the distal dorsal aorta, which does not regress.

GAS 215-216; N 219; McM 196

157 A. During embryonic development the left dorsal aorta gives rise to the thoracic aorta. The aortic

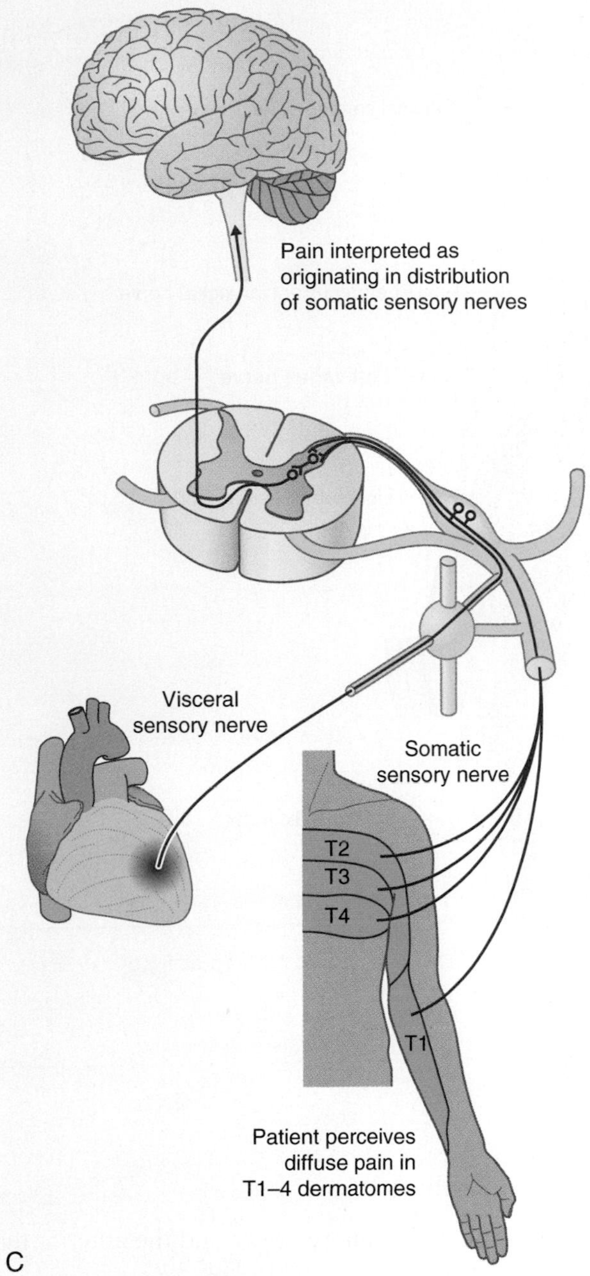

GAS **Fig. 3-108, cont'd**

arch is formed by the aortic sac and the fourth pharyngeal artery. The third pharyngeal artery will give rise to the common carotid artery. The fifth pharyngeal arch artery will disappear bilaterally, and the sixth will form the ductus arteriosus on the left and part of the pulmonary trunk. In this case the region of the arch of the aorta between the subclavian artery and the left common carotid artery is formed by the fourth aortic arch.

GAS 210-216; N 229; McM 196

158 C. The septum secundum develops from the dorsal endocardial cushion and the wall of the primitive atria ventrally. It overgrows the septum primum, which becomes a one-way valve during intrauterine development. The foramen primum is the space between the endocardial cushion and the developing septum primum. The truncus arteriosus will give rise to the ascending aorta and pulmonary trunk. The bulbus cordis will give rise to the smooth parts (arterial outflow) of both the left and right ventricles.

GAS 203; N 226; McM 187

159 A. The phrenic nerve passes anterior to the hilum of the lung on both the left and right sides and wraps around the hilar structures inferiorly. The phrenic nerve innervates the diaphragm and if damaged causes dyspnea. The vagus nerve passes along the esophagus as the left and right trunks and is posterior to the hilum on both sides. The intercostal nerves are separated from the tumor by muscle, fat, and fascia. Cardiopulmonary plexus is arranged around the trachea and is located posterior to the hilum of the lung. Wrapping around the arch of the aorta on the left and the subclavian artery on the right, the recurrent laryngeal nerve is far too superior to be affected. None of the other structures cause breathing difficulties.

GAS 218-222; N 190; McM 207

160 C. The left atrium lies directly anterior to the esophagus and compresses it when enlarged, resulting in difficulty swallowing. Nausea and vomiting may be present but is a symptom of a wide array of dysfunctions and are not a direct result of the enlarged atrium. Pain and tenderness over the thoracic vertebral spinous processes will not result because there is no compression of sensory nerves. Epigastric pain resulting from eating fatty foods is an indication of acute cholelithiasis, which is due to gallstones. Increased coughing could only result from irritation of the vagus nerves above the larynx, which is above the level of the left atria.

GAS 215-216; N 219; McM 196

161 D. The apex of the heart is typically visualized and palpated in the fifth intercostal space of the midclavicular line. This is termed the "apex beat" and is the result of blood being forced against it during atrial contraction. The atria should not give a visible pulsation on the thoracic wall unless there is atrial fibrillation. In atrial fibrillation the right atrium may give visible pulsations but not the left because it is located posteriorly. Pulsations from the aortic arch will only be present if there is an aneurysm of the aortic arch.

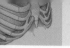

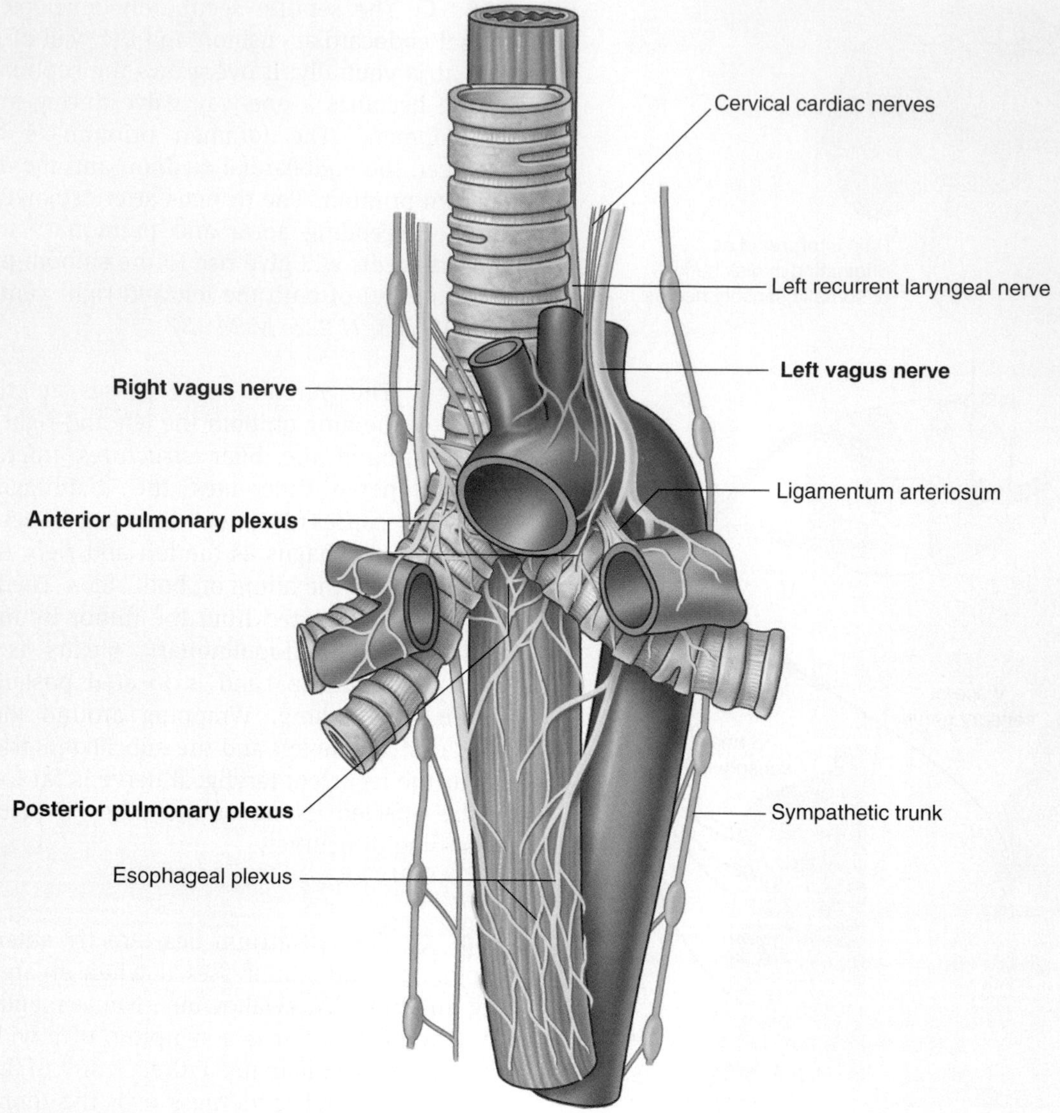

GAS Fig. 3-46

The mitral valve may be auscultated at this location and is one of the reasons why the physician would locate the apex beat.

GAS 190-196, 236; N 209; McM 178

162 B. The great cardiac vein accompanies the anterior interventricular artery, and the middle accompanies the posterior interventricular artery. The small cardiac vein accompanies the right coronary artery as it wraps around the right coronary sulcus. This is the external demarcation of the atrioventricular septum and on the left contains the coronary sinus. On the anterior and posterior aspect of the right and left ventricles the anterior and posterior cardiac veins are found. The posterior accompany the circumflex branch of the left coronary artery and the anterior the small unnamed branches (*GAS* Fig. 3-75).

GAS 197-205; N 215; McM 186

163 E. Thoracocentesis is a procedure whereby a needle is inserted into the pleural space to evacuate air or fluid that has become trapped. The pleural reflection lines posteriorly extend as far as T12 and will contain the fluid that has accumulated. To drain all of the fluid efficiently the needle must be placed into this costodiaphragmatic recess, which represents the lowest point of the pleura. Inserting the needle into the eleventh space ensures that the lung is not damaged, as it does not reach that low under normal circumstances. All of the other levels stand the risk

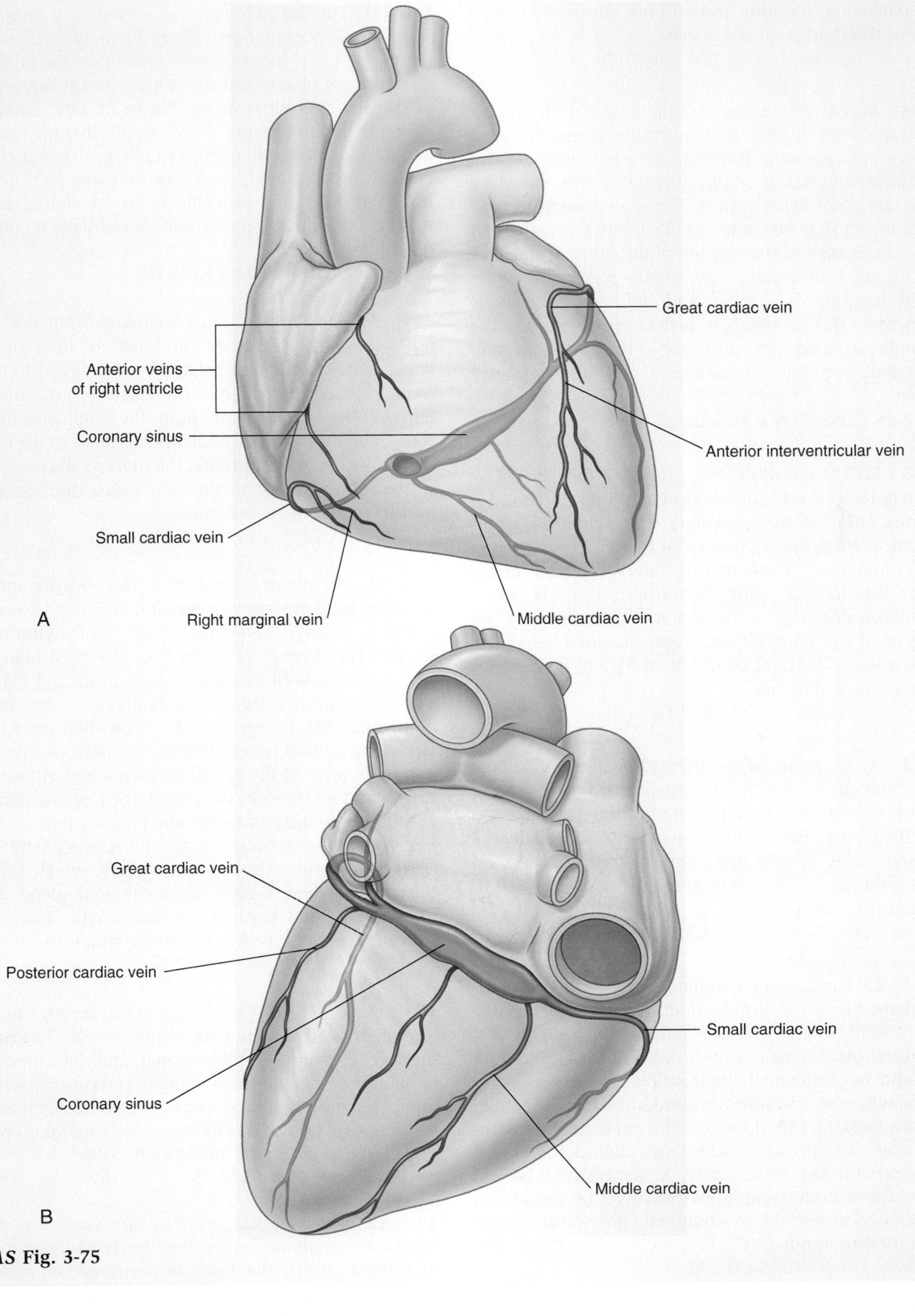
Great cardiac vein
Anterior veins of right ventricle
Coronary sinus
Anterior interventricular vein
Small cardiac vein
A
Right marginal vein
Middle cardiac vein
Great cardiac vein
Posterior cardiac vein
Small cardiac vein
Coronary sinus
Middle cardiac vein
B

GAS **Fig. 3-75**

of damaging, the lung and will not effectively extract all of the fluid from the space.
GAS 162-166; N 193, 194; McM 180

164 E. The esophageal hiatus creates a physiological sphincter during diaphragmatic contraction. As the esophagogastric junction does not have a valve either anatomically or physiologically this would be the last point of resistance. The area posterior to the left atrium may be compressed slightly but would not give resistance to the passing of the tube. At the level of the superior thoracic opening the pharyngoesophageal junction is located and will give resistance; however, this is the first resistance offered by the esophagus. The areas posterior to the aortic arch and left main bronchus are the second and third resistance sites.
GAS 222-225; N 230; McM 214

165 E. The question of dominance is determined by where the posterior interventricular artery arises. If it arises from the right coronary it is a right dominant heart; if from the circumflex of the left coronary it is left dominant. The anterior interventricular artery may anastomose with the posterior but is not a common origin or a determinant of dominance. The artery of the SA node and right marginal artery are branches of the right coronary artery and do not contribute to dominance.
GAS 197-205; N 215; McM 190

166 A. Murmurs of the tricuspid valve can be best auscultated in the fourth intercostal space at the left border of the sternum. The fifth intercostal space midclavicular line is the best site to auscultate the mitral valve. Second and third intercostal spaces on the right side of the sternum are the areas to listen to the aortic valve.
GAS 204, 234; N 210; McM 178

167 E. The patient exhibits signs of cardiac tamponade, known as Beck's triad: hypotension, muffled or absent heart sounds, and jugular-venous distension. As a result, a pericardiocentesis procedure should be performed. Pericardiocentesis is a procedure whereby a needle is inserted into the pericardial space to extract fluid. Inserting a chest tube and thoracocentesis are done to alleviate a pneumothorax and pleural effusion, respectively. A nasogastric tube will not alleviate any symptoms produced by pericardial fluid, and a central line would only provide access for intravenous fluids.
GAS 184 N 213; McM 185

168 D. The SA node receives information from the sympathetic preganglionic fibers T1 to T4 to increase the heart rate. If these fibers are damaged the preganglionic vagal fibers from the cardiac plexus are unopposed and will slow down the heart rate. Somatic efferents in the phrenic nerve supply the diaphragm and have no effect on cardiac function. Visceral afferents in the cardiopulmonary nerve carry pain fibers from the heart and bronchi. T1 to T4 ventral horn neurons are somatic motor nerves and have no effect on cardiac function.
GAS 206-209; N 224; McM 195

169 A. The thoracic duct originates from the cisterna chyli in the abdomen and ascends through the aortic hiatus in the diaphragm. It ascends in the posterior mediastinum among the thoracic aorta on its left, the azygos vein on its right, the esophagus anteriorly, and the vertebral bodies posteriorly. At the level of the T4, T5, or T6 vertebra, the thoracic duct crosses to the left, posterior to the esophagus, and ascends into the superior mediastinum.
GAS 227-228; N 235; McM 209

170 C. The major structures in the superior mediastinum, from anterior to posterior, are thymus, veins, arteries, airway, alimentary tract, and lymphatic trunks. The thymus develops from the third pharyngeal pouch as well as the inferior parathyroid gland. The first pharyngeal pouch derivatives are the endoderm lines the future auditory tube (pharyngotympanic, eustachian tube), middle ear, mastoid antrum, and inner layer of the tympanic membrane. Although the second pharyngeal pouch is largely obliterated, it contributes to the middle ear and palatine tonsils. The fourth pharyngeal pouch forms the superior parathyroid glands and ultimobranchial body, which forms the parafollicular C-cells of the thyroid gland and musculature and cartilage of the larynx. The fifth pharyngeal pouch is a rudimentary structure.
GAS 210-211; N 208; McM 206

171 D. A tension pneumothorax occurs when intrapleural air accumulates progressively, exerting positive pressure on mediastinal and intrathoracic structures. It is a life-threatening occurrence requiring rapid recognition and treatment if cardiac arrest is to be avoided. Pericardial effusion is an abnormal accumulation of fluid in the pericardial cavity.
GAS 242; N 193; McM 184

172 C. With ectopia cordis, a rare condition, the heart is in an abnormal location. In the thoracic form of ectopia cordis, the heart is partly or completely exposed on the surface of the thorax. It is usually associated with widely separated halves of the sternum (nonfusion) and an open pericardial sac. The pleuropericardial folds split into two layers, the somatopleuric layer forms the future body wall and the he splanchnopleuric layer forms the circulatory system and future gut wall. Failure of fusion of the pleuroperitoneal will lead to a diaphragmatic hernia.

GAS 191-193, 262; N 208; McM 184

173 A. There are four clinically significant types of ASD: ostium secundum defect, endocardial cushion defect with ostium primum defect, sinus venosus defect, and common atrium. The first two types of ASD are relatively common. Endocardial cushion defects with ostium primum occur in approximately 20% of persons with trisomy 21 (Down syndrome); otherwise, it is a relatively uncommon cardiac defect.

GAS 203; N 226; McM 187

174 D. VSDs are the most common type of coronary heart disease, accounting for approximately 25% of heart defects. A membranous VSD is the most common type but it may occur at any part of the interventricular septum. A bulbus cordis partitioning defect may lead to persistent truncus arteriosus or transposition of the great vessels. VSD is an acyanotic heart disease. Septum primum and septum secundum may close after birth. Failure of closure will lead to patent foramen ovale.

GAS 203; N 221; McM 188

175 D. With isolated dextrocardia, the abnormal position of the heart is not accompanied by displacement of other viscera. This defect is usually complicated by severe cardiac anomalies (e.g., single ventricle and transposition of the great vessels).

GAS 217; N 214; McM 184

176 A. The thoracic duct originates from the cisterna chyli in the abdomen and ascends through the aortic hiatus in the diaphragm. It ascends in the posterior mediastinum among the thoracic aorta on its left, the azygos vein on its right, the esophagus anteriorly, and the vertebral bodies posteriorly. At the level of the T4, T5, or T6 vertebra, the thoracic duct crosses to the left, posterior to the esophagus, and ascends into the superior mediastinum.

GAS 227-228; N 235; McM 209

177 E. Tetralogy of Fallot consists of four cardiac defects: pulmonary artery stenosis, VSD, dextroposition of aorta (overriding or straddling aorta), and right ventricular hypertrophy. The pulmonary trunk is usually small and there may be various degrees of pulmonary artery stenosis. Cyanosis (deficient oxygenation of blood) is an obvious sign of the tetralogy but is not usually present at birth. Persistent truncus arteriosus is present at birth. ASD, VSD, and PDA contribute to acyanotic heart disease.

GAS 203; N 221; McM 188

178 C. Patent ductus arteriosus (PDA), a common birth defect, is two to three times more common in females than males. If it remains patent, aortic blood is shunted into the pulmonary trunk. Aortic atresia is present when obstruction of the aorta or its valve is complete. Patent ductus venosus shunts a portion of the left umbilical vein blood flow directly to the inferior vena cava. In VSD the shunt will from the right to the left ventricle. Tetralogy of Fallot consists of four cardiac defects: pulmonary artery stenosis, VSD, dextroposition of aorta (overriding or straddling aorta), and right ventricular hypertrophy.

GAS 203; N 226; McM 195

179 B. Congenital diaphragmatic hernia is usually unilateral and results from defective formation and/or fusion of the pleuroperitoneal membranes with the other three parts of the diaphragm. This results in a large opening in the posterolateral region of the diaphragm. As a result, the peritoneal and pleural cavities are continuous with one another along the posterior body wall. In septum transversum defect the patient presents with midline diaphragmatic hernia. Tracheoesophageal septum defect can lead to esophageal atresia or tracheoesophageal fistula. The lesser omentum and falciform ligament form from the ventral mesogastrium, which is formed by the septum transversum.

GAS 262-263; N 191; McM 213

180 A. A tension pneumothorax occurs when intrapleural air accumulates progressively, exerting positive pressure on mediastinal structures and leading to mediastinal shift to the opposite side. It is a life-threatening occurrence requiring rapid recognition and treatment if cardiorespiratory arrest is to be avoided. Cardiac tamponade is pressure on the heart that occurs when blood or fluid builds up in the space between the visceral and parietal layers of the pericardium. Classical cardiac tamponade includes three signs, known as Beck's triad: hypotension, muffled heart sounds, and jugular-venous distension.

GAS 242; N 193; McM 207

181 A. The patient has hemothorax, which can be seen in the left hemithorax on the radiograph. A flail chest by itself will just show minimal soft tissue opacification without any lung field involvement and will not cause cyanosis. Paralysis of the diaphragm will likewise not cause opacification of the lung fields. Tension pneumothorax and spontaneous pneumothorax will not cause opacification of the lung fields but loss of vascular markings and there is loss of pleural integrity even if not observable.

GAS 162-167; N 193; McM 184

182 **A.** Pleuritic pain is due to inflammation of the parietal pleura which is mainly supplied by the intercostal nerves. The phrenic nerve only supplies the central and diaphragmatic parts of the visceral pleura which are not typically affected and not amenable to nerve blocks. The vagus nerve supplies visceral efferents and afferents to the lungs and visceral pleura but not the parietal pleura. Likewise the cardiopulmonary nerves do not carry somatic afferent fibers. The recurrent laryngeal nerve is a branch of the vagus nerve and does not innervate the lungs.

GAS 162-167; N 188; McM 182

183 **E.** Due to the long looping course of the left recurrent laryngeal nerve and its location in the superior mediastinum it is more easily damaged during thoracoscopic procedures than the other nerves, which are more posterior and protected from introduction of the thoracoscope. Increased pulmonary vascular markings indicate the presence of a left-to-right shunt. A systolic murmur crossing the S_2 heart sound characterizes the continuous (machinery) murmur heard in PDA. Prematurity increases the risk of a PDA. The blood shunt through the patent duct increases with physiological decline in the pulmonary artery pressure towards the end of first month of life.

GAS 218-222; N 208; McM 195

184 **B.** Any pneumothorax may cause hyperresonance to percussion, decrease breath sounds, and reduce vascular markings, but tracheal deviation to the opposite side accompanied by distended jugular veins can only be caused by a tension pneumothorax. Cardiac tamponade will cause muffled heart sounds, decreased blood pressure, and distended jugular veins. Pneumonia will not cause tracheal deviation or hyperresonance but lung dullness to percussion. Lung contusion will not cause any of the above signs but may produce some soft tissue edema and minor lung inflammation. Tracheal deviation to the opposite side of the affected lung is a result of a tension pneumothorax. Spontaneous pneumothorax normally causes tracheal deviation to the same side of the collapsed lung to fill the pleural space now unused by the lung. Tension pneumothorax is typically caused by injuries to the chest wall that cause defects in either the parietal or visceral pleurae.

GAS 242; N 193; McM 184

185 **D.** The right and left main coronary arteries arise directly from the root of the aorta. The left main coronary artery divides into the anterior interventricular (left anterior descending: LAD) and circumflex coronary artery. The anterior interventricular artery supplies the anterior 2/3 of the interventricular septum through septal perforating branches and the anterior wall of the left ventricle with diagonal branches. The circumflex coronary artery supplies most of the anterior and left lateral surfaces of the heart via obtuse marginal branches. The right coronary artery gives rise to the artery to the SA node and artery to the AV node. It also gives rise to the coronal artery supplying the area of the subpulmonary infundibulum or anterior ventricular wall and to the acute marginal artery that supplies the lower portion (closer to the diaphragm) of the anterior ventricular wall. In 85-90% of individuals, the right coronary artery gives rise to the posterior interventricular (posterior descending) artery. This artery supplies the posterior or diaphragmatic surface of the heart.

GAS 197-205; N 216; McM 190

186 **A.** The embryological basis of the combination of lesions is anterosuperior deviation (malalignment) of the developing outlet ventricular septum (subpulmonary infundibulum) and hypertrophied septoparietal trabeculations. The deviation of the muscular outlet septum (not to be confused with the aorticopulmonary septum) is also responsible for creating the malalignment type of ventricular septal defect and results in the aortic override. The associated hypertrophy of the right ventricular myocardium is the hemodynamic consequence of the anatomical lesions created by the deviated outlet septum. The cause of the abnormal anterosuperior deviation of the outlet ventricular septum is the abnormal neural crest cell migration. In contrast an endocardial cushion defect will be responsible for defects in the atrioventricular septum and atrioventricular valves. The endocardial cushion defects do not produce cyanosis.

187 **E.** The main structure immediately posterior to the esophagus is the descending aorta, and anterior to the esophagus is the left atrium, which is adjacent to the esophagus at this point. The left atrium forms the majority of the posterior surface of the heart and resides adjacent to the esophagus. Enlargement of the left atrium can compress the esophagus and cause dysphagia. The pulmonary veins are too lateral at this point, whereas the right atrium and right ventricle are more anterior.

GAS 222-230; N 233; McM 195

188 **C.** The defects in the diaphragm are at T8 for IVC/phrenic nerve, T10 for esophagus, and T12 for aorta/thoracic duct. T7 and T8 vertebra levels do not have any major diaphragmatic openings.

GAS 222-230; N 192; McM 213

189 **C.** Cardiac tamponade will cause muffled heart sounds, decreased blood pressure, and distended jugular veins (Beck's triad). Pneumothorax will cause hyperresonance to percussion, decreased breath sounds, reduced vascular markings, tracheal deviation to the opposite side, and distended jugular veins. Deep vein thrombosis may lead to pulmonary embolus, which can cause shortness of breath and even death but not Beck's triad. Hemothorax presents with dullness to percussion and lung field opacification.

GAS 184; N 208; McM 184

190 **A.** The pulmonic valve is auscultated at the left parasternal area in the second intercostal space, whereas the aortic valve is best heard at the right parasternal area in the second intercostal space. The mitral (bicuspid) valve is auscultated at the apex of the heart, which is typically the fourth or fifth intercostal space at the midclavicular line, to the right of the sternum. The tricuspid valve is auscultated at the fourth intercostal space right parasternal border.

GAS 236; N 210; McM 178

191 **C.** Since the sternal angle (of Louis) is in the transverse plane the best plane to view both the anterior and posterior mediastinum, as well as superior mediastinal structures, would be a lateral view. Anteroposterior or posteroanterior would make it difficult separating anterior and posterior structures. Since the sternal angle (of Louis) is in the axial plane an axial cut may miss the level completely.

GAS 128-129; N 213; McM 194

192 **E.** The order traversed is skin, external intercostal muscles, internal intercostal muscles, innermost intercostal muscle, and parietal pleura. The chest tube should not traverse the visceral pleura because this could cause a pneumothorax when it is removed.

GAS 152-160; N 213; McM 195

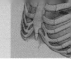

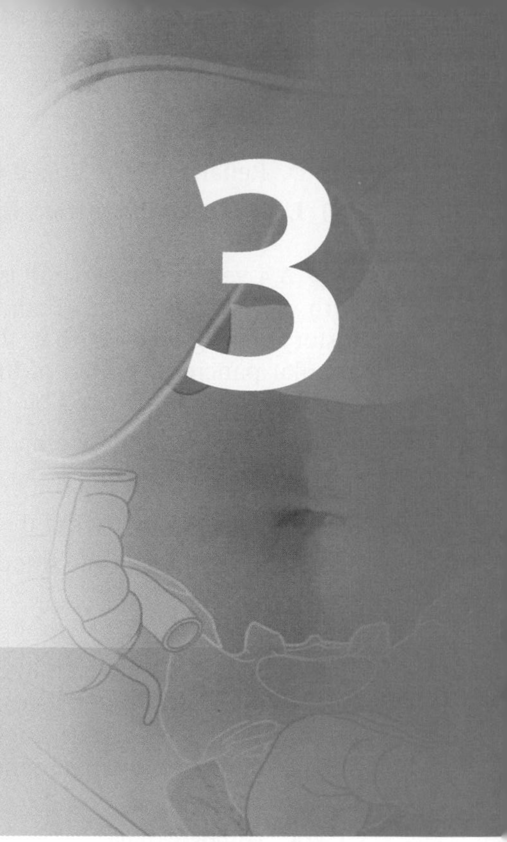

3

ABDOMEN

QUESTIONS

1 A 1-year-old girl is admitted to the hospital with a palpable mass in her labia majora. Radiographic examination reveals that a loop of intestine has herniated into the visibly enlarged labium majus. This condition is due to failure of the processus vaginalis to close off. From which of the following tissue layers is the processus derived?

- ▢ **A.** Parietal peritoneum
- ▢ **B.** Extraperitoneal tissue
- ▢ **C.** Transversalis fascia
- ▢ **D.** Dartos fascia
- ▢ **E.** Internal abdominal oblique aponeurosis

2 A 3-year-old boy is admitted to the hospital with signs of acute renal failure. Radiologic studies reveal that the boy has bilateral masses involving both kidneys. Examination of biopsy material confirms the diagnosis of Wilms tumor. Which of the following gene mutations is the most common in Wilms tumor?

- ▢ **A.** The gene responsible for *WT1*
- ▢ **B.** The gene responsible for *HGF*
- ▢ **C.** The gene responsible for *VEGF*
- ▢ **D.** The gene responsible for *GDNF*
- ▢ **E.** The gene responsible for *FGF-2*

3 Fusion of the caudal portions of the kidneys during embryonic development is most likely to result in which of the following congenital conditions?

- ▢ **A.** Bicornuate uterus
- ▢ **B.** Cryptorchidism
- ▢ **C.** Horseshoe kidney
- ▢ **D.** Hypospadias
- ▢ **E.** Renal agenesis

4 Which of the following congenital malformations will most predictably result in oligohydramnios?

- ▢ **A.** Anencephaly
- ▢ **B.** Pyloric stenosis
- ▢ **C.** Renal agenesis
- ▢ **D.** Tracheoesophageal fistula
- ▢ **E.** Urethral atresia

5 Failure to urinate during embryonic or fetal life usually causes respiratory difficulties postnatally. Which of the following relationships best describes this situation?

- ▢ **A.** Oligohydramnios linked with hypoplastic lungs
- ▢ **B.** Polycystic kidneys linked to tracheoesophageal fistula
- ▢ **C.** Polyhydramnios

- ▢ **D.** Renal agenesis linked to insufficient surfactant
- ▢ **E.** Urethral obstruction linked to ectopic viscera

6 A 4-year-old male child is admitted to the hospital with severe vomiting. Radiologic examination and history taking reveals that the boy suffers from an annular pancreas. Which of the following structures is most typically obstructed by this condition?

- ▢ **A.** Pylorus of the stomach
- ▢ **B.** First part of the duodenum
- ▢ **C.** Second part of the duodenum
- ▢ **D.** Third part of the duodenum
- ▢ **E.** Jejunum

7 A 3-year-old male child is admitted to the pediatric clinic. Diagnosis reveals that the intermediate portion of the processus vaginalis is not obliterated. Which of the following conditions will most likely result from this?

- ▢ **A.** Hypospadias
- ▢ **B.** Sterility
- ▢ **C.** Congenital hydrocele
- ▢ **D.** Ectopic testis
- ▢ **E.** Epispadias

8 Testicles are absent from the scrotum of a 1-year-old male admitted to the pediatric clinic. The pediatrician examined the infant and palpated the testes in the inguinal canal. Which of the following terms is used to describe this condition?

- ▢ **A.** Pseudohermaphroditism
- ▢ **B.** True hermaphroditism
- ▢ **C.** Cryptorchism
- ▢ **D.** Congenital adrenal hyperplasia
- ▢ **E.** Chordee

9 A 28-year-old woman who is 8 months pregnant goes to the outpatient clinic for her prenatal checkup. Ultrasound examination of the fetus reveals gastroschisis, with herniation of the small bowel into the amniotic cavity. Failure of proper formation of which of the following structure(s) has resulted in this condition?

- ▢ **A.** Head fold
- ▢ **B.** Tail fold
- ▢ **C.** Neural folds
- ▢ **D.** Lateral folds
- ▢ **E.** Amnion

10 Rotation of the stomach during development results in movement of the left vagus nerve from its original position. Through approximately how many degrees of rotation does the nerve move, and what is its final position?

- ▢ **A.** 90 degrees to become the anterior vagal trunk
- ▢ **B.** 90 degrees to become the posterior vagal trunk
- ▢ **C.** 270 degrees to become the anterior vagal trunk
- ▢ **D.** 270 degrees to become the posterior vagal trunk
- ▢ **E.** 180 degrees to become the right vagal trunk

11 A newborn baby was diagnosed with eventration of the diaphragm, wherein one half of the diaphragm ascends into the thorax during inspiration, but the other half contracts normally. What is the most likely cause of this condition?

- ▢ **A.** Absence of a pleuropericardial fold
- ▢ **B.** Absence of musculature in one half of the diaphragm
- ▢ **C.** Failure of migration of the diaphragm
- ▢ **D.** Failure of development of the septum transversum
- ▢ **E.** Absence of a pleuroperitoneal fold

12 A 2-day-old newborn male is cyanotic after attempts to swallow milk result in collection of the milk in his mouth. After 2 days he develops aspiration pneumonia. A tracheoesophageal fistula is suspected. Which of the following structures has most likely failed to develop properly?

- ▢ **A.** Esophagus
- ▢ **B.** Trachea
- ▢ **C.** Tongue
- ▢ **D.** Tracheoesophageal septum
- ▢ **E.** Pharynx

13 A 3-day-old newborn male has difficulties in breathing. A computed tomography (CT) scan of his chest and abdomen reveals the absence of the central tendon of the diaphragm. Which of the following structures most likely failed to develop properly?

- ▢ **A.** Pleuroperitoneal folds
- ▢ **B.** Pleuropericardial folds
- ▢ **C.** Septum transversum
- ▢ **D.** Cervical myotomes
- ▢ **E.** Dorsal mesentery of the esophagus

14 A 1-month-old infant with bilious vomiting and feeding intolerance is examined by the pediatric team. Imaging reveals malrotation of the small intestine without fixation of the mesenteries. The vessels around the duodenojejunal junction are obstructed and the intestine is at risk of becoming gangrenous. Which of the following has occurred to cause the obstruction?

- ▢ **A.** Diaphragmatic atresia
- ▢ **B.** Subhepatic cecum
- ▢ **C.** Midgut volvulus
- ▢ **D.** Duplication of the intestine
- ▢ **E.** Congenital megacolon

15 A 5-day-old male infant is diagnosed with Hirschsprung disease. CT scan examination reveals an abnormally dilated colon. Which of the following is the most likely embryologic mechanism responsible for Hirschsprung disease?

- ▢ **A.** Failure of neural crest cells to migrate into the walls of the colon
- ▢ **B.** Incomplete separation of the cloaca
- ▢ **C.** Failure of recanalization of the colon
- ▢ **D.** Defective rotation of the hindgut
- ▢ **E.** Oligohydramnios

16 A 1-day-old female infant has a mass protruding through her umbilicus. Physical examination reveals an umbilical hernia. A CT scan reveals that part of another organ is attached to the inner surface of the hernia. What portion of the gastrointestinal tract is most likely to be attached to the inner surface of the umbilical hernia?

- ▢ **A.** Anal canal
- ▢ **B.** Appendix
- ▢ **C.** Cecum
- ▢ **D.** Ileum
- ▢ **E.** Stomach

17 A 38-year-old pregnant woman is admitted to the emergency department with severe vaginal bleeding. Ultrasound examination confirms the initial diagnosis of ectopic pregnancy. Which of the following is the most common site of an ectopic pregnancy?

- ▢ **A.** Uterine tubes
- ▢ **B.** Cervix
- ▢ **C.** Mesentery of the abdominal wall
- ▢ **D.** Lower part of uterine body overlapping the internal cervical os
- ▢ **E.** Fundus of the uterus

18 A 23-year-old woman is admitted with severe abdominal pain, nausea, and vomiting. History taking shows that the pain is severe and has been constant for 4 days. The pain began in the epigastric region and radiated bilaterally around the chest to just below the scapulae. Currently the pain is localized in the right hypochondrium. A CT scan examination reveals calcified stones in the gallbladder. Which of the following nerves carries the afferent fibers of the referred pain?

- ▢ **A.** Greater thoracic splanchnic nerves
- ▢ **B.** Dorsal primary rami of intercostal nerves
- ▢ **C.** Phrenic nerves
- ▢ **D.** Vagus nerves
- ▢ **E.** Pelvic splanchnic nerves

19 A 32-year-old man is admitted to the emergency department with groin pain. Examination reveals that the patient has an indirect inguinal hernia. Which of the following nerves is compressed by the herniating structure in the inguinal canal to give the patient pain?

- ▢ **A.** Iliohypogastric
- ▢ **B.** Lateral femoral cutaneous
- ▢ **C.** Ilioinguinal
- ▢ **D.** Subcostal
- ▢ **E.** Pudendal

20 A 54-year-old man is admitted to the emergency department with severe upper abdominal pain. Gastroscopy reveals a tumor in the antrum of the stomach. A CT scan is ordered to evaluate lymphatic drainage of the stomach. Which of the following lymph nodes is most likely to be involved in a malignancy of the stomach?

- ▢ **A.** Celiac
- ▢ **B.** Superior mesenteric
- ▢ **C.** Inferior mesenteric
- ▢ **D.** Lumbar
- ▢ **E.** Hepatic

21 During a scheduled laparoscopic cholecystectomy in a 47-year-old female patient, the resident accidentally clamped the hepatoduodenal ligament instead of the cystic artery. Which of the following vessels would most likely be occluded in this iatrogenic injury?

- ▢ **A.** Superior mesenteric artery
- ▢ **B.** Proper hepatic artery
- ▢ **C.** Splenic artery
- ▢ **D.** Common hepatic artery
- ▢ **E.** Inferior vena cava

22 A 45-year-old man was admitted to the hospital with groin pain and a palpable mass just superior to the inguinal ligament. The patient was diagnosed with an inguinal hernia and a surgical repair was performed. During the operation the surgeon found a loop of intestine passing through the deep inguinal ring. Which of the following types of hernia was this?

- ▢ **A.** Direct inguinal
- ▢ **B.** Umbilical
- ▢ **C.** Femoral
- ▢ **D.** Lumbar
- ▢ **E.** Indirect inguinal

23 A 55-year-old man was admitted to the hospital with severe abdominal pain. Gastroscopy and CT scan examinations revealed a perforating ulcer in the posterior wall of the stomach. Where would peritonitis most likely develop initially?

- ▢ **A.** Right subhepatic space
- ▢ **B.** Hepatorenal space (of Morison)
- ▢ **C.** Omental bursa (lesser sac)
- ▢ **D.** Right subphrenic space
- ▢ **E.** Greater sac

24 A 58-year-old male alcoholic is admitted to the hospital after vomiting dark red blood (hematemesis). Endoscopy reveals ruptured esophageal varices, most likely resulting from portal hypertension. Which of the following venous tributaries to the portal system anastomoses with caval veins to cause the varices?

- ▢ **A.** Splenic
- ▢ **B.** Left gastro-omental
- ▢ **C.** Left gastric
- ▢ **D.** Left hepatic
- ▢ **E.** Right gastric

25 A 45-year-old man entered the emergency department with a complaint of severe abdominal pain. During physical examination it is observed that his cremasteric reflex is absent. Which of the following nerves is responsible for the efferent limb of the cremasteric reflex?

- ▢ **A.** Ilioinguinal
- ▢ **B.** Iliohypogastric
- ▢ **C.** Genitofemoral
- ▢ **D.** Pudendal
- ▢ **E.** Ventral ramus of T12

26 The decision is made by emergency department surgeons to perform an exploratory laparotomy on a 32-year-old female with severe abdominal pain. Where would the incision most likely be made to separate the left and right rectus sheaths?

- ▢ **A.** Midaxillary line
- ▢ **B.** Arcuate line
- ▢ **C.** Semilunar line
- ▢ **D.** Tendinous intersection
- ▢ **E.** Linea alba

27 After a "tummy-tuck" (abdominoplasty) procedure is performed on a 45-year-old man, which of the following layers of the abdominal wall will hold the sutures?

- ▢ **A.** Scarpa's fascia (membranous layer)
- ▢ **B.** Camper's fascia (fatty layer)
- ▢ **C.** Transversalis fascia
- ▢ **D.** Extraperitoneal tissue
- ▢ **E.** External abdominal oblique aponeurosis

28 A 49-year-old man presents with acute abdominal pain and jaundice. Radiologic studies reveal a tumor in the head of the pancreas. Which of the following structures is most likely being obstructed?

- ▢ **A.** Common bile duct
- ▢ **B.** Common hepatic duct
- ▢ **C.** Cystic duct
- ▢ **D.** Accessory pancreatic duct
- ▢ **E.** Proper hepatic artery

29 A 44-year-old man is admitted to the emergency department with excessive vomiting and dehydration. Radiologic images demonstrate that part of the bowel is being compressed between the abdominal aorta and the superior mesenteric artery, the so-called "nutcracker syndrome." Which of the following intestinal structures is most likely being compressed?

- ▢ **A.** Second part of duodenum
- ▢ **B.** Transverse colon
- ▢ **C.** Third part of duodenum
- ▢ **D.** First part of duodenum
- ▢ **E.** Jejunum

30 During the surgical repair of a perforated duodenal ulcer in a 47-year-old male patient, the gastroduodenal artery is ligated. A branch of which of the following arteries will continue to supply blood to the pancreas in this patient?

- ▢ **A.** Inferior mesenteric
- ▢ **B.** Left gastric
- ▢ **C.** Right gastric
- ▢ **D.** Proper hepatic
- ▢ **E.** Superior mesenteric

31 A 70-year-old man is admitted to the emergency department with severe diarrhea. An arteriogram reveals 90% blockage at the origin of the inferior mesenteric artery from the aorta. Which of the following arteries would most likely provide collateral supply to the descending colon?

- ☐ **A.** Left gastroepiploic artery
- ☐ **B.** Middle colic artery
- ☐ **C.** Sigmoid artery
- ☐ **D.** Splenic artery
- ☐ **E.** Superior rectal artery

32 A 24-year-old woman has a dull aching pain in the umbilical region, and flexion of the hip against resistance (psoas test) causes a sharp pain in the right lower abdominal quadrant. Which of the following structures is most likely inflamed to cause the pain?

- ☐ **A.** Appendix
- ☐ **B.** Bladder
- ☐ **C.** Gallbladder
- ☐ **D.** Pancreas
- ☐ **E.** Uterus

33 A 35-year-old man is admitted to the hospital from the emergency department because of excruciating pain in the back and left shoulder. A CT scan reveals an abscess in the upper part of the left kidney, but no abnormality is detected in the shoulder region. The shoulder pain may be caused by the spread of the inflammation to which of the following neighboring structures?

- ☐ **A.** Descending colon
- ☐ **B.** Diaphragm
- ☐ **C.** Duodenum
- ☐ **D.** Spleen
- ☐ **E.** Pancreas

34 A 62-year-old man is admitted to the hospital with dull, diffuse abdominal pain. A CT scan reveals a tumor at the head of the pancreas. The abdominal pain is mediated by afferent fibers that travel initially with which of the following nerves?

- ☐ **A.** Greater thoracic splanchnic
- ☐ **B.** Intercostal
- ☐ **C.** Phrenic
- ☐ **D.** Vagus
- ☐ **E.** Subcostal

35 A 52-year-old man with a history of smoking and hypercholesterolemia is diagnosed with severe atherosclerosis affecting the arteries of his body. Laboratory examination reveals extremely low sperm count. Which of the following arteries is most likely occluded?

- ☐ **A.** External iliac
- ☐ **B.** Inferior epigastric
- ☐ **C.** Umbilical
- ☐ **D.** Testicular
- ☐ **E.** Deep circumflex iliac

36 In a routine visit to the outpatient clinic for his annual checkup, a 42-year-old man is informed that ultrasound examination has given strong evidence that he has a tumor of his scrotum that appears not to be in a testes. Which of the following nodes are the first lymph nodes that drain the affected area?

- ☐ **A.** Superficial inguinal
- ☐ **B.** Internal iliac
- ☐ **C.** Lumbar
- ☐ **D.** Presacral
- ☐ **E.** Axillary

37 A 35-year-old man is admitted to the hospital with an indirect inguinal hernia. During an open hernioplasty (in contrast to a laparoscopic procedure), the spermatic cord and the internal abdominal oblique muscles are identified. Which component of the spermatic cord is derived from the internal abdominal oblique muscle?

- ☐ **A.** External spermatic fascia
- ☐ **B.** Cremaster muscle
- ☐ **C.** Tunica vaginalis
- ☐ **D.** Internal spermatic fascia
- ☐ **E.** Dartos fascia

38 A 63-year-old man with a history of alcoholism is brought to the emergency department with hematemesis (vomiting blood). Findings on endoscopic examination suggest bleeding from esophageal varices. The varices are most likely a result of the anastomoses between the left gastric vein and which other vessel or vessels?

- ☐ **A.** Azygos system of veins
- ☐ **B.** Inferior vena cava
- ☐ **C.** Left umbilical vein
- ☐ **D.** Superior mesenteric vein
- ☐ **E.** Subcostal veins

39 A 34-year-old man is undergoing an emergency appendectomy. After the appendectomy has been performed successfully, the patient undergoes an exploratory laparoscopy. Which of the following anatomic features are the most useful to distinguish the jejunum from the ileum?

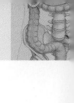

- ▢ **A.** Jejunum has thinner walls compared with the ileum
- ▢ **B.** Jejunum has less mesenteric fat compared with the ileum
- ▢ **C.** Jejunum has more numerous vascular arcades compared with the ileum
- ▢ **D.** Jejunum has more numerous lymphatic follicles beneath the mucosa compared with the ileum
- ▢ **E.** Jejunum has fewer villi compared with the ileum

40 After a mastectomy, a musculocutaneous flap is used to restore the thoracic contour in a 34-year-old female patient. The ipsilateral (same side) rectus abdominis muscle was detached carefully from the surrounding structures and transposed to the thoracic wall. Which of the following landmarks is most often used to locate the inferior end of the posterior, tendinous layer of the rectus sheath?

- ▢ **A.** Intercristal line
- ▢ **B.** Linea alba
- ▢ **C.** Arcuate line
- ▢ **D.** Pectineal line
- ▢ **E.** Semilunar line

41 An anteroposterior radiograph is taken of the lumbar region in a 31-year-old female patient who had been treated for tuberculous spondylitis at vertebral levels T12 to L1. The patient has been asymptomatic for 10 years. A density is detected; a calcified tuberculous abscess is suspected. Which of the following is the most likely site of the calcified tuberculous abscess?

- ▢ **A.** Body of pancreas
- ▢ **B.** Cecum
- ▢ **C.** Fundus of stomach
- ▢ **D.** Psoas fascia
- ▢ **E.** Suspensory ligament of the duodenum

42 A 45-year-old woman is admitted to the hospital with symptoms of an upper bowel obstruction. Upon CT examination it is found that the third (transverse) portion of the duodenum is being compressed by a large vessel. Which of the following vessels will most likely be causing the compression?

- ▢ **A.** Inferior mesenteric artery
- ▢ **B.** Superior mesenteric artery
- ▢ **C.** Inferior mesenteric vein
- ▢ **D.** Portal vein
- ▢ **E.** Splenic vein

43 A 61-year-old woman had been scheduled for a cholecystectomy. During the operation the scissors of the surgical resident accidentally entered the tissues immediately posterior to the epiploic (omental) foramen (its posterior boundary). The surgical field was filled immediately by profuse bleeding. Which of the following vessels was the most likely source of bleeding?

- ▢ **A.** Aorta
- ▢ **B.** Inferior vena cava
- ▢ **C.** Portal vein
- ▢ **D.** Right renal artery
- ▢ **E.** Superior mesenteric vein

44 A 32-year-old woman was admitted to the hospital with a complaint of pain over her umbilicus. Radiographic examination revealed acute appendicitis. The appendix was removed successfully in an emergency appendectomy. One week postoperatively the patient complained of paresthesia of the skin over the pubic region and the anterior portion of her perineum. Which of the following nerves was most likely injured during the appendectomy?

- ▢ **A.** Genitofemoral
- ▢ **B.** Ilioinguinal
- ▢ **C.** Subcostal
- ▢ **D.** Iliohypogastric
- ▢ **E.** Spinal nerve T9

45 Exploratory laparoscopy was performed on a 34-year-old man, following a successful emergency appendectomy. Which of the following anatomic relationships would be seen clearly, without dissection, when the surgeon exposes the beginning of the jejunum?

- ▢ **A.** The second portion of the duodenum is related anteriorly to the hilum of the right kidney.
- ▢ **B.** The superior mesenteric artery and vein pass posterior to the third part of the duodenum.
- ▢ **C.** The portal vein crosses anterior to the neck of the pancreas.
- ▢ **D.** The second part of the duodenum is crossed anteriorly by the attachment of the transverse mesocolon.
- ▢ **E.** The third part of the duodenum is related anteriorly to the hilum of the left kidney.

46 A 30-year-old female patient complains that she has been weak and easily fatigued over the past 6 months. She has a 3-month acute history of severe hypertension that has required treatment with antihypertensive medications. She has recently gained 4.5 kg

(10 lb) and currently weighs 75 kg (165 lb). Her blood pressure is 170/100 mm Hg. Purple striae are seen over the abdomen on physical examination and she possesses a "buffalo hump." Fasting serum glucose concentration is 140 mg/dL. A CT scan of the abdomen shows a 6-cm mass immediately posterior to the inferior vena cava. Which of the following organs is the most likely origin of the mass?

- ▢ **A.** Suprarenal (adrenal) gland
- ▢ **B.** Appendix
- ▢ **C.** Gallbladder
- ▢ **D.** Ovary
- ▢ **E.** Uterus

47 An obese 45-year-old female patient with an elevated temperature comes to the physician's office complaining of nausea and intermittent, acute pain in the right upper quadrant of the abdomen during the past 2 days. She has a 24-hour history of jaundice. She has a history of gallstones. Which of the following structures has most likely been obstructed by a gallstone?

- ▢ **A.** Common bile duct
- ▢ **B.** Cystic duct
- ▢ **C.** Left hepatic duct
- ▢ **D.** Pancreatic duct
- ▢ **E.** Right hepatic duct

48 A 67-year-old man has severe cirrhosis of the liver. He most likely has enlarged anastomoses between which of the following pairs of veins?

- ▢ **A.** Inferior phrenic and superior phrenic
- ▢ **B.** Left colic and middle colic
- ▢ **C.** Left gastric and esophageal
- ▢ **D.** Lumbar and renal
- ▢ **E.** Sigmoid and superior rectal

49 A 45-year-old man is admitted to the hospital with a massive hernia that passes through the inguinal triangle (of Hesselbach). Which of the following structures is used as a landmark to distinguish a direct inguinal hernia from an indirect inguinal hernia?

- ▢ **A.** Inferior epigastric vessels
- ▢ **B.** Femoral canal
- ▢ **C.** Inguinal ligament
- ▢ **D.** Rectus abdominis muscle (lateral border)
- ▢ **E.** Pectineal ligament

50 A 36-year-old man was brought to the emergency department with a bullet wound to the abdomen. The bullet penetrated the anterior abdominal wall superior to the umbilicus. If the bullet passed directly posterior in the midline, which of the following structures was most likely to have been struck first by the bullet?

- ▢ **A.** Abdominal aorta
- ▢ **B.** Transverse colon
- ▢ **C.** Stomach
- ▢ **D.** Gallbladder
- ▢ **E.** Pancreas

51 A 48-year-old man has had three episodes of upper gastrointestinal bleeding from esophageal varices. He has a history of chronic alcoholism but has recently been rehabilitated. Further evaluation shows ascites and splenomegaly. Which of the following surgical venous anastomoses is most commonly used to relieve these symptoms and signs before a liver transplant is attempted?

- ▢ **A.** Left gastric to splenic vein
- ▢ **B.** Right gastric to left gastric vein
- ▢ **C.** Right renal to right gonadal vein
- ▢ **D.** Splenic to left renal vein
- ▢ **E.** Superior mesenteric to inferior mesenteric vein

52 A 55-year-old man is admitted to the hospital with nausea, vomiting, and hematuria. A CT scan reveals a neoplasm in the posterior surface of the inferior pole of the left kidney that has invaded through the renal pelvis, renal capsule, ureter, and fat. To which of the following regions will pain most likely be referred?

- ▢ **A.** Skin of the anterior and lateral thighs and femoral triangle
- ▢ **B.** Skin over the gluteal region, pubis, medial thigh, and scrotal areas
- ▢ **C.** Skin over the medial, anterior, and lateral side of the thigh
- ▢ **D.** Skin over the pubis and umbilicus
- ▢ **E.** Skin over the pubis, umbilicus, and posterior abdominal wall muscles

53 A 30-year-old female patient has complained of weakness and fatigue over the past 6 months. She has a 3-month acute history of severe hypertension that has not responded to antihypertensive medications. Fasting serum glucose concentration is 140 mg/dL. A CT scan of the abdomen shows a 6-cm mass in the adrenal gland affecting the secretory cells of the adrenal medulla. Which of the following structures is most likely releasing products into the bloodstream to produce the hypertension and other signs?

- ▢ **A.** Preganglionic sympathetic axons in thoracic splanchnic nerves

- ▢ **B.** Cells of neural crest origin that migrated to the adrenal medulla
- ▢ **C.** Preganglionic parasympathetic branches of the posterior vagal trunk
- ▢ **D.** Postganglionic parasympathetic branches of the left or right vagus nerves
- ▢ **E.** Postganglionic fibers from pelvic splanchnic nerves

54 A 48-year-old man is admitted to the hospital with severe abdominal pain. Radiologic examination reveals a tumor in the tail of the pancreas. A diagnostic arteriogram shows that the tumor has compromised the blood supply to another organ. Which of the following organs is most likely to have its blood supply compromised by this tumor?

- ▢ **A.** Duodenum
- ▢ **B.** Gallbladder
- ▢ **C.** Kidney
- ▢ **D.** Liver
- ▢ **E.** Spleen

55 A 57-year-old man is admitted to the emergency department with left flank pain. Blood tests indicate hematuria and anemia. A magnetic resonance scan reveals that blood flow in the left renal vein is being occluded by an arterial aneurysm where the vein crosses the aorta. The aneurysm is most likely located in which of the following arteries?

- ▢ **A.** Celiac
- ▢ **B.** Inferior mesenteric
- ▢ **C.** Left colic
- ▢ **D.** Middle colic
- ▢ **E.** Superior mesenteric

56 A 57-year-old man is admitted to the emergency department with pain in his left flank and testicles. Laboratory tests indicate hematuria and anemia. A CT scan examination provides evidence that blood flow in the left renal vein is being occluded where it crosses anterior to the aorta. Which of the following is the most likely cause of the testicular pain?

- ▢ **A.** Compression of the testicular artery
- ▢ **B.** Occlusion of flow of blood in the testicular vein
- ▢ **C.** Compression of the afferent fibers in the lumbar splanchnic nerves
- ▢ **D.** Compression of the sympathetic fibers in the preaortic plexus
- ▢ **E.** Compression of the posterior vagus nerve

57 A 51-year-old woman is admitted to the hospital with an acutely painful abdomen. Radiographic examination reveals penetration of the fundic region of the stomach by an ulcer, resulting in intraabdominal bleeding. Which of the following arteries is the most likely source of the bleeding?

- ▢ **A.** Common hepatic artery
- ▢ **B.** Inferior phrenic artery
- ▢ **C.** Left gastroepiploic artery
- ▢ **D.** Short gastric artery
- ▢ **E.** Splenic artery

58 A 39-year-old woman is admitted to the hospital with pain radiating to her inguinal region. Radiologic and physical examination reveal a herniation. Which of the following is the most common type of hernia in a female patient?

- ▢ **A.** Femoral hernia
- ▢ **B.** Umbilical hernia
- ▢ **C.** Direct inguinal hernia
- ▢ **D.** Indirect inguinal hernia
- ▢ **E.** Epigastric hernia

59 Radiologic examination of a 42-year-old woman reveals penetration of the duodenal bulb by an ulcer, resulting in profuse intraabdominal bleeding. Which of the following arteries is the most likely source of the bleeding?

- ▢ **A.** Posterior superior pancreaticoduodenal
- ▢ **B.** Superior mesenteric
- ▢ **C.** Inferior mesenteric
- ▢ **D.** Inferior pancreaticoduodenal
- ▢ **E.** Right gastric

60 A 23-year-old man is admitted to the hospital with a bulge in his scrotum. Physical examination reveals an indirect inguinal hernia. During the open hernia repair the internal spermatic fascia is identified and reflected to expose the ductus deferens and testicular vessels. From which of the following does the internal spermatic fascial layer of the spermatic cord develop?

- ▢ **A.** External abdominal oblique aponeurosis
- ▢ **B.** Internal abdominal oblique aponeurosis
- ▢ **C.** Transversus abdominis aponeurosis
- ▢ **D.** Transversalis fascia
- ▢ **E.** Processus vaginalis

61 A 45-year-old woman is admitted to the emergency department with a complaint of severe abdominal pain. CT scan and MRI examinations reveal a tumor of the head of the pancreas involving the uncinate process. Which of the following vessels is most likely to be occluded?

- ▢ **A.** Common hepatic artery
- ▢ **B.** Cystic artery and vein
- ▢ **C.** Superior mesenteric artery
- ▢ **D.** Inferior mesenteric artery
- ▢ **E.** Portal vein

62 A 35-year-old obese man is admitted to the hospital with jaundice and complaints of abdominal pain. Physical examination reveals an epigastric pain that migrates toward the patient's right side and posterior toward the scapula. Radiographic examination reveals multiple gallstones, consistent with the patient's jaundice and typical pains of cholecystitis. Which of the following structures is most likely obstructed by the gallstones?

- ▢ **A.** Common bile duct
- ▢ **B.** Cystic duct
- ▢ **C.** Left hepatic duct
- ▢ **D.** Pancreatic duct
- ▢ **E.** Right hepatic duct

63 A 36-year-old woman is admitted to the hospital for the imminent birth of her baby. The decision is made to perform an emergency cesarean section. A Pfannenstiel incision is used to reach the uterus by making a transverse incision through the external sheath of the rectus muscles, about 2 cm above the pubic bones. It follows natural folds of the skin and curves superior to the mons pubis. Which of the following nerves is most at risk when this incision is made?

- ▢ **A.** T10
- ▢ **B.** T11
- ▢ **C.** Iliohypogastric
- ▢ **D.** Ilioinguinal
- ▢ **E.** Lateral femoral cutaneous

64 A 37-year-old woman was admitted to the emergency department with high fever (39.5° C), nausea, and vomiting. Physical examination revealed increased abdominal pain in the paraumbilical region, rebound tenderness over McBurney's point, and a positive psoas test. Blood tests showed marked leukocytosis. Which of the following is the most likely diagnosis?

- ▢ **A.** Ectopic pregnancy
- ▢ **B.** Appendicitis
- ▢ **C.** Cholecystitis
- ▢ **D.** Kidney stone
- ▢ **E.** Perforation of the duodenum

65 A 56-year-old man is admitted to the hospital with severe abdominal pain. The patient has a history of "irritable bowel syndrome" affecting his rectum. Which of the following nerves will most likely be responsible for the transmission of pain in this case?

- ▢ **A.** Lumbar sympathetic trunks
- ▢ **B.** Pelvic splanchnic nerves
- ▢ **C.** Pudendal nerves
- ▢ **D.** Sacral sympathetic trunks
- ▢ **E.** Vagus nerves

66 A 42-year-old woman is admitted to the hospital due to blood in her stools. Physical examination reveals no signs of inflammation, infection, or tumor. An endoscopic examination of the distal segment of the ileum reveals a lesion of the intestinal wall. Biopsy gives histologic evidence that the lesion contains gastric mucosa. Which of the following clinical conditions will most likely explain the symptoms and signs?

- ▢ **A.** Internal hemorrhoids
- ▢ **B.** External hemorrhoids
- ▢ **C.** Diverticulosis
- ▢ **D.** Meckel's diverticulum
- ▢ **E.** Borborygmi

67 An 80-year-old man is admitted to the hospital with hypertension. His history includes a notation that he has had a poor appetite for some time. During physical examination it is observed that his blood pressure is 175/95 mm Hg and that he has a marked pulsation in his epigastric region. Which of the following diagnoses will most likely explain the symptoms and signs?

- ▢ **A.** Hiatal hernia
- ▢ **B.** Splenomegaly
- ▢ **C.** Cirrhosis of the liver
- ▢ **D.** Aortic aneurysm
- ▢ **E.** Kidney stone

68 A 48-year-old woman is admitted to the hospital with a distended abdomen. A CT scan examination provides evidence of the presence of ascites (Fig. 3-1). In which of the following locations will an ultrasound machine most likely confirm the presence of the ascitic fluid with the patient in the supine position?

- ▢ **A.** Subphrenic recess
- ▢ **B.** Hepatorenal recess (pouch of Morison)
- ▢ **C.** Rectouterine recess (pouch of Douglas)
- ▢ **D.** Vesicouterine recess
- ▢ **E.** Subhepatic recess

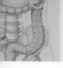

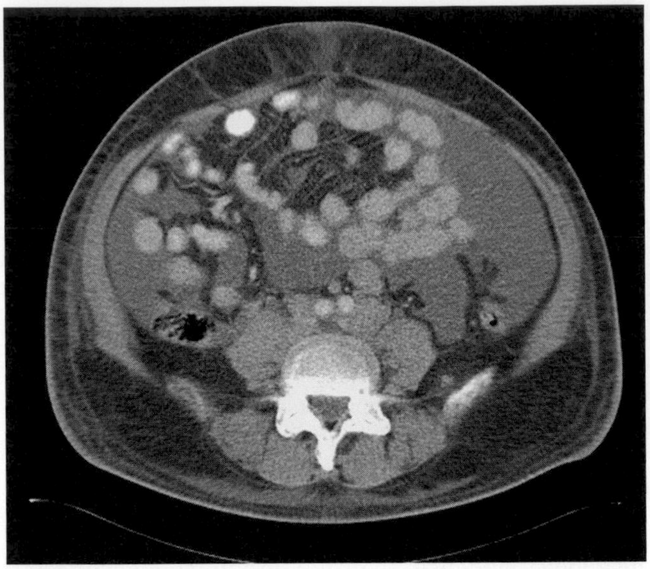

Fig. 3-1

69 A 19-year-old man is admitted to the hospital after an automobile collision. An MRI examination reveals that the spinal cord has been transected at the L4 cord level. Which of the following portions of the intestine will most predictably lose parasympathetic innervation from the central nervous system?

- ▢ **A.** Jejunum
- ▢ **B.** Ascending colon
- ▢ **C.** Ileum
- ▢ **D.** Descending colon
- ▢ **E.** Transverse colon

70 A 55-year-old man is admitted to the hospital because of severe weight loss over the preceding 6-month period of time. Radiographic examination and other tests provide evidence that a tumor is causing portal hypertension. Laboratory studies reveal that the patient has fatty stool, malnutrition, and liver hypoxia. At which of the following locations is the tumor most likely located?

- ▢ **A.** Right lobe of the liver
- ▢ **B.** Left lobe of the liver
- ▢ **C.** Porta hepatis
- ▢ **D.** Falciform ligament
- ▢ **E.** Hepatogastric ligament

71 During a laparoscopic cholecystectomy on a 61-year-old man, which of the following arteries must be clamped to remove the gallbladder safely?

- ▢ **A.** Common hepatic
- ▢ **B.** Proper hepatic
- ▢ **C.** Right hepatic
- ▢ **D.** Left hepatic
- ▢ **E.** Cystic

72 A 45-year-old woman is admitted to the hospital after her automobile left the highway in a rainstorm and hit a tree. She had been wearing a seat belt. On radiographic examination, it is observed that she has suffered fractures of the ninth and tenth rib on her left side and that she has intraabdominal bleeding. Physical examination reveals hypovolemic shock and progressive hypotension. Which of the following organs is most likely injured to result in these clinical signs?

- ▢ **A.** Liver
- ▢ **B.** Pancreas
- ▢ **C.** Left kidney
- ▢ **D.** Spleen
- ▢ **E.** Ileum

73 Two days after an appendectomy a 45-year-old man has an elevated temperature (39° C), is hypotensive, and complains of abdominal pain. An exploratory laparotomy reveals large amounts of blood in the peritoneal cavity due to an injury to a vessel that occurred during the appendectomy. Which of the following vessel(s) must be ligated to stop the bleeding?

- ▢ **A.** Right colic artery
- ▢ **B.** Right colic artery and superior rectal artery
- ▢ **C.** Superior mesenteric artery
- ▢ **D.** Ileocolic artery
- ▢ **E.** Ileocolic artery and middle colic artery

74 A 42-year-old man is admitted to the hospital with severe hematemesis. Radiographic studies reveal hepatomegaly and esophageal varices. During physical examination it is observed that the patient is icteric (jaundiced) and dilated veins ("caput medusae") are seen on his anterior abdominal wall. Which of the following venous structures is most likely obstructed for the development of caput medusae?

- ▢ **A.** Portal vein
- ▢ **B.** Inferior vena cava
- ▢ **C.** Superior vena cava
- ▢ **D.** Lateral thoracic vein
- ▢ **E.** Superficial epigastric vein

75 A 58-year-old man was admitted to the hospital with complaints of pain in the right upper quadrant and jaundice. Ultrasound examination reveals numerous large gallstones in his gallbladder. Which of the following nerves would transmit the pain of cholecystitis?

- A. The right vagus nerve, with referral to the inferior angle of the scapula
- B. Afferent fibers in spinal nerves T1 to T4
- C. Visceral afferent fibers in the greater thoracic splanchnic nerve, with referral to the dermatomes from T6 to T8
- D. Sympathetic T10 to T12 portions of greater thoracic splanchnic nerve via celiac ganglion and celiac plexus
- E. Afferent fibers of dorsal primary rami of spinal nerves T6 to T8, with referral to the epigastric region

76 A 15-year-old woman is brought to the hospital with fever, nausea, and diffuse paraumbilical pain, which later becomes localized in the lower right quadrant. An appendectomy procedure is begun with an incision at McBurney's point. Which of the following landmarks best describes McBurney's point?

- A. The midpoint of the inguinal ligament in line with the right nipple
- B. Two thirds of the distance from the umbilicus to the anterior superior iliac spine
- C. A line that intersects the upper one third of the inguinal ligament
- D. A line that intersects the lower third of the inguinal ligament, about 2 cm from the pubic tubercle
- E. One third of the distance from the anterior inferior iliac spine to the umbilicus

77 A 41-year-old woman is admitted to the hospital with upper abdominal pain. A gastroscopic examination reveals multiple small ulcerations in the body of the stomach. Which of the following nerves transmits the sensation of pain from this region?

- A. Spinal nerves T5 to T12
- B. Greater thoracic splanchnic nerves
- C. Lesser thoracic splanchnic nerves
- D. Lumbar splanchnic nerves
- E. Spinal nerves T12 to L2

78 A 68-year-old woman is admitted to the hospital with severe pain radiating from her lower back toward her pubic symphysis. Ultrasound examination reveals that a renal calculus (kidney stone) is partially obstructing her right ureter. At which of the following locations is the calculus most likely to lodge?

- A. Major calyx
- B. Minor calyx
- C. Pelvic brim
- D. Midportion of the ureter
- E. Between the pelvic brim and the uterine cervix

79 A 42-year-old woman is admitted to the hospital after a traumatic landing while skydiving. Radiographic examination reveals a ruptured spleen. An emergency splenectomy is performed. Which of the following peritoneal structures must be carefully manipulated to prevent intraperitoneal bleeding?

- A. Coronary ligament
- B. Gastrocolic ligament
- C. Splenorenal ligament
- D. Phrenocolic ligament
- E. Falciform ligament

80 A 74-year-old woman is admitted to the hospital with complaints of abdominal pain. Radiologic examination reveals diverticulosis and diverticulitis of the lower portion of the descending colon, with diffuse ulcerations. It is determined that the involved area of the bowel should be removed. If the patient's anatomy follows the most typical patterns, which vessels and nerves will be cut during the operation?

- A. Branches of the vagus nerve and middle colic artery
- B. Superior mesenteric plexus and superior rectal artery
- C. Branches of pelvic splanchnic nerves and left colic artery
- D. Branches of vagus nerve and ileocolic artery
- E. Left lesser thoracic splanchnic nerve and inferior mesenteric artery

81 A 15-year-old boy underwent an appendectomy. Two weeks postoperatively the patient complains of numbness of the skin over the pubic region and anterior portion of his genitals. Which of the following nerves was most likely iatrogenically injured during the operation?

- A. Pudendal
- B. Genitofemoral
- C. Spinal nerve T10
- D. Subcostal
- E. Ilioinguinal

82 A 5-year-old boy is admitted to the hospital with failure to thrive, dysphagia, and history of recurrent chest infections. Two days later the boy develops aspiration pneumonia. Esophagographic examination shows webs and strictures in the distal third of the thoracic esophagus. Which of the following developmental conditions will most likely explain the symptoms?

- ▢ **A.** Incomplete recanalization of the esophagus during the eighth week
- ▢ **B.** Tracheoesophageal fistula
- ▢ **C.** Esophageal atresia
- ▢ **D.** Duodenal atresia
- ▢ **E.** Duodenal stenosis

83 The vomitus of a 5-day-old infant contains stomach contents and bile. The vomiting has continued for 2 days. Radiographic examinations reveal stenosis of the fourth part of the duodenum. The child cries almost constantly, appearing to be hungry all of the time, yet does not gain any weight. Which of the following developmental conditions will most likely explain the symptoms?

- ▢ **A.** Patent bile duct
- ▢ **B.** Duodenal stenosis
- ▢ **C.** Hypertrophied pyloric sphincter
- ▢ **D.** Atrophied gastric antrum
- ▢ **E.** Tracheoesophageal fistula

84 A 4-day-old male infant vomits the contents of his stomach, but the vomitus does not appear to contain bile. The baby is obviously distressed and makes sucking movements of his lips in response to offerings to suckle by his mother or of the bottle, but he is failing to thrive. Which of the following conditions will best explain the symptoms?

- ▢ **A.** Duodenal stenosis
- ▢ **B.** Duodenal atresia
- ▢ **C.** Hypertrophied pyloric sphincter
- ▢ **D.** Atrophied gastric fundus
- ▢ **E.** Tracheoesophageal fistula

85 The vomit of a 5-day-old female infant contains stomach contents and bile. The vomiting continues for 2 days. Radiologic examinations reveal stenosis of the third part of the duodenum. The child cries consistently and is constantly hungry, but she does not gain any weight. Which of the following conditions will most likely explain her symptoms?

- ▢ **A.** Incomplete recanalization of the esophagus during the eighth week
- ▢ **B.** Incomplete recanalization of the duodenum
- ▢ **C.** Esophageal atresia
- ▢ **D.** Duodenal atresia
- ▢ **E.** Tracheoesophageal fistula

86 A 2-hour-old male infant had been diagnosed in utero with polyhydramnios. Now he is vomiting stomach contents and bile. The vomiting continues for 2 days. Radiographic examination reveals a "double bubble" sign on the ultrasound scan. The child cries consistently and is constantly hungry but has lost 300 g in weight. Which of the following conditions will most likely explain the symptoms?

- ▢ **A.** Duodenal stenosis
- ▢ **B.** Duodenal atresia
- ▢ **C.** Hypertrophied pyloric sphincter
- ▢ **D.** Atrophied gastric antrum
- ▢ **E.** Tracheoesophageal fistula

87 A 4-year-old male child is admitted to the hospital with severe vomiting. Radiologic examination and history taking reveal that the boy suffers from an annular pancreas. Which of the following conditions will most typically explain the symptoms?

- ▢ **A.** The main pancreatic duct persisted as an accessory duct that opened at the minor papilla.
- ▢ **B.** Bile ducts failed to canalize.
- ▢ **C.** The bifid ventral bud fused with the dorsal bud.
- ▢ **D.** Only the dorsal pancreatic bud formed a ring of pancreatic tissue.
- ▢ **E.** Dorsal pancreatic bud developed around the third part of the duodenum.

88 The surgeon decided that a 35-year-old male patient must undergo an emergency appendectomy due to rupture of his appendix. A midline incision was made for greater access to the peritoneal cavity. The surgeon noted a 5-cm-long fingerlike pouch on the anterior border of the ileum about 60 cm away from the ileocecal junction. Such a pouch is a remnant of which of the following developmental structures?

- ▢ **A.** Omphaloenteric duct (yolk stalk)
- ▢ **B.** Branch of superior mesenteric artery
- ▢ **C.** Umbilical vesicle (yolk sac)
- ▢ **D.** Cecal diverticulum
- ▢ **E.** Umbilical cord

89 A 3-month-old boy is admitted to the hospital with an abnormal mass of tissue protruding from his abdomen. An MRI examination reveals that the mass contains some greater omentum and some small intestine. The abnormal mass protrudes when the infant cries, strains, and coughs. Which of the following conditions will most likely explain the symptoms?

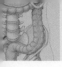

- ▢ **A.** Umbilical hernia
- ▢ **B.** Omphalocele
- ▢ **C.** Gastroschisis
- ▢ **D.** Epigastric hernia
- ▢ **E.** Indirect inguinal hernia

90 Ultrasound examinations of a male fetus in the seventh month of gestation indicate a defect on his right side, lateral to the median plane, in which the viscera protrude into the amniotic cavity. Which of the following conditions will most likely explain these findings?

- ▢ **A.** Nonrotation of the midgut
- ▢ **B.** Patent urachus
- ▢ **C.** Abdominal contents have not returned from the umbilical cord
- ▢ **D.** Incomplete closure of the lateral folds
- ▢ **E.** Persistent cloacal membrane

91 A 2-hour-old male infant vomits stomach contents and bile. The vomiting continues for 2 days. In addition, abdominal distension is noted, and he is unable to pass meconium (the earliest feces to be eliminated after birth). Which of the following is the most common cause of this condition?

- ▢ **A.** Infarction of fetal bowel due to volvulus
- ▢ **B.** Incomplete closure of the lateral folds
- ▢ **C.** Failure of recanalization of the ileum
- ▢ **D.** Remnant of the proximal portion of the omphaloenteric duct
- ▢ **E.** Nonrotation of the midgut

92 A 5-year-old male infant is admitted to the hospital with signs of appendicitis. An operation is performed and an ileal (Meckel's) diverticulum is discovered. Which of the following is the most common cause of this condition?

- ▢ **A.** Infarction of fetal bowel due to volvulus
- ▢ **B.** Incomplete closure of the lateral folds
- ▢ **C.** Failure of recanalization of the ileum
- ▢ **D.** Remnant of the proximal portion of the omphaloenteric duct
- ▢ **E.** Nonrotation of the midgut

93 A newborn male infant has no passage of first stool (meconium) for 48 hours after birth. Physical examination reveals that the young patient has anal agenesis with a perineal fistula. Which of the following is the most common cause of this condition?

- ▢ **A.** Incomplete separation of the cloaca by the urorectal septum
- ▢ **B.** Dorsal deviation of the urorectal septum
- ▢ **C.** Failure of the anal membrane to perforate
- ▢ **D.** Abnormal recanalization of the colon
- ▢ **E.** Remnant of the proximal portion of the omphaloenteric duct

94 A 3-month-old female infant is diagnosed with anal stenosis after several periods of stool infrequency, two of which lasted 10 days without a bowel movement. Which of the following is the most likely cause of this condition?

- ▢ **A.** Incomplete separation of the cloaca by the urorectal septum
- ▢ **B.** Dorsal deviation of the urorectal septum
- ▢ **C.** Failure of the anal membrane to perforate
- ▢ **D.** Abnormal recanalization of the colon
- ▢ **E.** Remnant of the proximal portion of the omphaloenteric duct

95 A 2-month-old male infant presents with a fecal discharge from his umbilicus. Which of the following diagnoses will best explain this condition?

- ▢ **A.** Enterocystoma
- ▢ **B.** Vitelline cyst
- ▢ **C.** Ileal (Meckel's) diverticulum
- ▢ **D.** Vitelline fistula
- ▢ **E.** Volvulus

96 A 5-day-old male infant is diagnosed with anorectal agenesis. An ultrasound study reveals a rectourethral fistula. Which of the following is the most likely embryologic cause of this condition?

- ▢ **A.** Failure of the proctodeum to develop
- ▢ **B.** Agenesis of the urorectal septum
- ▢ **C.** Failure of fixation of the hindgut
- ▢ **D.** Abnormal partitioning of the cloaca
- ▢ **E.** Premature rupture of the anal membrane

97 A 12-year-old boy was admitted to the hospital with massive rectal bleeding. Upon inspection, the color of the blood ranged from bright to dark red. The child appeared to be free of any pain. Radiographic examination revealed an ileal (Meckel's) diverticulum. Which of the following is the underlying embryologic cause of this condition?

- ▢ **A.** Failure of yolk stalk to regress
- ▢ **B.** Duplication of the intestine
- ▢ **C.** Malrotation of the cecum and appendix
- ▢ **D.** Nonrotation of the midgut
- ▢ **E.** Herniation of the intestines

98 A 23-year-old pregnant woman visits her gynecologist for her routine ultrasound checkup. Ultrasound of the fetus reveals unilateral renal agenesis and oligohydramnios. Which of the following conditions most likely occurred?

- ▢ **A.** Polycystic kidney disease
- ▢ **B.** Degeneration of the mesonephros
- ▢ **C.** Ureteric duplication
- ▢ **D.** Failure of a ureteric bud to form
- ▢ **E.** Wilms tumor

99 A 15-year-old girl was admitted to the hospital with bilateral inguinal masses. Physical examination revealed that she had not begun to menstruate but showed normal breast development for her age. Her external genitalia were female, the vagina was shallow, but no uterus could be palpated. Laboratory examination revealed that her sex chromatin pattern was negative. Which of the following is the most likely diagnosis?

- ▢ **A.** Male pseudohermaphroditism
- ▢ **B.** Female pseudohermaphroditism
- ▢ **C.** Androgen insensitivity syndrome
- ▢ **D.** Inguinal hernias
- ▢ **E.** Turner syndrome

100 An 18-year-old female gymnast is admitted to the hospital with pelvic pain. Physical examination reveals that the patient has a history of primary amenorrhea and an imperforate hymen. Which of the following is the most likely explanation for this condition?

- ▢ **A.** Failure of the vaginal plate to canalize
- ▢ **B.** Cervical atresia
- ▢ **C.** Patent processus vaginalis
- ▢ **D.** Androgen insensitivity syndrome
- ▢ **E.** Failure of the sinovaginal bulbs to develop

101 During a routine gynecologic visit, a 22-year-old woman complains of having dyspareunia (pain during sexual intercourse). During a pelvic examination a mass of tissue is detected on the lateral wall of the vagina. An ultrasound examination reveals that the abnormal structure is a Gartner duct cyst. From which of the following embryonic structures does this cyst take origin?

- ▢ **A.** Mesonephric tubules
- ▢ **B.** Paramesonephric duct
- ▢ **C.** Urogenital folds
- ▢ **D.** Mesonephric duct
- ▢ **E.** Sinovaginal bulbs

102 A 2-day-old male infant is hospitalized in the intensive care unit with acute respiratory distress. The patient is found to have anuria, oligohydramnios, and hypoplastic lungs. Facial characteristics are consistent with Potter syndrome. Which of the following is the most likely explanation for these initial findings?

- ▢ **A.** Multicystic dysplastic kidney
- ▢ **B.** Polycystic kidney
- ▢ **C.** Renal agenesis
- ▢ **D.** Wilms tumor
- ▢ **E.** Extrophy of the bladder

103 A 58-year-old male bricklayer is admitted to the hospital with severe pain that radiates from his lower back to the pubic region. Ultrasound examination reveals that a kidney stone is partially obstructing his right ureter; the examination also indicates the presence of a second ureter on the right side. Which of the following is the most likely cause of this latter finding?

- ▢ **A.** Failure of ureteric bud to form
- ▢ **B.** Early splitting of the ureteric bud
- ▢ **C.** Failure of urorectal septum to develop
- ▢ **D.** Persistent urachus
- ▢ **E.** Failure of ureteric bud to branch

104 A 50-year-old woman with a long history of heartburn (self-treated with various over-the-counter medications) develops severe epigastric pain and is urgently admitted to the hospital. A gastroscopic examination reveals a small, perforated ulceration in the posterior wall of the stomach body. At surgery, with the patient in the supine position, 150 mL of blood-tinged, frothy gray liquid is aspirated from the peritoneal cavity. Where in the peritoneal cavity would liquid most likely first collect when the patient is supine?

- ▢ **A.** Right subphrenic space
- ▢ **B.** Hepatorenal pouch (of Morison)
- ▢ **C.** Left paracolic gutter
- ▢ **D.** Vesicouterine pouch
- ▢ **E.** Rectouterine pouch (of Douglas)

105 A 43-year-old female accountant complains of severe epigastric pain and is admitted to the hospital. A gastroscopic examination reveals a small, perforated ulceration in the posterior wall of the greater curvature of her stomach. An upright chest radiograph reveals a small amount of free air in the peritoneal cavity. Where is the air most likely located?

- ▢ **A.** Right subphrenic space
- ▢ **B.** Supravesical space
- ▢ **C.** Paracolic gutters

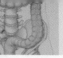

- ☐ **D.** Vesicouterine pouch
- ☐ **E.** Rectouterine pouch (of Douglas)

106 A 25-year-old woman is admitted to the hospital with sharp pain in the left lower quadrant. Patient history reveals that her last menstrual period was 10 days ago. Transvaginal ultrasound reveals a ruptured cyst on the left ovary. The sonogram also reveals approximately 100 mL of fluid in the pelvis, which is presumed to represent cyst contents and bleeding from the rupture site. Where is this fluid most likely located?

- ☐ **A.** Right subphrenic space
- ☐ **B.** Hepatorenal pouch (of Morison)
- ☐ **C.** Paracolic gutters
- ☐ **D.** Vesicouterine pouch
- ☐ **E.** Rectouterine pouch (of Douglas)

107 A 60-year-old man is admitted to the emergency department with severe abdominal pain. Physical examination reveals guarding and rigidity in the abdominal wall. An abdominal CT scan shows a thrombus in an intestinal artery supplying the ileum. Which of the following layers of peritoneum will have to be entered by the surgeon to access the affected vessel?

- ☐ **A.** Parietal peritoneum and the greater omentum
- ☐ **B.** Greater and lesser omentum
- ☐ **C.** Lesser omentum and the gastrosplenic ligament
- ☐ **D.** Parietal peritoneum and the mesentery
- ☐ **E.** Greater omentum and the transverse mesocolon

108 A 52-year-old man presents to the emergency department complaining of persistent severe right upper quadrant pain for the past 2 hours. During that period of time he felt nauseated, was sweating profusely, and also experienced pain in the posterior aspect of his right shoulder. The pain began shortly after a lunch consisting of "fast food." Ultrasound examination reveals multiple stones in an inflamed gallbladder with a normal bile duct. Which of the following spinal nerve segments are involved in the shoulder pain, associated with cholecystitis?

- ☐ **A.** C3 to C5
- ☐ **B.** C5 to C8
- ☐ **C.** T1 to T4
- ☐ **D.** T5 to T9
- ☐ **E.** T10, T11

109 During a cholecystectomy on a 64-year-old woman, the right hepatic artery was accidentally injured. In addition to bleeding profusely, the lacerated artery was hidden from view by overlying connective tissue and fat plus pooling blood. Which of the following procedures would most likely be performed by the surgeon to slow, or perhaps arrest, the blood loss?

- ☐ **A.** Pringle maneuver
- ☐ **B.** Kocher maneuver
- ☐ **C.** Valsalva maneuver
- ☐ **D.** Heimlich maneuver
- ☐ **E.** Placement of a vascular clamp on the porta hepatis

110 A 53-year-old quality control engineer is admitted to the hospital with severe abdominal pain. The patient's history and physical examination indicate chronic colonic diverticulitis, with tachycardia and hypotension at the present time. An ultrasonographic examination reveals massive bleeding from the descending colon. Which of the following arteries is most likely to be the source of the hemorrhage?

- ☐ **A.** Branch of the inferior mesenteric
- ☐ **B.** Middle colic
- ☐ **C.** Superior rectal
- ☐ **D.** Inferior rectal
- ☐ **E.** Left gastroepiploic

111 The gallbladder of a 51-year-old female patient is characterized by the presence of multiple gallstones, consistent with the diagnosis of cholecystitis. Which of the following tests would be anticipated to be positive in this patient?

- ☐ **A.** Rebound tenderness
- ☐ **B.** Iliopsoas test
- ☐ **C.** Obturator sign
- ☐ **D.** Murphy's sign
- ☐ **E.** Cough tenderness

112 A 35-year-old man is admitted to the hospital with a small-caliber bullet wound to the left upper quadrant of the abdomen. Radiographic examination reveals profuse intraperitoneal bleeding. An emergency laparotomy is performed, and the source of bleeding appears to be a vessel within the lesser sac. Which of the following ligaments would most likely be transected to gain adequate entry to the lesser sac?

- ☐ **A.** Coronary
- ☐ **B.** Gastrosplenic
- ☐ **C.** Splenorenal
- ☐ **D.** Gastrocolic
- ☐ **E.** Hepatoduodenal

113 A 45-year-old woman is admitted to the hospital with rectal bleeding. Physical examination, including a rectal examination, reveals an abnormal mass of tissue protruding below the pectinate line. Biopsy reveals the presence of an adenocarcinoma. Which of the following groups of lymph nodes would first receive lymph from the area of pathology?

- ☐ **A.** Internal iliac
- ☐ **B.** External iliac
- ☐ **C.** Middle rectal
- ☐ **D.** Superficial inguinal
- ☐ **E.** Deep inguinal

114 A 53-year-old man is admitted to the hospital with rectal bleeding. Physical examination, including a rectal examination, reveals an abnormal mass of tissue protruding from an area superior to the external anal sphincter, superior to the pectinate line. Biopsy reveals the presence of an adenocarcinoma. Which of the following groups of lymph nodes would first receive lymph from the cancerous area?

- ☐ **A.** Internal iliac
- ☐ **B.** External iliac
- ☐ **C.** Middle rectal
- ☐ **D.** Superficial inguinal
- ☐ **E.** Deep inguinal

115 A 32-year-old man is admitted to the emergency department with severe esophageal reflux. Radiographic examination reveals that the patient has a hiatal hernia, and a surgical procedure is scheduled. Which of the following landmarks would be the most useful to distinguish between sliding and paraesophageal hiatal hernias?

- ☐ **A.** Sliding hernias possess a normal gastroesophageal junction.
- ☐ **B.** In sliding hernias the gastroesophageal junction is displaced.
- ☐ **C.** Paraesophageal hernias have a displaced gastroesophageal junction.
- ☐ **D.** In paraesophageal hernias the antrum moves into the stomach corpus.
- ☐ **E.** In paraesophageal hernias the antrum and the cardia move into the body of the stomach.

116 A 43-year-old man is admitted to the emergency department with complaints of intense abdominal pain. Radiographic examination reveals a right subphrenic abscess that extends to the midline. Which of the following structures would most likely be in a position to retard the spread of the abscess across the midline?

- ☐ **A.** Round ligament
- ☐ **B.** Falciform ligament
- ☐ **C.** Coronary ligament
- ☐ **D.** Hepatoduodenal ligament
- ☐ **E.** Gastroduodenal ligament

117 A 21-year-old male football player is admitted to the emergency department with intense back pain. Physical examination shows that his left lower back is bruised and swollen. He complains of sharp pain during respiration. A radiograph reveals a fracture of the eleventh rib on the left side. Which of the following organs would be the most likely to sustain injury at this site?

- ☐ **A.** Spleen
- ☐ **B.** Lung
- ☐ **C.** Kidney
- ☐ **D.** Liver
- ☐ **E.** Pancreas

118 A 46-year-old man is admitted to the hospital with a rather large but painless mass on his right groin. During physical examination it is noted that the inguinal lymph nodes are hard and palpable. A lymph node biopsy reveals the presence of malignant cells. Which of the following locations would be the most likely primary source of carcinoma?

- ☐ **A.** Prostate
- ☐ **B.** Bladder
- ☐ **C.** Testis
- ☐ **D.** Anal canal
- ☐ **E.** Sigmoid colon

119 A 54-year-old man is admitted to the hospital with vomiting and severe weight loss. Physical examination reveals that the umbilical and epigastric regions are tender and painful. A CT scan examination reveals a massive tumor originating from the third part of the duodenum. Which of the following structures is most likely to be compressed or invaded by the tumor?

- ☐ **A.** Common bile duct
- ☐ **B.** Portal vein
- ☐ **C.** Superior mesenteric artery
- ☐ **D.** Gastroduodenal artery
- ☐ **E.** Posterior superior pancreaticoduodenal artery

120 A 24-year-old woman is admitted to the hospital with lower abdominal pain. A CT examination reveals an abnormal mass occupying the left adnexa in the pelvis. During the surgical procedure the ureter and the structures immediately medial to the ureter are identified. Which of the following vascular structures crosses the ureter just lateral to the cervix of the uterus?

- ☐ **A.** Middle rectal artery
- ☐ **B.** Superior vesical artery
- ☐ **C.** Internal pudendal vein
- ☐ **D.** Uterine artery
- ☐ **E.** Gonadal vein

121 A 32-year-old woman is admitted to the hospital with cramping abdominal pain around her umbilicus and vomiting for the previous 2 days. Radiologic studies indicate numerous stones in the gallbladder and air accumulation in the gallbladder and biliary tree. At which of the following places will an obstructive stone most likely be found?

- ☐ **A.** Jejunum
- ☐ **B.** Terminal ileum
- ☐ **C.** Common bile duct
- ☐ **D.** Duodenum
- ☐ **E.** Hepatic duct

122 A 37-year-old woman is admitted to the hospital with signs of cholecystitis. A physical examination confirms the initial diagnosis and a cholecystectomy is planned. Which of the following landmarks will best describe the precise location of the gallbladder with respect to the body wall?

- ☐ **A.** The intersection of the right linea semilunaris with the ninth costal cartilage
- ☐ **B.** The intersection of the right linea semilunaris with the intertubercular plane
- ☐ **C.** To the right of the epigastric region
- ☐ **D.** Superiorly to the umbilical region
- ☐ **E.** Upper right quadrant

123 A 45-year-old man is admitted to the hospital with a palpable and painful mass at his groin that is exacerbated when he stands erect or physically exerts himself. Physical examination indicates the probability of a direct inguinal hernia, a diagnosis that is confirmed laparoscopically. Which of the following is the most likely cause of this type of inguinal hernia?

- ☐ **A.** Defective transversalis fascia around the deep inguinal ring
- ☐ **B.** Defective peritoneum around the deep inguinal ring
- ☐ **C.** Defective aponeurosis of external abdominal oblique muscle
- ☐ **D.** Defective extraperitoneal connective tissue
- ☐ **E.** Defective aponeurosis of transversus abdominis muscle

124 A 22-year-old woman is admitted to the hospital with a complaint of intense periumbilical pain. Physical examination indicates a strong possibility of appendicitis. Shortly before an appendectomy is to be performed, the inflamed appendix ruptures. In which area would the extravasating blood and infectious fluids from the appendiceal region most tend to collect if the patient was sitting upright?

- ☐ **A.** Subphrenic space
- ☐ **B.** Hepatorenal recess (pouch of Morison)
- ☐ **C.** Rectouterine recess (pouch of Douglas)
- ☐ **D.** Vesicouterine space
- ☐ **E.** Subhepatic space

125 A 22-year-old woman complains of severe pain in the epigastric region. A CT scan reveals that the source of the pain is an inflamed appendix. Which of the following structures contain the nerve cell bodies from the appendix that are causing the referred pain in the epigastrium?

- ☐ **A.** Sympathetic trunk ganglia
- ☐ **B.** Celiac ganglion
- ☐ **C.** Lateral horn of the spinal cord
- ☐ **D.** Dorsal root ganglia of spinal nerves T8 to T10
- ☐ **E.** Dorsal root ganglia of spinal nerves L2 to L4

126 A 30-year-old woman complains of weakness and fatigability over the past 6 months. She has a 3-month acute history of severe hypertension that has required treatment with antihypertensive medications. Radiographic examination reveals a tumor of her right suprarenal gland. The patient is diagnosed with a pheochromocytoma (tumor of the adrenal medulla) and is scheduled for a laparoscopic adrenalectomy. Which of the following nerve fibers will need to be cut when the adrenal gland and tumor are removed?

- ☐ **A.** Preganglionic sympathetic fibers
- ☐ **B.** Postganglionic sympathetic fibers
- ☐ **C.** Somatic motor fibers
- ☐ **D.** Postganglionic parasympathetic fibers
- ☐ **E.** Preganglionic parasympathetic fibers

127 A 55-year-old man is admitted to the hospital for his annual checkup. An ultrasound examination reveals a tumor that has incorporated the right common iliac artery and compressed the vein that lies posterior to it. Doppler ultrasound studies give evidence of the development of a deep venous thrombosis that could block venous return from the left lower limb, causing ischemia and pain. Which of the following vessels is most likely to be involved in the production of the deep venous thrombosis?

- ▢ **A.** Inferior vena cava
- ▢ **B.** Right renal vein
- ▢ **C.** Left testicular vein
- ▢ **D.** Left common iliac vein
- ▢ **E.** Right common iliac vein

128 A 48-year-old woman is admitted to the emergency department with a complaint of severe abdominal pain. Radiographic examination reveals advanced carcinoma of the head of the pancreas. A celiac plexus block is performed to relieve her pain. Which of the following best describes the nerve structures that are most likely to be present in the celiac ganglion?

- ▢ **A.** Preganglionic parasympathetic and somatic motor fibers
- ▢ **B.** Postganglionic parasympathetic and visceral afferent fibers
- ▢ **C.** Postganglionic sympathetic and visceral afferent fibers
- ▢ **D.** Pre- and postganglionic sympathetic, preganglionic parasympathetic, and visceral afferent fibers
- ▢ **E.** Preganglionic sympathetic, preganglionic parasympathetic, and visceral afferent fibers

129 A 21-year-old woman is admitted to the hospital with a complaint of severe pain radiating from her lower back toward and above the pubic symphysis. Ultrasound examination reveals that a kidney stone is partially obstructing her right ureter. Which of the following nerves is most likely responsible for conducting the sensation of pain?

- ▢ **A.** Subcostal
- ▢ **B.** Iliohypogastric
- ▢ **C.** Ilioinguinal
- ▢ **D.** Lateral femoral cutaneous
- ▢ **E.** Obturator

130 A 42-year-old woman is admitted to the hospital with an acutely painful abdomen and vomiting bright red blood. Radiographic examination reveals penetration of a posterior duodenal ulcer resulting in intraabdominal bleeding. Which of the following arteries is most commonly eroded by this type of ulcer?

- ▢ **A.** Gastroduodenal artery
- ▢ **B.** Superior mesenteric
- ▢ **C.** Posterior superior pancreaticoduodenal
- ▢ **D.** Posterior inferior pancreaticoduodenal
- ▢ **E.** Right gastric

131 A 37-year-old female court stenographer is admitted to the hospital with a complaint of intense pain in her abdomen. Radiologic examination reveals penetration of an anterior duodenal ulcer. Which of the following conditions will most probably occur?

- ▢ **A.** Bleeding from gastroduodenal artery
- ▢ **B.** Bleeding from superior mesenteric artery
- ▢ **C.** Bleeding from posterior superior pancreaticoduodenal artery
- ▢ **D.** Bleeding from posterior inferior pancreaticoduodenal artery
- ▢ **E.** Peritonitis

132 A 56-year-old man is diagnosed with midgut volvulus and intestinal ischemia. A laparotomy is performed to release the obstruction of the intestines. Which of the following structures is used as a landmark to determine the position of the duodenojejunal junction?

- ▢ **A.** Superior mesenteric artery
- ▢ **B.** Inferior mesenteric artery
- ▢ **C.** Vasa recta
- ▢ **D.** Suspensory ligament of the duodenum (ligament of Treitz)
- ▢ **E.** Phrenocolic ligament

133 A 4-month-old female infant is admitted to the hospital with cyanosis. Physical examination reveals decreased breath sounds, abdominal sounds in the thorax, and respiratory distress. A radiographic examination reveals a posterolateral defect of the diaphragm and abdominal contents in the left pleural cavity. Which of the following is the most likely cause of this defect?

- ▢ **A.** Absence of a pleuropericardial fold
- ▢ **B.** Absence of musculature in one half of the diaphragm
- ▢ **C.** Failure of migration of diaphragm
- ▢ **D.** Failure of the septum transversum to develop
- ▢ **E.** Failure of pleuroperitoneal fold to close

134 A 58-year-old man complains of sharp epigastric pain, most commonly felt just after a large meal. He is tender to palpation at the xiphisternal junction. Barium swallow exams and dye injections (HIDA scan) to test gallbladder functions are negative. Ultrasound reveals that a portion of the greater omentum is trapped at its entry to the thorax between the xiphoid process and the costal margin on the right. What is the most likely diagnosis of this condition?

- ▢ **A.** Bochdalek hernia
- ▢ **B.** Sliding esophageal hernia

- ▢ **C.** Morgagni hernia
- ▢ **D.** Cholecystitis
- ▢ **E.** Hiatal hernia

135 A 62-year-old woman is admitted to the emergency department with abdominal pains of uncertain origin. A CT scan reveals an aortic aneurysm affecting the origin of the superior mesenteric artery, resulting in ischemia to an abdominal organ. Which of the following organs is most likely affected?

- ▢ **A.** Ileum
- ▢ **B.** Transverse colon
- ▢ **C.** Spleen
- ▢ **D.** Stomach
- ▢ **E.** Duodenum

136 A 41-year-old man entered the emergency department with abdominal trauma after his motorcycle was struck by a hit-and-run automobile driver. One week following emergent surgery the patient was released from the hospital. Two months postoperatively the patient complained of abdominal pain. A CT scan examination demonstrated an internal hernia in which the hepatic flexure of the colon had herniated through the epiploic (omental) foramen (of Winslow). Gastrointestinal veins appeared to be markedly dilated, including the veins forming anastomoses between the portal and caval systems (veins of Retzius). Which of the following structures is most likely compressed?

- ▢ **A.** Portal vein
- ▢ **B.** Inferior vena cava
- ▢ **C.** Hepatic artery
- ▢ **D.** Common bile duct
- ▢ **E.** Cystic duct

137 A 48-year-old woman visited the outpatient clinic with a complaint of lower left quadrant pain that had persisted for the previous 3 months. Laboratory examinations revealed that the patient had blood in her stools. A colonoscopy gave evidence of diverticulosis that had been affecting the distal part of the descending colon. To which of the following dermatomes would pain have most likely been referred?

- ▢ **A.** T5 to T9
- ▢ **B.** T10 to L1
- ▢ **C.** L1, L2
- ▢ **D.** L1 to L4
- ▢ **E.** T10 to L2

138 A 61-year-old man is admitted to the emergency department with abdominal pain and a 2-day history of vomiting. Physical examination reveals a colicky abdominal pain in the right lower quadrant, with abdominal distention. Upon auscultation, episodes of pain were associated with rushes, gurgling, and tinkling sounds. A CT scan examination reveals a mechanical obstruction of the bowel. Which of the following parts of the gastrointestinal tract is most likely obstructed?

- ▢ **A.** Hepatopancreatic ampulla of Vater
- ▢ **B.** Duodenal bulb
- ▢ **C.** Proximal ileum
- ▢ **D.** Pyloric sphincter
- ▢ **E.** Ileocecal junction

139 A 43-year-old woman is admitted to the emergency department with esophageal pain and hematemesis after swallowing a fish bone. An endoscopic examination reveals perforation of the intraabdominal portion of the esophageal wall. Which of the following arteries is most likely injured?

- ▢ **A.** Branches of left gastric
- ▢ **B.** Bronchial
- ▢ **C.** Thoracic intercostal
- ▢ **D.** Branches of right gastric
- ▢ **E.** Right inferior phrenic

140 A 42-year-old patient is admitted to the hospital after suffering a ruptured spleen in a skiing accident. Physical examination reveals intense pain that radiates to the region of the left shoulder, presumably due to irritation of the diaphragm. Which of the following signs best describes this condition?

- ▢ **A.** Mittelschmerz
- ▢ **B.** Kerh's sign
- ▢ **C.** Rovsing's sign
- ▢ **D.** Psoas sign
- ▢ **E.** Obturator sign

141 A 43-year-old man is admitted to the hospital with a knife wound to the right lobe of the liver. After a laparotomy is performed, digital pressure (Pringle's maneuver) is applied to the hepatoduodenal ligament, but brisk bleeding continues, indicating a variation in the origin of the right hepatic artery. Which of the following is the most common variation in the arterial supply to the right lobe of the liver?

- ▢ **A.** The right hepatic originates from the gastroduodenal
- ▢ **B.** The right hepatic originates from the superior mesenteric

- ▢ **C.** The right hepatic originates from the left gastric
- ▢ **D.** The right hepatic originates from the left hepatic
- ▢ **E.** The right hepatic originates directly from the aorta

142 A 38-year-old woman is admitted to the hospital with signs of cholecystitis and gallbladder stones. During cholangiography, the catheter is inserted with difficulty into the gallbladder. Which of the following structures is most likely to interfere with the passage of the catheter into the cystic duct?

- ▢ **A.** Cystic duct compression by a hepatic artery
- ▢ **B.** Spiral valve (of Heister)
- ▢ **C.** Tortuosity of the cystic duct
- ▢ **D.** Adhesions from the hepatoduodenal ligament
- ▢ **E.** Portal vein compression of the cystic duct

143 A 57-year-old woman is admitted to the hospital with symptoms and signs of acute cholecystitis. Radiographic and physical examinations confirm the initial diagnosis, and a cholecystectomy is performed. On the fifth postoperative day the patient develops bile peritonitis. Which of the following conditions would most likely be responsible for such an outcome, assuming the cholecystectomy had been performed correctly?

- ▢ **A.** The common bile duct is leaking
- ▢ **B.** The ducts of Luschka are leaking
- ▢ **C.** The right hepatic duct is leaking
- ▢ **D.** The cystic duct is leaking
- ▢ **E.** The left hepatic duct is leaking

144 A 64-year-old man is admitted to the hospital with intense abdominal pain from a pancreatic tumor. A neurectomy is performed to interrupt the neural fibers supplying the pancreas. Which of the following neural fibers would be the most likely objective of the neurectomy?

- ▢ **A.** Sympathetic preganglionic
- ▢ **B.** Sympathetic postganglionic
- ▢ **C.** Visceral afferent
- ▢ **D.** Preganglionic parasympathetics
- ▢ **E.** Postganglionic parasympathetics

145 A 54-year-old man is admitted to the emergency department with a 2-day history of mild abdominal pain, in addition to bloating, nausea, vomiting, and poor appetite. Past medical history reveals that the patient has just recovered from a pneumonia infection. Radiographic examination reveals a paralytic ileus. Which of the followings signs would most likely be found during a physical examination?

- ▢ **A.** Increased bowel sounds
- ▢ **B.** Absent bowel sounds
- ▢ **C.** Borborygmi
- ▢ **D.** Crampy abdominal pain
- ▢ **E.** Localized tenderness

146 A 65-year-old man is admitted to the emergency department with complaints of nonspecific abdominal pain. Physical and radiographic examinations reveal mild intestinal ischemia due to atherosclerotic occlusion of the midproximal part of the superior mesenteric artery, but collateral blood supply has delayed the onset of necrosis. What vessels provide collateral channels between the celiac trunk and the superior mesenteric artery?

- ▢ **A.** Superior and inferior pancreaticoduodenal
- ▢ **B.** Left gastric and hepatic
- ▢ **C.** Cystic and gastroduodenal
- ▢ **D.** Right and left colic
- ▢ **E.** Right and left gastro-omental

147 A 22-year-old man is admitted to the emergency department with acute abdominal pain at his right lower quadrant. Radiographic and physical examinations provide evidence of acute appendicitis. An appendectomy is performed, beginning with an incision at the McBurney's point. Through which of the following abdominal layers must the surgeon pass to reach the appendix through this incision?

- ▢ **A.** External abdominal oblique muscle, internal oblique muscle, transversalis fascia, and parietal peritoneum
- ▢ **B.** Aponeurosis of the external abdominal oblique muscle, internal oblique muscle, transversus abdominis muscle, transversalis fascia, and parietal peritoneum
- ▢ **C.** Aponeurosis of the external abdominal oblique muscle, internal oblique muscle, transversus abdominis muscle, and parietal peritoneum
- ▢ **D.** Aponeurosis of the external abdominal oblique muscle, aponeurosis of internal oblique muscle, transversus abdominis muscle, transversalis fascia, and parietal peritoneum
- ▢ **E.** Aponeurosis of the external abdominal oblique muscle, aponeurosis of internal oblique muscle, aponeurosis of transversus abdominis muscle, transversalis fascia, and parietal peritoneum

148 A 12-year-old boy is admitted to the hospital with profuse rectal bleeding but appears to be free of any associated pain. Which of the following is the most common cause of severe rectal bleeding in the pediatric age group?

- ☐ **A.** Internal hemorrhoids
- ☐ **B.** External hemorrhoids
- ☐ **C.** Diverticulosis
- ☐ **D.** Ileal (Meckel's) diverticulum
- ☐ **E.** Borborygmi

149 A 48-year-old man is admitted to the hospital with abdominal distension and pain. The radiographic image is shown in Fig. 3-2. In which of the following locations will blood be detected with an ultrasound machine if the patient stands upright?

- ☐ **A.** Subphrenic space
- ☐ **B.** Hepatorenal space (pouch of Morison)
- ☐ **C.** Rectouterine space (pouch of Douglas)
- ☐ **D.** Rectovesical space
- ☐ **E.** Subhepatic space

150 A 27-year-old woman is admitted to the emergency department with markedly elevated temperature and abdominal pain. Physical examination initially indicates paraumbilical pain, but the site of origin of pain soon shifts to the right lower quadrant. A CT scan is shown in Fig. 3-3. Which of the following structures is affected?

- ☐ **A.** Right ovary
- ☐ **B.** Appendix
- ☐ **C.** Ileocecal junction
- ☐ **D.** Ascending colon
- ☐ **E.** Ileum

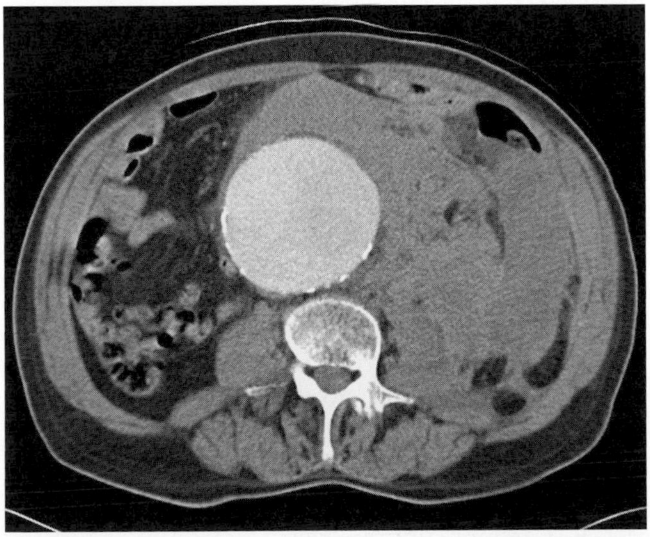

Fig. 3-2

151 A 51-year-old man complains of abdominal pain of 2-month duration. A CT scan of the patient's abdomen is shown in Fig. 3-4. An angiogram indicates that several arteries of the gastrointestinal tract are occluded due to atherosclerosis, producing bowel ischemia. Which of the following arteries is most likely occluded in the CT scan?

- ☐ **A.** Middle colic
- ☐ **B.** Right colic
- ☐ **C.** Left colic
- ☐ **D.** Ileocolic
- ☐ **E.** Marginal

152 A 53-year-old man visits the outpatient clinic because of an abnormal mass developing in his anal canal. An image from the physical examination is seen in Fig. 3-5. A biopsy of the tissue reveals squamous cell carcinoma of the anus. Which of the following lymph nodes will most typically first receive cancerous cells from the anal tumor?

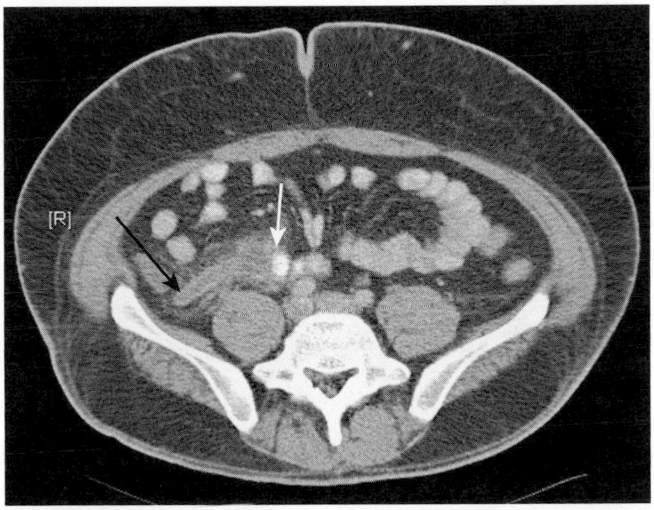

Fig. 3-3

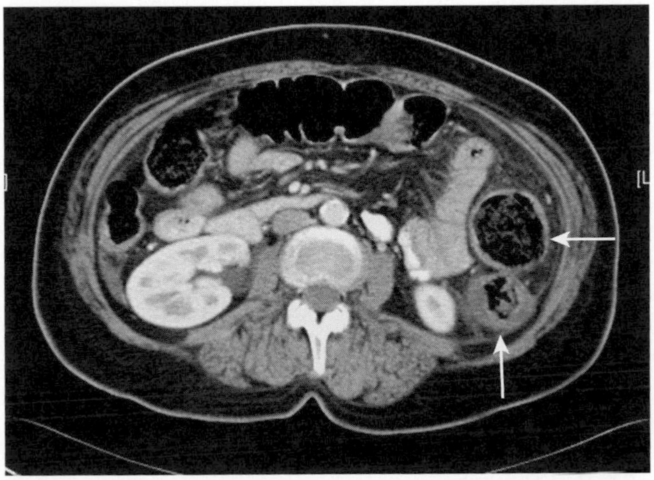

Fig. 3-4

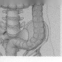

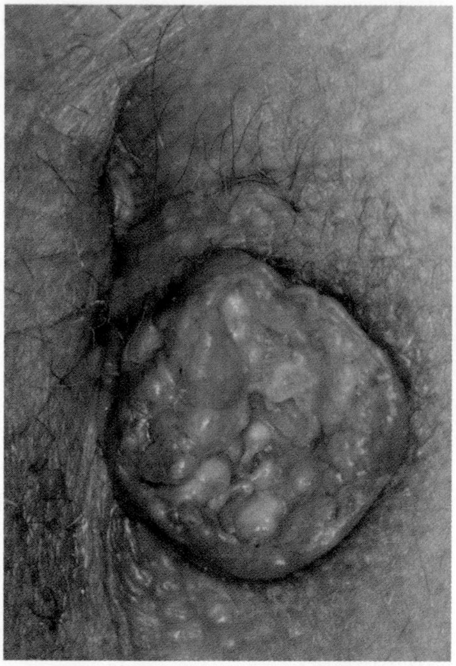

Fig. 3-5

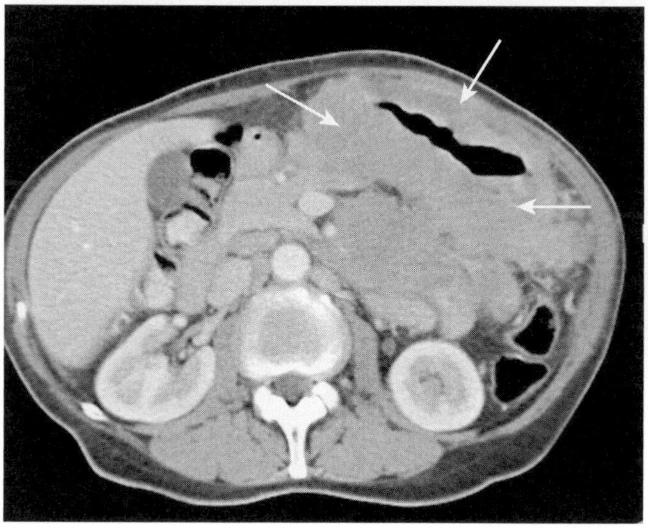

Fig. 3-6

- ▢ **A.** Deep inguinal lymph nodes
- ▢ **B.** Superficial inguinal lymph nodes
- ▢ **C.** Internal iliac nodes
- ▢ **D.** External iliac nodes
- ▢ **E.** Para-aortic nodes

153 A 49-year-old man comes to the outpatient clinic with complaints of bloating, gas, and a sense of fullness for the preceding 2 years. A CT scan examination is shown in Fig. 3-6. Which of the following structures is affected?

- ▢ **A.** Spleen
- ▢ **B.** Stomach

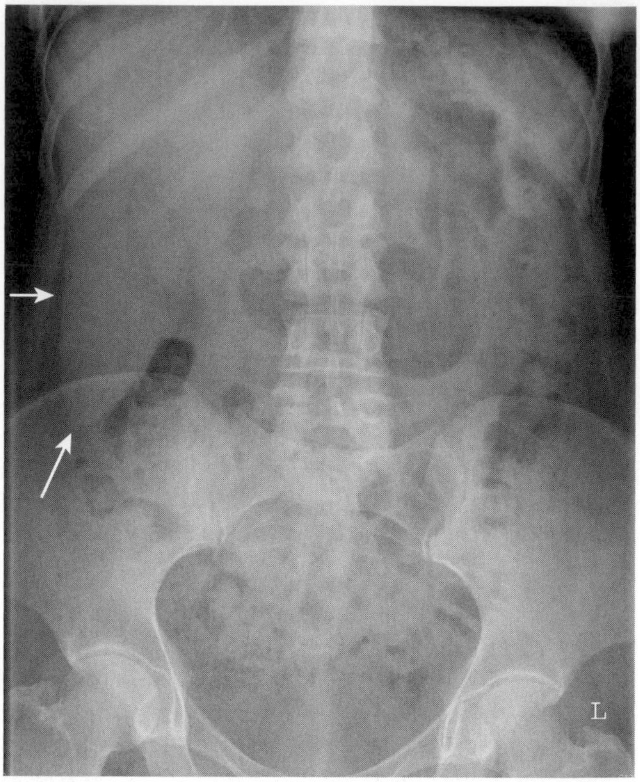

Fig. 3-7

- ▢ **C.** Duodenum
- ▢ **D.** Pancreas
- ▢ **E.** Descending colon

154 An endoscopic examination is performed on a 49-year-old patient with a preliminary diagnosis of a gastrointestinal cancer, and a tissue sample is sent for histopathologic examination. Biopsy reveals a gastric adenocarcinoma, and a total gastrectomy is performed. Which of the following lymph nodes will most likely first receive metastatic cells?

- ▢ **A.** Celiac
- ▢ **B.** Splenic
- ▢ **C.** Suprapancreatic
- ▢ **D.** Right gastric
- ▢ **E.** Cisterna chyli

155 A 28-year-old woman visits the outpatient clinic to receive the required physical examination for an insurance policy. Physical and laboratory examinations give evidence that she is probably a normal, healthy woman. A radiograph of the patient is shown in Fig. 3-7. Which of the following is the most likely diagnosis?

- ▢ **A.** Cholecystitis
- ▢ **B.** Carcinoma of the liver

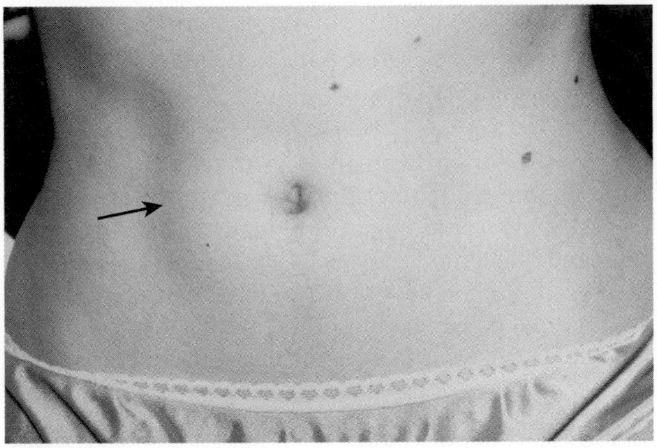

Fig. 3-8

- ▢ **C.** A caudal extension of the right hepatic lobe (Riedel's lobe)
- ▢ **D.** Pancreatic carcinoma
- ▢ **E.** Carcinoma of the stomach

156 A 35-year-old woman is admitted to the hospital with a mass protruding through her skin at the right lower quadrant. Physical examination reveals intestinal herniation, as shown in Fig. 3-8. Which of the following is the most likely diagnosis?

- ▢ **A.** Richter's hernia
- ▢ **B.** Spigelian hernia
- ▢ **C.** Paraumbilical
- ▢ **D.** Incisional hernia
- ▢ **E.** Ventral hernia

157 A 3-year-old boy is admitted to the pediatric clinic with a palpable mass in the right side of his scrotum, and a preliminary diagnosis is made of a congenital, indirect inguinal hernia. Which of the following is the most likely cause of an indirect inguinal hernia in this patient?

- ▢ **A.** The deep inguinal ring opens into an intact processus vaginalis
- ▢ **B.** Congenital hydrocele
- ▢ **C.** Ectopic testis
- ▢ **D.** Epispadias
- ▢ **E.** Rupture of the transversalis fascia

158 A 43-year-old woman visits the outpatient clinic with complaints of chronic dysphagia and gastroesophageal reflux. An endoscopic examination reveals achalasia of the cardia of the stomach. Which of the following is the most likely cause of this condition?

- ▢ **A.** Failure of relaxation of the lower esophageal sphincter
- ▢ **B.** Dyspepsia
- ▢ **C.** Gastritis
- ▢ **D.** Gastroparesis
- ▢ **E.** Peptic ulcer

159 A 21-year-old man is admitted to the hospital with periumbilical pain. A CT scan examination reveals internal bleeding about 2 feet proximal to the ileocecal junction. Which of the following is the most likely diagnosis?

- ▢ **A.** Ruptured appendix
- ▢ **B.** Volvulus
- ▢ **C.** Diverticulosis
- ▢ **D.** Ileal (Meckel's) diverticulum
- ▢ **E.** Borborygmi

160 A 45-year-old man is admitted to the hospital with pain in the right upper quadrant, with radiation to the tip of his scapula. Radiographic examination reveals gallbladder stones, with associated cholecystitis. An open cholecystectomy is performed, using a Kocher incision (along the right costal margin). Which of the following nerves are most likely at risk during this incision?

- ▢ **A.** T5, T6
- ▢ **B.** T6 to T8
- ▢ **C.** T7, T8
- ▢ **D.** T9 to L1
- ▢ **E.** T5 to T9

161 A 3-year-old girl is admitted to the pediatric clinic because of a palpable right inguinal mass. An open surgical procedure is performed. Digital pressure is used to return organ contents of the hernia to the abdomen. A sac of peritoneum can be seen clearly, protruding from the internal ring. Which of the following terms is most accurate for the origin of this structure?

- ▢ **A.** A patent processus vaginalis (canal of Nuck)
- ▢ **B.** Congenital hydrocele
- ▢ **C.** Ectopic uterus
- ▢ **D.** Femoral hernia
- ▢ **E.** Rupture of the transversalis fascia

162 A 48-year-old woman was scheduled for radiographic examination because of severe abdominal pain. The imaging gave evidence of a pancreatic pseudocyst. Which of the following is the typical topographic location for this type of pseudocyst?

- ▢ **A.** Right subhepatic space
- ▢ **B.** Hepatorenal space
- ▢ **C.** Omental bursa

- ☐ **D.** Right subphrenic space
- ☐ **E.** Greater sac

163 A 38-year-old man is examined in the outpatient clinic because of his complaint of mild abdominal pain of 2 years' duration. Upon examination, it is observed that the pain is dull and located principally in the left upper quadrant around the xiphoid process. An endoscopic examination reveals that the patient suffers from a gastric ulcer. At which of the following spinal nerve levels are the neuronal cell bodies located for the sensory fibers in such a case of gastric ulcer?

- ☐ **A.** T5, T6
- ☐ **B.** T6 to T8
- ☐ **C.** T7, T8
- ☐ **D.** T9 to L1
- ☐ **E.** T5 to T9

164 A 43-year-old man is admitted to the hospital with abdominal pain and vomiting. A CT scan examination reveals that the patient has an internal hernia involving his duodenum at the fossa of Landzert. An exploratory laparotomy reveals a paraduodenal hernia. Which of the following arteries is most at risk during the repair of this hernia?

- ☐ **A.** Middle colic
- ☐ **B.** Sigmoidal
- ☐ **C.** Ileocolic
- ☐ **D.** Ileal
- ☐ **E.** Ascending branches of left colic

165 A 42-year-old man with jaundice is admitted to the hospital with severe pain that radiates to his back. A CT scan examination reveals a tumor at the neck of the pancreas. A biopsy reveals a ductular adenocarcinoma. Which of the following structures will first receive metastatic cells?

- ☐ **A.** Stomach
- ☐ **B.** Spleen
- ☐ **C.** Duodenum
- ☐ **D.** Liver
- ☐ **E.** Vertebral column

166 A major vessel appears to be nearly occluded in a 42-year-old male patient diagnosed with ductular adenocarcinoma. A CT scan examination has clearly demonstrated the tumor is at the neck of the pancreas. Which of the following vessels would be the most likely to be obstructed?

- ☐ **A.** Inferior mesenteric vein
- ☐ **B.** Portal vein
- ☐ **C.** Celiac trunk
- ☐ **D.** Posterior superior pancreaticoduodenal artery
- ☐ **E.** Greater pancreatic artery

167 A 49-year-old woman is admitted to the hospital with abdominal pain. Physical examination reveals epigastric pain that migrates toward the patient's right side and posteriorly toward the scapula. She is not jaundiced. Radiologic examination reveals cholecystitis with a large gallstone and no jaundice. In which of the following structures is the gallstone most likely located?

- ☐ **A.** Common bile duct
- ☐ **B.** Hartmann's pouch
- ☐ **C.** Left hepatic duct
- ☐ **D.** Pancreatic duct
- ☐ **E.** Right hepatic duct

168 A 47-year-old woman is admitted to the hospital with jaundice and epigastric pain that migrates toward the patient's right side and posteriorly toward the scapula. Radiographic examination reveals cholecystitis with a large gallstone. Which of the following is the most likely site for a gallstone to lodge?

- ☐ **A.** Common bile duct
- ☐ **B.** Hepatopancreatic ampulla (of Vater)
- ☐ **C.** Left hepatic duct
- ☐ **D.** Pancreatic duct
- ☐ **E.** Right hepatic duct

169 A 40-year-old man of nine children agrees with his wife to have a vasectomy. During the operation the urologist separates the layers of the spermatic cord to expose the ductus deferens so that it can be ligated and cut. From what structure is the internal spermatic fascial covering derived?

- ☐ **A.** Internal oblique muscle
- ☐ **B.** Cremaster muscle
- ☐ **C.** External abdominal oblique muscle fascia
- ☐ **D.** Transversus abdominis aponeurosis
- ☐ **E.** Transversalis fascia

170 A 26-year-old woman has a nonpainful hernia in the midline of the abdominal wall, several inches above the level of the umbilicus. Which of the following hernias will most likely characterize this condition?

- ☐ **A.** Umbilical hernia
- ☐ **B.** Spigelian hernia
- ☐ **C.** Epigastric hernia
- ☐ **D.** Femoral hernia
- ☐ **E.** Omphalocele

171 A 23-year-old man suffered a knife wound to the epigastric region. At laparotomy, when the abdomen is opened for inspection, it is seen that an injury to the liver occurred between the bed of the gallbladder and the falciform ligament, and the wound is bleeding profusely. The Pringle maneuver is performed with a non-traumatic vascular clamp, but blood continues spurting from the surface of the liver. Which part of the liver and which artery is most likely injured?

- ☐ **A.** Lateral segment of the left lobe and the left hepatic artery
- ☐ **B.** Caudate segment of the liver, with injury both to right and left hepatic arteries
- ☐ **C.** Anterior segment of the right lobe, with injury to the right hepatic artery
- ☐ **D.** Medial segment of the left lobe, with injury to an aberrant left hepatic artery
- ☐ **E.** Quadrate lobe, with injury to the middle hepatic branch of the right hepatic artery

172 A 47-year-old male patient had undergone bilateral vagotomy, with division of both vagus trunks at the esophageal hiatus, to relieve his chronic difficulty with peptic ulcers. Which of the following conditions will most likely occur?

- ☐ **A.** Parasympathetic supply to the descending colon is lost.
- ☐ **B.** The patient would no longer have contraction of the urinary bladder.
- ☐ **C.** The patient would become impotent.
- ☐ **D.** The patient would be sterile because of paralysis of the ductus deferens and ejaculatory duct.
- ☐ **E.** Parasympathetic supply to the ascending colon would be reduced or absent.

173 A 35-year-old male accountant was brought to the emergency department with the complaint of intense abdominal pain of 1-hour duration. His abdomen was distended, rigid, did not move in respiration, and was painful to palpation. He had adynamic (paralytic) ileus resulting from a peptic ulcer, although there was very little bleeding into the peritoneal cavity. He complained that he had pain in his right shoulder. Which of the following conditions will most likely occur?

- ☐ **A.** Radiographs would not reveal the presence of air under his diaphragm.
- ☐ **B.** Borborygmi would be decreased in frequency and amplitude.
- ☐ **C.** He probably suffered from a posterior penetrating ulcer rather than from an anterior perforating ulcer.
- ☐ **D.** The patient's ulcer probably occurred in the second part of the duodenum.
- ☐ **E.** The patient probably had acute appendicitis.

174 A 68-year-old woman had been suffering long-term effects of diverticulosis and inflammation of the transverse colon. To permit operating on a patient with severe diverticulosis of the transverse colon, it would be necessary to first ligate (tie off) or clamp the source of arterial supply. Which of the following arteries will most likely be ligated?

- ☐ **A.** Middle colic
- ☐ **B.** Right colic
- ☐ **C.** Superior mesenteric
- ☐ **D.** Ileocolic
- ☐ **E.** Left colic

175 A hard mass (a fecalith) in the ostium of a 27-year-old patient's appendix had led to a local infection (appendicitis) with a slightly elevated temperature and a moderate increase in WBC count. The initial pain from the infection was dull and difficult to localize, but the patient placed his hand in the periumbilical area to indicate the general area of discomfort. The region of the umbilicus receives its sensory supply, classically, from which of the following spinal nerves?

- ☐ **A.** T7
- ☐ **B.** T8
- ☐ **C.** T10
- ☐ **D.** T12
- ☐ **E.** L1

176 A 55-year-old man had been unsuccessfully treated for alcoholism for 3 years. He was admitted to the hospital for emergency medical treatment for severe portal hypertension. Which of the following is a feature of the development of severe portal hypertension?

- ☐ **A.** Esophageal varices—from increased pressure in the right gastric vein
- ☐ **B.** Ascites—from effusion of fluid from the inferior mesenteric vein
- ☐ **C.** Internal hemorrhoids—from increased pressure within the superior mesenteric vein and its tributaries
- ☐ **D.** Expansion of veins within the falciform ligament, which anastomose with veins of the umbilical region
- ☐ **E.** Recanalization and expansion of the vessels within the medial umbilical ligaments

177 In performing a laparoscopic hernia repair on a 24-year-old female gymnast, the surgical resident observed the bright reflection provided by the tissues of the iliopubic tract. The iliopubic tract could be traced medially to the site of the femoral herniation. The iliopubic tract is best characterized by which of the following statements?

- ▢ **A.** The iliopubic tract represents the aponeurotic origin of the transversus abdominis.
- ▢ **B.** The iliopubic tract forms the lateral border of the inguinal triangle (of Hesselbach).
- ▢ **C.** The iliopubic tract forms the lateral border of the femoral ring.
- ▢ **D.** The iliopubic tract is the part of the inguinal ligament that attaches to the pectineal ligament.
- ▢ **E.** The iliopubic tract is the lateral extension of the pectineal ligament.

178 A 47-year-old man had been scheduled for an appendectomy. During the open operative procedure it was discovered that atypical embryologic rotation of the intestine, adhesions, and adipose tissue made it somewhat difficult to find the appendix. Most commonly, the vermiform appendix is best located by locating and tracing which of the following?

- ▢ **A.** Anterior cecal artery
- ▢ **B.** Descending branch of the right colic artery
- ▢ **C.** Ileum to the ileocecal juncture
- ▢ **D.** Posterior cecal artery
- ▢ **E.** Taeniae coli of the ascending colon

179 A 5-day-old male infant presents with abdominal distention, constipation, and vomiting. A CT scan reveals an abnormally dilated descending colon and a diagnosis of Hirschsprung's disease (megacolon) is made. What is the embryologic mechanism responsible for Hirschsprung's disease?

- ▢ **A.** Failure of neural crest cells to migrate into the walls of the colon
- ▢ **B.** Incomplete separation of the cloaca
- ▢ **C.** Failure of recanalization of the colon
- ▢ **D.** Defective rotation of the hindgut
- ▢ **E.** Oligohydramnios

180 A 32-year-old man visits his family physician complaining of groin pain. Examination reveals that the patient has an indirect inguinal hernia. Which nerve is most likely responsible for the pain transmission?

- ▢ **A.** Iliohypogastric
- ▢ **B.** Lateral femoral cutaneous
- ▢ **C.** Ilioinguinal
- ▢ **D.** Lumbar splanchnic
- ▢ **E.** Greater splanchnic

181 A 35-year-old immune-compromised woman is suffering from herpes zoster (shingles). She presents with a severe sharp burning pain and vesicular eruption on the skin around the umbilicus. Which spinal nerve contributes to this dermatome?

- ▢ **A.** T8
- ▢ **B.** T9
- ▢ **C.** T10
- ▢ **D.** T11
- ▢ **E.** T12

182 A 68-year-old woman is diagnosed with a posterior abdominal wall tumor that has invaded the superior mesenteric plexus. Which structure will most likely be affected?

- ▢ **A.** Ascending colon
- ▢ **B.** Rectum
- ▢ **C.** Stomach
- ▢ **D.** Descending colon
- ▢ **E.** Kidney

183 A 35-year-old woman visits her general practitioner after an appendectomy complaining of paresthesia (numbness) over the anterior part of her right labium majus. Which nerve was most likely traumatized during the procedure?

- ▢ **A.** Iliohypogastric and ilioinguinal
- ▢ **B.** Ilioinguinal
- ▢ **C.** Genital branch of genitofemoral
- ▢ **D.** Subcostal
- ▢ **E.** Obturator

184 A 54-year-old man underwent a gastroscopy, which revealed a tumor in the pyloric antrum of the stomach. A CT scan was ordered to evaluate lymph node involvement. Which of the following nodes initially drain the pyloric antrum?

- ▢ **A.** Celiac
- ▢ **B.** Superior mesenteric
- ▢ **C.** Inferior mesenteric
- ▢ **D.** Lumbar
- ▢ **E.** Hepatic

185 A 21-year-old football player is admitted to the emergency department with severe back pain. A radiograph reveals a fractured angle of the eleventh rib on the left side. Which of the following organs is most likely at risk for injury?

- ▢ **A.** Stomach
- ▢ **B.** Descending colon
- ▢ **C.** Kidney
- ▢ **D.** Liver
- ▢ **E.** Pancreas

186 A 32-year-old woman is admitted to the hospital for complaints of upper abdominal pain. A CT scan shows evidence of an ulcer in the posterior wall of the duodenal cap. Which structure will most likely be affected if the ulcer perforates?

- ▢ **A.** Hepatic portal vein
- ▢ **B.** Superior mesenteric artery
- ▢ **C.** Bile duct
- ▢ **D.** Proper hepatic artery
- ▢ **E.** Gastroduodenal artery

187 A 45-year-old man is admitted to the hospital with groin pain and a palpable mass just superior to the inguinal ligament. The patient is diagnosed with a hernia and surgical repair is performed. During the operation, the surgeon found a loop of intestine in the deep inguinal ring. Which type of hernia is this?

- ▢ **A.** Direct inguinal
- ▢ **B.** Umbilical
- ▢ **C.** Femoral
- ▢ **D.** Lumbar
- ▢ **E.** Indirect inguinal

188 A 67-year-old woman is admitted to the hospital with severe abdominal pain. Gastroscopy and a CT scan reveal a perforating ulcer in the posterior wall of the stomach, spilling stomach contents and blood directly into which of the following areas?

- ▢ **A.** Right subhepatic space
- ▢ **B.** Hepatorenal space
- ▢ **C.** Omental bursa (lesser sac)
- ▢ **D.** Right subphrenic space
- ▢ **E.** Greater sac

189 A 55-year-old woman is admitted to the emergency department with severe abdominal pain. She had a history of peptic ulcer disease and recently resumed a course of nonsteroidal antiinflammatory drugs for arthritis pain of her knees. During physical examination the abdomen is flat, firm, and generally tender with guarding and rebound tenderness. An ultrasound examination of the abdomen reveals intraperitoneal fluid. A diagnosis of perforated peptic ulcer is established and the patient is undergoing a laparotomy. Which of the following sites is least likely to show fluid collection in this patient?

- ▢ **A.** Morison's pouch
- ▢ **B.** The rectouterine pouch
- ▢ **C.** The right paracolic gutter
- ▢ **D.** The greater sac
- ▢ **E.** The omental bursa

190 A 45-year-old woman is admitted to the emergency department with severe right sided lower abdominal pain for 1 day. Two days ago the pain was poorly localized to the umbilical region. During physical examination the abdomen is flat, firm, and tender maximally at McBurney's point. There is guarding and rebound tenderness and bowel sounds are decreased. Ultrasound examination reveals fluid in the right paracolic gutter. Which mechanism best explains the initial periumbilical pain this patient experienced?

- ▢ **A.** Sympathetic supply to the appendix and somatic sensation to the umbilicus share the same spinal cord levels.
- ▢ **B.** Parasympathetic supply to the appendix share the same spinal cord levels with the umbilicus.
- ▢ **C.** Somatic afferents of the peritoneum were stimulated by the inflamed appendix.
- ▢ **D.** Somatic afferents travel with visceral afferents to T10 spinal cord level.
- ▢ **E.** Somatic afferents synapse with visceral afferents of T10 spinal cord level.

191 A 45-year-old woman is admitted to the emergency department with abdominal pain and vomiting for the past day. She has a history of gastroesophageal reflux disease and was previously diagnosed with gallstones. Initially, her pain was poorly localized at the epigastric region, but became sharp and well localized in the right hypochondrium. Physical examination elicits a positive Murphy's sign. What mechanism best explains the initial pattern of pain?

- ▢ **A.** Visceral afferent fibers synapse with sympathetic fibers at T7 to T9 spinal cord levels
- ▢ **B.** Visceral afferent and sympathetic fibers to the gallbladder share T7 to T9 spinal cord levels
- ▢ **C.** Gallbladder inflammation spread to diaphragmatic peritoneum supplied by phrenic nerve
- ▢ **D.** The inflamed gallbladder contacted the abdominal peritoneum at dermatomes T7 to T9

- ☐ **E.** Visceral afferents travel with intercostal nerves back to T7 to T9 spinal cord levels

192 A 28-year-old woman delivers an infant boy at term after an uneventful pregnancy. The intern on call reported that there was clear fluid draining from the umbilicus of the infant. The nurse is asked to collect some of the fluid and performed a urine dipstick test on the same. The fluid was determined to be urine. Which of the following developmental defects is most likely to explain this finding?

- ☐ **A.** Obliterated distal end of the urachus
- ☐ **B.** Obliterated proximal end of the urachus
- ☐ **C.** Completely patent urachus
- ☐ **D.** Patent urachus at one point along its length
- ☐ **E.** Completely obliterated urachus

193 A 33-year-old woman is admitted to the emergency department with complaints of sharp, well demarcated, right-sided abdominal pain for one day, associated with fever, vomiting, and loose stools. During physical examination her abdomen is flat, firm, and generally tender. Maximal tenderness and pain occurred at the McBurney's point, and a rebound tenderness test was performed. A urine human chorionic gonadotropin (HCG) test was negative. What mechanism correctly explains the distribution of pain in this patient?

- ☐ **A.** Visceral afferents of the appendix travel with sympathetics to T10 spinal cord level
- ☐ **B.** Inflamed visceral peritoneum stimulates somatic intercostal nerves
- ☐ **C.** The appendix is a midgut structure, thus, pain is referred to T10 and T11 dermatomes
- ☐ **D.** Contact of inflamed appendix with visceral peritoneum stimulates visceral afferents
- ☐ **E.** Contact of inflamed appendix with parietal peritoneum stimulates somatic afferents

194 An 81-year-old man is admitted to the emergency department with complaints of left side abdominal pain and fever for the past 2 days. Physical examination reveals a soft and tender abdomen but in the left lumbar region there is a firm mass. The psoas sign was negative and bowel sounds were decreased. CT scan of the abdomen showed evidence of a large perinephric abscess. Which of the following will most likely describe the fluid location?

- ☐ **A.** Between renal fascia and transversalis fascia
- ☐ **B.** Between the renal capsule and renal fascia
- ☐ **C.** Between transversalis fascia and peritoneal fascia
- ☐ **D.** Between the renal cortex and renal capsule
- ☐ **E.** Within the paranephric fat

195 A 55-year-old woman is admitted to the emergency department with complaints of abdominal pain. The pain was epigastric, burning in nature, and occurred after eating spicy or greasy foods. It improved with chewable antacids and was not associated with shortness of breath, or diaphoresis. The physician diagnosed the patient with gastroesophageal reflux disease. Which of the following organs is not derived from the same embryological structure as this patient's stomach?

- ☐ **A.** Spleen
- ☐ **B.** Right bronchus
- ☐ **C.** Second part of the duodenum
- ☐ **D.** Tail of the pancreas
- ☐ **E.** Right lobe of the liver

196 A 45-year-old woman presented to the ER with a one-day history of severe abdominal pain, vomiting, and fever. Two days previously the pain was poorly localized to the epigastrium but became sharp in nature and located in the right hypochondrium region. She now complains of the pain radiating to the right shoulder and scapular region. On physical examination, she is febrile (T 40°C), with dry mucous membranes, icteric, with a soft and tender abdomen and a positive Murphy's sign. Abdominal ultrasound reveals thickening of the wall of the gallbladder but no free fluid in the abdomen. Blood chemistry shows elevation of serum bilirubin. Endoscopic retrograde cholangiopancreatography shows an obstruction along the extrahepatic biliary tree with normal pancreatic duct flow. Which structure is most likely to be obstructed in this patient's condition?

- ☐ **A.** The infundibulum of the gallbladder
- ☐ **B.** The cystic duct
- ☐ **C.** The common bile duct
- ☐ **D.** The hepatopancreatic ampulla
- ☐ **E.** The left hepatic duct

197 A 72-year-old woman has abdominal pain, fever, vomiting, diarrhea, and anorexia. She had a history of atrial fibrillation but refused to take warfarin because it made her feel unwell. She is admitted to the emergency department looking ill, pale, and with dry mucous membranes. Vital signs: P140 bpm, BP 90/50, RR 20/min, T 40°C. The abdomen was distended and tender in the epigastrium and umbilical areas. There was guarding and rebound tenderness. Bowel sounds were absent. An erect abdominal radiograph showed dilated small bowel with air-fluid levels with a "stacked coins" appearance. A diagnosis of mesenteric ischemia secondary to embolus to intestinal vessel(s) was made. If the superior mesenteric artery was occluded, how could the midgut receive its blood supply?

- ▢ **A.** Anastomosis between left and right gastric arteries
- ▢ **B.** Anastomosis between left and right gastroepiploic arteries
- ▢ **C.** Anastomosis between left and right gastro-omental arteries
- ▢ **D.** Anastomosis between superior and inferior pancreaticoduodenal arteries
- ▢ **E.** Anastomosis between adjacent short gastric arteries

198 A 72-year-old woman is admitted to the emergency department with complaints of abdominal pain. The onset of pain was sudden and severe about 1 hour before presentation. The patient had a history of diverticular disease, cigarette smoking, and alcohol abuse. On examination, he was in painful distress and diaphoretic. Vital signs: P110 bpm, BP 100/50, RR 30/min, afebrile. The abdomen was firm with tenderness in the epigastrium, guarding, and rebound tenderness. A CT abdomen showed pneumoperitoneum under the diaphragm. Laparotomy revealed a perforation of the posterior wall of the third part of the duodenum. Which of the following structure(s) are most likely in immediate danger in this patient?

- ▢ **A.** Aorta and inferior vena cava
- ▢ **B.** Superior mesenteric artery and vein
- ▢ **C.** Head of the pancreas
- ▢ **D.** Transverse colon
- ▢ **E.** Greater curvature of the stomach

199 A 51-year-old man is admitted to the emergency department after a 2-month history of difficulty swallowing, vomiting, and weight loss. The patient had a history of gastroesophageal reflux disease and was treated with antibiotics for *Helicobacter pylori* 10 years previously. He also had a 20-pack year history of cigarette smoking. On physical examination, the abdomen was soft and nontender. An ultrasound examination revealed a 4 × 6 cm hard, irregular nonpulsatile and nontender mass resembling a Sister Mary Joseph nodule in the umbilical area. An abdominal CT scan revealed a large mass involving the stomach in the region of the lesser curvature. What other structure(s) are most likely at immediate risk of damage by the tumor in this patient?

- ▢ **A.** Right and left gastroepiploic vessels
- ▢ **B.** Right and left pancreaticoduodenal vessels
- ▢ **C.** Right and left gastric vessels
- ▢ **D.** The portal triad
- ▢ **E.** Short gastric vessels

200 A 55-year-old woman presents with complaints of weight loss, pale colored stool, and tea-colored urine to the emergency department. Lab blood tests are as follows: serum bilirubin = 5 mg/dL, elevated alanine aminotransferase (ALT), aspartate aminotransferase (AST), alkaline phosphatase (ALP), gamma-glutamyl transferase (GGT), and increased prothrombin time. Physical examination reveals yellowing of the sclerae. She is diagnosed with cholestasis. An ultrasound performed reveals dilation of the biliary tree. During laparoscopic cholecystectomy, it is found that the patient has an aberrant cystic artery. What are the boundaries of the triangle of Calot?

- ▢ **A.** Inferior border of the left ventricle (LV), cystic duct, common hepatic duct
- ▢ **B.** Gallbladder, hepatic duct, bile duct
- ▢ **C.** Inferior border of LV, bile duct, common hepatic duct
- ▢ **D.** Cystic artery, inferior border of LV, bile duct
- ▢ **E.** Cystic artery, common hepatic duct, bile duct

201 A 10-year-old boy is imaged following an injury while camping. A laceration of the body of the pancreas is seen with hemorrhage around the vessel traveling along the superior border of the pancreas. Which vessel is this?

- ▢ **A.** Superior mesenteric artery
- ▢ **B.** Portal vein
- ▢ **C.** Left gastric artery
- ▢ **D.** Splenic artery
- ▢ **E.** Left gastro-omental artery

202 A 5-year-old girl is brought to the emergency department because of fever and severe abdominal pain. Acute appendicitis is diagnosed. In the emergency department, she keeps her right thigh flexed and resists extension at the hip. If the thigh is extended there is severe pain caused by stretching the irritated parietal peritoneum lying over which muscle?

- ▢ **A.** Psoas major
- ▢ **B.** External abdominal oblique
- ▢ **C.** Obturator internus
- ▢ **D.** Transversus abdominis
- ▢ **E.** Quadratus lumborum

203 A 40-year-old woman with a history of obesity and diabetes develops abdominal pain. Lab results and ultrasound examination support a diagnosis of acute cholecystitis. The patient undergoes a laparoscopic cholecystectomy. Which of the following structures would most likely be identified and ligated within the triangle of Calot?

- ▢ **A.** Bile duct
- ▢ **B.** Right hepatic duct
- ▢ **C.** Cystic duct
- ▢ **D.** Right hepatic artery
- ▢ **E.** Cystic artery

204 A 34-year-old man is admitted to the hospital after a car crash. A CT scan reveals a lacerated spleen which requires an urgent splenectomy. During the procedure, the surgeon ligates the blood supply of the spleen at its hilum. Improper placement of the ligature may occlude the artery that supplies which of the following structures?

- ▢ **A.** Fundus of the stomach
- ▢ **B.** Kidney
- ▢ **C.** Pyloric sphincter
- ▢ **D.** Head of the pancreas
- ▢ **E.** Splenic flexure of the colon

205 A 55-year-old man with a history of portal hypertension is brought to the emergency department with severe abdominal pain. A CT scan of his chest, at the vertebra level T7, reveals a circular grey structure immediately anterior to the vertebral bodies and just to the right of midline. The structure appears to be much larger than usual. Given the location and the patient's history what is this structure?

- ▢ **A.** Inferior vena cava
- ▢ **B.** Superior vena cava
- ▢ **C.** Esophagus
- ▢ **D.** Azygos vein
- ▢ **E.** Pulmonary vein

206 A 45-year-old man is admitted to the surgical ward for a scheduled procedure to remove a renal cell carcinoma. The CT scan reveals the renal cell carcinoma is confined within the renal fascia of the right kidney. Using a posterolateral approach to reach the kidney which of the following layers will most likely have to be incised?

- ▢ **A.** Parietal pleura
- ▢ **B.** Diaphragmatic pleura
- ▢ **C.** Parietal peritoneum
- ▢ **D.** Transversalis fascia
- ▢ **E.** Visceral peritoneum

207 A 43-year-old man is admitted to the emergency department with a severe upper right quadrant abdominal pain. An ultrasonographic examination reveals thickened inflamed gallbladder walls and several large echogenic gallstones. During laparoscopic cholecystectomy the scope is passed into the greater sac through a small port in the anterior abdominal wall. Which organ is the surgeon unable to view directly?

- ▢ **A.** Ileum
- ▢ **B.** Jejunum
- ▢ **C.** Pancreas
- ▢ **D.** Stomach
- ▢ **E.** Transverse colon

208 A 25-year-old man visits the gastroenterology outpatient clinic because of several episodes of dark blood in his stools for the past 2 weeks. A stool examination confirms blood. A CT scan shows no tumors in the abdomen or rectum. A technetium-99 scan shows a 2-inch long spot of radioactive accumulation in the midabdomen. Which of the following is the most likely diagnosis?

- ▢ **A.** Gastritis
- ▢ **B.** Hirschsprung's disease
- ▢ **C.** Hemorrhoids
- ▢ **D.** Meckel diverticulum
- ▢ **E.** Anal fissure

209 A 21-year-old man presents to the emergency department with fever and a high white blood cell count. He reports having suffered a small stab wound in his back a few months ago. Because it was a shallow wound, he did not seek medical attention. The physician states that he has a retroperitoneal abdominal infection. Which of the following structures is most likely to be affected?

- ▢ **A.** Descending colon
- ▢ **B.** Jejunum
- ▢ **C.** Stomach
- ▢ **D.** Transverse colon
- ▢ **E.** Appendix

210 A 68-year-old man complained of acute onset low back pain on the right with concomitant loss of sensation of the skin in the posterolateral gluteal and anterior pubic regions on the right side. During the physical examination, the patient experienced severe pain inferior to the twelfth rib at the right costovertebral angle when the physician palpated there. The physician also found that the patient had paralysis of the right internal oblique and transversus abdominis muscles. An abdominal CT scan revealed a tumor that originated in the right kidney, broke through the center of the posterior renal capsule and pressed on the ipsilateral quadratus lumborum muscle. Which of the following nerves was most likely compressed by the tumor?

- ☐ **A.** Subcostal
- ☐ **B.** Lateral cutaneous nerve of thigh
- ☐ **C.** Ilioinguinal
- ☐ **D.** Femoral
- ☐ **E.** Iliohypogastric

211 A 15-year-old boy who is an amateur bodybuilder has dreams of one day becoming a professional bodybuilder. To that end, he begins an intensive abdominal workout routine consisting of sit-ups and crunches to develop his "6-pack." The muscle that this adolescent is isolating in his workout to get the "6-pack" look attaches to which of the following skeletal areas?

- ☐ **A.** Iliac crest
- ☐ **B.** Ribs 10 to 12
- ☐ **C.** Pubic crest
- ☐ **D.** Costal cartilages 7 to 12
- ☐ **E.** Xiphoid process

212 A 52-year-old man with a long history of alcoholic cirrhosis complained of severe dysphagia and retrosternal "burning" pain. During esophagoscopy, the endoscopist advanced the endoscope until its tip reached the esophageal hiatus of the diaphragm. At which of the following vertebral levels did the tip of the endoscope most likely end?

- ☐ **A.** T7
- ☐ **B.** T8
- ☐ **C.** T10
- ☐ **D.** T11
- ☐ **E.** T12

213 The following statement was written in an abdominal surgery report: "The patient's abdominal aortic aneurysm was repaired using an endovascular graft where the center of the graft was in-line with the subcostal plane." Based on this information, the center of the graft was most likely anterior to which of the following vertebrae?

- ☐ **A.** L1
- ☐ **B.** L2
- ☐ **C.** L3
- ☐ **D.** L4
- ☐ **E.** L5

214 A 59-year-old man with a long history of alcoholism and cirrhosis underwent a right hepatectomy. During the surgery the surgeon divided the liver in the principal plane. Which of the following liver segments were most likely removed by the surgeon?

- ☐ **A.** V, VI, VII, VIII
- ☐ **B.** IV, V, VI, VII
- ☐ **C.** III, IV, V, VI
- ☐ **D.** II, III, IV, V
- ☐ **E.** I, II, III, IV

215 A 50-year-old man with a long history of alcohol abuse staggers into the emergency department and complains of severe abdominal pain. Physical examination of his abdomen reveals caput medusae. The blood vessel that is obstructed in this patient is most likely formed by the union of which of the following vessels?

- ☐ **A.** Right and left common iliac arteries
- ☐ **B.** Superior mesenteric and left gastric veins
- ☐ **C.** Inferior mesenteric and left gastric veins
- ☐ **D.** Inferior mesenteric and paraumbilical veins
- ☐ **E.** Superior mesenteric and splenic veins

216 A patient was found to have a tumor in the middle of the posterior wall of the stomach that perforated the stomach at this location. Diagnostic imaging revealed that stomach fluid had traversed the resultant aperture. Which of the following spaces did the fluid most likely first enter after it traversed the aperture?

- ☐ **A.** Supracolic compartment
- ☐ **B.** Omental foramen
- ☐ **C.** Infracolic compartment
- ☐ **D.** Paracolic gutter
- ☐ **E.** Omental bursa

217 An abdominal computed tomography scan of a 68-year-old woman revealed complete occlusion of her inferior vena cava at the L3 vertebral level. As a result of the occlusion, which of the following veins most likely acted as collateral channels to allow blood to flow from the lower to upper parts of her body?

- ☐ **A.** Left common iliac
- ☐ **B.** Hemiazygos
- ☐ **C.** Ascending lumbar
- ☐ **D.** Azygos
- ☐ **E.** Left renal

218 A 19-year-old gang member was shot with a 9-mm bullet in his right lower quadrant. The bullet entered and traversed the anterolateral abdominal wall. The following structures form the layers of this wall.

- ☐ **1.** Internal oblique muscle
- ☐ **2.** Transversalis fascia

- ▢ **3.** Transversus abdominis muscle
- ▢ **4.** Camper fascia
- ▢ **5.** Scarpa fascia
- ▢ **6.** External oblique muscle

Which of the following best represents the order of structures traversed by the bullet?

- ▢ **A.** 4-5-6-1-3-2
- ▢ **B.** 4-5-2-6-1-3
- ▢ **C.** 4-5-1-6-3-2
- ▢ **D.** 4-2-6-1-3-5
- ▢ **E.** 5-4-6-1-3-2

219 A 72-year-old man with a family history of colon cancer is referred for colonoscopy. The scope typically passes through the entire colon in order to examine for any abnormal surface changes in the lumen of the colon. Which of the following colonic landmark is indicative that the end of the colon has been reached?

- ▢ **A.** Hepatic flexure
- ▢ **B.** Splenic flexure
- ▢ **C.** Paracolic gutter
- ▢ **D.** Ileocecal valve
- ▢ **E.** Gastroesophageal (GE) junction

220 A 55-year-old man who has cirrhosis of the liver due to a chronic hepatitis B infection is brought to the emergency department because he has been vomiting blood for 2 hours. He has a 2-month history of abdominal distention, dilated veins over the anterior abdominal wall, and internal hemorrhoids. The anastomosis of which portal system vein with the esophageal veins can result in the hematemesis?

- ▢ **A.** Right gastric
- ▢ **B.** Periumbilical
- ▢ **C.** Left gastric
- ▢ **D.** Splenic
- ▢ **E.** Left gastroomental

221 A 55-year-old man complained of nausea and abdominal pain around his umbilical area. Examination revealed that he had an inflamed appendix, which was subsequently surgically removed. Which nerve fibers carried the pain from the inflamed appendix?

- ▢ **A.** Somatic afferents
- ▢ **B.** Preganglionic sympathetic
- ▢ **C.** Preganglionic parasympathetic
- ▢ **D.** Postganglionic sympathetic
- ▢ **E.** Visceral afferent

222 A 32-year-old man presents to the emergency department with severe pain in the left lower quadrant radiating over his lower back. Blood was found in the urine. Ultrasound examination revealed that the ureters were of normal size, but the left renal pelvis appeared enlarged and the renal calyces were rounded or blunted. Assuming that his symptoms and anatomical changes are due to a urinary stone, where is the most likely location for this stone to be lodged?

- ▢ **A.** Urethra
- ▢ **B.** Bladder
- ▢ **C.** Ureter at the uretero-vesical junction
- ▢ **D.** Ureter at the pelvic brim
- ▢ **E.** Ureter at the uretero-pelvic junction

223 A 49-year-old man presents with acute abdominal pain and jaundice resulting from a tumor at the head of the pancreas. The tumor will most likely obstruct which of the following structures?

- ▢ **A.** Bile duct
- ▢ **B.** Common hepatic duct
- ▢ **C.** Left hepatic duct
- ▢ **D.** Cystic duct
- ▢ **E.** Right hepatic duct

224 A 44-year old man is admitted to the emergency department with severe vomiting. Examination of the vomitus reveals the presence of bile. Imaging reveals part of the bowel being compressed between the abdominal aorta and superior mesenteric artery. Which part is being compressed?

- ▢ **A.** Second part of duodenum
- ▢ **B.** Ileum
- ▢ **C.** Thirds part of duodenum
- ▢ **D.** First and second part of duodenum
- ▢ **E.** Proximal part of jejunum

225 A 47-year-old man is undergoing surgical repair of a perforated duodenal ulcer. During the procedure the gastroduodenal artery is ligated. A branch of which artery will continue to supply blood to the duodenum in this patient?

- ▢ **A.** Splenic
- ▢ **B.** Left gastric
- ▢ **C.** Right gastric
- ▢ **D.** Proper hepatic
- ▢ **E.** Superior mesenteric

226 A 14-year-old girl presents to the emergency department complaining of severe difficulty breathing. On physical examination it is noted that she has a prolonged expiratory phase due to bronchospasm leading to the diagnosis of asthma. Which of the following nerves is responsible for the constriction of the bronchial smooth muscle cells?

- ▢ **A.** Vagus
- ▢ **B.** Phrenic
- ▢ **C.** Greater thoracic splanchnic
- ▢ **D.** Cardiopulmonary
- ▢ **E.** Intercostal

227 A 70-year-old woman is admitted to the hospital with intense abdominal pain from a pancreatic tumor. A neurectomy is performed to interrupt the neural pathway carrying pain from the pancreas. Which structure was severed?

- ▢ **A.** Vagus nerve
- ▢ **B.** Phrenic nerve
- ▢ **C.** Celiac ganglion
- ▢ **D.** Aorticorenal ganglion
- ▢ **E.** Inferior mesenteric ganglion

228 A 39-year-old woman presents to the emergency department with pain in her right side that radiates to the suprapubic region. She also has hematuria and a history of urinary tract infections. A CT scan reveals polycystic kidney disease with stretched capsule. Which nerve will convey the pain to the central nervous system (CNS)?

- ▢ **A.** Greater thoracic splanchnic nerve
- ▢ **B.** Lesser thoracic splanchnic nerve
- ▢ **C.** Pelvic splanchnic nerve
- ▢ **D.** Celiac plexus
- ▢ **E.** Iliohypogastric nerve

229 A 21-year-old woman is admitted to the hospital with pain radiating from her lower back towards her pubic symphysis. A kidney stone is suspected and ultrasound reveals a stone partially obstructing the lower part of her right ureter. The stone is probably lodged where the ureter crosses which structure?

- ▢ **A.** Inferior vena cava
- ▢ **B.** Internal iliac artery
- ▢ **C.** Common iliac artery
- ▢ **D.** Fourth lumbar artery
- ▢ **E.** Inferior mesenteric artery

230 A 40-year-old woman with jaundice and epigastric pain was taken to the emergency department where examination showed stones in the bile duct and gallbladder. During laparoscopic cholecystectomy the surgeon had to ligate and cut the cystic artery. A branch from which nervous structure traveling along the artery was also cut?

- ▢ **A.** Inferior mesenteric plexus
- ▢ **B.** Superior mesenteric plexus
- ▢ **C.** Celiac plexus
- ▢ **D.** Aorticorenal plexus
- ▢ **E.** Superior hypogastric plexus

231 Seven hours after delivery a baby began crying and started to vigorously vomit. On physical examination his abdomen appeared distended and it was noted that he had passed small amounts of meconium. Two abdominal radiographs are shown below (Fig. 3-9). Which of the following embryological abnormalities is the most likely cause of the baby's condition?

- ▢ **A.** Defect in the tracheoesophageal septum
- ▢ **B.** Failure of the muscular tissue from the body wall to extend into the pleuroperitoneal membrane
- ▢ **C.** Failure of recanalization of the duodenum
- ▢ **D.** Malrotation of the intestines
- ▢ **E.** Defective fusion of the pleuroperitoneal membranes

232 Autopsy of a newborn boy reveals multiple congenital heart defects in addition to absence of kidneys and poorly developed ureters bilaterally. Ultrasonography at 28 weeks' gestation would most likely have shown which of the following?

- ▢ **A.** Polyhydramnios
- ▢ **B.** Annular pancreas
- ▢ **C.** Malrotation of the gut
- ▢ **D.** Bilateral gonadal dysgenesis
- ▢ **E.** Oligohydramnios

233 A 35-year-old man is in surgery for a ruptured appendix. A midline incision was made for greater access to the peritoneal cavity. The surgeon noted a 2-inch long finger-like pouch on the anterior border of the ileum about 2 feet away from the ileocecal junction. This is a remnant of which developmental structure?

- ▢ **A.** Omphaloenteric duct
- ▢ **B.** Branch of superior mesenteric artery
- ▢ **C.** Connecting stalk
- ▢ **D.** Cecal diverticulum
- ▢ **E.** Umbilical cord

234 A neonate was born at 34 weeks of gestation and was admitted for pneumonitis. A CT scan reveals that the upper segment of the esophagus ends blindly and the presence of an abnormal communication between

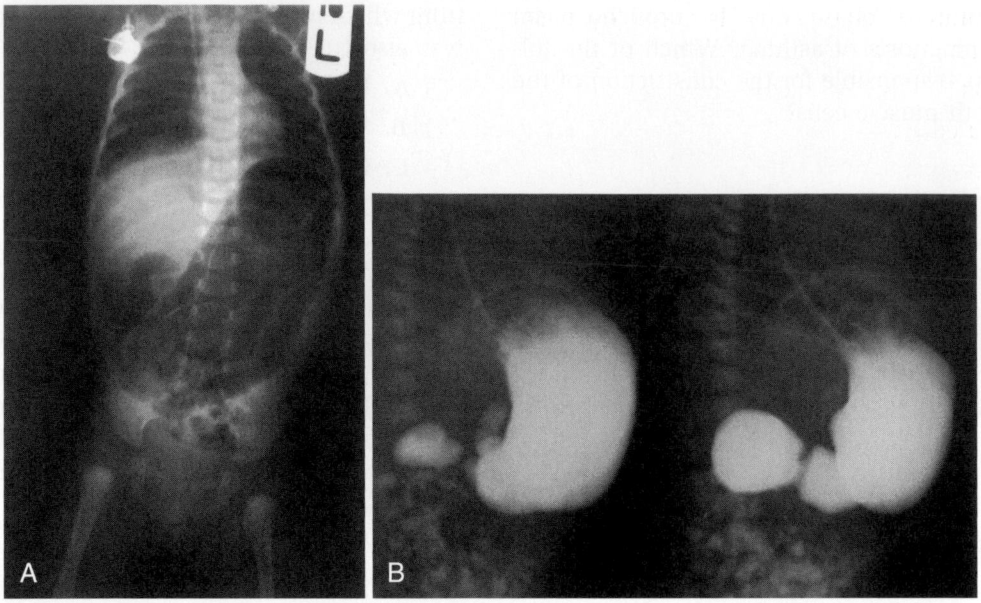

Fig. 3-9

trachea and the lower segment of esophagus. Which of the following clinical conditions is most likely seen with this congenital anomaly?

- ☐ **A.** Polyhydramnios
- ☐ **B.** Oligohydramnios
- ☐ **C.** Anhydramnios
- ☐ **D.** Umbilicoileal fistula
- ☐ **E.** Down syndrome

235 A newborn boy has a foul-smelling yellow-brown discharge from his umbilicus. A catheter was inserted into a small opening in the umbilicus and contrast material was injected before acquiring an abdominal radiograph. The radiograph demonstrated that the contrast material filled the loops of ileum through a small (4 to 5 cm) connection between the ileum and the umbilicus. Based on these findings, which of the following is the most likely diagnosis?

- ☐ **A.** Ileal diverticulum
- ☐ **B.** Ileal diverticulum with ulceration
- ☐ **C.** Omphaloenteric fistula
- ☐ **D.** Omphaloenteric cyst
- ☐ **E.** Persistent vitelline artery

236 A 4-year-old boy is admitted to the hospital with severe bile-stained vomiting. Radiographic examination and history taking reveals that the boy suffers from an annular pancreas. Which structure is most likely obstructed by this condition?

- ☐ **A.** Pylorus of the stomach
- ☐ **B.** First part of the duodenum
- ☐ **C.** Second part of the duodenum
- ☐ **D.** Third part of the duodenum
- ☐ **E.** Jejunum

237 A 2-year-old boy is seen by the pediatrician because his parents notice a gradually enlarging scrotal mass. Transillumination and scrotal ultrasound reveal a large fluid collection around a normally developed testis. Which of the following structures has most likely developed abnormally?

- ☐ **A.** Deep inguinal ring
- ☐ **B.** Tunica albuginea
- ☐ **C.** Processus vaginalis
- ☐ **D.** Gubernaculum
- ☐ **E.** Dartos tunic

238 A 1-year-old boy is seen in the pediatric clinic because the mother has noticed only one testis in the scrotum of her child. The pediatrician examined the infant and palpated the testis in the inguinal canal. Which condition is this?

- ☐ **A.** Pseudohermaphroditism
- ☐ **B.** True hermaphroditism
- ☐ **C.** Cryptorchidism
- ☐ **D.** Retractile testes
- ☐ **E.** Chordee

239 A 25-year-old woman in the 8th month of pregnancy went to the outpatient clinic for her prenatal checkup. Ultrasound examination of the fetus showed part of the small bowel herniating into the amniotic cavity due to failure of fusion of the lateral folds in the abdominal region. Which condition is this?

- ▢ **A.** Volvulus
- ▢ **B.** Nonrotated gut
- ▢ **C.** Situs inversus
- ▢ **D.** Gastroschisis
- ▢ **E.** Ileal diverticulum

240 A newborn girl with Down's syndrome begins vomiting shortly after her first feeding. The vomitus is stained with bile. Which condition is most likely causing the vomiting?

- ▢ **A.** Atresia of the third part of the duodenum
- ▢ **B.** Atresia of the first part of the duodenum
- ▢ **C.** Congenital hypertrophic pyloric stenosis
- ▢ **D.** Esophageal stenosis
- ▢ **E.** Tracheoesophageal fistula

241 A 2-day-old girl with fever is examined by the pediatric team. Imaging reveals malrotation of the small intestine with unfixed mesenteries. The vessels around the duodenojejunal junction are obstructed and gangrene of the intestine is developing. Which condition has probably caused this?

- ▢ **A.** Diaphragmatic atresia
- ▢ **B.** Subhepatic cecum
- ▢ **C.** Midgut volvulus
- ▢ **D.** Duplication of the intestine
- ▢ **E.** Congenital megacolon

242 A 5-day-old infant boy presents with abdominal distention, constipation, and vomiting. A CT scan reveals an abnormally dilated descending colon and a diagnosis of Hirschsprung disease (megacolon) is made. What is the embryologic mechanism responsible for Hirschsprung disease?

- ▢ **A.** Failure of neural crest cells to migrate into the walls of the colon
- ▢ **B.** Incomplete separation of the cloaca
- ▢ **C.** Failure of recanalization of the colon
- ▢ **D.** Defective rotation of the hindgut
- ▢ **E.** Oligohydramnios

243 A 32-year-old man visits his family physician complaining of groin pain. Examination reveals that the patient has an indirect inguinal hernia. Which nerve is most likely responsible for the pain transmission?

- ▢ **A.** Iliohypogastric
- ▢ **B.** Lateral femoral cutaneous
- ▢ **C.** Ilioinguinal
- ▢ **D.** Lumbar splanchnic
- ▢ **E.** Greater thoracic splanchnic

244 A 26-year-old man visits his family physician complaining of a number of areas of thickened scaly skin on his abdominal wall below the level of the umbilicus. The physician suspected actinic keratosis, which is a premalignant condition and can progress to squamous cell carcinoma. Which lymph nodes will first receive drainage from this area of skin?

- ▢ **A.** Deep inguinal
- ▢ **B.** External iliac
- ▢ **C.** Internal iliac
- ▢ **D.** Lateral aortic
- ▢ **E.** Superficial inguinal

245 A 33-year-old man requests a vasectomy. During the procedure the urologist separates the various layers of the spermatic cord to expose the ductus deferens so that it can be ligated and cut. From which structure is the internal spermatic fascia derived?

- ▢ **A.** Internal abdominal oblique muscle
- ▢ **B.** Cremaster muscle
- ▢ **C.** External abdominal oblique muscle
- ▢ **D.** Transversus abdominis aponeurosis
- ▢ **E.** Transversalis fascia

246 A 45-year-old man presents to the emergency department with severe nausea and recurrent bilious vomiting. Past medical history reveals that his symptoms initially began 1 month ago as postprandial epigastric pain, but have worsened during the past week. Physical examination shows a slightly tender and distended abdomen with high-pitched bowel sounds. A CT scan reveals that the angle between the superior mesenteric artery and the aorta is significantly decreased. Which of the following structures is most likely to be obstructed by the artery?

- ▢ **A.** Ascending portion of the duodenum
- ▢ **B.** Descending portion of the duodenum
- ▢ **C.** Duodenal bulb
- ▢ **D.** Duodenojejunal flexure
- ▢ **E.** Transverse portion of the duodenum

247 A 70-year-old man is admitted to the emergency department complaining of cramping midabdominal pain, abdominal distention, and vomiting for the past 24 hours. History reveals that the patient suffers from gallstones. Abdominal radiograph reveals air in the gallbladder and biliary tree. In which of the following sites is a gallstone most likely lodged?

- ▢ **A.** Cystic duct
- ▢ **B.** Bile duct
- ▢ **C.** Duodenum
- ▢ **D.** Jejunum
- ▢ **E.** Ileum

248 Which of the following age ranges best represents when the bones that form the acetabulum fuse?

- ▢ **A.** 13 to 15 years
- ▢ **B.** 16 to 18 years
- ▢ **C.** 19 to 21 years
- ▢ **D.** 22 to 24 years
- ▢ **E.** 25 to 27 years

249 A 68-year-old man was found to have a tumor that originated from the lining of the urinary bladder. During transurethral resection to remove the tumor, the cystoscope entered the urinary bladder. Which of the following structures did the cystoscope traverse immediately before entering the urinary bladder?

- ▢ **A.** Intramural part of urethra
- ▢ **B.** Intermediate part of urethra
- ▢ **C.** Prostatic urethra
- ▢ **D.** Spongy urethra
- ▢ **E.** Paraurethral part

250 A 38-year-old man was diagnosed with metastatic cancer of the left testes. Which of the following most likely represents the route by which the cancer spread from the left testes to the rest of the body?

- ▢ **A.** Left testicular vein; inferior vena cava; left renal vein
- ▢ **B.** Right testicular vein; left testicular vein; inferior vena cava
- ▢ **C.** Left testicular vein; left common iliac vein; inferior vena cava
- ▢ **D.** Left testicular vein; median sacral vein; inferior vena cava
- ▢ **E.** Left testicular vein; left renal vein; inferior vena cava

251 A gynecology resident physician was performing a pelvic examination on a 25-year-old woman who was in the lithotomy position during a physical examination. In order to palpate the patient's uterus, the index and middle fingers of the resident's right hand were inside her vagina while the fingers of his left hand were pressing on the abdomen inferior to the umbilicus. The resident concomitantly lowered his left palm onto the patient's skin and felt a bony structure in the lower midline. Which of the following structures did the resident most likely feel on the palm of his left hand?

- ▢ **A.** Ilium
- ▢ **B.** Coccyx
- ▢ **C.** Sacrum
- ▢ **D.** Ischium
- ▢ **E.** Pubis

252 A 21-year-old man presents to the emergency department with fever and a high white blood cell count. He reports having suffered a small stab wound in his back a few months ago. Because it was a shallow wound, he did not seek medical attention. The physician states that he has a retroperitoneal infection. Which of the following structures is most likely to be affected?

- ▢ **A.** Descending colon
- ▢ **B.** Jejunum
- ▢ **C.** Stomach
- ▢ **D.** Transverse colon
- ▢ **E.** Appendix

253 A 67-year-old man complained of the acute onset of lower back pain on the right with concomitant loss of sensation of the skin in the posterolateral gluteal and anterior pubic regions on the right side. During the physical examination, the patient experienced severe pain inferior to the twelfth rib at the right costovertebral angle with palpation. The physician also found that the patient had paralysis of the right internal oblique and transversus abdominis muscles. An abdominal CT scan revealed a tumor that originated in the right kidney, entered the posterior renal capsule, and pressed on the ipsilateral quadratus lumborum muscle. Which of the following nerves was most likely compressed by the tumor?

- ▢ **A.** Subcostal
- ▢ **B.** Lateral cutaneous nerve of thigh
- ▢ **C.** Ilioinguinal
- ▢ **D.** Femoral
- ▢ **E.** Iliohypogastric

ANSWERS

1 A. The processus vaginalis (meaning sheathlike process) is composed of parietal peritoneum that precedes the testis as it "migrates" from a position in the upper lumbar wall to a position outside the abdomen. This process usually obliterates, leaving only a distal portion that surrounds most of the testis as the tunica vaginalis. Whereas these features are typical of development in the male, females also have a processus vaginalis that extends into the labia majus, although congenital inguinal hernias are more common in males than females. The other listed structures are not involved in congenital inguinal hernias.
GAS 293; N 257; McM 272, 275

2 A. Wilms tumor is a kidney malignancy that usually occurs in children. It has recently been shown that it can be caused by mutations in the *WT1* gene, behaving according to the Knudson two-hit model for tumor suppressor genes.
GAS 373; N 308; McM 255, 258

3 C. During development, the kidneys typically "ascend" from a position in the pelvis to a position high on the posterior abdominal wall. Although the kidneys are bilateral structures, occasionally the inferior poles of the two kidneys fuse. When this happens, the "ascent" of the fused kidneys is arrested by the first midline structure they encounter, the inferior mesenteric artery. The incidence of horseshoe kidney is about 0.25% of the population.
GAS 373; N 309; McM 259, 250

4 C. In normal kidney development the kidneys function during the fetal period with the resulting urine contributing to the fluid in the amniotic cavity. When the kidneys fail to develop (renal agenesis), this contribution to the fluid is missing and decreased amniotic fluid (oligohydramnios) results.
GAS 373; N 309; McM 255, 256

5 A. There is some evidence that oligohydramnios is linked to hypoplastic lungs. This is apparently not a genetic link but rather related to the importance of adequate amniotic fluid in normal lung development.
GAS 167, 373; N 208; McM 199

6 C. In normal pancreatic development a bifid ventral pancreatic bud rotates around the dorsal side of the gut tube and fuses with the dorsal pancreatic bud. Rarely, a portion of the ventral bud rotates around the ventral side of the gut tube, resulting in an annular pancreas. The portion of the gut tube is the same where the main pancreatic duct enters the second part of the duodenum (along with the common bile duct). The incidence of annular pancreas is about 1 in 7000.
GAS 336; N 281; McM 235

7 C. The distal portion of the processus vaginalis contributes to the tunica vaginalis that is related to the testis. If an intermediate portion of the processus vaginalis persists, it often fills with fluid, creating a hydrocele. If the entire processus vaginalis persists, the patient is likely to develop a congenital inguinal hernia.
GAS 269; N 365; McM 265, 266

8 C. Cryptorchism, often called an undescended testis, is the result of incomplete migration of the gonad from the abdomen to a location in the scrotum where it is exposed to temperatures slightly lower than core body temperature. This is important for spermatogenesis and testicular function. A testis that cannot be surgically relocated into the scrotum is usually removed because it would otherwise be prone to develop testicular cancer.
GAS 293; N 364; McM 265, 266

9 D. The lateral folds are key structures in forming the muscular portion of the anterior abdominal wall. Failure of the lateral folds can cause a minor defect, such as an umbilical hernia, or a major defect, such as gastroschisis.
GAS 265, 311; N 247; McM 222

10 A. Rotation of the gut tube is a major event in the development of the gastrointestinal system. Parts of the tube rotate 270 degrees, but the proximal foregut, specifically that portion that forms the esophagus, rotates only 90 degrees. Looking from below (the standard CT or MRI view), this rotation is counterclockwise. This brings the left vagus nerve onto the anterior surface of the esophagus as it passes through the thorax.
GAS 265, 363-364; N 263; McM 241, 257

11 B. The diaphragm develops from several components. Initially, the septum transversum (which will become the central tendon) forms in the cervical region, gaining innervation from C3, C4, and C5. Later, myoblasts migrate in from the body wall to form the muscular part of the diaphragm, often considered to be two bilateral hemidiaphragms. These muscles are innervated by the phrenic nerves that are derived from C3, C4, and C5. Eventration of the diaphragm occurs when one muscular hemidiaphragm fails to develop. With positive pressure in the abdominal cavity, and low or negative pressure in the thoracic cavity, abdominal organs are pushed into the thorax. The pleuroperitoneal folds contribute to a portion of the diaphragm posteriorly.

GAS 371; N 191, 192; McM 213, 260

12 D. The tracheoesophageal septum is the downgrowth that separates the ventral wall of the foregut (esophagus) from the laryngotracheal tube. The presence of a fistula would result in passage of fluid from the esophagus into the trachea and could cause aspiration pneumonia. If the esophagus did not develop correctly, as in esophageal atresia, it would end as a blind tube. This kind of defect, although associated with tracheoesophageal fistula, is not the result of an opening into the trachea, and pneumonia would not result. Abnormal tracheal development can be associated with tracheoesophageal fistula, therefore, but it is not the direct cause of it. Abnormal tongue development does not result in a tracheoesophageal fistula. Abnormal development of the pharynx is not associated with a tracheoesophageal fistula.

GAS 172; N 230; McM 196

13 C. The septum transversum forms the central tendon of the diaphragm. The pleuroperitoneal folds form the posterolateral part of the diaphragm. The pleuropericardial folds separate the pericardial cavity from the pleural cavity and form the fibrous pericardium. The cervical myotomes form the musculature of the diaphragm. The dorsal part of the dorsal mesentery of the esophagus forms the crura of the diaphragm.

GAS 161; N 191, 192; McM 213, 260

14 C. Midgut volvulus is a possible complication of malrotation of the midgut loop without fixed mesentery. The small intestines twist around the vasculature that is providing support for them. This can cause ischemic necrosis of the intestine, resulting in gangrene. Diaphragmatic atresia is not a cause of volvulus. Subhepatic cecum is due to failure of the descent of the cecal bud and results in the absence of an ascending colon. Duplication of the intestine would not cause volvulus because there would still be a fixed mesentery and no free movement of the intestines. Congenital aganglionic megacolon is due to faulty migration of neural crest cells into the wall of the colon, resulting in a lack of parasympathetic postganglionic neurons and creating a functional blockage and an enlarged colon proximal to the block.

GAS 311; N 263; McM 277

15 A. Congenital megacolon (Hirschsprung's disease) results from the failure of neural crest cells to migrate into the walls of the colon. Incomplete separation of the cloaca would result in anal agenesis either with or without the presence of a fistula. The failure of recanalization of the colon results in rectal atresia, wherein both the anal canal and rectum exist but are not connected due to incomplete canalization or no recanalization. Defective rotation of the hindgut can cause volvulus or twisting of its contents. Oligohydramnios is a deficiency of amniotic fluid, which can cause pulmonary hypoplasia but would not cause Hirschsprung disease.

GAS 323; N 264; McM 239

16 D. The ileum is the most common site of Meckel's diverticulum. This outpouching is a persistence of the vitelline duct and it can be attached to the umbilicus. The other answer choices are not correlated with the vitelline duct and therefore will not result in the condition discussed here.

GAS 318; N 274; McM 223

17 A. The most common site of ectopic pregnancy is in the uterine (fallopian) tubes. Implantation in the internal os of the cervix can result in placenta previa, but the internal os of the cervix is not the most common site. The other choices listed are not the most common sites of ectopic pregnancy. The endometrium in the fundus of the uterus is the normal site of implantation.

GAS 477, 530; N 301; McM 274

18 A. The greater thoracic splanchnic nerve carries general visceral afferent fibers from abdominal organs, specifically the foregut, and can be involved in the occurrence of referred pain. The dorsal primary rami of intercostal nerves carry general somatic afferent fibers. Pain from these fibers would result in sharp, localized pain not dull and diffuse as occurs in referred pain. Although the phrenic nerve carries visceral afferent fibers, it does not innervate the gallbladder. The vagus nerve carries visceral afferent fibers that are important for visceral reflexes, but they do not transmit pain. The pelvic splanchnic nerves are parasympathetic nerves from S2 to S4 and contain visceral afferent fibers that transmit pain from the pelvis but not from the gallbladder.

GAS 358-365, 38; N 303; McM 236

19 C. An indirect inguinal hernia occurs when a loop of bowel enters the spermatic cord through the

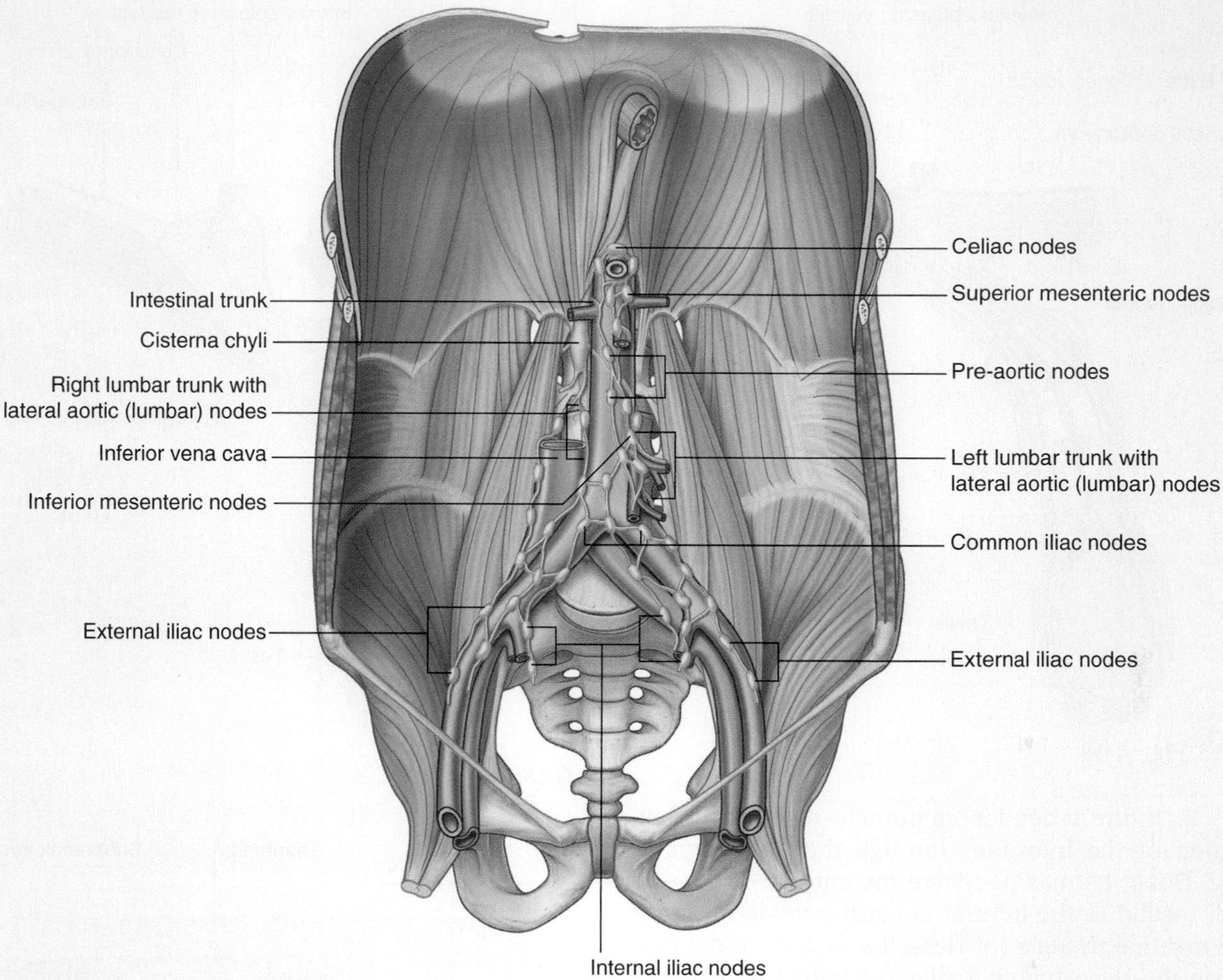

***GAS* Fig. 4-155**

deep inguinal ring (lateral to the inferior epigastric vessels). The ilioinguinal nerve runs with the spermatic cord to innervate the anterior portion of the scrotum and proximal parts of the genitals and could be compressed during an indirect inguinal hernia. The other nerves listed are not likely to be compressed by the hernia. The iliohypogastric nerve innervates the skin of the suprapubic region. The lateral femoral cutaneous nerve innervates the skin over the lateral thigh. The subcostal nerve innervates the band of skin superior to the iliac crest and inferior to the umbilicus. The pudendal nerve innervates the musculature and skin of the perineum.

GAS 301-302; N 256; McM 224

20 **A.** The celiac lymph nodes receive lymph drainage directly from the stomach before they drain into the cisterna chyli. The superior and inferior mesenteric lymph nodes receive drainage below the stomach and not from the stomach itself. The lumbar lymph nodes receive drainage from structures inferior to the stomach and not the stomach directly. Hepatic lymph nodes are associated with liver drainage and not drainage from the stomach (*GAS* Fig. 4-155).

GAS 358; N 261; McM 235

21 **B.** The proper hepatic artery is the only artery typically within the hepatoduodenal ligament and therefore would be occluded. This artery lies within the right anterior free margin of the omental (or epiploic) foramen (of Winslow). The superior mesenteric artery branches from the abdominal aorta inferior to the hepatoduodenal ligament. The splenic artery runs behind the stomach and is not located in the hepatoduodenal ligament. The common hepatic artery gives origin to the proper hepatic artery but does not run within the hepatoduodenal ligament. The inferior vena cava is located at the posterior margin of the omental foramen and therefore would not be clamped.

GAS 343; N 284; McM 224

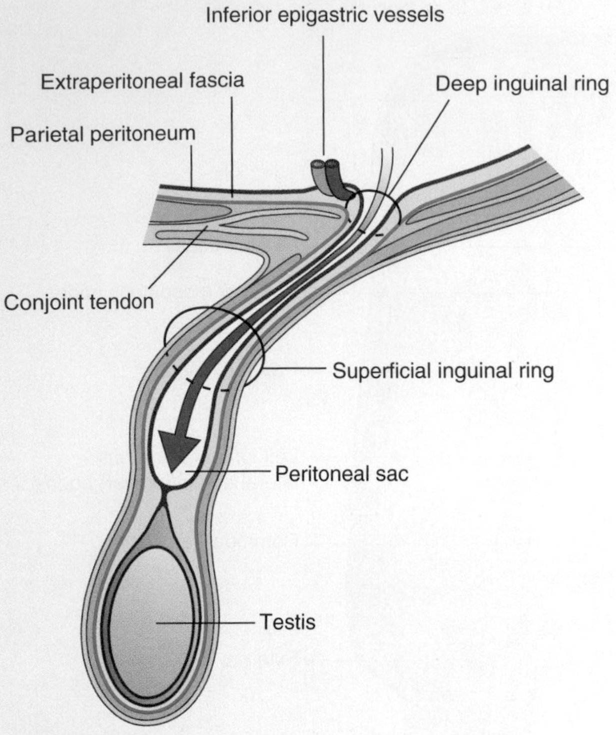

GAS **Fig. 4-48**

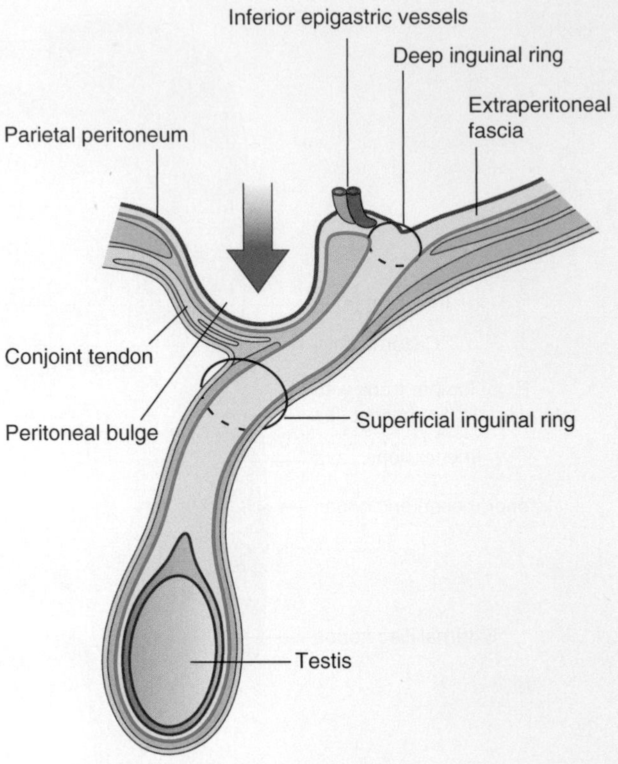

GAS **Fig. 4-49**

22 E. Indirect hernias commonly result from herniation of the intestines through the deep inguinal ring. Direct hernias penetrate the anterior abdominal wall medial to the inferior epigastric vessels through the inguinal triangle (of Hesselbach) and do not penetrate the deep inguinal ring. Umbilical hernias exit through the umbilicus, not the deep inguinal ring. Femoral hernias exit through the femoral ring inferior to the inguinal ligament. Lumbar hernias can penetrate through superior (Grynfeltt) or inferior (Petit) lumbar triangles. (*GAS* Figs. 4-48 and 4-49)
GAS 301-302; N 256; McM 225

23 C. The omental bursa is located directly posterior to the stomach and therefore would be the most likely space to develop peritonitis initially. The right subhepatic space (also called the hepatorenal space, or pouch of Morison) is the area posterior to the liver and anterior to the right kidney. This space can potentially accumulate fluid and may participate in peritonitis but primarily when the patient is in the supine position. The right subphrenic space lies just inferior to the diaphragm on the right side and is not likely to accumulate fluid from a perforated stomach ulcer. Peritonitis could develop in this area only when the patient is in the supine position. Fluid from a perforated ulcer on the posterior aspect of the stomach is not likely to enter the greater sac (*GAS* Fig 4-93).
GAS 307; N 266; McM 231

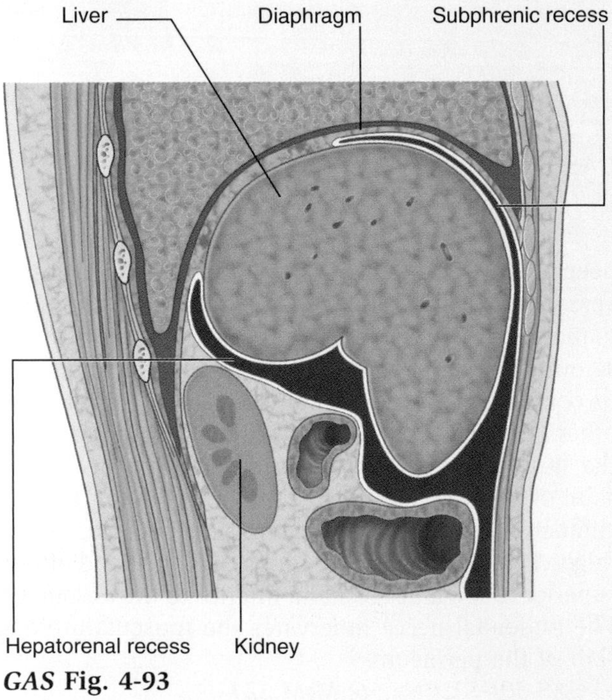

GAS **Fig. 4-93**

24 C. The left gastric vein carries blood from the stomach to the portal vein. At the esophageal-gastric junction the left gastric vein (portal system) anastomoses with esophageal veins (caval system). High blood pressure in the portal system causes high

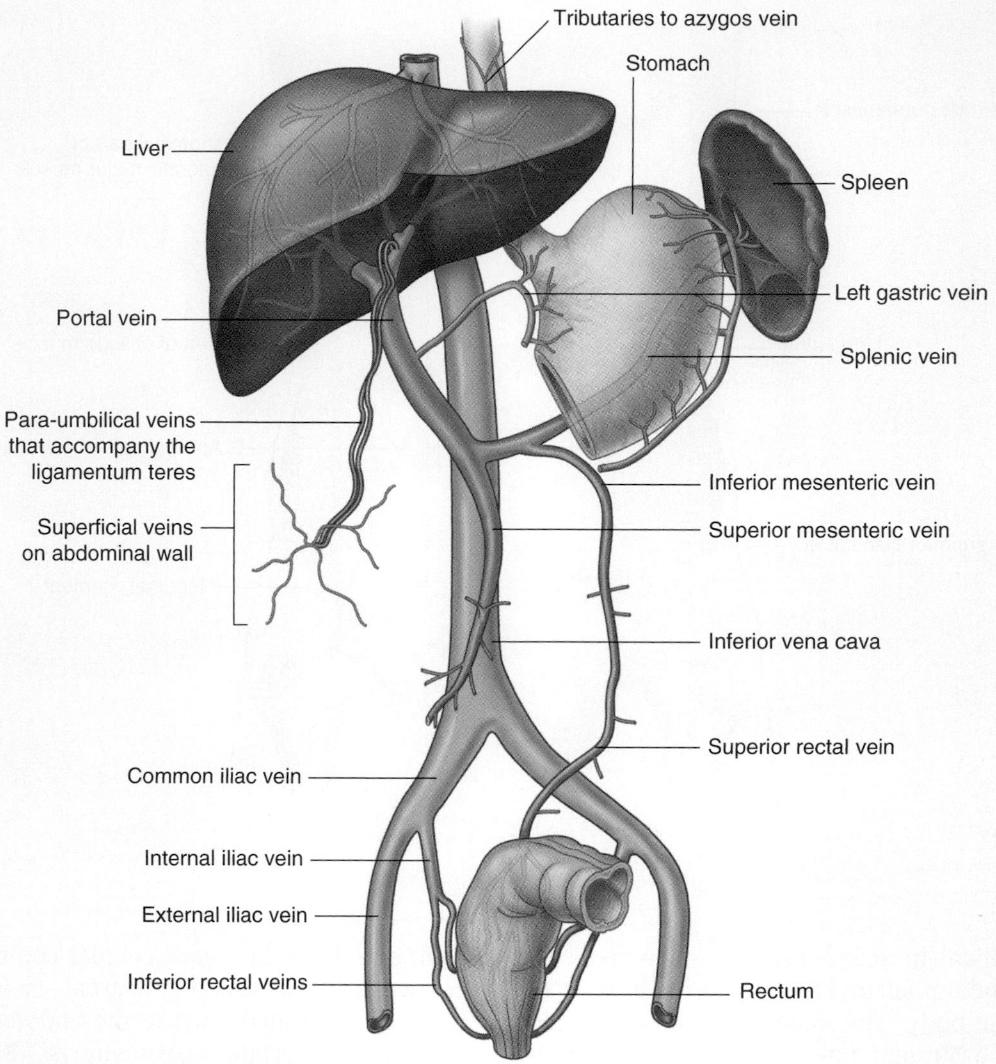

***GAS* Fig. 4-122**

pressure in this anastomosis, causing the ruptured esophageal varices. The splenic vein and its tributaries carry blood away from the spleen and do not form a caval-portal anastomosis. The left gastro-omental vein accompanies the left gastro-omental artery and joins the splenic vein with no direct anastomosis with caval veins. The left hepatic vein is a caval vein and empties into the inferior vena cava. The right gastric vein drains the lesser curvature of the stomach and is part of the portal system but does not have any caval anastomosis (*GAS* Fig. 4-122).

GAS 273, 354; N 289; McM 248

25 **C.** The genitofemoral nerve originates from the ventral rami of L1 and L2. The "femoral" part supplies skin to the femoral triangle area, whereas the "genito" part in males travels with the spermatic cord and supplies the cremaster muscle and scrotal skin. The ilioinguinal nerve arises from L1 and supplies the skin over the root of the penis and upper part of the scrotum in the male. The iliohypogastric nerve arises from L1 (and possibly fibers from T12) and supplies skin innervation over the hypogastric region and anterolateral gluteal region. The pudendal nerve provides innervation to the external genitalia for both sexes but does not innervate the cremaster muscle in males. The ventral ramus of T12 is also associated with the lower portion of the anterior abdominal wall and the iliohypogastric nerve; it does not contribute to the cremasteric reflex.

GAS 299-301; N 253; McM 261

26 **E.** The linea alba is formed by the intersection of aponeurotic tissues between the right and left

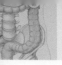

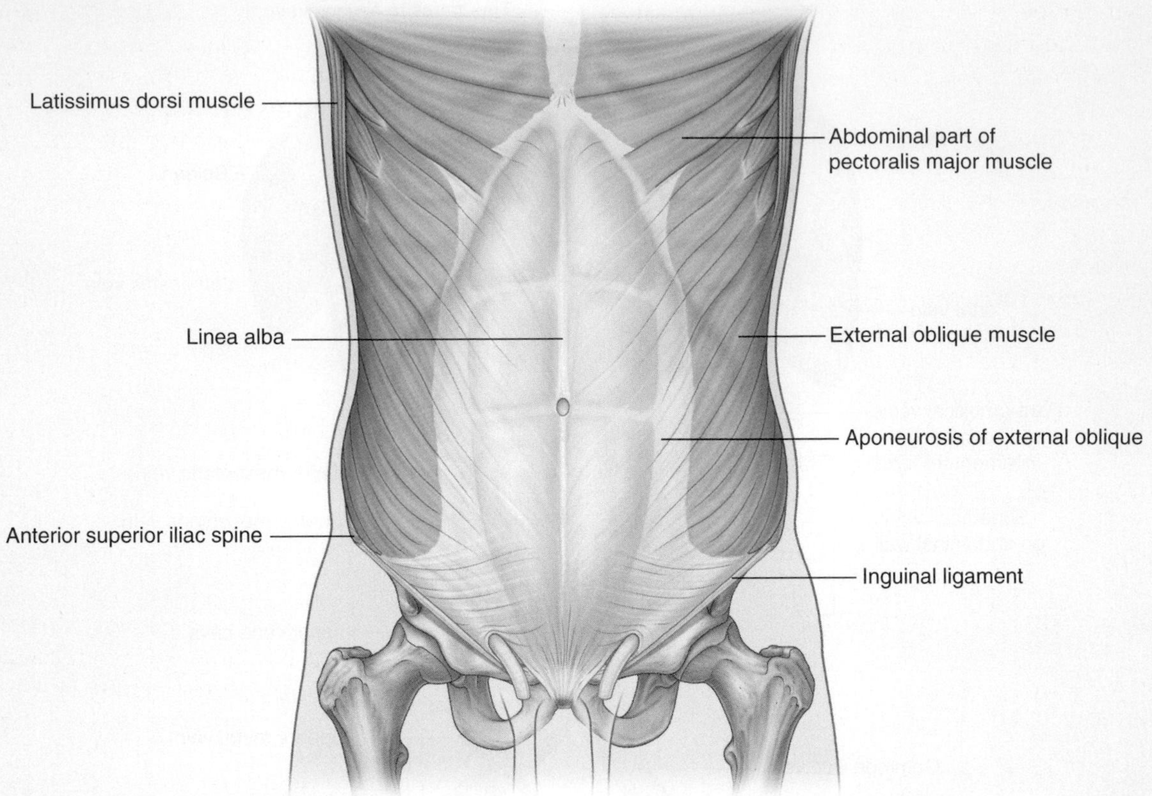

***GAS* Fig. 4-27**

rectus abdominal muscles. It contains the aponeuroses of the abdominal muscles and is located at the midline of the body. The midaxillary line is oriented vertically in a straight line inferior to the shoulder joint and axilla. The arcuate line (of Douglas) is a curved horizontal line that represents the lower edge of the posterior tendinous portion of the rectus abdominis sheath. An incision at this line will not separate the rectus abdominis sheaths. The semilunar line is represented by an imaginary vertical line below the nipples and usually parallels the lateral edge of the rectus sheath. The tendinous intersections of the rectus abdominis muscles divide the muscle into sections and are usually not well defined. An incision along these intersections would not divide the two rectus sheaths (*GAS* Fig. 4-27).

GAS 282; N 245; McM 219

27 A. Scarpa's fascia is the thick, membranous layer deep to the Camper's adipose fascia in the anterior abdominal wall (subcutaneous). Because of the relatively thick, tough nature of connective tissue that makes up Scarpa's fascia, this layer is typically the site to maintain sutures. Camper's fascia is a fatty layer (subcutaneous) and tends not to hold sutures as well, due to the increased cellular content versus the connective tissue found in Scarpa's layer. Transversalis fascia is located deep to the abdominal musculature and associated aponeurosis. Extraperitoneal fascia is the deepest layer, adjacent to the parietal peritoneum of the anterior abdominal wall. The anterior wall of the rectus sheath is the layer just deep to Scarpa's fascia and superficial to the rectus abdominis muscle anteriorly. The latter three layers are not considered to be superficial fascia.

GAS 280; N 321; McM 223

28 A. The common bile duct is located at the head of the pancreas and receives contents from the cystic duct and hepatic duct. An obstruction at this site causes a backup of bile back through the common bile duct and hepatic duct, with resulting pain and jaundice. The common hepatic duct is located more superior to the head of the pancreas and leads into the cystic duct. The cystic duct allows bile to enter the gallbladder from the hepatic duct (draining the liver) and releases bile to the hepatic duct. The accessory pancreatic duct is not affected by an obstruction of the common bile duct due to a lack of any connections between the two ducts. The proper hepatic artery will not be obstructed, for it carries blood from the liver to the inferior vena cava.

GAS 296; N 280; McM 246

29 C. The third part of the duodenum takes a path situated anterior to the abdominal aorta and inferior to the superior mesenteric artery (a major ventral branch of the abdominal aorta). Because the third part of the duodenum lies in the angle between ("sandwiched") these two structures, constrictions of this portion of the duodenum can occur readily. The second part of the duodenum lies parallel with, and to the right of, the abdominal aorta and is not normally in close proximity to the superior mesenteric artery. The transverse colon takes a horizontal path through the anterior abdominal cavity but travels superior or anterior to the superior mesenteric artery. The first part of the duodenum continues from the pylorus, flexing to lead to the second part of the duodenum; thus, it is not located near the superior mesenteric artery or abdominal aorta. The jejunum is an extension of the small intestine after the duodenum and is further removed from the superior mesenteric artery.

GAS 346; N 281; McM 238

30 E. The superior mesenteric artery will supply the pancreas if the gastroduodenal artery is ligated. It arises immediately inferior to the celiac trunk from the thoracic aorta. Its first branches are the anterior and posterior inferior pancreaticoduodenal arteries, which anastomose with the superior pancreaticoduodenal arteries (which take origin from the gastroduodenal branch of the celiac trunk) in supplying the pancreas with oxygenated blood. The inferior mesenteric artery is the most inferior of the three main arterial branches supplying the gastrointestinal tract. It supplies the hindgut from the left colic flexure to the rectum. The left gastric artery is the smallest branch of the celiac trunk and supplies the cardioesophageal junction, the inferior esophagus, and the lesser curvature of the stomach. The right gastric artery arises from the common hepatic artery, which is a branch from the celiac trunk. It supplies the lesser curvature of the stomach and anastomoses with the left gastric artery. The proper hepatic artery arises from the common hepatic artery and ascends to supply the liver and gallbladder. It is one of three structures forming the portal triad and is found in the free edge of the hepatoduodenal ligament.

GAS 348; N 284; McM 238

31 B. The middle colic artery can provide collateral supply to the descending colon when the inferior mesenteric artery is blocked or ligated. It is one of the first branches of the superior mesenteric artery and supplies the transverse colon. It provides collateral blood supply both to the ascending colon and descending colon by anastomosing with the right colic branch of the superior mesenteric artery and with the left colic artery, a branch from the inferior mesenteric artery. The left gastroepiploic artery, also known as the left gastro-omental artery, is a branch of the splenic artery and supplies the greater curvature of the stomach along with the right gastro-omental branch of the gastroduodenal artery. The sigmoid arteries are branches from the inferior mesenteric artery and supply the inferior portion of the descending colon, the sigmoid colon, and the rectum. The sigmoid arteries have no contributing branches to the foregut or midgut. The splenic artery is the largest artery arising from the celiac trunk. It supplies the spleen and the neck, body, and tail of the pancreas and also provides short gastric branches to the stomach. It supplies no structures in the midgut or hindgut. Finally, the superior rectal artery is the terminal branch of the inferior mesenteric artery and supplies only the rectum.

GAS 348; N 288; McM 238

32 A. The appendix is the most likely structure that is inflamed. It lies in the right lower quadrant, and of the choices provided, it is most closely associated with the umbilical region by way of referral of pain. The patient also exhibited a positive psoas sign when flexion of the hip against resistance was attempted. This is because the iliopsoas muscle lies directly beneath the appendix, and upon flexion of this muscle, contact and direct irritation to the appendix can occur. The bladder lies inferior to the umbilicus within the pelvis and is not related to the site of pain or with a positive psoas sign. The gallbladder lies inferior to the liver and is positioned in the upper right abdominal quadrant, which is superior to the umbilicus. It is not associated with a positive psoas sign. The pancreas lies behind the stomach and is positioned between the spleen and the duodenum. It therefore lies in the upper left quadrant and is superior to the umbilicus. The uterus is located within the pelvis and is positioned anteflexed and anteverted over the bladder. It lies inferior and medial to the iliopsoas group and would not be affected by flexion of these muscles (*GAS* Fig. 4-22).

GAS 322; N 273; McM 251

33 B. The abscess may have spread to the diaphragm and be causing the referred shoulder pain. This is because the diaphragm lies in close proximity

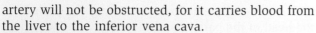

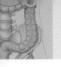

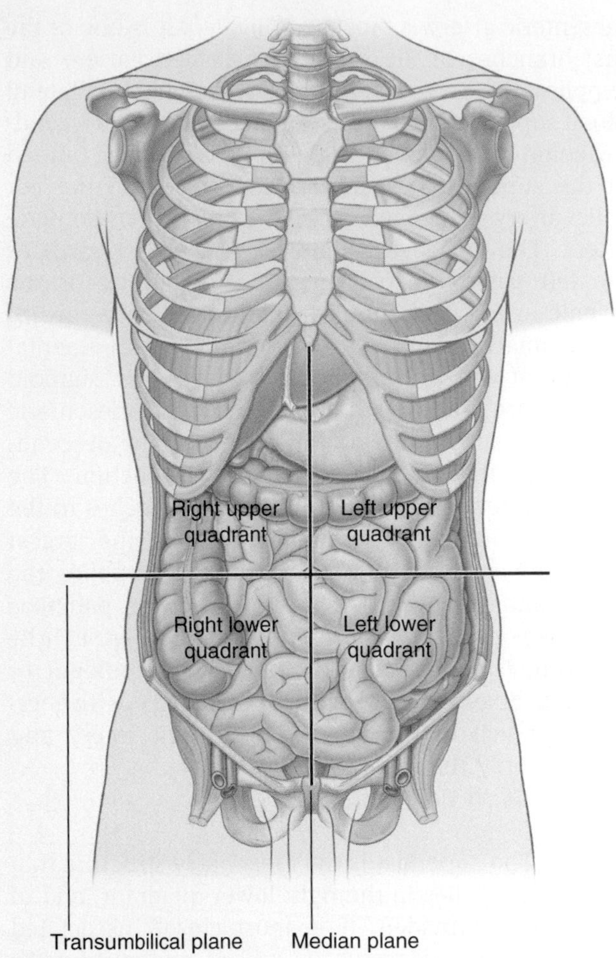

***GAS* Fig. 4-22**

to the superior poles of the kidneys. The diaphragm is innervated by the phrenic nerves, bilaterally, which descend to the diaphragm from spinal nerve levels C3, C4, and C5. It is probably at the spinal cord that the referral of pain occurs between the phrenic nerve and somatic afferents entering at those levels. The descending colon is innervated by parasympathetic nerves from S2 to S4 and visceral afferents, which do not carry pain. The duodenum is innervated by the vagus nerve, which innervates the gastrointestinal tract to the left colic flexure. The liver is innervated sympathetically from the celiac ganglion; the parasympathetic nerves to the liver are by the vagus nerve. Neither of these two sources of innervation enters the spinal cord at the level of the shoulder and therefore could not cause referred pain to the shoulder. The pancreas is innervated by the vagus nerve, branches from the celiac ganglion, and the pancreatic plexus. None of these nerves enters the spinal cord at the level of the shoulder and therefore cannot facilitate referral of pain to the shoulder.

GAS 373; N 259; McM 260

34 A. The afferent fibers mediating the pain from the head of the pancreas run initially with the greater thoracic splanchnic nerves. The greater thoracic splanchnic nerves arise from sympathetic ganglia at the levels of T5 to T9 and innervate structures of the foregut and thus the head of the pancreas. Running within these nerves are visceral afferent fibers that relay pain from foregut structures to the dorsal horn of the spinal cord. Also entering the dorsal horn are the somatic afferents from that vertebral level, which mediate pain from the body wall. Intercostal nerves T1 to T12 provide the terminal part of the pathway to the spinal cord of visceral afferents for pain from the thorax and much of the abdomen. Therefore, pain fibers from the pancreas pass by way of the splanchnic nerves to the sympathetic trunks and then, by way of communicating rami, to ventral rami of intercostal nerves, finally entering the spinal cord by way of the dorsal roots. The phrenic nerve innervates the diaphragm and also carries visceral afferents from mediastinal pleura and the pericardium, but it does not carry with it any visceral afferent fibers from the pancreas. The vagus nerve innervates the pancreas with parasympathetic fibers and ascends all the way up to the medulla where it enters the brain. It has no visceral afferent fibers for pain. The subcostal nerve is from the level of T12 and innervates structures below the pancreas and carries no visceral afferents from the pancreas.

GAS 333, 358-364; N 300; McM 237

35 D. The testicular artery originates from the abdominal aorta and travels with the spermatic cord, supplying the testes in the male. The external iliac artery is located "downstream" to the origin of the testicular artery from the aorta and would not cause any problems in sperm count. The inferior epigastric artery originates close to the deep inguinal ring (spermatic cord exit) as a branch of the external iliac artery and is not associated with the testicular production of sperm. The umbilical artery originates from the internal iliac artery and is divided in adults: one part is obliterated (medial umbilical artery), and the other part gives origin to superior vesical arteries to the urinary bladder. The umbilical artery plays no role in sperm production.

GAS 387-388; N 259; McM 261

36 A. The lymph drainage of the scrotum is into the superficial inguinal nodes. The internal iliac lymph nodes drain the pelvis, perineum, and gluteal region. The lumbar nodes drain lymph from kidneys, the adrenal glands, testes or ovaries, uterus, and uterine tubes. They also receive lymph from the common

internal or external nodes. Axillary lymph nodes drain the anterior abdominal wall above the umbilicus.
GAS 519; N 261; McM 265

37 B. The contents of the spermatic cord include ductus deferens; testicular, cremasteric, and deferential arteries; the pampiniform plexus of testicular veins; the genital branch of the genitofemoral nerve; the cremasteric nerves; and the testicular sympathetic plexus and also lymph vessels. The cremaster muscle and fascia originate from the internal abdominal oblique muscle. The external spermatic fascia is derived from the aponeurosis and fascia of the external oblique muscle. The tunica vaginalis is a continuation of the processus vaginalis (from parietal peritoneum) that covers the anterior and lateral sides of the testes and epididymis. The internal spermatic fascia is derived from the transversalis fascia. The dartos tunic consists of a blending of the adipose (Camper's) and membranous (Scarpa's) layers of the superficial fascia, with interspersed smooth muscle fibers.
GAS 279; N 365; McM 265

38 A. Esophageal varices are dilated veins in the submucosa of the lower esophagus. They often result from portal hypertension due to liver cirrhosis. The left gastric vein and the esophageal veins of the azygos system form an important portal-caval anastomosis when pressure in the portal vein, and in turn the left gastric vein, is increased. None of the other choices forms important portal-caval anastomoses.
GAS 275, 356; N 234; McM 209

39 B. The jejunum makes up the proximal two fifths of the small intestine. There are several ways in which the ileum and jejunum differ. During surgery the easiest way to distinguish the two based on appearance is the relative amount of mesenteric fat. The jejunum has less mesenteric fat than the ileum. Although the jejunum does have thicker walls, more villi, and higher plicae circulares compared with the ileum, these distinctions are not visible unless the intestinal wall is incised. The jejunum has fewer vascular arcades in comparison with the ileum. Lymphatic follicles are visible, usually only histologically, in the ileum.
GAS 313; N 263; McM 252

40 C. The arcuate line is a horizontal line that demarcates the lower limit of the posterior aponeurotic portion of the rectus sheath. It is also where the inferior epigastric vessels perforate the sheath to enter the rectus abdominis. The intercristal line is an imaginary line drawn in the horizontal plane at the upper margin of the iliac crests. The linea alba is a tendinous, median raphe running vertically between the two rectus abdominis muscles from the xiphoid process to the pubic symphysis. The pectineal line is a feature of the superior ramus of the pubic bone; it provides an origin for the pectineus muscle of the thigh and medial insertions for the abdominal obliques and transversus muscles. The semilunar line is the curved, vertical line along the lateral border of the sheath of the rectus abdominis.
GAS 287; N 247; McM 220

41 D. The psoas muscles (covered in psoas fascia) originate from the transverse processes, intervertebral disks, and bodies of the vertebral column at levels T12 to L5. In the image, this fascia contains a calcified tuberculous abscess. The pancreas is an elongated organ located across the back of the abdomen, behind the stomach. The tapering body extends horizontally and slightly upward to the left and ends near the spleen. The cecum is the blind-ending pouch of the ascending colon, lying in the right iliac fossa. The fundus of the stomach lies inferior to the apex of the heart at the level of the fifth rib. The suspensory ligament of the duodenum is a fibromuscular band that attaches to the right crus of the diaphragm.
GAS 371; N 258; McM 257

42 B. The superior mesenteric artery arises from the aorta, behind the neck of the pancreas, and descends across the uncinate process of the pancreas and the third part of the duodenum before it enters the root of the mesentery behind the transverse colon. It can compress the third part of the duodenum. The inferior mesenteric artery passes to the left behind the horizontal portion of the duodenum. The inferior mesenteric vein is formed by the union of the superior rectal and sigmoid veins and it does not cross the third part of the duodenum. The portal vein is formed by the union of the splenic vein and the superior mesenteric vein posterior to the neck of the pancreas. It ascends behind the bile duct and the hepatic artery within the free margin of the hepatoduodenal ligament. The splenic vein is formed by the tributaries from the spleen and is superior to the third part of the duodenum.
GAS 348; N 259; McM 235

43 B. The omental (epiploic) foramen (of Winslow) is the only natural opening between the lesser and greater sacs of the peritoneal cavity. It is bounded superiorly by the visceral peritoneum (liver capsule of Glisson) on the caudate lobe of the liver, inferiorly by the peritoneum on the first part of the duodenum, anteriorly by the free edge of the hepatoduodenal ligament, and posteriorly by the parietal peritoneum covering the inferior vena cava. Therefore, the inferior vena cava would be the most likely source of bleeding. The aorta lies to the left of the inferior vena cava in the abdomen. The portal vein, right renal artery, and superior mesenteric vein are not borders of the epiploic foramen.

GAS 304-307; N 266; McM 231

44 B. The ilioinguinal nerve, which arises from the L1 spinal nerve, innervates the skin on the medial aspect of the thigh, scrotum (or labia majora), and the mons pubis. It has been injured in this patient. The genitofemoral nerve splits into two branches: The genital branch supplies the scrotum (or labia majora) whereas the femoral branch supplies the skin of the femoral triangle. The subcostal nerve has a lateral cutaneous branch that innervates skin in the upper gluteal region, in addition to distribution over the lower part of the anterior abdominal wall. The iliohypogastric nerve innervates the skin over the iliac crest and the hypogastric region. Spinal nerve T9 supplies sensory innervation to the dermatome at the level of T9, above the level of the umbilicus.

GAS 398; N 253; McM 220

45 D. The second part of the duodenum is crossed anteriorly by the transverse mesocolon, a relationship that can be seen when the beginning of the jejunum is exposed by lifting the transverse colon superiorly. The posterior relationships of the second part of the duodenum and the portal vein cannot be seen without some dissection. The third part of the duodenum is not related anteriorly to the hilum of the left kidney.

GAS 312; N 271; McM 239

46 A. The right adrenal gland is a retroperitoneal organ on the superomedial aspect of the right kidney, partially posterior to the inferior vena cava. The appendix is a narrow, hollow tube that is suspended from the cecum by a small mesoappendix. The gallbladder is located at the junction of the ninth costal cartilage and the lateral border of the rectus abdominis, quite anterior to the pathologic mass. The ovaries and uterus are both inferior to the confluence of the inferior vena cava.

GAS 386; N 321; McM 258

47 A. The symptoms of yellow eyes and jaundice would be caused by reversal of flow of bile into the bloodstream. The common bile duct, if obstructed, allows no collateral pathway for drainage of bile from the liver or gallbladder. The cystic duct would block gallbladder drainage but allow for bile flow from the liver. Obstruction of either the right or left hepatic duct would still allow for drainage from the liver, as well as the gallbladder. The pancreatic duct is not involved in the path of bile flow from the liver to the duodenum. It drains pancreatic enzymes from the pancreas to the duodenum.

GAS 331, 341; N 280; McM 246

48 C. Cirrhosis of the liver would lead to inability of the portal system to accommodate blood flow. Blood backs up toward systemic circulation, draining to the inferior vena cava, with pooling at areas of portal-caval anastomoses. The left gastric vein (portal) anastomoses with the esophageal vein (caval) and enlarges or expands in instances of cirrhosis. The left colic and middle colic veins are both simply tributaries to the portal system. The inferior phrenic and superior phrenic veins are both systemic veins and would not be affected by portal hypertension. The same can be said for the renal and lumbar veins, both components of the caval-systemic venous system. The sigmoidal and superior rectal veins are both components of the portal venous system and would not engorge due to the portal-caval hypertension experienced in cirrhosis. (The anastomoses between the superior rectal veins and middle or inferior rectal veins can expand in portal hypertension as hemorrhoids.)

GAS 356; N 292; McM 237

49 A. The key distinguishing feature of a direct inguinal hernia is that it does not pass through the deep inguinal ring; it passes through the lower portion of the inguinal triangle (of Hesselbach). This triangle is bordered laterally by the inferior epigastric artery and vein; medially, it is bordered by the lateral edge of rectus abdominis; inferiorly, it is bordered by the iliopubic tract and inguinal ligament. An indirect hernia passes through the deep inguinal ring and into the inguinal canal. It often descends through the superficial ring into the scrotum or labium, a feature less common in a direct inguinal hernia. If the tip of the examiner's little finger is inserted into the superficial ring and the patient is asked to cough, an indirect inguinal hernia may be felt hitting the very tip of the examining finger. A direct inguinal hernia will be felt against the side of the digit. Both types of inguinal hernias occur above the inguinal ligament, and both are present lateral to the lateral border of the rectus abdominis. The pubic symphysis, a midline joint between the two pubic bones, provides no information for distinguishing types of hernias. The femoral

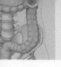

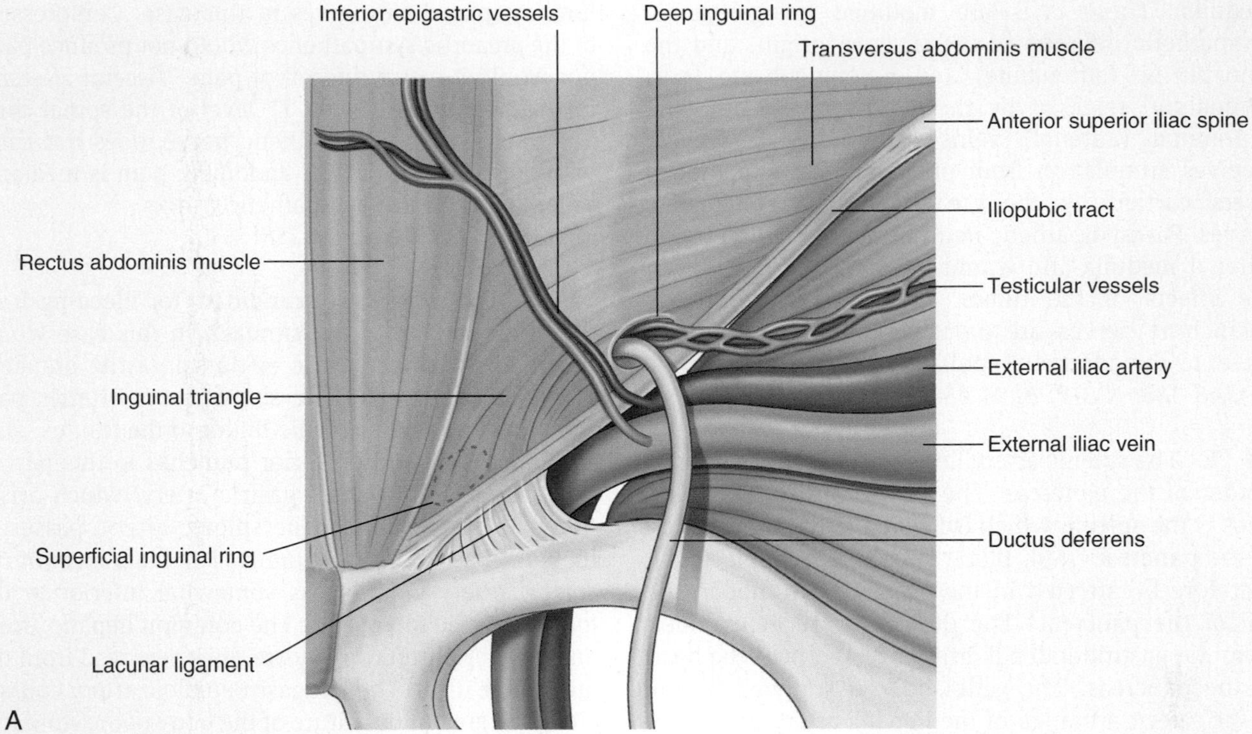

GAS **Fig. 4-50A**

canal, a feature of the femoral sheath, passes beneath the inguinal ligament into the thigh, providing the pathway taken by a femoral hernia. The pectineal ligament lies behind, or deep to, the proximal end of the femoral canal (*GAS* Fig. 4-50A).

GAS 299-301; N 257; McM 220

50 B. The bullet would probably first penetrate the transverse colon because it is the most superficial structure located slightly superior to the umbilicus. The abdominal aorta is located deep, on the left side of the vertebral column, and would not be encountered first. The stomach is located more superior, to the left, and posterior to the transverse colon and would not be affected by the anterior-posterior trajectory of the bullet. The pancreas is located deep to the stomach and duodenum. The gallbladder is located superiorly in the upper right quadrant of the abdomen, largely under cover of the liver. This would exclude its possibility of being penetrated by the midline bullet.

GAS 277, 322; N 291; McM 219

51 D. Surgical anastomoses to alleviate symptoms of portal hypertension are rooted in the premise that connection of a large portal vein to a large systemic vein allows for collateral drainage of the portal system. The splenic vein, a major tributary component of the portal venous system, and the left renal vein, a component of the caval-systemic venous system, are ideally located to allow for a low-resistance, easily performed anastomosis. Anastomosing the left gastric vein to the splenic vein, the right gastric vein to the left gastric vein, or the superior mesenteric vein to the inferior mesenteric vein would all be ineffectual because each of these veins is a component of just the portal venous system. In addition, the right renal and right gonadal veins are both tributaries of the caval system, and surgical connection would provide no benefit.

GAS 356-357; N 292; McM 236

52 B. Visceral pain from the kidneys and the ureter at the point of the neoplasm is mediated via T11 and T12 spinal cord levels. Therefore, pain is referred to these dermatomes leading to pain in the upper gluteal, pubic, medial thigh, scrotal, and labial areas (from subcostal and iliohypogastric nerves, in particular). In contrast, the umbilical region, the T10 dermatome, is supplied by the T10 spinal nerve. The dermatomes that supply the anterior and lateral thighs are of upper lumbar origin and would not receive pain referred from the kidneys.

GAS 379-380; N 318; McM 261

53 B. The mass leads to increased stimulation and secretions of the chromaffin cells of the adrenal medulla. These cells are modified postganglionic sympathetic neurons of neural crest origin, and the epinephrine (adrenaline) and norepinephrine (noradrenaline) released by these cells passes into the suprarenal (adrenal) veins. The adrenal medulla receives stimulation from preganglionic sympathetic fibers carried by the greater thoracic splanchnic nerves. Parasympathetic neurons are not found in the adrenal medulla and would have no participation in the effects of the tumor. In addition, the pelvic splanchnic nerves are parasympathetic and do not travel to the adrenal medulla.

GAS 386; N 319; McM 258

54 E. The splenic artery lies adjacent to the superior border of the pancreas. The organ it principally supplies is the spleen, which is located at the termination of the pancreatic tail. Blood supply to the spleen can therefore be affected in the event of a tumor in the tail of the pancreas. The duodenum receives blood from the gastroduodenal artery, located near the head of the pancreas. The gallbladder is supplied by the cystic artery, a branch of the hepatic artery and is not in contact with the pancreas. The liver is also supplied by the hepatic artery. The kidneys are supplied by the right and left renal arteries. The left renal artery lies deep and medial to the pancreatic tumor, and blood supply would proceed uninterrupted.

GAS 338-346; N 284; McM 234

55 E. The superior mesenteric artery lies just superior and anterior to the left renal vein as the vein passes to its termination in the inferior vena cava. The celiac artery is located superiorly and would not compress the left renal vein. The inferior mesenteric artery and its left colic branch are located too inferiorly to occlude the left renal vein. The middle colic artery arises from the anterior aspect of the superior mesenteric artery inferior to the position of the left renal vein. An aneurysm of the superior mesenteric artery would therefore be most likely to occlude the left renal vein.

GAS 348, 378; N 288; McM 238

56 B. Blood flow would be impeded or greatly reduced in the left testicular vein because of the occlusion of the left renal vein—into which the left testicular vein drains. This would result in pain as the testicular venous vessels become swollen. The testicular artery originates from the abdominal aorta more inferiorly and is not being compressed. Pain mediated from the renal organs would pass to the T11 and T12 spinal cord levels via the least thoracic splanchnic nerves. There would be no compression of lumbar splanchnic nerves in this case. Compression of the preaortic sympathetics would not produce pain, nor would it cause referral of pain. Visceral afferents for pain terminate at the T7 level of the spinal cord. The vagus, a parasympathetic nerve, does not carry visceral pain fibers in the abdomen; pain is mediated by branches of the sympathetic trunks.

GAS 516; N 310; McM 258

57 D. The most likely candidate for bleeding from the fundic region of the stomach in this case would be either the short gastric or dorsal gastric branches of the splenic artery. The short gastric arteries pass from the area of the splenic hilum to the fundus, supplying anterior and posterior branches to this part of the stomach. The dorsal gastric artery, which arises from the midportion of the splenic artery, passes to the dorsal aspect of the fundus. The main stem of the splenic artery would pass somewhat inferior to the location of the ulceration. The common hepatic artery and inferior phrenic artery are quite removed from the area of the ulcer. The left gastroepiploic artery courses along the greater curvature of the body of the stomach, distal to the fundus.

GAS 346; N 283; McM 241

58 D. Indirect inguinal hernia is the most common groin hernia in females. Although femoral hernias occur more commonly in females than in males, the occurrence of indirect inguinal hernias in women is greater. Inguinal hernias are much more common in males than in females. Epigastric and umbilical hernias would not present with pain to the inguinal region. Direct inguinal hernias, while exhibiting equal incidence in both sexes, are not the most common female hernia.

GAS 299-301; N 257; McM 225

59 A. The posterior superior pancreaticoduodenal artery arises from the gastroduodenal artery and travels behind the first part of the duodenum, supplying the proximal portion, with branches to the head of the pancreas. Duodenal ulcers commonly arise within the first portion of the duodenum, thus making the posterior superior pancreaticoduodenal artery one of the more frequently injured vessels. The superior mesenteric artery supplies derivatives of the midgut from the distal half of the duodenum to the left colic flexure. It lies inferior to the region of ulceration. The inferior pancreaticoduodenal artery arises from the superior mesenteric artery and supplies the distal portion of the second part of the duodenum, with anastomoses with its superior counterparts. The inferior mesenteric artery is responsible for supplying

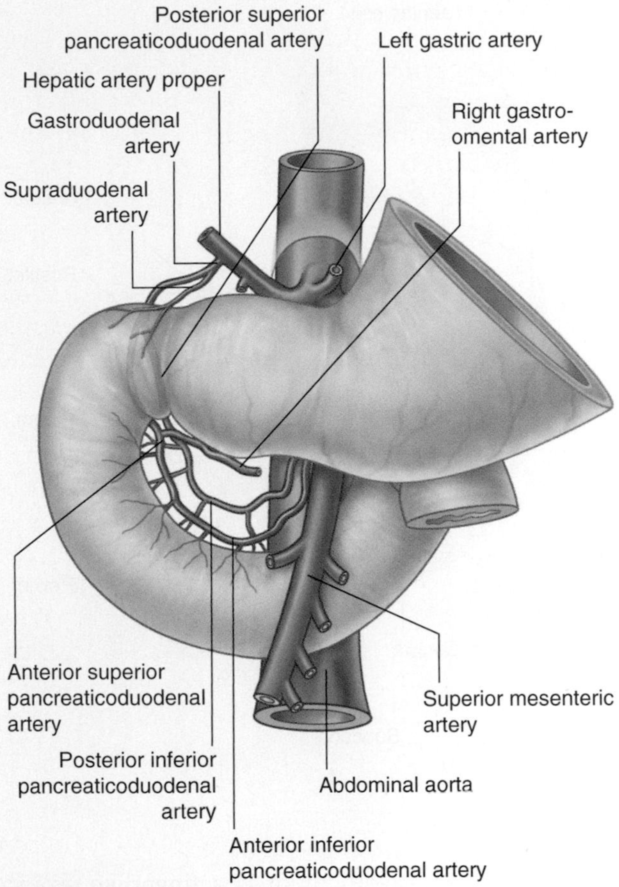

***GAS* Fig. 4-64**

most of the hindgut derivatives, generally supplying intestine from the left colic flexure to the superior aspect of the rectum. The right gastric artery is responsible for supplying the pyloric portion of the lesser curvature of the stomach (*GAS* Fig. 4-64).

GAS 347; N 284; McM 237

60 D. The transversalis fascial layer is the source of the internal spermatic fascia. The walls of the spermatic cord consist of three layers: external spermatic fascia, cremaster muscle, and the internal spermatic fascia. The external spermatic fascia is an extension of the external oblique fascia and aponeurosis. The cremaster muscle is a derivative of the internal oblique abdominal muscle and its fascia. The processus vaginalis is a pouch of peritoneum that precedes the testis as it descends through the deep inguinal ring and inguinal canal in the seventh month of development. That portion of the processus that is normally retained forms the tunica vaginalis of the testis. Retention of the proximal part of the processus provides a pathway for a congenital indirect inguinal hernia. If a portion of the intermediate part of the processus remains, it can form a fluid-filled hydrocele.

GAS 296-297; N 257; McM 220

61 C. The superior mesenteric artery arises from the aorta, deep to the neck of the pancreas, then crosses the uncinate process and third part of the duodenum. An uncinate tumor can cause compression of the superior mesenteric artery. The common hepatic artery arises superior to the body of the pancreas and is unlikely to be affected by a tumor in the uncinate region of the pancreas. The cystic artery and vein, supplying the gallbladder, are also superior to the pancreas. The inferior mesenteric artery arises at the level of L3, which is thus situated deep to and inferior to the head of the pancreas. The portal vein, formed by the confluence of the superior mesenteric vein and splenic vein, passes deep to the neck of the pancreas.

GAS 348; N 259; McM 238

62 A. The common bile duct is occluded. The pattern of pain of cholecystitis (and other signs), combined with jaundice, indicates blockage of release of bile into the duodenum. The cystic duct joins the common hepatic duct to form the common bile duct. Bile is released from the gallbladder into the cystic duct in response to cholecystokinin. From the cystic duct, bile flows normally through the common bile duct and the hepatopancreatic ampulla (of Vater) to enter the descending duodenum. Patients will often present with multiple gallstones. Cholecystitis is an inflammation of the gallbladder, most frequently in association with the presence of gallstones, and often resulting from a blocked cystic duct. Increasing concentration of bile in the gallbladder can precipitate a bout of inflammation. Blockage of the cystic duct, with concomitant cholecystitis, is not necessarily associated with jaundice. An obstruction in the common hepatic duct and subsequently the common bile duct would thus prevent communication between the duodenum and the liver, causing obstructive jaundice. An occlusion in either the left or right hepatic duct might cause mild jaundice; however, gallstones might not be present. An occlusion in the pancreatic duct would result in neither gallstones nor jaundice but may cause pancreatitis.

GAS 331, 341; N 280; McM 246

63 C. The anterior cutaneous branch of the iliohypogastric nerve is responsible for the innervation of the skin above the mons pubis. This nerve arises from the T12 and L1 spinal nerves and runs transversely around the abdominal wall and over the lowest portion of the rectus sheath. It is the first cutaneous nerve situated superior to the mons pubis. Nerves from the T11 and the T12 ventral rami terminate below the umbilicus but superior to the mons pubis. The ilioinguinal nerve courses through the inguinal canal, commonly on the lateral side of the spermatic cord and is therefore typically inferior to the incision. The lateral femoral cutaneous nerve travels lateral to the psoas muscle and emerges from the abdomen about an inch medial to the anterior superior iliac spine, passing thereafter to the lateral aspect of the thigh.

GAS 398; N 253; McM 253

64 B. Appendicitis is often characterized by acute inflammation and is indicated with both a positive psoas test and rebound pain over McBurney's point. McBurney's point lies 1 inch lateral to the midpoint of an imaginary line in the right lower quadrant, joining the anterior superior iliac spine and the umbilicus. In patients with appendicitis, rebound tenderness may be felt over McBurney's point after quick, deep compression of the left lower quadrant. An ectopic pregnancy would be associated with generalized abdominal pain instead of the localized pain felt over McBurney's point. Cholecystitis results from an inflammation of the gallbladder and would result in pain over the epigastric region shifting to the right hypochondriac region. Kidney stones result in referred pain to the lumbar or possibly inguinal regions. Perforation of the duodenum could result in pain to palpation of the abdomen, together with adynamic (paralytic) ileus, rigidity of the abdominal wall, and referral of pain to the shoulder (*GAS* Fig. 4-79).

GAS 322; N 273; McM 251

65 B. The visceral afferent innervation of the rectum is transmitted by way of the pelvic splanchnic nerves, which also provide the parasympathetic supply to this organ. The lumbar sympathetic trunk receives sensory fibers from the fundus and body of the uterus. The pudendal nerve provides origin for the inferior rectal nerve, the perineal nerve, and the dorsal nerve of the penis. The inferior rectal nerve supplies somatosensory fibers to the anal canal below the pectinate line and the perianal skin; the perineal nerve and dorsal nerve of the penis innervate structures of the urogenital region. The vagus nerve provides parasympathetic supply and afferent innervation (excluding pain) to the intestine proximal to the left colic flexure. The lumbar and sacral sympathetic trunks contribute sympathetic fibers for innervation of smooth muscle and glands of certain pelvic viscera, but not sensory fibers for the rectum.

GAS 358-364; N 388; McM 268

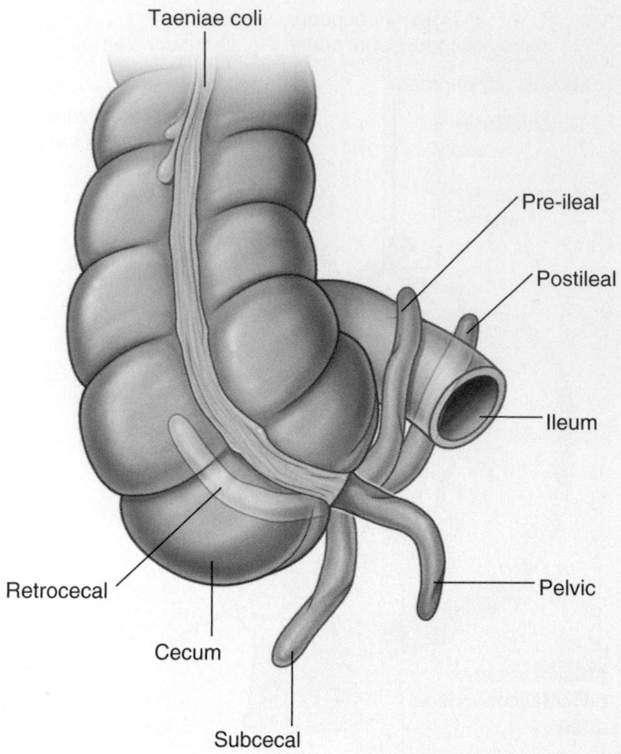

***GAS* Fig. 4-79**

66 D. Meckel's diverticulum is a fingerlike projection of the ileum that is generally remembered by the "rule of 2s": It occurs in about 2% of the population, is approximately 2 feet proximal from the ileocecal junction, is about 2 inches long, occurs 2 times as often in males as in females, may contain 2 types of ectopic tissue, and may be confused often with 2 different clinical conditions. The two types of ectopic tissue are gastric mucosa and pancreatic tissue. These, along with bleeding and pain, may give indications of peptic ulcer or appendicitis. Internal and external hemorrhoids involve the rectoanal area, not the ileum, in addition to which biopsy of hemorrhoids would not reveal the presence of gastric mucosa. Borborygmi are bowel sounds that occur with the passage of gas and bowel contents through the intestines. Diverticuloses are outpouchings of the colon and would therefore be lined with colic mucosa.

GAS 318; N 274; McM 232

67 D. The aortic aneurysm often occurs between L3 and L4, below the bifurcation of the aorta, resulting in significant increase in pressure, creating the marked abdominal pulsation. The remaining answer choices would be associated with referred pain and would not be likely to result in elevated blood pressure.

GAS 388; N 259; McM 258

68 **B.** In a supine patient, fluid accumulation will often occur in the hepatorenal pouch (of Morison), which is the lowest space in the peritoneal cavity in the supine position. The hepatorenal space is located behind the liver and in front of the parietal peritoneum covering the right kidney. The vesicouterine and rectouterine spaces are also potential areas of fluid accumulation; however, fluid accumulation in these spaces occurs when the patient is in an erect position rather than a supine position.
GAS 322; N 340; McM 266

69 **D.** Descending colon. Below the left colic flexure, innervation of the gastrointestinal tract is supplied by parasympathetic fibers of the pelvic splanchnic nerves. The parasympathetic innervation of the midgut up to the descending colon is supplied by the vagus nerve. A hematoma occurring below L4 would affect innervation of the descending colon because the pelvic splanchnic nerves arise from spinal nerve levels S2 to S4. The jejunum, ascending colon, ileum, and transverse colon are all innervated by the vagus nerve.
GAS 322; N 303; McM 239

70 **C.** The porta hepatis (transverse fissure of liver) transmits the proper hepatic artery, portal vein, common hepatic duct, autonomic nerves, and lymph vessels. A tumor in this region would be most detrimental because of its abundance of vessels and lymphatics that could lead to all of these symptoms when they are compromised functionally. A tumor in either the right or left lobes would not be as serious because it would not completely obstruct all of these vessels. The falciform ligament does not carry any vessels (except some small periumbilical veins), so a tumor in this area would not lead to the symptoms described. The hepatogastric ligament is the bilaminar peritoneal connection between the liver and the lesser curvature of the stomach and is unrelated to the symptoms and signs here.
GAS 330; N 277; McM 245

71 **E.** The cystic artery is the only artery listed that goes directly to the gallbladder. It is often a branch of the right hepatic artery and must be clamped before the gallbladder is cut free from its attachments. The common hepatic artery provides origin to the proper hepatic artery, which divides into right and left hepatic arteries supplying the liver, gallbladder, and biliary tree (*GAS* Fig. 4-97A).
GAS 331; N 280; McM 246

72 **D.** The spleen is a large lymphatic organ that rests against the diaphragm and ribs 9, 10, and 11 in the left hypochondriac area. A laceration of this friable organ is often associated with severe blood loss and shock. Almost all of the liver is located in the right hypochondrium and epigastrium, although some protrudes into the left hypochondrium below the diaphragm. The left kidney lies retroperitoneally approximately at the level of the T11 to L3 vertebrae on the left side of the body. The ilium is the upper portion of the hip bone and contributes to the bony pelvis. Ileum is the distal portion of the small intestine and is pronounced the same as "ilium."
GAS 338; N 281; McM 235

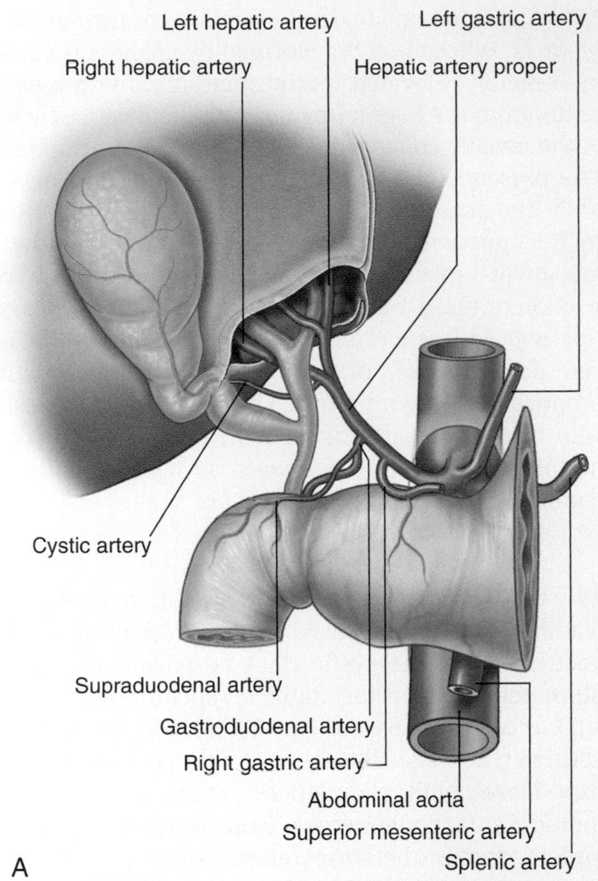

***GAS* Fig. 4-97A**

73 **D.** The ileocolic artery is the only artery listed that directly supplies the appendix, giving off an appendicular branch. The superior mesenteric artery gives origin to the ileocolic, right colic, and middle colic arteries; however, the latter two lie superior to the site of the appendix. The superior rectal artery is the terminal branch of the inferior mesenteric artery and supplies the lower portion of the sigmoid colon and superior rectum.
GAS 350; N 287; McM 251

74 **A.** Caput medusae (referring to the head of Medusa, whose hair was formed by snakes) is caused by severely elevated portal pressure, with venous reflux from the liver to the periumbilical veins, by way of the usually collapsed veins in the ligamentum teres. The presence of caput medusae is usually associated with end-stage disease. Caput medusae is identified by the appearance of engorged veins radiating toward the lower limbs. The portal vein is the central connection of these anastomoses. Obstruction of the inferior vena cava, superior vena cava, and lateral thoracic vein do not cause portal hypertension and would not produce these symptoms. The superficial epigastric vein also is not associated with the development of portal hypertension but could provide a collateral channel for venous drainage.
GAS 275; N 292; McM 236

75 **C.** Cholecystitis is an inflammation of the gallbladder due to increased concentration of bile or obstruction of the cystic duct by gallstones. Pain is ultimately felt in the right hypochondriac region, which corresponds to the T6 to T8 dermatomes. Sensory afferents from the viscera carry pain fibers as they travel with sympathetic axons in the greater thoracic splanchnic nerves. Pain cannot be felt in the viscera and is therefore referred to the body wall. The vagus nerve carries visceral sensory fibers from the head, neck, and trunk, but these do not include pain fibers. Spinal nerves of T1 to T4 receive afferents for pain from thoracic viscera, including the heart, but not abdominal organs. Sympathetic neurons are autonomic motor nerves and therefore do not carry sensory information. Afferent fibers of the dorsal primary rami of spinal nerves T6 to T8 convey sensory fibers from the back but not from internal organs.
GAS 341; N 306; McM 237

76 **B.** McBurney's point usually corresponds to the location of the base of the appendix where it attaches to the cecum. It is found on the right side of the abdomen, about two thirds of the distance from the umbilicus to the anterior superior iliac spine. The inguinal ligament is localized lateral and inferior to the appendix and hence would not be used as a landmark.
GAS 321; N 275; McM 221

77 **B.** The greater thoracic splanchnic nerves arise from the levels of the T5 to T9 thoracic sympathetic ganglia and are responsible for carrying general visceral afferents from upper abdominal organs and, therefore, from the body of the stomach. The pain fibers pass from the sympathetic trunk to spinal nerves T5 to T9, thereafter to the spinal cord. Spinal nerves T1 to T5 do receive sensory afferents for pain but from thoracic organs. The vagus nerves do not carry afferents for pain. The lumbar splanchnic nerves are associated with the lower portion of the abdominopelvic area.
GAS 358-364; N 300; McM 210

78 **C.** The ureter is normally constricted to some degree as it crosses the pelvic brim from major to minor pelvis. The minor and major calyces are proximal to the ureter and not typical sites for obstruction by kidney stones. The midportion of the ureter is not a typical site for obstruction. The site of oblique entrance of the ureter into the urinary bladder is a common site for obstruction because it is compressed by bladder contents and the muscular wall as the bladder fills. There are no common sites of obstruction between the pelvic brim and the uterine cervix.
GAS 379; N 314; McM 259, 261

79 **C.** The splenorenal ligament is the attachment of the spleen to the left kidney and is the only ligament that contains the major branches of the splenic artery to the spleen and greater curvature of the stomach. The coronary ligament is the peritoneal reflection from the diaphragmatic surface of the liver onto the diaphragm that encloses the bare area of liver; it is not attached to the spleen. The falciform ligament is a peritoneal fold in contact with only the diaphragm and the liver. The gastrocolic ligament contains branches of the gastro-omental vessels but should not be a factor in the splenectomy (*GAS* Fig. 4-104).
GAS 338; N 266; McM 250

80 **C.** Pelvic splanchnic nerves and the left colic artery supply the descending colon. The vagus nerve supplies the bowel only to the left colic flexure, and the middle colic artery supplies the transverse colon. The superior rectal artery supplies the lower sigmoid and rectum. The ileocolic artery supplies the cecum, appendix, and ascending colon. The left lesser thoracic splanchnic nerve has nothing to do with the descending colon.
GAS 350, 358-364; N 303; McM 269

81 **E.** The ilioinguinal nerve is a terminal branch of ventral ramus of spinal nerve L1. It innervates the skin overlying the iliac crest; the anterior portion of the urogenital region; and the upper, inner thigh. Its usual pathway takes it below McBurney's point, but it can be injured with extension of an appendectomy incision. Spinal nerve T10, the genitofemoral nerve, and the pudendal nerve are not located in the area of

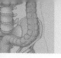

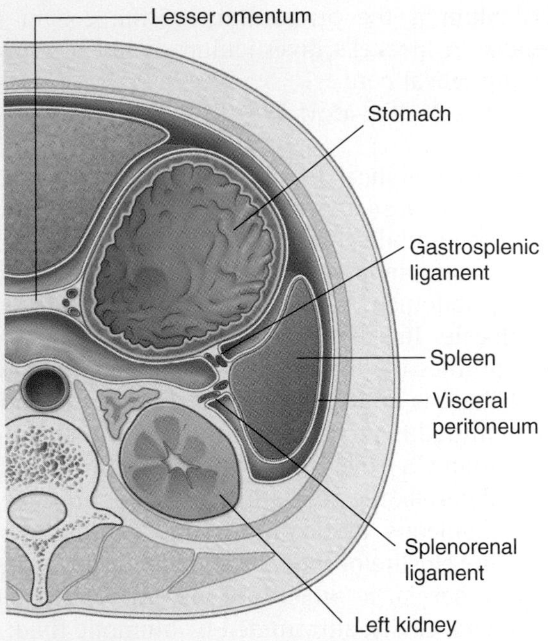

***GAS* Fig. 4-104**

the incision; what is more, the area of sensory deficit does not correlate well with their injury. The genitofemoral nerve leaves the body wall at the superficial inguinal ring, well below the appendectomy incision. The pudendal nerve is both motor and sensory to the perineum. The genitofemoral nerve provides motor supply to the cremaster, sensory fibers to the scrotum, and a femoral branch innervating only the skin over the femoral triangle. Spinal nerve T10 innervates the umbilical region. The subcostal nerve innervates the skin at the level of the costal margin and the lower portion of the abdominal wall above the pubic region.

GAS 290, 320; N 253; McM 220

82 A. Esophageal stenosis results from a failure of esophageal recanalization in the eighth week of development, which may also cause esophageal atresia. Webs and strictures are found in an examination of the esophagus in cases of stenosis, but they are not noticed in cases of atresia. A tracheoesophageal fistula is an abnormal passage between the trachea and the esophagus and is associated with esophageal atresia; therefore, webs and strictures would not be seen. Duodenal atresia and stenosis occur in the small intestine and would not cause aspiration pneumonia, and clinical manifestations would not be seen in the esophagus.

GAS 222; N 231; McM 214

83 B. Duodenal stenosis is caused by incomplete recanalization of the duodenum. The vomit contains bile in addition to the stomach contents because of the location of the occlusion, distal to the hepatopancreatic ampulla (of Vater) where the common bile duct enters the small intestine. Lack of weight gain is due to constant vomiting. A patent bile duct would not cause vomiting with bile. A hypertrophied pyloric sphincter would cause projectile vomiting without the presence of bile. An atrophied gastric antrum is caused by the removal of the membranous lining of the stomach and occurs proximal to the site of the entrance of the bile duct; therefore, the vomit would not contain bile. A tracheoesophageal fistula would not cause vomiting of stomach contents and bile because it is a defect of the respiratory system and occurs proximal to the site at which bile is added to stomach contents.

GAS 312; N 272; McM 236

84 C. With hypertrophy of the pyloric sphincter and the associated narrowing of the pyloric canal, there is projectile vomiting of stomach contents, but without bile, because bile enters the duodenum distal to the pyloric constriction. Duodenal atresia, like duodenal stenosis, causes vomiting of stomach contents and bile. Vomiting begins soon after birth in cases of atresia; vomiting due to stenosis does not begin necessarily immediately after birth and can occur days after delivery. Lack of weight gain is due to constant vomiting. An atrophied gastric fundus would not produce the signs seen here. A tracheoesophageal fistula would not cause vomiting of stomach contents and bile because it is a defect of the respiratory system and occurs proximal to the site at which bile is added to intestinal contents.

GAS 312; N 270; McM 236

85 B. Incomplete recanalization of the duodenum is caused either by duodenal stenosis or partial occlusion of the lumen of the duodenum and usually occurs in the distal third portion of the duodenum. This occlusion often results in vomiting of stomach contents plus bile later in life and is the reason the child was constantly hungry but did not gain weight. Incomplete recanalization of the esophagus during the eighth week of development causes esophageal stenosis and presents as webs and strictures. Esophageal atresia is generally seen with a tracheoesophageal fistula because it is caused by the tracheoesophageal septum deviating in the posterior direction. In some cases, it may result from a failure of recanalization during the eighth week of development and presents as a fetus with polyhydramnios due to an inability to swallow amniotic fluid. Duodenal atresia is the result of a failed reformation of the lumen of the duodenum and is associated with vomiting within the first few days of birth, polyhydramnios, and the "double bubble" sign. Tracheoesophageal fistula is an abnormal passage between the trachea and esophagus and would not be a cause for vomiting because it is associated with the respiratory system and also occurs proximal to the site of the defect.

GAS 265; N 272; McM 236

86 B. Duodenal atresia is the result of a failed reformation of the lumen of the duodenum and is associated with vomiting within the first few days of birth. Polyhydramnios is seen due to abnormal absorption of amniotic fluid by the intestines. Finally, radiographic or ultrasound examination would reveal the "double bubble" sign because of distended, gas-filled stomach. Duodenal stenosis is caused by incomplete recanalization of the duodenum and often results in vomiting of stomach contents plus bile later in life. Hypertrophied pyloric sphincter would cause projectile vomiting. An atrophied gastric antrum is caused by the removal of the membranous lining of the stomach and occurs proximal to the site of the entrance of the common bile duct; therefore, vomit would not contain bile. Tracheoesophageal fistula is an abnormal passage between the trachea and esophagus and would not be a cause for any of symptoms cited in the question.

GAS 312; N 272; McM 236

87 C. Annular pancreas causes duodenal obstruction due to the thick band of pancreatic tissue that surrounds and constricts the second part of the duodenum. This obstruction can be found shortly after birth or much later. Annular pancreas can result from the bifid ventral pancreatic bud wrapping around the duodenum during development and fusing with the dorsal pancreatic bud, thereafter forming a ring. Both the dorsal and bifid ventral pancreatic buds are involved in this process; therefore, answers A, D, and E cannot be correct because they refer to either the dorsal or ventral buds, not both. This anomaly is not involved with lack of canalization of the bile ducts.

GAS 336; N 294; McM 235

88 A. A remnant of the omphaloenteric duct generally presents as an ileal (Meckel's) diverticulum in the proximal portion of the omphaloenteric duct. It normally arises as a fingerlike pouch about 3 to 6 cm long from the antimesenteric border of the ileum and 40 to 50 cm from the ileocecal junction. The umbilical vesicle normally turns into a pear-shaped remnant about 5 mm in diameter by week 20. The cecal diverticulum is the primordium of the cecum and appendix. A Meckel's diverticulum is not a remnant of the umbilical cord.

GAS 318; N 263; McM 238

89 A. An umbilical hernia results when the body wall does not close appropriately at the site of attachment of the umbilical cord. In such cases, part of the greater omentum and small intestine can herniate from the abdomen. Umbilical herniation differs from omphalocele. In congenital omphalocele, there is a failure of intestine to return to the abdominal cavity so that there is an apparent herniation of abdominal viscera into the proximal portion of the umbilical cord, without a covering of the hernia by skin. In umbilical hernia, the herniating structures are covered by subcutaneous tissue and skin. Gastroschisis is incomplete closure of the lateral folds, resulting in an epigastric hernia, in which the viscera protrude into the amniotic cavity, surrounded by amniotic fluid. An epigastric hernia occurs through a defect in the linea alba superior to the level of the umbilicus and occurs far more commonly in adults. An indirect inguinal hernia is when the communication between the tunica vaginalis and the peritoneal cavity do not close, and a loop of intestine or a portion of another organ such as the cecum herniates through the deep inguinal ring into the inguinal canal, with possible further descent through the superficial inguinal ring into the scrotum or labium majus.

GAS 301-302; N 247; McM 223

90 D. Gastroschisis results from an incomplete closure of the lateral folds during the fourth week of development from a defect in the medial plane of the abdominal wall. This results in an epigastric hernia, with viscera that protrude into the amniotic cavity without a peritoneal covering and are covered by amniotic fluid. Nonrotation of the midgut results in the lower portion of the loop returning to the abdomen first, the small intestine passing to the right side of the abdomen, and the large intestine lying entirely on the left. Most cases are asymptomatic; however, obstruction of the superior mesenteric artery can cause infarction and gangrene of the part of the intestine it supplies. An umbilical hernia results when an abdominal organ herniates through an umbilical ring that does not close perfectly. Such a hernia often contains part of the greater omentum and small intestine. The cloacal membrane usually ruptures during the eighth week of development, creating a communication between the anal canal and the amniotic cavity.

GAS 265; N 247; McM 222

91 **A.** The inability to pass meconium denotes an obstruction of the fetal bowel. Midgut volvulus results in the twisting of the intestines and ultimately obstruction of the small and/or large intestines. Gastroschisis results from an incomplete closure of the lateral folds during the fourth week of development from a defect in the medial plane of the abdominal wall. This results in an epigastric hernia, with viscera that protrude into the amniotic cavity and are covered by amniotic fluid. Failure of recanalization of the ileum is seen with 50% of obstructive lesions of the intestine. This obstruction is caused by stenosis or atresia of the intestines. A remnant of the omphaloenteric duct generally presents as an ileal (Meckel's) diverticulum in the proximal portion of the omphaloenteric duct. It normally arises as a fingerlike pouch about 3 to 6 cm long from the antimesenteric border of the ileum and 40 to 50 cm from the ileocecal junction. Nonrotation of the midgut results in the lower portion of the loop returning to the abdomen first, the small intestine sitting on the right side of the abdomen, and the large intestine lying entirely on the left. Most cases are asymptomatic; however, obstruction of the superior mesenteric artery can cause infarction and gangrene of the part of the intestine it supplies.

GAS 325; N 321; McM 229

92 **D.** A remnant of the proximal portion of the omphaloenteric duct generally presents as an ileal (Meckel's) diverticulum. It normally arises as a fingerlike pouch about 3 to 6 cm long from the antimesenteric border of the ileum and 40 to 50 cm from the ileocecal junction. Midgut volvulus results from a twisting of the intestines and, ultimately, obstruction of the small and large intestines. Infarction of fetal bowel is seen and would not be the cause of the signs of appendicitis. Gastroschisis results from an incomplete closure of the lateral folds during the fourth week of development from a defect in the medial plane of the abdominal wall. This results in an epigastric hernia, with viscera that protrude into the amniotic cavity and are covered by amniotic fluid. Failure of recanalization of the ileum is seen in 50% of obstructive lesions of the intestine. This obstruction is caused by stenosis or atresia of the intestines. Nonrotation of the midgut results in the lower portion of the loop returning to the abdomen first so that the small intestine becomes fixed on the right side of the abdomen, with the large intestine lying entirely on the left. Most cases are asymptomatic; however, obstruction of the superior mesenteric artery can cause infarction and gangrene of the part of the intestine it supplies.

GAS 314; N 263; McM 238

93 **A.** Incomplete separation of the cloaca by the urorectal septum results in anal agenesis. Dorsal deviation of the urorectal septum would result in anal stenosis. Failure of the anal membrane to perforate externally results in imperforate anus, not anal agenesis. Abnormal recanalization of the colon results in rectal atresia, in which there is no connection between the rectum and anal canal. Remnants of the proximal portion of the omphaloenteric duct would result in a Meckel diverticulum, not anal agenesis.

GAS 504; N 308; McM 267

94 **B.** Dorsal deviation of the urorectal septum results in anal stenosis. Incomplete separation of the cloaca by the urorectal septum results in anal agenesis. Failure of the anal membrane to perforate results in imperforate anus. The anal canal exists but is obstructed by a layer of tissue. Abnormal recanalization of the colon results in rectal atresia, in which there is no connection between the rectum and anal canal. Remnants of the proximal portion of the omphaloenteric duct would result in a Meckel diverticulum, not anal stenosis.

GAS 485; N 308; McM 267

95 **D.** A vitelline fistula is caused by the persistence of the vitelline duct, which can, by its connections with the umbilicus, cause the symptoms described. An enterocystoma is a tumor and would not result in the symptoms described. A vitelline cyst is a persistence of the vitelline duct; however, it would not open directly to the outside so would not cause the symptoms. Meckel diverticulum can result in a vitelline fistula, but it is simply the persistence of the vitelline duct that can appear in different forms (such as cyst or fistula). Volvulus is the twisting of the small intestines around their suspending vasculature. It can result from malrotation of the midgut loop and would not result in the symptoms described.

GAS 318; N 247; McM 223

96 **D.** Anorectal agenesis is due to abnormal partitioning of the cloaca and is often associated with a rectourethral, rectovaginal, or rectouterine fistula. Failure of fixation of the hindgut can result in volvulus. Failure of the proctodeum to develop will result in an imperforate anus. Agenesis of the urorectal septum would most likely lead to a fistula but would not cause anorectal agenesis. Premature rupture of the anal membrane would not cause anorectal agenesis.

GAS 504; N 308; McM 266

97 **A.** Meckel's diverticulum is a remnant of the yolk stalk. It is usually 2 inches long and 2 feet proximal from the ileocecal junction. Meckel's diverticulum is prone to ulceration (possibly leading to perforation) that can result in gastrointestinal bleeding. Duplication of the intestine does not predispose the patient to GI bleeding. A subhepatic cecum and appendix is due to failure of the cecal bud to form and results in the absence of an ascending colon. Nonrotation of the midgut could lead to volvulus but is not the most likely cause for GI bleeding. Herniation of intestines can exist without any symptoms; however, if the loop of intestine becomes strangulated, it can lead to gangrene.

GAS 318; N 263; McM 232

98 **D.** Failure of the ureteric bud to form results in renal agenesis and oligohydramnios, that is, deficient production of amniotic fluid. Polycystic kidney disease is an autosomal recessive disease characterized by spongy kidneys with a multitude of cysts. Degeneration of the mesonephros occurs during normal development; however, a small portion of the mesonephric tubules may go on to form parts of the urogenital system. Ureteric duplication occurs due to premature division of the ureteric bud and can result in either a double kidney or a duplication of the ureter. Wilms tumor is a malignancy of the kidney that is more common in children than it is in adults; it does not cause renal agenesis.

GAS 373; N 308; McM 253

99 **C.** Androgen insensitivity syndrome involves the development of testes and female external genitalia, with a blind-ending vagina and absence of the uterus and uterine tubes. This is consistent with the presenting symptoms. Male pseudohermaphroditism and female pseudohermaphroditism have different presentations from those described and result from 46XY and 46XX genotypes, respectively. Inguinal hernias have nothing to do with absence of the uterus and a negative sex chromatin pattern. Turner syndrome results from a 45X genotype and presents with short stature, webbed neck, congenital hypoplasia of the lymphatics, and shield chest—among other symptoms—and is not consistent with the symptoms described.

GAS 476; N 367; McM 272

100 **A.** The vaginal plate, which arises from the sinovaginal bulbs, undergoes canalization during embryonic development. Failure of canalization results in a persistent vaginal plate and thus imperforate hymen. The hymen is a fold of mucous membrane that covers the opening of the vaginal canal. It is often torn early in life. The processus vaginalis is a tubelike projection of the peritoneum into the inguinal canal that precedes the descent of the testis or round ligament. Both cervical atresia and androgen insensitivity syndrome would result in amenorrhea; however, neither disorder would present with an imperforate hymen because the vaginal canal would still undergo canalization. The sinovaginal bulbs are responsible for the development of the vaginal plate. Failure of development would result in complete absence of the vagina.

GAS 480; N 366; McM 272

101 **D.** Gartner ducts cysts, which often appear in the lateral wall of the vagina, are the result of remnants of the mesonephric (Wolffian) duct. The mesonephric duct gives rise to a variety of structures, including the ureter and collecting tubules. In males, the duct eventually forms the ductus deferens and ejaculatory ducts, whereas it often disappears in females. The only remaining traces of the mesonephric ducts are the epoophoron, paroophoron, and Gartner's duct, which can form a cyst. The mesonephric tubules are elongations of the mesonephric vesicles. These tubules are subsequently invaginated by the glomeruli to form a component of the renal corpuscle. The paramesonephric ducts are responsible for formation of the uterus, cervix, and uppermost aspect of the vagina. The urogenital folds form the labia minora in females and the spongy urethra in males. Sinovaginal bulbs are responsible for the development of the vaginal plate in embryonic development.

GAS 480; N 367; McM 273

102 **C.** Potter sequence, or Potter syndrome, is a rare autosomal recessive trait and is associated with renal agenesis or hypoplasia. Altered facial characteristics include flattened nasal bridge, mandibular micrognathia, malformed low-set ears, etc. Absence or lack of proper development of the kidneys causes oligohydramnios, or possibly anhydramnios. Multicystic dysplastic kidney and polycystic kidney are usually secondary to Potter sequence and are therefore not the cause of Potter sequence or oligohydramnios. Wilms tumor is a relatively common renal tumor that presents in children; it is not associated with oligohydramnios and Potter sequence. Extrophy of the bladder is a congenital defect that exposes the posterior surface of the bladder on the exterior of the abdominal wall; there is no indication of this defect in the patient.

GAS 373; N 308; McM 258

103 **B.** The ureteric bud is responsible for the development of the ureter, and thus an early splitting of the ureteric bud would result in formation of a second ureter on the ipsilateral side. Failure of the ureteric bud to form would cause a complete absence of the ureter, whereas failure of the ureteric bud to branch occurs normally during embryonic development and results in one ureter joined to each kidney. The urorectal septum is a section of tissue of mesenchymal origin that develops between the allantois and hindgut. Failure of this structure to develop would not result in an additional ureter. Finally, a persistent patent urachus acts as an abnormal fistula that runs from the bladder to the umbilicus, resulting in urine leaking from the anterior abdominal wall.

GAS 373; N 314; McM 261

104 **B.** The hepatorenal pouch (or recess or space of Morison) is situated between the liver and both the parietal peritoneum covering the right kidney and suprarenal gland. This recess is the lowest space in the peritoneal cavity in supine patients. Accumulation of fluid in the peritoneal cavity will ordinarily collect in this pouch. The right subphrenic space is located between the liver and diaphragm. Although this recess is positioned in the appropriate abdominal quadrant, it is not the deepest space within the peritoneal cavity. Fluid may reach the right subphrenic space, but it will not accumulate in this region. The paracolic gutters are grooves lateral to the ascending and descending colons. Though these recesses are potential spaces for fluid accumulation, they are located inferior to the hepatorenal recess and would not collect fluid while the patient is supine. The vesicouterine and rectouterine pouch would not be potential spaces for fluid accumulation in a supine patient, although they provide predictable sites when the patient is upright or ambulating.

GAS 328; N 269; McM 272

105 **A.** The right subphrenic space is located between the inferior aspect of the diaphragm and the superior surface of the liver. An ulceration in the posterior stomach wall would allow the passage of air from the stomach into the right subphrenic space through an open communication in the omental bursa. The remaining answer choices are located inferior to the site of ulceration and would not accumulate air. The paracolic gutters traverse lateral to the ascending and descending colons. The vesicouterine and rectouterine pouches are located in the pelvic cavity; air would not accumulate in these spaces.

GAS 328; N 277; McM 244

106 **E.** The most likely location of fluid to accumulate is the rectouterine pouch (of Douglas) because it is the lowest point in the pelvis when a patient is standing erect. Additionally, fluid would accumulate here because the mesovarian ligament causes the ovary to be located on the posterior aspect of the board ligament. This allows for communication between the fluid of the ovary and the rectouterine pouch. The right subphrenic space is located inferior to the right side of the diaphragm and superior to the liver. The paracolic gutters are located lateral to the ascending and descending colons. Neither of these locations is a likely site of fluid accumulation when the patient is standing. The hepatorenal recess is situated between the liver and both the right kidney and suprarenal gland. This recess, also known as Morison's pouch, is the deepest space in the peritoneal cavity in a supine patient but not when the patient sits or stands. The vesicouterine pouch is located between the bladder and uterus and is separated from the ovaries by a double layer of mesentery also known as the broad ligament of the uterus.

GAS 381; N 346; McM 272

107 **D.** Parietal peritoneum and "the mesentery." The parietal peritoneum lines the abdominal wall, whereas the visceral peritoneum is in intimate contact with organs. The greater omentum extends from the greater curvature of the stomach and covers the midgut. Access to the ileum would require penetration of the parietal peritoneum to enter the peritoneal cavity and interruption of the visceral peritoneum of "the mesentery" covering the thrombosed vessel. Although it would probably be necessary to reflect the greater omentum for adequate exposure, it would not ordinarily require an incision.

GAS 387; N 257; McM 229

108 **D.** Referred pain from cholecystitis is generally referred to the region of the inferior angle of the right scapula. These fibers are generally from T5 to T9. These sensory fibers for pain are stimulated by the gallbladder inflammation because of the proximity of the adjacent structures. C3 to C5 sensory fibers innervate the shoulder area. The distribution of C5 to C8 is primarily to the upper limb, to the level of the hand; T1 to T4 distribution is to the upper thoracic wall and medial upper arm; T10 and T11 distribution is to the thoracic and abdominal wall. T1 to T4 visceral fibers for pain are generally associated with referred pain from the heart.

GAS 341, 358-364; N 306; McM 236

109 **A.** The Pringle maneuver is a surgical technique employed when the hepatic artery has been accidentally ligated. The hepatoduodenal ligament is clamped off to prevent the passage of blood flow through both the hepatic artery and the portal vein. The Kocher maneuver, in which the ascending colon and descending duodenum are reflected to the left, is often employed to expose and arrest a hemorrhage from the inferior vena cava. The Valsalva maneuver involves stopping the passage of air with the vocal folds to build up intrathoracic pressure, as for coughing or vocalization. The Heimlich maneuver involves sharp, rapid compressions of the xiphisternal region to expel foreign bodies from the trachea. Putting a clamp on the porta would not stop the bleeding but could certainly produce major injury to the numerous vascular elements there.

GAS 307; N 269; McM 237

110 A. The most likely source of this hemorrhage is from the left colic artery. Colonic diverticular disease is the development of blind end sacs from the wall of the colon. Of the selected choices the left colic artery is the only artery supplying a portion of the descending colon. The internal pudendal artery supplies the external genitalia and the perineum. The superior and inferior rectal (hemorrhoidal) arteries supply the rectum and anal canal. The left gastroepiploic artery arises from the splenic artery and supplies the greater curvature of the stomach (*GAS* Fig. 4-86).

GAS 350; N 288; McM 239

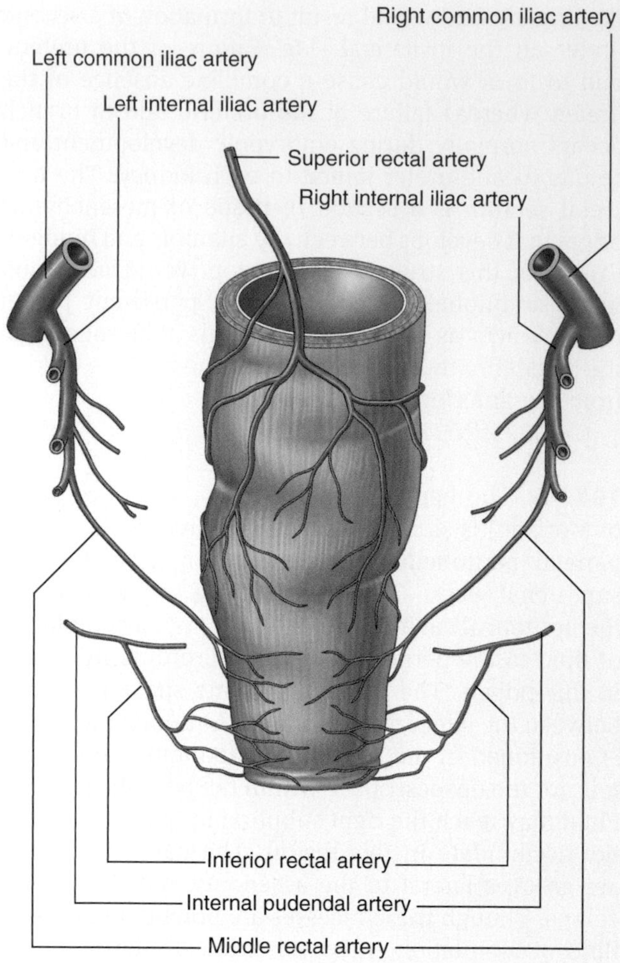

***GAS* Fig. 4-86**

111 D. Murphy's sign is a specific test designed to detect and diagnose problems in the upper right abdominal quadrant. It is classically used to diagnose diseases of the gallbladder by pressing deeply under the right costal margin and asking the patient to breathe deeply. This causes sharp pain in the patient with cholecystitis. Rebound tenderness is pain experienced when applied pressure is removed quickly from a location on the body. It is not specific to areas of the body and is not indicative of problems in the upper right quadrant. The iliopsoas test is generally used to diagnose appendicitis because flexing the iliopsoas muscle group applies pressure to the cecum and appendix. When the appendix is inflamed, this pressure elicits pain. The obturator sign is used to diagnose irritation of the obturator internus muscle and would not elicit a positive test with the patient's current symptoms. Finally, cough tenderness would not be present because it is generally associated with hernias and problems associated with rises in intraabdominal pressure.

GAS 331, 341; N 306; McM 236

112 D. The lowest point of the lesser sac occurs at the intersection of the gastrocolic ligament and transverse colon. Bleeding would travel to the lowest point of the lesser sac. Access to this area would require entry through the gastrocolic ligament, which extends from the greater curvature of the stomach to the transverse colon. The hepatogastric and hepatoduodenal ligaments attach between the liver and the lesser curvature of the stomach and the first part of the duodenum, respectively. Dividing the hepatogastric ligament provides entry through the lesser omentum, but this is not the most efficient access point because it does not provide the best exposure of the inferior aspect of the lesser sac (*GAS* Fig. 4-57).

GAS 303-309; N 268; McM 230

113 D. Superficial inguinal nodes. The external anal sphincter is skeletal muscle of the anal canal. This suggests that the carcinoma is originating from the anal canal. The results of the biopsy support the finding that the carcinoma most likely occurred below the pectinate line where squamous cells of the anal canal are found. The anal canal primarily drains to

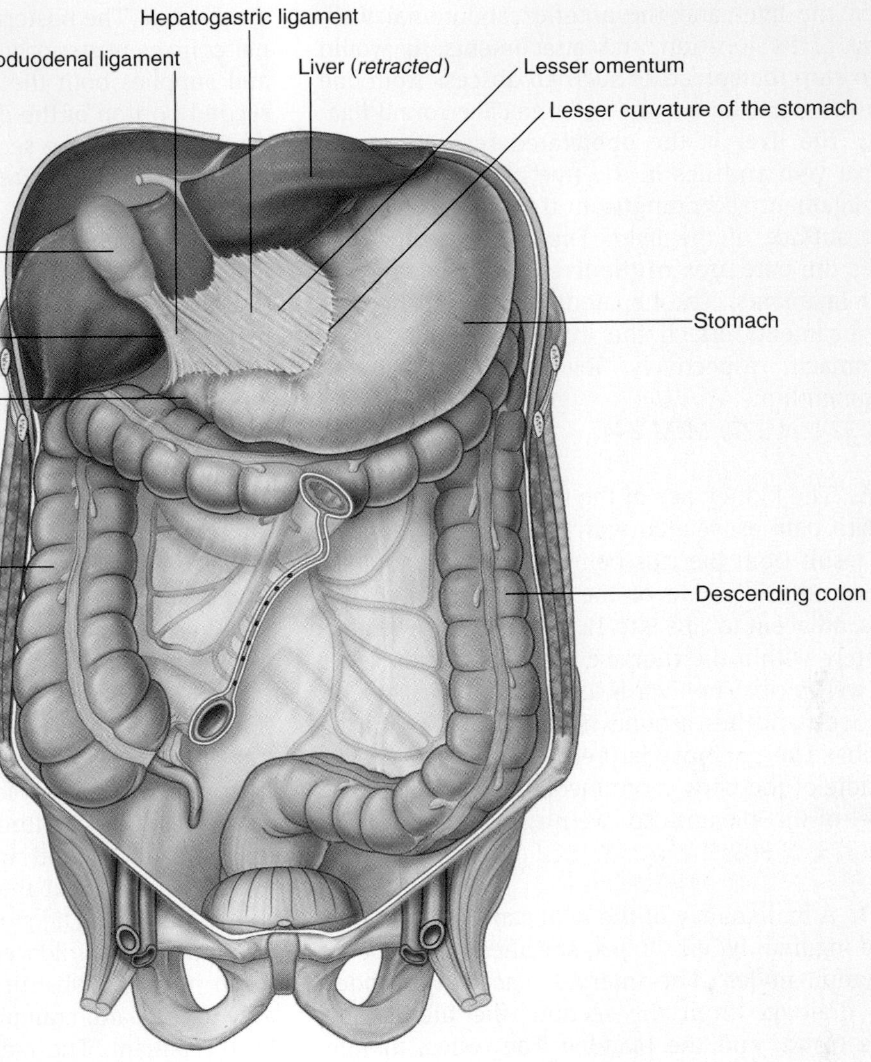

GAS Fig. 4-57

the superficial inguinal lymph nodes. The inferior rectum above the pectinate line drains into the internal iliac nodes. The superior aspect of the rectum drains into the middle rectal lymph nodes. The external iliac nodes primarily drain lower limb, pelvic, and deep peritoneal structures. The deep inguinal lymph nodes drain the glands of the clitoris and penis and the superficial inguinal nodes.

GAS 519; N 261; McM 224

114 A. The lymphatics of the inferior rectum above the pectinate line drain into the internal iliac nodes. Below the pectinate line, lymphatics of the anal canal will primarily drain into the superficial inguinal (horizontal) nodes. The external iliac nodes primarily drain lower limb, pelvic, and deep peritoneal structures. The deep inguinal lymph nodes primarily drain the glands of the clitoris and penis, receiving lymph also from the superficial inguinal nodes. The superior aspect of the rectum is drained by the middle rectal nodes, lymph from which eventually flows into the lumbar nodes.

GAS 519; N 386; McM 268

115 B. In sliding hernias the gastroesophageal junction is displaced. Diaphragmatic hernias of the esophagus can be characterized by analyzing the gastroesophageal junction. In sliding hernias the gastroesophageal junction is displaced anteriorly into the mediastinum. The paraesophageal hernia is generally characterized by herniation of the stomach into the mediastinum; however, the gastroesophageal junction remains fixed. In paraesophageal hernias the fundus herniates into the stomach, but the antrum does not.

GAS 372; N 258; McM 260

116 B. The falciform ligament separates the subphrenic spaces into right and left recesses and extends between the liver and the anterior abdominal wall. Because of its location and attachments, it would serve to stop the spread of such an abscess from one side to the other across the midline. The round ligament of the liver is the obliterated remains of the umbilical vein and lies in the free margin of the falciform ligament ascending from the umbilicus to the inferior surface of the liver. The coronary ligament encloses the bare area of the liver and forms the triangular ligaments. The hepatoduodenal and hepatogastric ligaments attach the liver to the duodenum and stomach, respectively. Together they form the lesser omentum.

GAS 328; N 277; McM 244

117 A. The kidney lies at the twelfth rib, and problems with pain associated with respiratory processes would result from the ribs being injured. The spleen lies under the left side of the liver superior to the kidneys, adjacent to ribs 9 to 11. The lungs are located completely within the thoracic cavity above the level of the twelfth rib. The liver is located on the right side of the body and lies around the level of the fifth to tenth ribs. The pancreas is predominantly located in the middle of the body more medial to the kidneys at the level of the eleventh to twelfth ribs.

GAS 373; N 309; McM 253

118 D. A malignancy of the anal canal would drain into the inguinal lymph nodes, specifically the superficial lymph nodes. The internal iliac lymph nodes receive drainage from the rectum, the uterus, the prostate gland, and the bladder. The testes, though located in the scrotum, external to the abdominopelvic cavities, drain into the lumbar nodes located on the anterior aspect of the aorta. The sigmoid colon drains into the inferior mesenteric lymph nodes.

GAS 519; N 386; McM 268

119 C. The superior mesenteric artery arises from the aorta, behind the neck of the pancreas, at the level of L1 within the abdominal cavity, and traverses inferiorly across the anterior surface of the third part of the duodenum. As it crosses the uncinate process of the pancreas and duodenum, this artery could readily be affected by a tumor in the immediate area. The common bile duct and the portal vein course anteriorly from the head of the pancreas and therefore are associated with the first part of the duodenum. The gastroduodenal artery supplies the duodenum, the head of the pancreas, and the greater curvature of the stomach and is a branch of the common hepatic artery. This artery does not cross the third part of the duodenum. The posterior superior pancreaticoduodenal courses posteriorly over the head of the pancreas and supplies both the head of the pancreas and the second portion of the duodenum. It is therefore more associated with the second part of the duodenum.

GAS 343, 353; N 288; McM 238

120 D. Vascular structures situated immediately medial to the ureter are often subject to ligation during surgical procedures. The ureter is crossed by the uterine artery an inch or so lateral to the cervix and must be identified and avoided when ligating the uterine vessels. The middle rectal artery arises from the internal iliac artery and passes dorsal to the uterus and the rectum. The superior vesical artery arises from the umbilical artery anteriorly in the pelvis. The internal pudendal vein enters the pelvis through the greater sciatic foramen and terminates in the internal iliac vein, laterally at the pelvic wall. The gonadal vein in the female passes to the ovary by way of the infundibulopelvic ligament, near the pelvic brim.

GAS 379; N 314; McM 261

121 B. Pain in the umbilical region can be indicative of referred pain from the large intestine. Gallstones can ulcerate through the wall of the fundus of the gallbladder and into the transverse colon, or through the wall of the body of the gallbladder into the duodenum. The stone would then most likely be entrapped at the ileocecal junction, possibly leading to an intestinal obstruction. This could lead predictably to the pain, cramping, and vomiting experienced by the patient. The radiographic results suggest that the biliary trees are clear (indicated by the presence of air) and rule out the common bile duct or hepatic duct as potential sites of gallstone obstruction. Because the gallstones would pass thereafter through the duodenum, this would not be the site of blockage. Because the gallstones could pass freely through the intestine as far distally as the ileocecal junction, it would be unlikely that they would accumulate in the jejunum.

GAS 331, 341; N 306; McM 238

122 A. The intersection of the right linea semilunaris with the ninth costal cartilage in the right upper quadrant is associated typically with the point of contact of the gallbladder fundus with the anterior abdominal wall. The anatomic quadrants provide a useful tool for understanding the location of various anatomic structures and viscera located within the body. The linea semilunaris runs parallel with the lateral border of the rectus sheath and is a prominent landmark for surface anatomy. The upper right quadrant is the correct anatomic region for the location of the gallbladder as mentioned earlier; however, this is too general and would not be the best answer. Similarly, the intersection of the right semilunaris with the right intertubercular plane is situated in the upper right quadrant; however, this is not the most precise location of the gallbladder. The epigastric region is located superior to the umbilical region. The contents of the epigastric region are the left portion of the liver and a portion of the stomach. The right hypochondriac region, the anatomic region situated to the right of the epigastric region, is located superior and lateral to the gallbladder.

GAS 407; N 244; McM 217

123 E. The transversus abdominis aponeurosis and transversalis fascia form a significant portion of the posterior wall of the inguinal canal and the lower part of the inguinal triangle (of Hesselbach). Gradual weakness or attrition of tissues in the posterior wall provides the likelihood of egress of a direct inguinal hernia. A patent processus vaginalis at the deep inguinal ring, or expansion of the deep inguinal ring, with stretching of the transversalis fascia there, can contribute to the formation of indirect inguinal hernias. Weakness of the transversalis fascia by itself is not a key feature of inguinal herniation, nor is weakness of the peritoneum, or defects in the aponeuroses of the external or internal oblique muscles.

GAS 301; N 257; McM 222

124 C. The rectouterine pouch (of Douglas) is the lowest recess of the female abdominopelvic cavity when the woman is standing or sitting upright. Any fluid accumulation in this cavity will settle in the rectouterine pouch due to it being the most dependent or inferior space. The subphrenic space would likely not collect fluid because of its location in the superior abdominal cavity, which does not tend to collect fluid from the pelvis. The hepatorenal pouch (of Morison) is located in the right posterosuperior aspect of the abdominal cavity, far from the pelvic cavity. The vesicouterine space is a recess that is similarly located in the lower portion of the abdomen between the urinary bladder and uterus, but it is slightly superior to the pouch of Douglas and separated from it and the pathway of the leaking fluid by the broad ligament of the uterus. The broad ligament tends to prevent the collection of fluids in the vesicouterine pouch.

GAS 481; N 346; McM 272

125 D. The dorsal root ganglia contain all cell bodies of sensory neurons from the body wall and limbs. Afferent fibers from the appendix travel in the dorsal root ganglia of T8 to T10. The sympathetic trunk contains postganglionic sympathetic cell bodies that are targeted to smooth muscle and glands of the viscera and heart muscle. The greater thoracic splanchnic nerve (T5 to T9) carries preganglionic sympathetic axons to the celiac ganglion, which is formed by postganglionic sympathetic neurons. The lateral horn of the spinal cord is found in levels T1 to L2 and contains preganglionic sympathetic cell bodies.

GAS 314; N 303; McM 210

126 A. The preganglionic sympathetic fibers running to the adrenal gland would be cut during adrenalectomy for they synapse on catecholamine-secreting cells within the adrenal medulla. Unlike the normal route of sympathetic innervation, which is to first synapse in a sympathetic ganglion and then send postganglionic fibers to the target tissue, the chromaffin cells of the adrenal gland are innervated directly by preganglionic sympathetic fibers. This is because the chromaffin cells are embryologically postganglionic neurons that migrate to the medulla and undergo differentiation. The adrenal gland receives no other recognized types of innervation.

GAS 394; N 319; McM 258

127 D. The left common iliac vein lies posterior to the right common iliac artery. Compression of the vein in this location is a frequent cause of deep venous thrombosis of the left lower limb; that is, the venous drainage of the lower limb is obstructed. This can cause extreme pain, together with ischemia of the limb that, in some untreated cases, can lead to amputation of the limb or gangrene leading to death. The inferior vena cava would not be compressed, for it has branched superior to the location of the tumor. The renal veins would not be compromised because these veins extend from the kidneys to the inferior vena cava quite far above the blockage. The testicular veins pass lateral to the area of obstruction, with the right gonadal vein passing superiorly to join the inferior vena cava, and the left gonadal vein terminating in the left renal vein. The right common iliac vein passes freely about the pelvic brim after taking origin from the inferior vena cava and would not be subjected to compression by the right common iliac artery. The subcostal nerve exits the spinal cord at the level of T12 and runs into the abdominal cavity behind the diaphragm on top of the quadratus lumborum.

GAS 272; N 288; McM 261

128 D. Preganglionic and postganglionic sympathetics, preganglionic parasympathetic, and visceral afferent fibers are present within the celiac ganglion. The cell bodies of postganglionic sympathetic fibers are contained within the celiac ganglion and their axons pass to upper abdominal organs (foregut). Preganglionic parasympathetic nerves also run through the ganglion but do not synapse within the ganglion; therefore, there are no postganglionic parasympathetic nerves in the ganglion. The preganglionic parasympathetic fibers are extensions from the right vagal trunk and run within the preaortic plexus. No somatic motor fibers are present within this ganglion. Running through all of the abdominal ganglia are also visceral afferent fibers passing superiorly to reach the spinal cord at spinal nerve levels T5 to L2. There are no postganglionic parasympathetic fibers running within the ganglion or the celiac plexus. Postganglionic parasympathetic nerves arise from terminal ganglia located upon, or within the wall of, target organs. Answers C and E are incorrect because they do not include postganglionic sympathetic cell bodies and their axons, which also run through the celiac ganglion.

GAS 359; N 307; McM 242

129 C. The ureter is innervated by sympathetic and parasympathetic fibers in the ureteric plexus. General visceral afferent fibers in the ureteric plexus follow sympathetic fibers from spinal cord levels T11 to L2; therefore, pain from these fibers will be referred to nerves at these levels. The iliohypogastric nerve receives fibers from T12 and L1 and innervates the skin over the pubic symphysis. The ilioinguinal nerve receives fibers from L1 and innervates the skin from the iliac crest to the upper portions of the labia. The subcostal nerve innervates skin at the T12 dermatome level. The lateral cutaneous branch of the iliohypogastric nerve contains fibers from T12-L1 and supplies the anterior superior gluteal skin. The lateral femoral cutaneous nerve contains fibers from L2 and L3 spinal cord levels and innervates the skin over the lateral thigh. The obturator nerve contains fibers from L2 to L4 spinal cord levels and innervates the adductors of the thigh.

GAS 290, 380; N 318; McM 220

130 C. Perforation of a posterior duodenal ulcer most commonly damages the posterior superior pancreaticoduodenal artery. This artery branches from the inferior aspect of the gastroduodenal artery. The superior mesenteric artery does not lie directly beneath the duodenum and is not likely to be damaged. The posterior inferior pancreaticoduodenal artery branches from the superior mesenteric artery and lies too far inferior to be damaged. The right gastric artery branches from the proper hepatic artery and runs along the pyloric portion of the lesser curvature of the stomach.

GAS 315; N 284; McM 236

131 E. A perforating ulcer in the anterior wall of the duodenum is likely to cause peritonitis. The duodenum is covered anteriorly by a layer of peritoneum, and an erosion would allow intestinal contents into the greater peritoneal sac. The gastroduodenal and posterior superior pancreaticoduodenal arteries lie posterior to the duodenum and are not likely to be damaged. The posterior inferior pancreaticoduodenal artery is a branch of the superior mesenteric artery and neither of these arteries is likely to be damaged because they lie inferior to the duodenum. Perforating ulcers pierce the duodenum or stomach anteriorly; penetrating ulcers pierce the duodenum or stomach posteriorly.

GAS 315; N 284; McM 236

132 D. The suspensory ligament of the duodenum (ligament of Treitz) originates from the right crus of the diaphragm and is attached to the fourth part of the duodenum at the duodenojejunal junction. This ligament is commonly used as a palpable landmark during abdominal surgeries. The superior and inferior mesenteric arteries and the vasa recta are highly variable and cannot be used as reliable landmarks. Ladd bands connect the cecum to the abdominal wall and can obstruct the duodenum in cases of malrotation of the intestine. These bands can be surgically divided to treat malrotation of the intestine, but Ladd bands are not used as a common landmark (*GAS* Fig. 4-66).

GAS 313; N 264; McM 234

133 E. Failure of fusion of the pleuroperitoneal folds can cause herniation of abdominal contents into the thorax (congenital diaphragmatic hernia), most commonly on the left side. This defect can impair lung function, causing respiratory distress and cyanosis. The absence of the pleuropericardial fold would cause communication between the pericardial sac and the pleural cavity of the lung and would not lead to the symptoms described. The musculature of the diaphragm is derived from the third to fifth cervical myotomes. Absence of musculature in one half of the diaphragm (eventration of the diaphragm) would cause paradoxical respiration. The downward migration of the diaphragm is due to the elongation of the posterior body wall and is not likely to lead to this patient's condition. Failure of the septum transversum to develop would cause an absence of the central

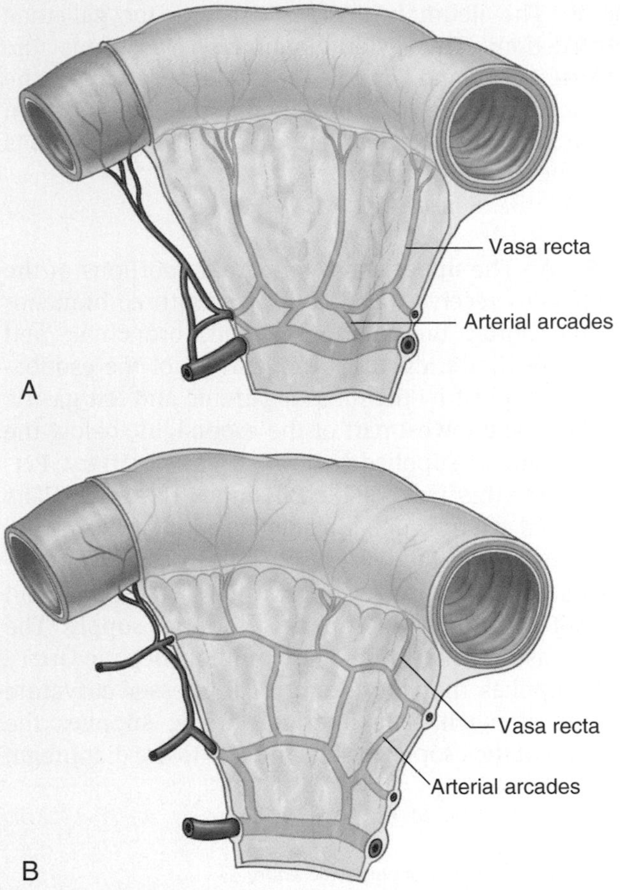

GAS **Fig. 4-66**

tendon of the diaphragm and is not normally associated with congenital diaphragmatic hernia.

GAS 373; N 191; McM 260

134 C. Both Morgagni and Bochdalek hernias are due to defects in the pleuroperitoneal membrane. Morgagni hernia is normally found retrosternally just lateral to the xiphoid process and, if severe, can cause respiratory distress. More commonly, it is perceived as a sharp, epigastric pain that can be confused with several other maladies. In this case, the barium test rules out esophageal problems; the HIDA scan injection to study the gallbladder and biliary apparatus is negative also. Bochdalek hernia can cause similar symptoms but is due to a posterolateral herniation and would not be near the xiphoid process. A congenital hiatal hernia occurs when part of the stomach herniates into the thoracic cavity and can be caused by a shortened esophagus. This type of hernia would not present between the xiphoid process and costal margin.

GAS 372; N 191; McM 260

135 A. The ileum can become ischemic when arterial supply from the superior mesenteric artery is compromised. The superior mesenteric artery arises from the aorta posterior to the neck of the pancreas. It descends across the third part of the duodenum and enters the root of the mesentery behind the transverse colon. This artery gives origin to the following branches: inferior pancreaticoduodenal artery, middle colic artery, ileocolic artery, right colic artery, and intestinal arteries. The ileocolic artery descends behind the peritoneum toward the right and ends by dividing into the ascending colic artery, anterior and posterior cecal arteries, the appendicular artery, and ileal branches. The ileum is supplied by the ileal branches, which do not have any anastomoses with another major source vessel. The transverse colon is supplied by the marginal artery (of Drummond), which possesses anastomoses of the right colic artery arising from the superior mesenteric artery, and the left colic artery arising from the inferior mesenteric artery. The spleen, stomach, and duodenum are all supplied by branches of the celiac trunk, which arise from the abdominal aorta just below the aortic hiatus of the diaphragm.

GAS 354; N 287; McM 238

136 A. The portal vein is compressed in its passage through the hepatoduodenal ligament because it is the anterior border of the omental (epiploic) foramen (of Winslow). The veins of Retzius are located along the sides of the abdominal walls and communicate between tributaries of retroperitoneal parts of the gastrointestinal tract and veins of the body wall. In portal hypertension the portal blood cannot pass freely through the liver, and the portal-caval tributaries and their anastomoses become dilated. The inferior epigastric veins anastomose with the paraumbilical veins, which is the first branch off the hepatic portal vein. These would be the first affected in portal hypertension. The inferior vena cava is the main route of blood return to the right atrium and is posterior to the omental (epiploic) foramen (of Winslow); it would not likely be compressed due to herniation through the foramen. Compression of the proper hepatic artery in the hepatoduodenal ligament would not result in dilation of veins of Retzius but could conceivably diminish blood supply to the gallbladder and liver. Common bile duct compression would result in jaundice and increased serum bilirubin. The cystic duct joins with the hepatic duct to form the common bile duct. Compression of this would lead to an inflamed gallbladder (cholecystitis).

GAS 354-357; N 289; McM 236

137 C. A dermatome is an area of skin that is supplied by a single spinal nerve. The descending colon receives its visceral sensory supply for pain from spinal segments L1 and L2. Injury to the descending colon can cause referral of pain to the corresponding dermatomes. Spinal segments T6 to T10 supply upper abdominal organs, including the pancreas and the duodenum. L1 to L4 supply the rectum, bladder, and uterus. T6 to L2 supply portions of all abdominal viscera.

GAS 405; N 303; McM 97

138 E. A gallstone ileus occurs when a gallstone (cholelith) ulcerates through the wall of the body of the gallbladder and into the duodenum. In this case, gallstones became lodged in the ileocecal region. Obstruction in the ileocecal junction can produce pain that mimics appendicitis. However, bowel sounds will be exaggerated above the obstruction and absent distal to the obstruction. This obstruction would require surgical correction. The hepatopancreatic ampulla (of Vater) is the location where the pancreatic and bile ducts join before entering the duodenum. An obstruction here would cause jaundice, and radiating pain would be localized into the right upper quadrant, with referred pain to the scapula. The duodenal cap, or bulb, is proximal to the entrance of the common bile duct, and any obstruction would be distal to this point. The ileum is not a likely site for gallstone obstruction. The pyloric sphincter surrounds the pyloric orifice and controls the rate of emptying of the stomach contents into the duodenum. This location is proximal to the entrance of gallbladder contents into the small intestine.

GAS 331, 341; N 273; McM 232

139 A. The upper and intermediate portions of the esophagus receive blood supply from three branches of the aorta: the inferior thyroid, bronchial, and esophageal arteries; the lower portion of the esophagus is supplied by the inferior phrenic and left gastric arteries. The lowest part of the esophagus, below the diaphragm, is supplied by the left gastric artery. Perforation to this area could easily injure this artery. The bronchial artery supplies a small section of the esophagus inferior to the level of the carina (T4). The thoracic intercostal arteries supply intercostal spaces and do not contribute to esophageal arterial supply. The right gastric arises from the common hepatic artery and supplies the pyloric part of the lesser curvature of the stomach. The inferior phrenic supplies the portion of the esophagus just inferior to the diaphragm (*GAS* Fig. 4-132).

GAS 343-344; N 233; McM 241

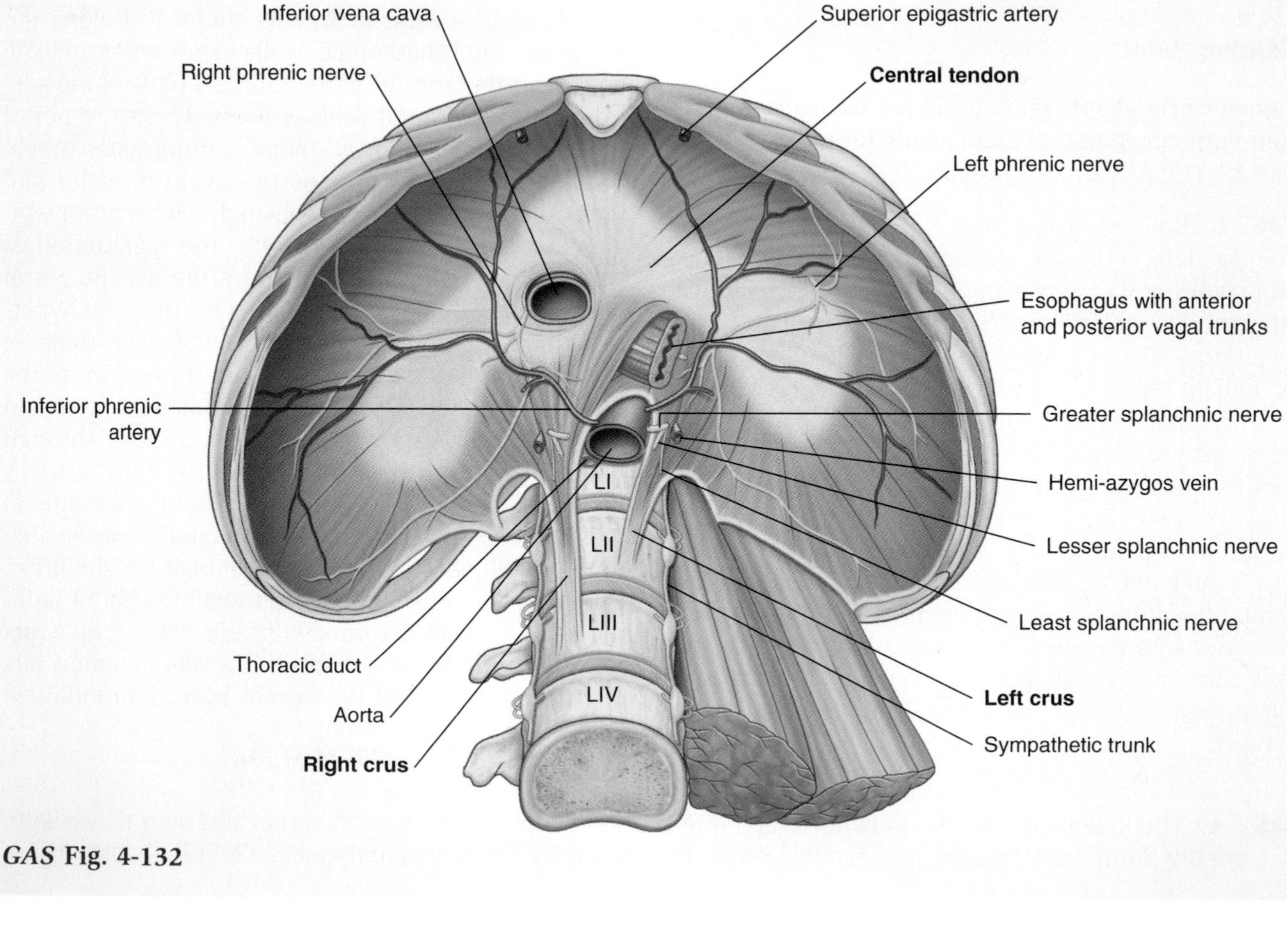

***GAS* Fig. 4-132**

140 **B.** Kerh's sign is a clinical indication of a ruptured spleen and is characterized by intense radiating pain to the top of the left shoulder. Mittelschmerz can occur in the middle of a woman's menstrual cycle when the Graafian follicle ruptures and the ovum is released from the ovary. Rovsing's sign is a clinical indicator of gallbladder inflammation and pain referred to the right shoulder, also owing to diaphragmatic irritation. The iliopsoas muscle has clinically important relations to the kidneys, ureters, cecum, appendix, sigmoid colon, pancreas, lumbar lymph nodes, and nerves to the posterior abdominal wall. If any of these structures is diseased, a positive psoas sign will be observed. The obturator sign may cause painful spasms of the adductor muscles of the thigh and sensory deficits in the medial thigh.

GAS 342; N 284; McM 249

141 **B.** The most common variation in hepatic artery supply to the right lobe of the liver is the right hepatic artery originating from the superior mesenteric artery, occurring in approximately 18% of cases.

GAS 347; N 284; McM 236

142 **B.** The gallbladder consists of a fundus, body, and neck. The fundus is the rounded, blind end that comes in contact with the transverse colon. The body is the major part and rests on the upper part of the duodenum and transverse colon. The neck is the narrowest part and gives rise to the cystic duct. This duct contains the spiral valve (of Heister), which is a redundant mucosal fold that maintains patency of the duct. This is not actually a valve and does not determine the direction of flow of bile. This could potentially be a point of constriction that could present difficulty with insertion of a catheter. The cystic duct comes into contact only with the cystic artery and is not particularly tortuous. The hepatoduodenal ligament is the thickened free edge of the lesser omentum, and it conducts the portal triad (portal vein, hepatic artery, and bile duct) and encloses structures that pass through the porta hepatis. This ligament is unlikely to compress the cystic duct. Though the cystic duct is in close relation to the portal vein and the hepatic artery, the most likely cause of difficulty would be potential constriction by the spiral valve.

GAS 331; N 280; McM 246

143 **B.** The ducts of Luschka are accessory biliary ducts that are not present in all individuals. During a cholecystectomy the cystic duct and cystic artery are ligated and the gallbladder is removed, using sharp dissection to separate the gallbladder from the liver. Routinely, the right hepatic duct and left hepatic duct are not encountered directly. If the surgeon was unaware that ducts of Luschka were present in the patient, they would not have been ligated or clipped and their leakage would result in bile peritonitis. The common bile duct and hepatic ducts are left intact during the surgery and should not leak. The cystic duct is ligated during the surgery and with proper ligation would not produce bile peritonitis.

GAS 335; N 280; McM 246

144 **C.** Visceral afferents are nerve fibers that transmit the sensation of visceral pain. The target of the neurectomy would be to eradicate visceral pain. One would not want to interfere with sympathetic and parasympathetic nerves, as these provide motor innervation to viscera.

GAS 394; N 307; McM 235

145 **B.** Adynamic ileus is essentially paralysis of the bowel. It can result from many causes, including kidney stone, spinal injury, peritonitis, etc. Typically, bowel obstruction is characterized initially by increased borborygmi (bowel sounds, particularly the stomach). Mechanical obstruction can be caused by blockage within the bowel or compression of the bowel from an external source. Increased borborygmi usually follow such obstructions immediately. As the bowel muscle tires, however, bowel sounds can become reduced or absent. Although this patient might have peritonitis, with an abdomen tender to palpation, the data simply indicate generalized abdominal pain. Crampy pain has not been noted.

GAS 308; N 263; McM 252

146 **A.** Blood supply from the inferior pancreaticoduodenal artery via the superior mesenteric artery can provide collateral blood supply to the head of the pancreas and the first part of the duodenum in situations when the celiac trunk is occluded. Such anastomoses occur between the superior pancreaticoduodenal branches of the gastroduodenal artery (a derivative of the common hepatic branch of the celiac trunk) and the inferior pancreaticoduodenal (a branch of the superior mesenteric artery). The left gastric artery and hepatic artery are derivatives of the celiac trunk and do not anastomose with the superior mesenteric. The cystic artery and the gastroduodenal artery are derivatives of the common hepatic from the celiac trunk. They would not typically provide an anastomosis between the celiac trunk and superior mesenteric artery (unless there is an aberrant right hepatic branch from the superior mesenteric artery). The right colic artery and left colic artery anastomose via the marginal artery of the colon, but this provides collateral supply of the inferior mesenteric artery. The right and left gastro-omental arteries anastomose and provide collateral supply to the greater curvature of the stomach but are derived from the celiac trunk and thus do not provide communication between the celiac trunk and superior mesenteric artery.

GAS 344-350; N 284; McM 237

147 **B.** The incision and tissue separation at McBurney's point to reach the appendix will usually encounter the aponeurosis of the external abdominal oblique muscle, internal oblique muscle, transversus abdominis muscle, transversalis fascia, and parietal peritoneum. Muscle fibers of the internal oblique and transversus can be separated bluntly, without cutting them. The appendix is located intraperitoneally within the abdomen, thus it is covered with visceral peritoneum. The transversalis fascia separates the internal surface of the transversus abdominis from the parietal peritoneum. Thus, five layers must be penetrated to access the inflamed appendix.

GAS 389; N 275; McM 221

148 **D.** Ileal (Meckel's) diverticulum, which is an outpouching of the distal ileum, is twice as prevalent in males as in females. The diverticulum is clinically important because ulceration of the diverticulum with pain, bleeding, perforation, and obstruction is a complication that may require emergent surgery. Signs and symptoms frequently mimic appendicitis or peptic ulcer. Internal hemorrhoids are thrombosed tributaries of the middle rectal vein, which can prolapse into the anal canal. External hemorrhoids are thromboses in the veins of the external rectal venous plexus. Diverticulosis is ordinarily an outpouching of the wall of the large intestine. This primarily affects the aged and does not cause bleeding in most cases. Borborygmi are sounds created by gas and intestinal contents as they pass through the gastrointestinal tract.

GAS 318; N 273; McM 238

149 **D.** Fig. 3-2 is a CT scan that reveals an aortic aneurysm with hemorrhage. If the man stands in an erect position, the blood will be detected in the rectovesical space, which is a peritoneal recess between the bladder and the rectum in males and is the lowest space in the peritoneal cavity. The subphrenic space is a peritoneal pouch between the diaphragm and the anterior and superior part of the liver. The hepatorenal space (pouch of Morison) is a deep peritoneal pocket between the posterior surface of the liver and the right kidney and suprarenal gland. The rectouterine space (pouch of Douglas) is a sac in females formed by a peritoneal-lined recess between the rectum and uterus. The rectouterine space is found only in women. The subhepatic space is between the liver and the transverse colon.

GAS 479-480; N 369; McM 268

150 **B.** Paraumbilical pain progressing into the right iliac fossa is a sign of appendicitis. The CT scan is one of an inflamed appendix. The structures in the scan that lie to the right of the vertebral body are part of the psoas muscle. Transverse section of this muscle signifies that it is a cut from the lumbar region.

GAS 407; N 303; McM 251

151 **C.** The arrows in the CT scan point to the descending colon. Therefore, the left colic artery, which supplies the descending colon, is the one most likely occluded in the CT scan. The middle colic, right colic, and ileocolic artery supply the ascending colon, and the marginal artery provides an anastomosis between branches of the superior mesenteric artery and inferior mesenteric artery.

GAS 350; N 288; McM 229

152 **B.** The superficial inguinal lymph nodes are the first drainage site for superficial perineal structures like the skin of the perianal region, prepuce of penis, scrotum, and anal canal inferior to the pectinate line. The superficial inguinal nodes also drain structures of the inferolateral quadrant of the trunk, including the anterior abdominal wall inferior to the umbilicus, gluteal region, and the lower limb. The deep inguinal lymph nodes drain the glans of the penis and the distal spongy urethra and receive drainage from the superficial inguinal lymph nodes. The common iliac nodes drain the external and internal iliac lymph nodes. The internal iliac lymph nodes drain inferior pelvic structures and deep perineal structures and receive drainage from the sacral nodes. The para-aortic nodes are the final drainage site for all the above lymph nodes before they drain to the thoracic duct by way of the lumbar lymph trunks.

GAS 392; N 261; McM 368

153 **B.** The white arrows in the CT scan in Fig. 3-6 point to the stomach. The spleen would not be in this CT slice because it is located more superiorly in the body than this section. Also, note that the psoas muscles are seen lying on the sides of the vertebral body, meaning that the section is in the lumbar region of the body. The duodenum is the structure located to the right of the stomach in the scan and is posterolateral to the aorta.

GAS 305-306; N 269; McM 219, 228

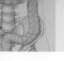

154 **A.** Cancerous cells in the stomach would metastasize first to the celiac nodes. The splenic nodes are located along the splenic artery and are related to drainage from the pancreas; therefore, they will not be the first to receive metastatic cells from a stomach cancer. The suprapancreatic nodes would be associated with pancreatic carcinoma. The right gastric lymph nodes may receive metastatic cells but would not be the first to receive this lymph because they are located along the lesser curvature of the stomach. The cisterna chyli, the proximal expanded portion of the thoracic duct, receives lymph drainage from the entire abdomen; therefore, it would not be first to receive cancerous cells.

GAS 318, 358; N 293; McM 236

155 **C.** Because physical and laboratory tests show a normal, healthy woman, the anomaly of the radiograph would be expected to be benign. Riedel's lobe is a normal variation of the liver, often an inferior extension of the right lobe of the liver, lateral to the gallbladder that extends about 4 or 5 cm below the rib cage. Carcinomas would present with abnormal laboratory examinations, and cholecystitis would present with an abnormal physical examination, as when the gallbladder is inflamed.

GAS 328; N 277; McM 235

156 **B.** A Spigelian hernia occurs along the semilunar line below the umbilical region and can protrude through the skin. A Richter hernia is a hernia that presents as a strangulated segment of part of the wall of an intestinal loop through any hernial opening. A paraumbilical hernia occurs at the level of the umbilicus, near the midline. An incisional hernia occurs with dehiscence (breakdown and reopening) of an operative incision after surgery. A ventral hernia is a type of incisional hernia located on the ventral surface of the abdomen, occurring only after surgery.

GAS 301; N 251; McM 219

157 **A.** Congenital inguinal hernias occur when a large patency of the processus vaginalis remains so that a loop of intestine herniates into the inguinal canal. A congenital hydrocele is also caused by a patent segment of a processus vaginalis filled with fluid, but it does not cause an indirect hernia. Ectopic testes occur when the gubernaculum does not migrate correctly during development and the testis does not reach the scrotum, but this does not cause a hernia. Epispadias occurs when the external urethral orifice opens onto the dorsal surface of the penis and is generally associated with exstrophy of the bladder. A rupture, or tear, of the transversalis fascia would not cause the intestines to herniate through the deep inguinal ring and therefore would not cause an indirect inguinal hernia.

GAS 299-301; N 257; McM 223

158 **A.** Failure of relaxation of the lower esophageal sphincter (also known as the cardiac sphincter) causes an accumulation of food in the esophagus. Achalasia is the failure of motility of food through the esophagus into the stomach. A constricted lower esophageal sphincter is the cause of these conditions. Dyspepsia is chronic pain or discomfort in the upper abdomen. This usually accompanies problems with digestion and is not associated with difficulty swallowing. Gastritis is inflammation of the mucosal lining of the stomach and would also not contribute to dysphagia. Gastroparesis is defined as delayed stomach emptying due to stomach paralysis, which would reveal chyme overloading in the stomach and esophagus (achalasia involves only the esophagus). Peptic ulcers mostly result in pain in the stomach, more commonly the duodenum, due to erosion of the mucosal lining.

GAS 310; N 230; McM 213

159 **D.** Meckel's diverticulum is an embryologic remnant of the vitelline duct in the embryo located on the distal ileum and proximal to the cecum. If this diverticulum becomes infected, it produces pain in the umbilical region of the abdomen, in addition to possible bleeding. A ruptured appendix usually presents with pain in the lower right quadrant of the abdomen, when the infective processes come in contact with adjacent parietal peritoneum. A volvulus is characterized by a twisted bowel, which causes obstruction of the bolus and/or ischemia as the blood supply is occluded. Diverticulosis is a condition that causes outpouchings of the wall of the gut tube, usually found in the sigmoid colon. Pain from this condition would usually present in the lower left quadrant. Borborygmi are sounds produced from gas and other contents moving through the bowels. This would not cause pain in one specific area because peristaltic activity moves the length of the GI tract.

GAS 318; N 273; McM 227

160 **C.** Pain from the gallbladder is sent to the spinal cord by visceral afferents and also is mediated (referred) by nerve fibers that provide pain sensation to the scapula. Open cholecystectomy would cause a risk to the T7 and T8 spinal nerves due to their close proximity to the gallbladder. These nerves are located below the associated rib and along the same horizontal plane as the gallbladder. T5 and T6 nerves are located superior to an incision and thus are not affected. For the same reason, nerves from T6 to T8 would not be the right choice due to T6 not being at risk during this procedure. Nerves from T9 to L1 are located inferior to the incision during this procedure. T5 to T9 is a broad range that includes many nerves that would not be affected by the incision.

GAS 341, 358-364; N 306; McM 217

161 A. The processus vaginalis is formed as the parietal peritoneum layer of the abdominal wall (inguinal region) evaginates through the deep inguinal ring and continues through the superficial inguinal ring. Normally, this evagination or outpouching is obliterated during development. A cyst can develop in a segment of the processus (which is also referred to as the canal of Nuck) if this processus is not obliterated. Congenital hydrocele would present at the base of the canal; in this case, the swelling would be in the labium majus. An ectopic uterus would present as a mass in the pelvis and not the inguinal region. A femoral hernia would be palpated below the inguinal ligament (usually) just medial to the femoral triangle. A defect of the transversalis fascia could result in inflammation in a specific area but would not be located along the inguinal ligament because this fascial layer is located deep to the inguinal ligament.

GAS 269; N 257; McM 223

162 C. The most likely place that a pancreatic pseudocyst will be formed is in the floor of the omental bursa, deep to the stomach. The omental bursa is a potential space behind the stomach and directly anterior to the pancreas. Pancreatic extravasations will fill this space. The right subhepatic space is the space in the peritoneal cavity between the inferior visceral surface of the liver and the transverse colon. The hepatorenal space of the subhepatic space, also known as the pouch of Morison, is located between the right lobe of the liver and the parietal peritoneum covering the superior pole of the right kidney and suprarenal gland. The right subphrenic space is the space directly inferior to the diaphragm and above the diaphragmatic surface of the liver. It is above the pancreas; therefore, fluid from the pancreas could not accumulate there. Finally, the greater sac is the general peritoneal cavity of the abdomen. The greater sac communicates with the omental bursa (lesser sac) by way of the omental (epiploic) foramen (of Winslow). The peritoneal cavity contains nothing except a very thin film of serous fluid that allows the organs to slip around relatively freely against one another and on the body wall.

GAS 307; N 281; McM 230

163 C. The spinal cord levels containing the soma of the sensory fibers transporting the sensation of pain are more than likely at the level of T7 and T8. This is because the xiphoid process is at these dermatome levels for somatic sensations of pain, and these same spinal nerves receive visceral afferents from the stomach.

GAS 358; N 300; McM 228

164 E. The fossa of Landzert is formed by two peritoneal folds enclosing the left colic artery and the inferior mesenteric vein, respectively, at the side of the duodenum. Herniation into the left paraduodenal fossa (fossa of Landzert) occurs more frequently than herniation into the right fossa (fossa of Kolb). The ascending branches of the left colic artery are at risk during repair of a paraduodenal hernia because the location of this hernia is in the upper left quadrant, adjacent to the junction of the terminal duodenum and the jejunum. The ascending branches of the left colic artery supply the upper segment of the descending colon and the splenic flexure of the transverse colon. The middle colic artery arises from the superior mesenteric artery and supplies the ascending colon and the transverse colon and anastomoses with the left colic artery. The right colic artery is a more inferior branch of the superior mesenteric artery and supplies the proximal ascending colon. The ileocolic artery supplies the ileum and large intestine in the area of the ileocecal junction. Finally, the ileal arteries are the small terminal branches of the superior mesenteric artery supplying blood to the ileum.

GAS 351; N 288; McM 239

165 D. The liver would be the first structure to receive these metastatic cells because they would flow through the portal venous system from the pancreas to the liver. The stomach would not receive these cells because there is no communication between the stomach and pancreas through circulatory or ductal pathways. The spleen also does not have direct communication with the pancreas and would not receive metastatic cells first. The duodenum is the site for pancreatic emptying, but as these metastases pass through venous circulation they would not pass into the duodenum. The vertebral column would not receive the metastases because they would not enter the vertebral venous plexus.

GAS 328, 354; N 294; McM 248

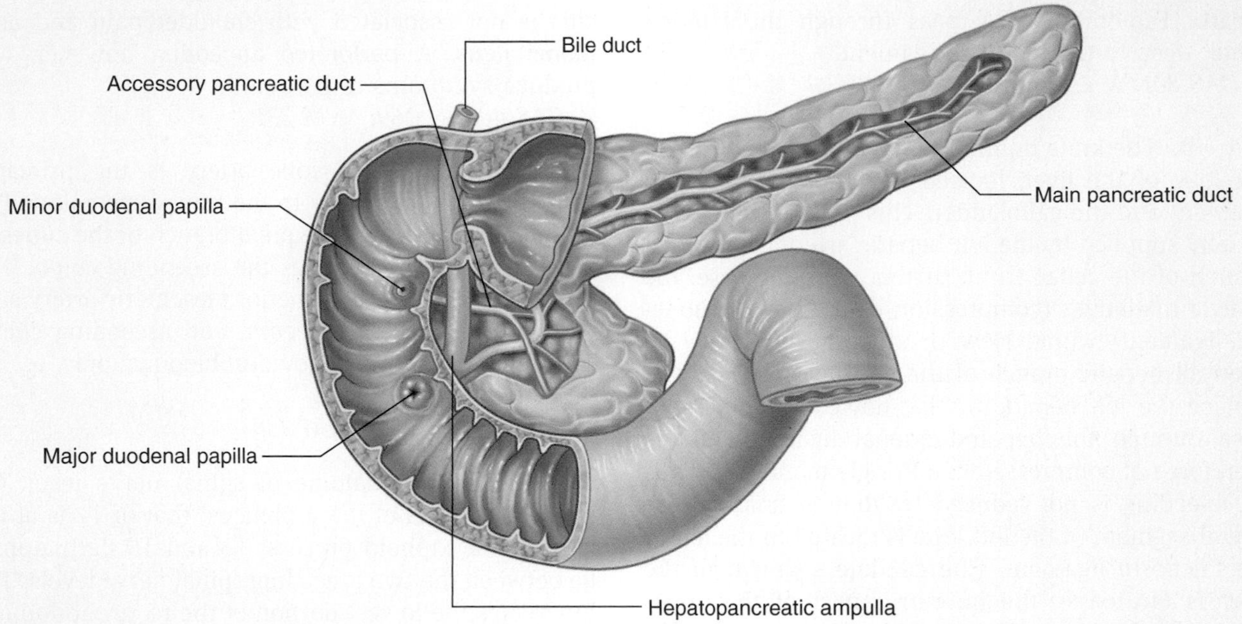

GAS **Fig. 4-100**

166 B. The portal vein is the most likely structure to be occluded by a large tumor at the neck of the pancreas due to its proximity. The pancreas is drained via the splenic vein and empties into the portal vein. The celiac trunk is superior to the tumor. The inferior mesenteric vein drains the distal part of the large intestine and is inferior to the tumor. The posterior superior pancreaticoduodenal artery would never receive these metastases, nor would the greater pancreatic artery. Similarly, the celiac trunk is outside the plane of the tumor.

GAS 354; N 292; McM 243

167 B. Hartmann's pouch is located in the gallbladder at the junction of the neck and the cystic duct. When a gallstone is located in this area, the patient will present with pain but usually no jaundice because the cystic duct is not occluded. A common bile duct and/or left and right hepatic duct obstruction would cause posthepatic jaundice due to bile obstructed in the duct system. Obstruction of the pancreatic duct would cause pain in the umbilical region, not in the right upper quadrant.

GAS 341; N 280; McM 246

168 B. The hepatopancreatic ampulla is also known as the ampulla of Vater and is located at the junction of the pancreatic duct and common bile duct. It is the narrowest part of the biliary duct system. The common bile duct, left hepatic duct, pancreatic duct, and right hepatic duct all have larger diameters than the ampulla of Vater (*GAS* Fig. 4-100).

GAS 333-337; N 280; McM 247

169 E. The innermost covering of the spermatic cord is the internal spermatic fascia. It originates from the transversalis fascia. The internal oblique muscle provides origin for the cremaster layer of the cord. The external spermatic fascia is continuous from the external oblique aponeurosis and its fascia. The transversus abdominis aponeurosis plays no part in the formation of the spermatic cord.

GAS 296-298; N 257; McM 224

170 C. An epigastric hernia is formed by a weakness in the intersecting fibers of the linea alba superior to the umbilicus. In most cases, herniation of fat and other tissue through the defect causes a palpable, but painless, mass. If a nerve branch also passes through the defect, it can be associated with local pain. Umbilical hernias are common in newborn babies and pregnant females in the third trimester of pregnancy. This kind of hernia usually represents a weakness in the wall structure at the level of the umbilicus. Omphaloceles are a more serious (but less common) defect, representing failure of the intestines to return to the abdominal cavity, associated with lack of proper growth of the body wall. Spigelian hernias occur through the semilunar lines, lateral to the rectus sheath. Femoral hernias pass through the femoral canal, deep to the inguinal ligament.

GAS 301; N 251; McM 218

171 **D.** The knife injured the medial segment of the left lobe of the liver, located between the falciform ligament and the gallbladder. This area of the liver is usually supplied by the left hepatic artery, an indirect branch of the celiac trunk. If this were the case, the Pringle maneuver (compression of the hepatoduodenal ligament) would slow or stop the bleeding. An aberrant hepatic branch of the left gastric artery can replace the left hepatic artery; however, it does not pass through the hepatoduodenal ligament and is therefore not compressed in a Pringle maneuver. Thus the bleeding is not reduced by that technique. The lateral segment of the left lobe is located to the left of the falciform ligament. The caudate segment of the liver is located in the inferior aspect of the upper portion of the liver, well above the site of injury. The anterior segment of the right lobe is located to the right of the gallbladder. The right lobe receives its arterial supply from the right hepatic artery.

GAS 328-332; N 244; McM 245

172 **E.** Interruption of both vagus nerves would deprive the abdominal viscera (foregut and midgut) of parasympathetic supply, that is, to the level of the splenic flexure of the colon. Distal to the splenic flexure, the colon receives parasympathetic nerves from pelvic splanchnic nerves. Pelvic splanchnic nerves supply the descending colon, the urinary bladder, and the erectile tissues of the penis. The innervation of the ductus deferens and ejaculatory duct is carried by sympathetic nerve supply through the pelvic plexuses. Parasympathetic supply to the ascending colon is carried by the vagus nerves and would be lost.

GAS 363; N 303; McM 241

173 **B.** Adynamic ileus is paralysis of the bowel. Peristaltic activity ceases. Borborygmi (bowel sounds) are absent when this occurs, as in peritonitis. Radiographs would indicate the presence of air under the diaphragm. Pain in the shoulder is due to air under the diaphragm from the perforated anterior duodenal wall; this air irritates somatic afferent pain fibers of the diaphragm, carried by the right phrenic nerve to spinal nerve levels C3 to C5. Referral of pain to the shoulder occurs because somatic sensory fibers from the shoulder enter the spinal cord at similar levels. A posterior penetrating ulcer would be associated usually with profuse bleeding, mostly from branches of the gastroduodenal artery that supply the duodenal bulb, the first part of the duodenum. Acute appendicitis is not associated with shoulder pain and adynamic ileus. A perforated appendix, however, will produce symptoms of peritonitis.

GAS 408; N 269; McM 231

174 **A.** The middle colic artery is the principal source of arterial supply to the transverse colon. The right colic artery, an infrequent branch of the superior mesenteric artery, supplies the ascending colon. The ileocolic branch of the superior mesenteric artery supplies the distal ileum, cecum, and ascending colon. The left colic artery provides blood supply to the descending colon.

GAS 348; N 288; McM 238

175 **C.** The dermatome of spinal nerve level T10 crosses the level of the umbilicus; that of T7 is at the level of the xiphoid process. T8 and T9 dermatomes lie between the two preceding spinal nerve levels. T12 innervates the lowest portion of the rectus abdominis and overlying skin with motor and sensory supply, respectively. L1 distribution by iliohypogastric and ilioinguinal nerves supplies the suprapubic region, the pubic area, and anterior portions of the urogenital region. Pain from appendicitis is most often perceived at first in the periumbilical region, reflecting the level of embryologic spinal nerve supply to the appendix, which is from T10. When the appendix swells and/or ruptures and contacts the body wall, somatic sensory fibers of the adjacent body wall cause the apparent site of pain to shift to the lower right abdominal quadrant.

GAS 289-290; N 303, 162; McM 215

176 **D.** Caput medusae is an end-stage characteristic of liver cirrhosis. The snakelike appearance of veins on the body wall results from anastomoses between tiny veins that accompany the ligamentum teres hepatis (that is within the falciform ligament) with veins of the anterior abdominal body wall. The umbilical veins are expanded, due to portal hypertension. Esophageal varices result from portal-systemic anastomoses between the left gastric vein and submucosal esophageal veins. Ascites is formed by fluid transudate from thin-walled and dilated anastomotic vessels joining retroperitoneal intestinal veins and veins of the body wall. Internal hemorrhoids result from expansion of anastomoses between superior rectal tributaries to the inferior mesenteric vein and middle rectal branches of the internal iliac vein. Anastomoses between middle rectal veins and inferior rectal branches of the internal pudendal vein of the perineum result in external hemorrhoids.

GAS 356; N 292; McM 280

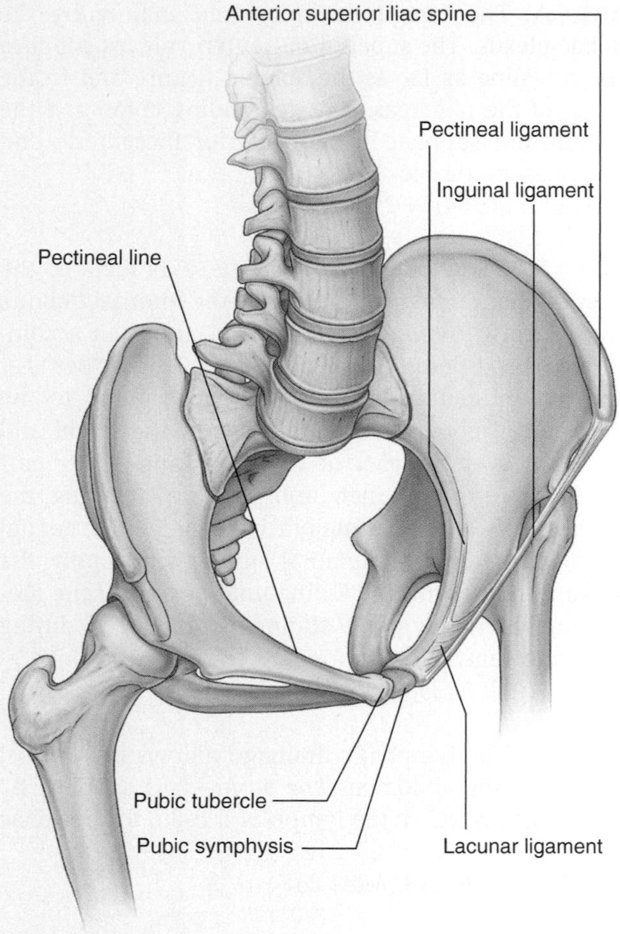

GAS **Fig. 4-29**

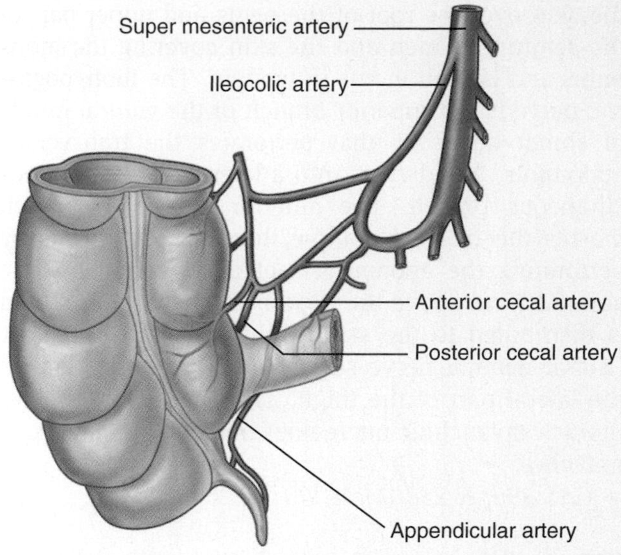

GAS **Fig. 4-80**

177 A. The iliopubic tract is a reflective band of aponeurotic tissue of the origin of the transversus abdominis, when visualized with the laparoscope. The lateral border of the inguinal triangle (of Hesselbach) is provided by the inferior epigastric artery and vein. The lateral border of the femoral ring is the femoral vein and connective tissue separating the vein from the femoral canal. The part of the inguinal ligament that attaches to the pectineal ligament is the lacunar ligament (of Gimbernat). The pectineal ligament becomes less dense and thinner as it is traced laterally from the femoral artery toward the iliopectineal portion of the inguinal ligament (*GAS* Fig. 4-29).

GAS 301; N 257; McM 225

178 E. Taeniae coli are three conspicuous bands that are a characteristic feature of the colon. Those of the ascending colon extend to the cecum and can be traced inferiorly to the base of the appendix, even when the appendix is retrocolic or retroileal in position, hidden thereby. The posterior cecal artery, although it provides origin to the appendicular artery, is very difficult to find quickly, especially in the presence of malrotation and much adipose tissue. The other structures listed do not lead easily to the location of the appendix (*GAS* Fig. 4-80).

GAS 319; N 276; McM 251

179 A. Infants with congenital aganglionic megacolon, or Hirschsprung's disease, lack autonomic ganglion cells in the myenteric plexus distal to the dilated segment of colon. The enlarged colon—megacolon—has the normal number of ganglion cells. The dilation results from failure of relaxation of the aganglionic segment, which prevents movement of the intestinal contents, resulting in a functional obstruction and dilation of the colon proximal to it. Megacolon results from failure of neural crest cells to migrate into the wall of the colon during the fifth to seventh weeks. This results in failure of parasympathetic ganglion cells to develop in the Auerbach and Meissner plexuses. Incomplete separation of the cloaca causes malformation of the hindgut like, imperforate anus or absent anus, insufficient anus and ectopic sinus. The cause of rectal atresia may be abnormal recanalization of the colon. The rotation happens at the midgut. Oligohydramnios can be associated with Hirschsprung's disease, but it's not one of the causes of it.

GAS 319; N 276; McM 240

180 C. The ilioinguinal nerve is a branch of the first lumbar nerve (L1). It pierces the internal oblique muscle, distributing filaments to it, and then accompanies the spermatic cord through the superficial inguinal ring. Its fibers are then distributed to the skin of the upper and medial parts of the thigh, and the skin over the root of the penis and upper part of the scrotum in men and the skin covering the mons pubis and labium majus in women. The iliohypogastric nerve is the superior branch of the ventral ramus of spinal nerve L1 that perforates the transversus abdominis, and divides into a lateral and an anterior cutaneous branch. The anterior cutaneous branch pierces the internal oblique, becomes cutaneous by perforating the aponeurosis of the external oblique about 2.5 cm above the superficial inguinal ring, and is distributed to the skin of the hypogastric region. Lateral femoral nerve supply innervates the skin on the lateral part of the thigh. The lumber and greater thoracic splanchnic nerve does not give off cutaneous branches.

GAS 398; N 253; McM 261

181 C. The unilateral area of skin innervated by the sensory fibers of a single spinal nerve is called a dermatome. The 7th thoracic spinal nerves supply the area of the xiphoid process. The 10th thoracic spinal nerves supply the area around the umbilicus. The 12th thoracic spinal nerves supply the hypogastric area (*GAS* Fig. 4-38).

GAS 289-290; N 162; McM 215

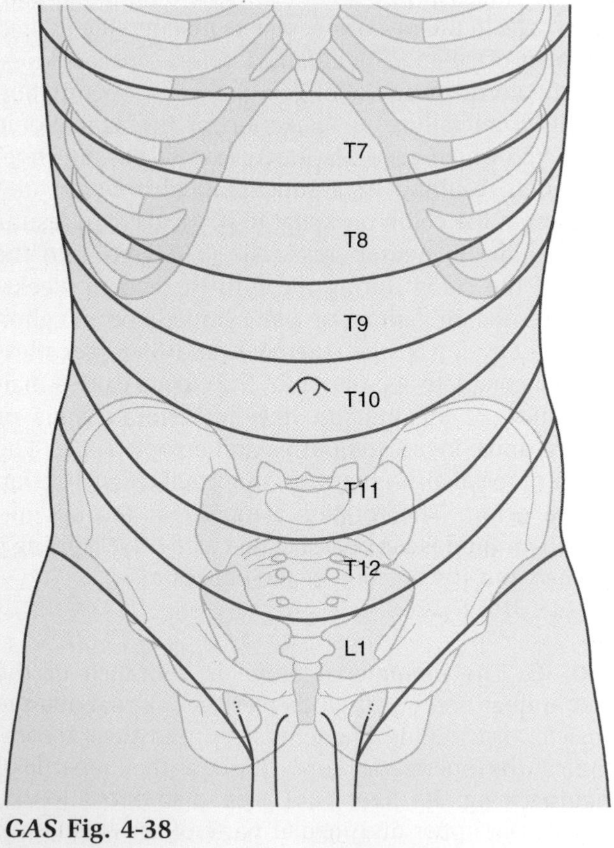

***GAS* Fig. 4-38**

182 A. The foregut is innervated mainly by the celiac plexus. The superior mesenteric plexus supplies the intestine as far as the splenic flexure and to the some of the pancreas. The descending colon and the rectum are supplied by the inferior mesenteric and intermesenteric plexuses.

GAS 358-364; N 298; McM 234

183 B. The ilioinguinal nerve is a branch of the first lumbar nerve (L1). It pierces the internal oblique muscle, distributing filaments to it, and then accompanies the spermatic cord through the superficial inguinal ring. Its fibers are then distributed to the skin of the upper and medial part of the thigh, and the skin over the root of the penis and upper part of the scrotum in men and the kin covering the mons pubis and labia majora in women. The genital branch of the genitofemoral nerve will supply the labium majus with the ilioinguinal nerve but the ilioinguinal nerve is more commonly damaged during appendectomy.

GAS 398; N 253; McM 261

184 A. The lymphatic drainage follows the arterial supply in the abdomen. The stomach is supplied by the celiac artery, so the lymph will drain to the celiac lymph nodes.

GAS 358; N 293; McM 237

185 C. They kidneys lie retroperitoneally on the posterior abdominal wall, one on each side of the vertebral column at the level of the T12–L3 vertebrae. The liver is found primarily on the right side. The pancreas and the descending colon are at the level of T12 and below. A fracture through the angle of the rib would be unlikely to injure the stomach, which can have a varied level.

GAS 373; N 309; McM 255

186 E. The duodenal cap and the first part of the duodenum are supplied by the gastroduodenal artery and the superior duodenal artery, which arise from the hepatic artery. The gastroduodenal artery descends retroperitoneally, posterior to the gastroduodenal junction and gives off two branches: right gastroepiploic artery and superior pancreaticoduodenal artery. The superior mesenteric artery usually arises from the abdominal aorta at the level of the L1 vertebra, approximately 1 cm inferior to the celiac trunk, will supply the derivatives of the midgut. The bile duct joined by the pancreatic duct usually combines to form the ampulla of Vater at the second the part of the duodenum.

GAS 312, 344; N 284; McM 236

187 E. The indirect inguinal hernia is the most common form of hernia and is believed to be congenital in origin. The hernia sac enters the inguinal canal through the deep inguinal ring and lateral to the inferior epigastric vessels. The direct inguinal hernia makes up about 15% of all inguinal hernias. The sac of a direct hernia bulges directly anteriorly through the posterior wall of the inguinal canal medial to the inferior epigastric vessels. The hernia sac descends through the femoral canal within the femoral sheath, creating a femoral hernia. Acquired umbilical hernia of adults is more correctly referred to as a paraumbilical hernia. The hernia sac does not protrude through the umbilical scar, but through the linea alba in the region of the umbilicus. The lumbar hernia occurs through the lumbar triangle and is rare. The lumbar triangle (Petit's triangle) is a weak area in the posterior part of the abdominal wall.

GAS 299-301; N 257; McM 225

188 C. The omental bursa is a potential space that lies posterior to the stomach, lesser omentum, and adjacent structures. The omental bursa has a superior recess, limited superiorly by the diaphragm and the posterior layers of the coronary ligament of the liver, and an inferior recess between the superior parts of the layers of the greater omentum. The omental bursa communicates with the greater sac through the omental foramen (epiploic foramen of Winslow). The hepatorenal space or subhepatic space is the space that separates the liver from the right kidney. Right and left subphrenic spaces lie between the diaphragm and liver and are separated by the falciform ligament.

GAS 307; N 266; McM 230

189 D. The greater sac encompasses the most space in the peritoneal cavity, beginning with the diaphragm and ending at the pelvic cavity. Morison's pouch, the rectouterine pouch (of Douglas), the right paracolic gutter, and the omental bursa are all dependent areas in the peritoneal sac, where fluid will collect if the patient is supine or standing.

GAS 307; N 321; McM 228

190 A. Visceral afferents that innervate the appendix will be stimulated by the inflammation. These visceral afferents return to the spinal cord by traveling with sympathetics. Since the appendix is a midgut structure, it receives major sympathetic supply from the lesser thoracic splanchnic nerve, which originates at T10. Therefore the patient will initially experience a visceral pain at the umbilicus, which is at the T10 level. Visceral afferents that travel with parasympathetics mediate unconscious sensations (that may reach conscious levels, such as nausea and the urge the defecate) and physiological reflexes and so are not involved in this patient's condition. The appendix is a visceral organ and is not innervated by somatic nerves.

GAS 358-364; N 303; McM 251

191 B. Visceral afferents that innervate the gallbladder will be stimulated by the inflammation. These visceral afferents return to the spinal cord by traveling with sympathetics. Since the gallbladder is a foregut structure, it receives major sympathetic supply from the greater thoracic splanchnic nerve, which originates from T5 to T9. Therefore the patient will initially experience a visceral pain at the epigastric region, which is at the T7 to T9 levels. The phrenic nerve innervates the diaphragmatic peritoneum and originates from C3, C4 and C5. If it were affected, the patient would complain of shoulder and neck pain corresponding to the dermatomes innervated by this spinal nerve. The sharp and well-localized pain in the right hypogastrium corresponds to the inflammation spreading to the abdominal peritoneum but does not explain the initial epigastric pain.

GAS 354-364; N 306; McM 233

192 C. The urachus is a thick fibrous cord that is a remnant of the allantois (a tube connecting the urinary bladder to the umbilicus in the fetus. It is involved in the processing of nutrition and the excretion of waste products in the embryo). In some cases a remnant of the lumen can persist leading to the development of urachal cyst and/or sinus. If the entire urachus remains patent, it forms a urachal fistula connecting the urinary bladder to the umbilicus. This allows urine to escape from the umbilical orifice.

GAS 302; N 321; McM 223

193 E. The anatomical location of the appendix is in the right lower quadrant at McBurney's point. When the inflamed appendix contacts the parietal peritoneum, it stimulates the somatic afferents that innervate the body wall. This results in sharp, localized pain in the right lower quadrant. Visceral afferents are stimulated by inflammation, not contact. They travel back to the spinal cord with sympathetics of the T10 dermatome. The patient will experience dull periumbilical pain, which is usually a prelude to the somatic pain.

GAS 322; N 303, 275; McM 221

194 B. Immediately external to the renal capsule is an accumulation of extraperitoneal fat called the perinephric fat. This completely surrounds the kidney.

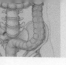

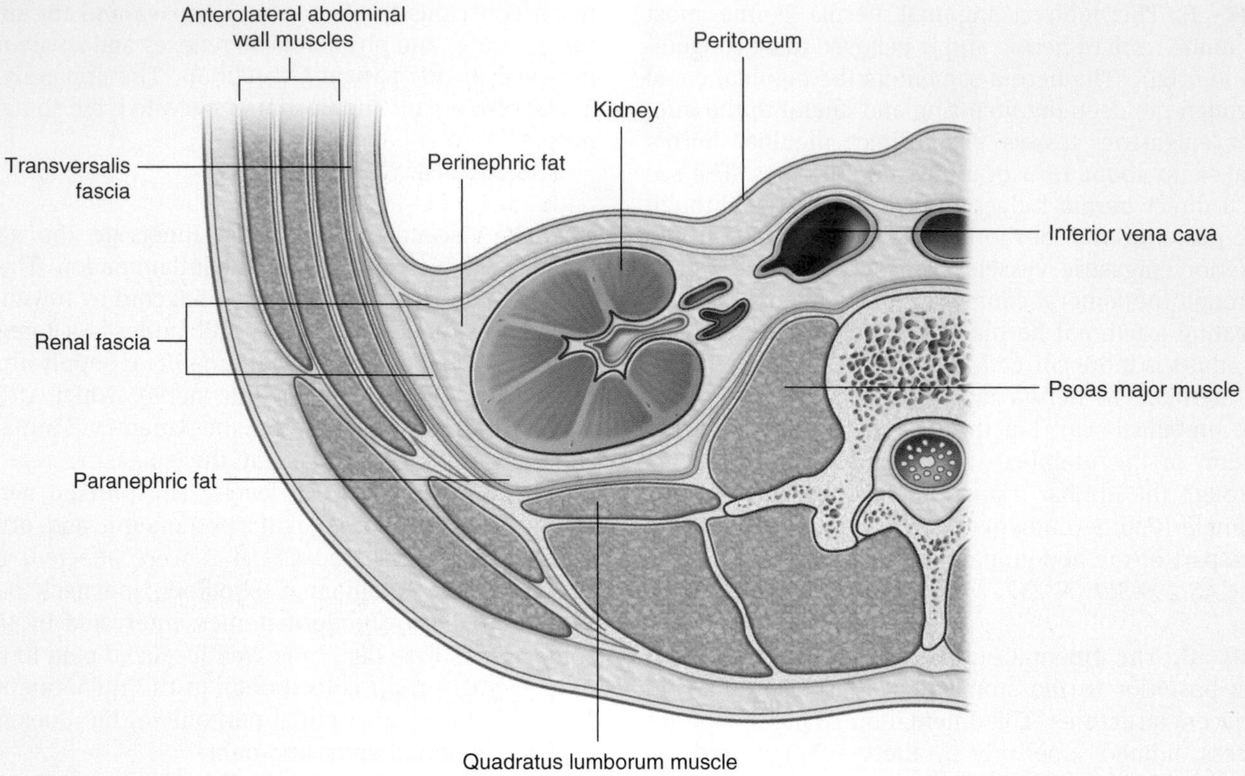

GAS **Fig. 4-140**

Surrounding the perinephric fat is a membranous condensation of extraperitoneal fascia called the renal fascia (of Gerota). A final external layer of paranephric fat completes the renal fat and fasciae. The patient is suffering from a perinephric abscess, which would be located in the perinephric fat between the renal capsule and renal fascia (*GAS* Fig. 4-140).

GAS 376; N 315; McM 257

195 A. The stomach is derived from the foregut. Other derivatives of the foregut include the upper and lower respiratory system, the pharynx, esophagus, the first and second parts of the duodenum up to the major duodenal papillae, the liver, the pancreas and the gallbladder. The spleen is derived from the dorsal mesogastrium of the stomach.

GAS 310; N 321; McM 236

196 C. Obstruction of the bile duct will result in stasis of bile. The bile duct receives the cystic duct from the gallbladder and the common hepatic duct from the liver. Therefore there will be backflow into the gallbladder leading to the symptoms of cholecystitis (fever, positive Murphy's sign, pain that began at the epigastrium then moved to the right hypogastrium). There will also be backflow into the liver leading to the increase in serum bilirubin. Obstruction of the infundibulum of the gallbladder or the cystic duct will affect the gallbladder but not the liver. Obstruction of the left hepatic duct will only affect the liver. Obstruction of the hepatopancreatic ampulla will not only lead to symptoms from the gallbladder and the liver, but also to the pancreas as the pancreatic duct will also be obstructed (*GAS* Fig. 4-102).

GAS 341; N 280; McM 246

197 D. The superior pancreaticoduodenal arteries are branches of the gastroduodenal artery, which is a branch of the celiac trunk. The inferior pancreaticoduodenal artery is a branch of the superior mesenteric artery. If the superior mesenteric artery was occluded, the anastomosis between these two vessels will allow blood to flow from the celiac trunk to the midgut to provide blood supply. The right and left gastric arteries, the left and right gastro-omental arteries, the short gastric arteries and the left and right gastroepiploic arteries all provide blood supply to the stomach (*GAS* Fig. 4-106).

GAS 347-348; N 284; McM 234

198 A. The third part (inferior part) of the duodenum is the longest section. It crosses over the inferior vena cava, aorta, and vertebral column. Any

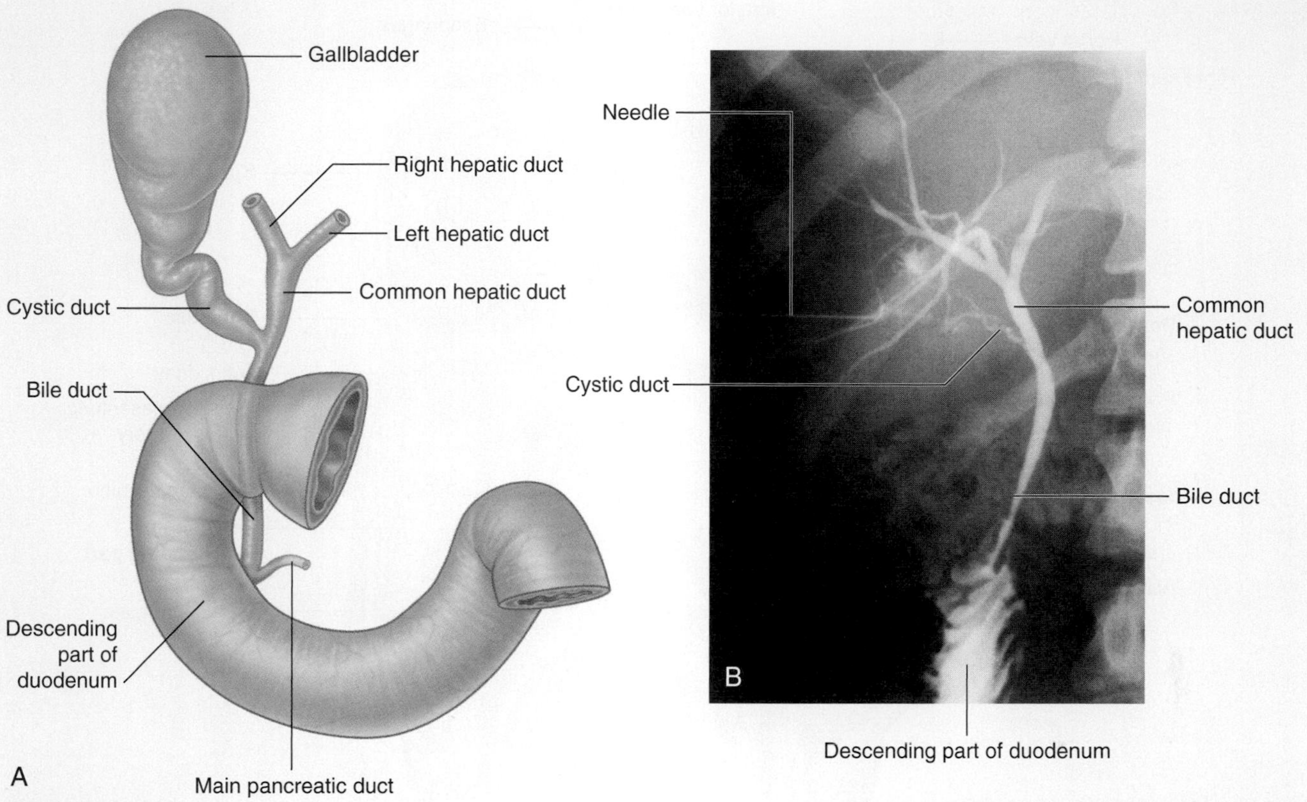

GAS Fig. 4-102

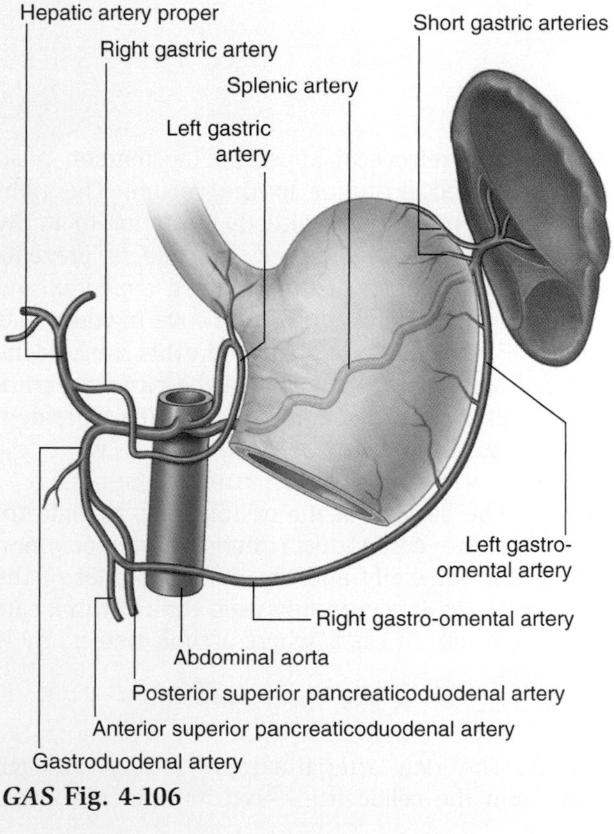

GAS Fig. 4-106

perforation to the posterior wall will immediately affect these structures. It is crossed anteriorly by the superior mesenteric artery and vein (*GAS* Fig. 4-63).
GAS 346-347; N 284; McM 235

199 C. The left gastric is a branch of the celiac trunk while the right gastric is a branch of the common (or occasionally proper) hepatic. They anastomose on the lesser curvature and provide it with blood supply. The right and left gastroepiploic vessels anastomose on the greater curvature and provide its blood supply. The pancreaticoduoduodenal vessels form and anastomosis between the celiac trunk and the superior mesenteric artery and supplies the pancreas and the duodenum, respectively. The short gastric vessel supplies the fundus of the stomach. The portal triad is located at the porta hepatis of the liver.
GAS 344; N 284; McM 234

200 A. The borders of the cystohepatic triangle (of Calot) are the cystic duct inferiorly, the common hepatic duct medially and the inferior border of the liver superiorly. It is currently used clinically to locate the cystic artery in cases where a cholecystectomy is performed. It is also the location of Calot's node,

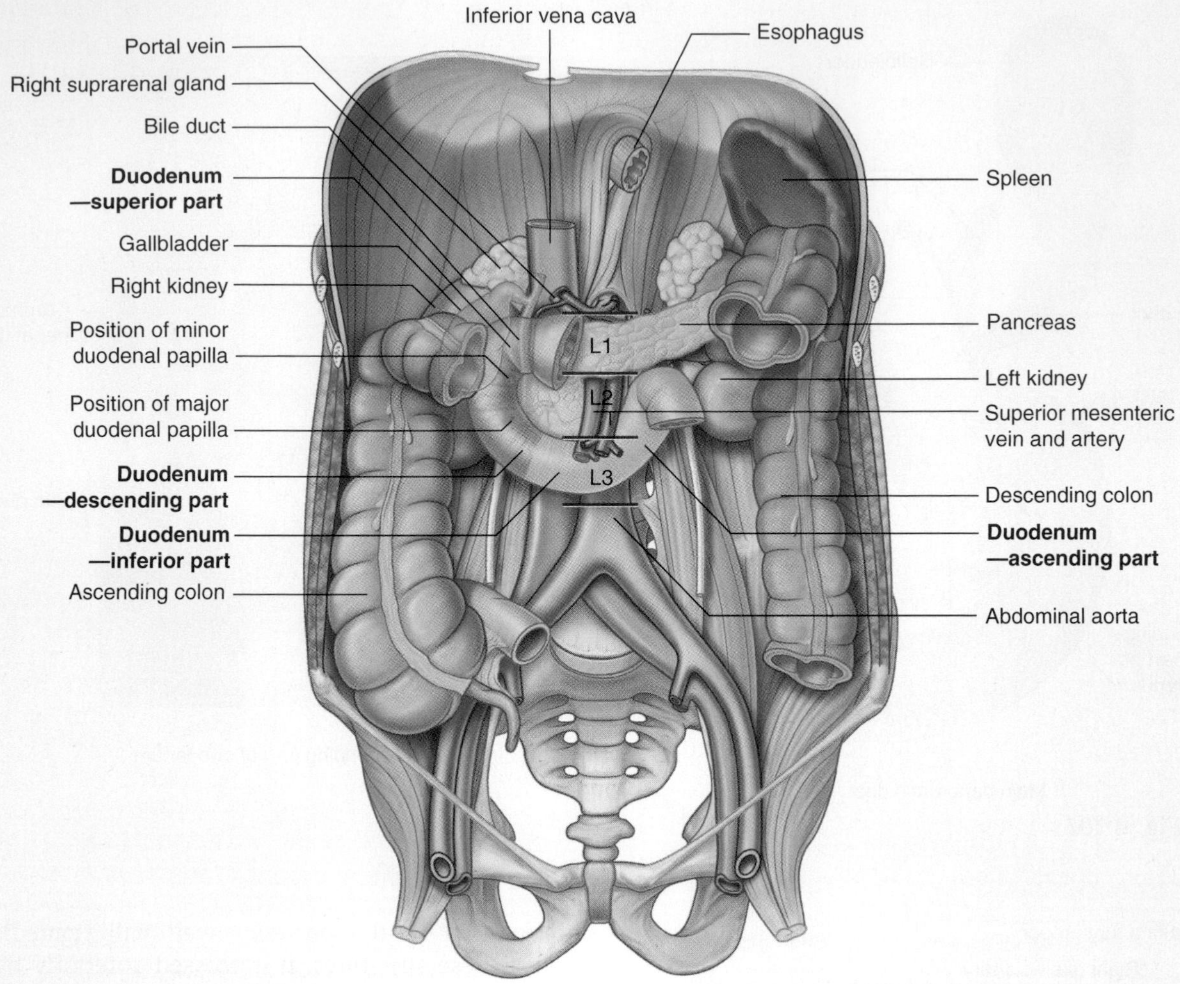

GAS **Fig. 4-63**

which directly drains the gallbladder. (Of note: Jean-Francois Calot originally described the cystic artery as one of the boundaries of the triangle.).

GAS 332, 347; N 284; McM 236

201 D. The splenic artery is the largest branch of the celiac trunk. It takes a tortuous course to the left along the superior border of the pancreas. As it passes along the superior border of the pancreas it gives off branches to the neck, body, and tail of the pancreas. The superior mesenteric artery is a direct branch of the abdominal aorta and runs anterior to the uncinate process of the liver before giving branches to the intestines. The portal vein is formed by the splenic and superior mesenteric veins posterior to the neck of the pancreas before ascending to the liver. The left gastric artery is located on and supplies the lesser curvature of the stomach. The left gastro-omental artery is located on and supplies the greater curvature of the stomach.

GAS 347; N 284; McM 235

202 A. The retrocecal appendix (a common position) is located posterior to the cecum. The right psoas major muscle lies directly posterior to it. By keeping her right thigh flexed, the patient prevents any excessive contact of the inflamed appendix and the underlying parietal peritoneum covering the psoas muscle. If the thigh is extended, this causes the inflamed appendix to rub against the parietal peritoneum resulting sharp somatic pain for the patient.

GAS 320; N 275; McM 251

203 E. The borders of the cystohepatic triangle (of Calot) are the cystic duct inferiorly, the common hepatic duct medially and the inferior border of the liver superiorly. It is currently used clinically to locate the cystic artery in cases where a cholecystectomy is performed.

GAS 332, 347; N 284; McM 236

204 A. The rich arterial supply of the stomach arises from the celiac trunk and its branches. Most blood is supplied by anastomoses formed along the lesser curvature by the right and left gastric arteries, and along the greater curvature by the right and left gastro-omental (gastroepiploic) arteries. The short gastric arteries arise from the splenic artery at the hilum of the spleen and pass forward in the gastrosplenic ligament to supply the fundus. The kidney is supplied by the renal arteries, which are branches of the abdominal aorta. The pyloric sphincter is supplied by the gastroduodenal artery and the supraduodenal artery. The left colic artery, which is a branch of the inferior mesenteric artery, supplies the splenic flexure of the colon.

GAS 344; N 283; McM 234

205 D. The azygos vein ascends in the posterior mediastinum, passing close to the right sides of the bodies of the inferior 8 thoracic vertebrae. It arches over the superior aspect of the root of the right lung to join the SVC, similar to the way the arch of the aorta passes over the root of the left lung. In portal hypertension (an abnormally increased blood pressure in the portal venous system), blood is unable to pass through the liver via the hepatic portal vein, causing a reversal of flow into the systemic tributaries of the azygos veins at the lower third of the esophagus. The large volume of blood causes the submucosal veins to enlarge markedly, forming esophageal varices.

GAS 356; N 203; McM 209

206 D. The kidneys lie retroperitoneally and therefore, of the layers listed, a posterior approach will only require transection of the transversalis fascia. The parietal peritoneum lies anterior to the kidneys and the visceral peritoneum covers the gastrointestinal tract forming the peritoneal cavity between them. The diaphragmatic pleura is located in the thoracic cavity and is a subdivision of the parietal pleura.

GAS 373; N 309; McM 250

207 C. The pancreas is located retroperitoneally and may only be visualized directly if the posterior parietal peritoneum is divided. The ileum, jejunum, stomach, and transverse colon are all intraperitoneal and therefore easily visualized with the scope.

GAS 333; N 266; McM 227

208 D. Meckel's diverticulum is a congenital condition where the proximal portion of the omphaloenteric (vitelline) duct does not completely regress, so it forms a fingerlike projection from the ileum. It may become filled with fecal material and subsequently obstructed with resulting inflammation. Gastritis is inflammation of the lining of the stomach and will not give the appearance of a 2-inch long structure in the midabdomen on radiographic studies. Hirschsprung's disease is a congenital disorder marked by difficulty in passing stool and may as a result produce a bloody sample. The blood will be bright red and the 2-inch structure will not be present on radiography. Hemorrhoids are varicose veins in the anal canal and rectum, which may protrude from the canal if very large and are typically the result of excessive straining while trying to pass stool. Anal fissures are tears that may result from straining excessively and trying to pass hard or dry stools.

GAS 318; N 273; McM 227

209 A. The descending colon is the only option listed which is a retroperitoneal organ. All the other organs are intraperitoneal and will therefore not be affected by a retroperitoneal infection.

GAS 322; N 288; McM 226

210 E. The ilioinguinal and iliohypogastric nerves are located directly posterior to the kidney. Much of the sensory distribution of the iliohypogastric nerve is to the skin over the posterolateral gluteal and pubic regions. The ilioinguinal nerve supplies the upper medial thigh and, specifically, the skin over the mons pubis and labia majora in women or skin over the root of the penis and anterior scrotum in men. The lateral cutaneous nerve of the thigh gives sensory innervation to the lateral thigh. The femoral nerve is the nerve of the anterior thigh and supplies muscles and skin of this region. The subcostal nerve runs just inferior to the 12th rib and supplies the muscles and skin of the surrounding area.

GAS 398; N 253; McM 253

211 C. The muscle that will provide the "6-pack" look is rectus abdominis, which runs between the pubic crest and the costal margin in the midline of the abdominal wall. The upper attachment is the lower border of the 7th costal cartilage and the muscle often covers the costal cartilages for a short distance anteriorly. Ribs 10-12 and the iliac crest are too far lateral for rectus abdominis to attach to it. The xiphoid process may be covered by the muscle but does not serve as an attachment.

GAS 286; N 246; McM 218

212 C. There are three major structures that pass through the diaphragm. At the level of T10 the esophagus will pass through while the inferior vena cava will traverse at T8 and the aorta at T12. The levels T7 and 11 are not associated with any particular structures passing through the diaphragm.

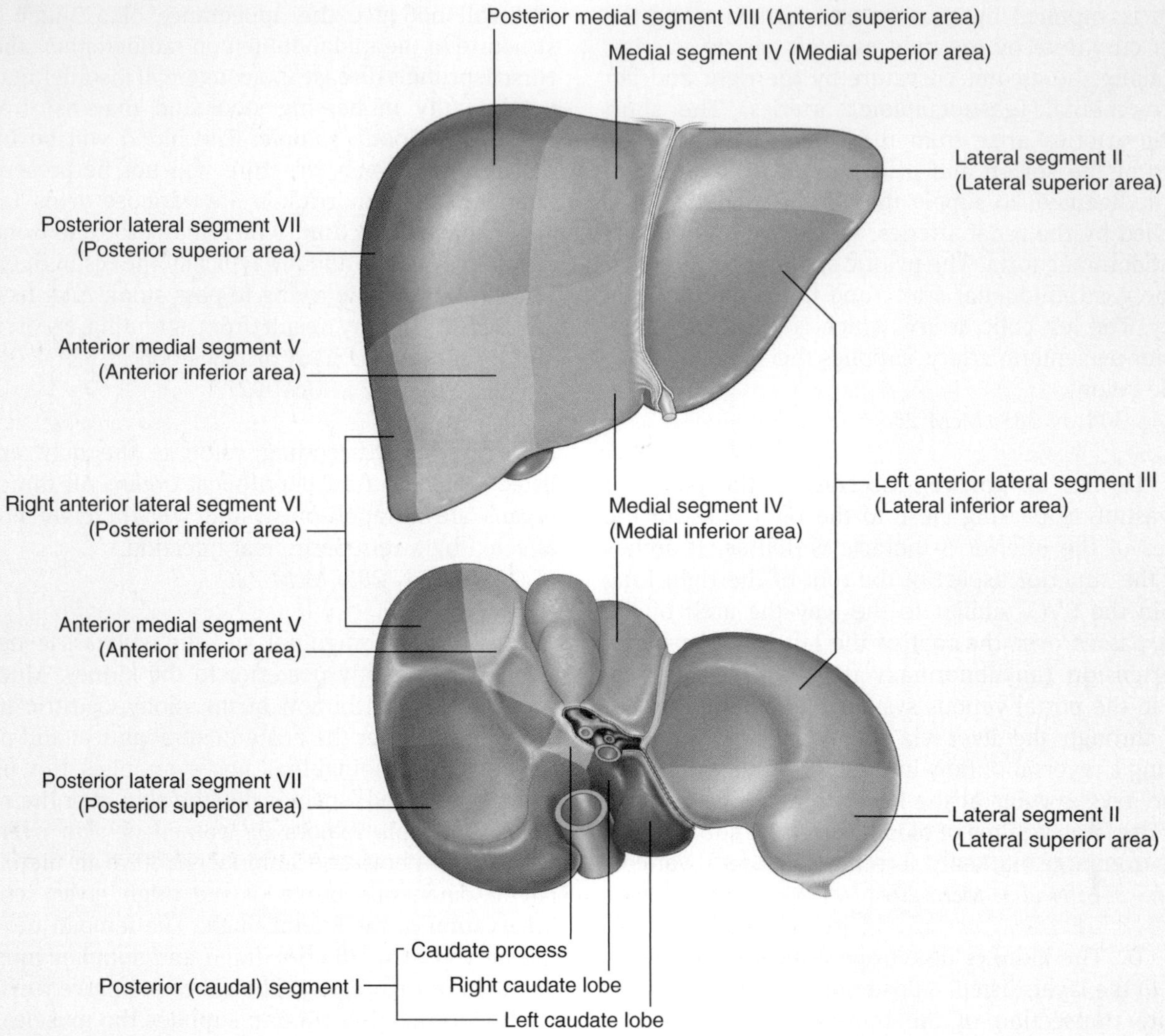

GAS **Fig. 4-107**

213 C. The ribs slope vertically downward as they move to attach to the sternum in the midline. This produces a thoracic cage with lowermost anterior point being several vertebral levels lower than that of the posterior part of the rib. The costal margin is therefore corresponding with the L3 vertebra. Vertebrae L1 and 2 are too high and correspond to the lower margin of the 11th and 12th ribs respectively. Levels L4 and 5 are close to the pelvic area and is therefore too low.

GAS 262; N 258; McM 213

214 A. The principle plane also known as Cantlie's line divides the liver into functional right and left lobes. This division makes the caudate and quadrate lobes part of the left lobe of the liver. The caudate lobe is segment I, the quadrate lobe segment IV and the left lobe consisting of segments II and III. Removing the right lobe according to this resection will therefore remove segments; V, VI, VII and VIII (*GAS* Fig. 4-107).

GAS 339; N 277; McM 245

215 E. Caput medusae is the appearance of enlarged veins radiating outward from the umbilical area and is a sign of increased pressure in the portal vein. The portal vein takes nutrient rich blood from the intestines to the liver and is formed by the fusion of the superior mesenteric and splenic veins. The right and left common iliac arteries are the terminal branches of the abdominal aorta and carry oxygen rich blood toward the lower limbs. The gastric veins drain into the splenic, superior mesenteric and portal veins and do not contribute to the formation of the portal vein. The inferior mesenteric vein drains typically into the splenic vein. The para-umbilical veins are the ones

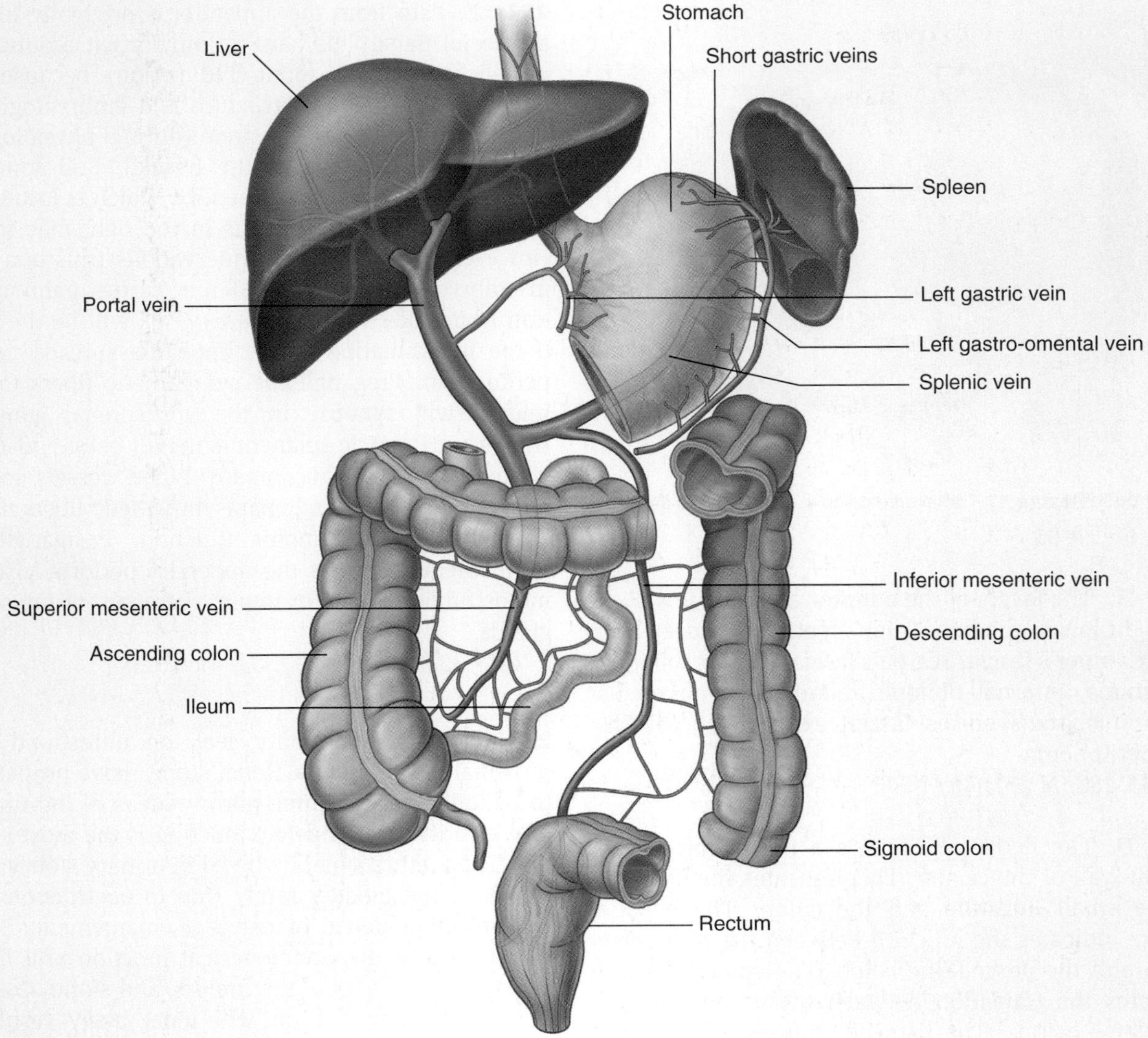

GAS **Fig. 4-121**

that take the blood toward the umbilicus as an alternative direction of blood flow back to the heart. This alternative route will bypass the liver entirely (*GAS* Fig. 4-121).

GAS 356; N 292; McM 248

216 E. The stomach forms part of the anterior boundary of the omental bursa. A perforated lesion in the posterior wall will result in stomach contents being expelled into the omental bursa also referred to as the lesser peritoneal sac. The omental (epiploic) foramen (of Winslow) is the space bounded by the portal triad and inferior vena cava, which is the only communication between the greater and lesser sacs. The paracolic gutters are spaces lateral to the ascending and descending colons in which fluid may accumulate when the patient is supine. The supracolic and infracolic compartments are spaces above and below the transverse colon and are located in the greater sac.

GAS 307; N 278; McM 230

217 C. The ascending lumbar vein connects the common iliac veins to the azygos system bilaterally and would provide an additional pathway for blood. The left common iliac will join with the right common iliac to give rise to the inferior vena cava. The azygos and hemiazygos veins drain the posterior thoracic walls of the right and left sides respectively and will receive the ascending lumbar veins in most instances. The left renal vein drains into the inferior vena cava superior to the L3 vertebra and although it receives the left gonadal vein it cannot provide an alternative pathway for blood.

GAS 390-391; N 189; McM 209

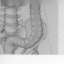

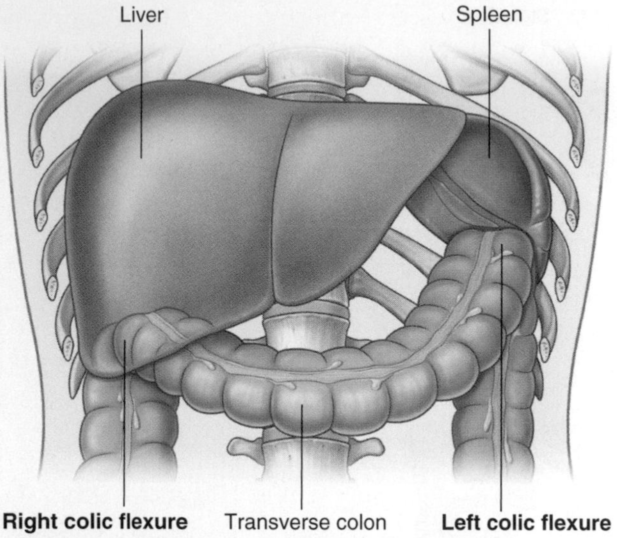

GAS Fig. 4-83

218 **A.** The layers of the anterior abdominal wall in the right lower quadrant from superficial to deep are; skin, Camper's fascia, Scarpa's fascia, external oblique abdominis, internal oblique abdominis, transversus abdominis, transversalis fascia, extra peritoneal fat, and peritoneum.
GAS 280; N 251; McM 220

219 **D.** The ileocecal valve is a narrowing in the medial wall of the cecum. This indicates the junction of the small intestine and the colon. The hepatic flexure indicates the junction between the transverse colon and the descending colon. The splenic flexure indicates the transition between the ascending and transverse colons. The paracolic gutters are external to the colon. The GE junction is located at the point where the esophagus joins the stomach and is not located in the colon (*GAS* Fig. 4-83).
GAS 320-322; N 274; McM 251

220 **C.** Left gastric vein anastomose with the esophageal branches of the azygos vein. Distension of this network in cases of obstruction results in esophageal varices at lower esophagus. A is incorrect because the right gastric vein drains directly to the hepatic portal vein and forms no communication with a systemic vein. B is incorrect because the periumbilical veins anastomose with the superficial epigastric vessels around the umbilicus. They form caput medusae when distended. The splenic vein joins the superior mesenteric vein and forms no clinically described disorder. The left gastro-omental vein drains into the superior mesenteric vein and is therefore not involved in hematemesis.
GAS 356; N 292; McM 241

221 **E.** Pain from the appendix is originally felt as a visceral pain. This pain is initially felt around the umbilical area (at about T10 region) because the appendix is a midgut structure and embryologically related to the umbilical area (during physiological hernia and reduction of the hernia). Subsequently during gut rotation, the appendix, which is located at the base of the cecum, rests in the right iliac fossa. However, it maintains its innervations (this is a rule in embryology). Somatic afferent carries pain sensation from body wall structures. This will be the case if the inflammation of the appendix spreads to the peritoneum. Preganglionic sympathetic fibers to the midgut will synapse in the aorticorenal ganglion (the lesser thoracic splanchnic nerve) before postganglionic fibers will accompany blood vessels to the appendix. Preganglionic parasympathetic fibers to the appendix perform motor function. Postganglionic sympathetic fibers to the appendix perform visceral motor functions, for example, secretion by intestinal glands.
GAS 322, 358-364; N 303; McM 251

222 **E.** The abnormality seen on ultrasound was proximal to the ureters. Renal stones have propensity to be lodged at the three narrow areas of the ureters of which the ureteropelvic junction is the most superior. The urethra is not involved in urinary stones, and stones in the bladder rarely lead to obstruction that will result in pelvic or calyceal enlargement. Stone obstruction at the ureterovesical junction will likely lead to enlargement of the ureters, and stone obstruction at the pelvic brim will most likely result in enlargement of the ureters.
GAS 380; N 314; McM 255, 259

223 **A.** The pancreatic head is related to the concavity of the duodenum. The bile duct and the main pancreatic duct join at the ampulla of Vater to open into the beginning portion of the second part of the duodenum. Carcinoma of the head of the pancreas can therefore obstruct the bile duct at this region. The common hepatic duct is proximal to the duodenum and not likely to be compressed by carcinoma of the pancreatic head. Similarly, the left hepatic duct is also proximal to the duodenal concavity and will not be obstructed in cancer of the head of pancreas. The cystic duct is above and to the right of the duodenum and pancreatic head and not likely to be compressed in cancer of the head of the pancreas. The right hepatic artery is proximal and above the duodenum and the head of the pancreas.
GAS 333; N 294; McM 247

224 C. is correct because the superior mesenteric artery crosses in front of the distal part of the third part of the duodenum with the abdominal aorta behind. The bile duct enters the duodenum at the beginning of the second part of the duodenum. Compression of the duodenum at the third part will therefore lead to back up of bile leading to the presence of bile in the vomitus of the patient. The second part of the duodenum is not crossed by the superior mesenteric artery, and the duodenum could not have been compressed at this point. The ileum is distal to the duodenum, and although it receives its blood supply from the superior mesenteric artery, it is not crossed by it. The first and second parts of the duodenum are located superior to the branch point of the superior mesenteric artery from the aorta. The proximal part of the jejunum is superior to the branch point of the superior mesenteric artery from the aorta.

GAS 348; N 284; McM 243

225 E. The inferior pancreaticoduodenal artery will continue to supply the pancreas, particularly the head of the pancreas, if the gastroduodenal artery is compromised. This artery is a branch of the superior mesenteric artery. The splenic artery does not supply the head of the pancreas. The left gastric artery gives off branches to the inferior esophagus and supplies the lesser curvature of the stomach together with the right gastric artery. The right gastric artery supplies the lesser curvature of the stomach, and the proper hepatic artery provides blood supply to the liver.

GAS 348; N 284; McM 243

226 A. Vagus nerve carries postganglionic parasympathetic fibers responsible for contracting the smooth muscles of the tracheobronchial tree. Since the patient suffers from asthma, a condition that the smooth muscles cells of the tracheobronchial tree are constricted, vagus nerve is the most likely correct answer. Vagus also be responsible for innervating the mucous gland found in the submucosa of the tracheobronchial tree, as well as being responsible for pain sensation. Phrenic nerve will provide motor supply to muscle of the diaphragm, greater splanchnic nerve will carry preganglionic sympathetic fibers from T5-T9 to the celiac ganglion in the abdomen, as well as carry visceral pain sensation from the abdomen back to the dorsal root ganglia of T5-T9, cardiopulmonary nerve will be mainly responsible for innervation of the heart and finally, intercostal nerve will be responsible for motor, sensory and sympathetic innervation of the dermatome that innervates.

GAS 358-364; N 207; McM 206

227 C. The visceral afferent fibers from the pancreas accompany sympathetic nerves. Postganglionic sympathetic nerves to the foregut, including the pancreas, are located in the celiac ganglion, as are visceral afferent fibers. Neurectomy of this ganglion will therefore interrupt the pain pathway from the pancreas by disrupting the afferent fibers. The nerve cell bodies of these fibers are located in the dorsal root ganglia of T5 to T9. Visceral pain fibers from the pancreas do not travel with the vagus nerve. The phrenic nerve supplies motor innervations to the diaphragm. The aorticorenal ganglion is the location of the postganglionic cell bodies of the least thoracic splanchnic nerve, which supplies sympathetic innervation to the midgut. The inferior mesenteric ganglion receives the intermesenteric plexus, which is mainly from the superior mesenteric ganglion. These ganglia mainly contain postganglionic sympathetic fibers to the midgut.

GAS 358-364; N 307; McM 235

228 E. The iliohypogastric nerve will receive sensation from the capsule of the kidney and is typically innervating the dermatome over the pubic symphysis. The dermatome below the pubic symphysis is innervated by the ilioinguinal nerve.

GAS 373, 394-401; N 253; McM 260

229 C. The ureter is narrowed at some regions, hence stones are more likely to be trapped at these areas of constriction. At the lower part of the ureter, the ureter is narrowed at the point where it crosses the common iliac artery and where it opens into the bladder at the vesicoureteric junction. The ureters do not cross the inferior vena cava in its path; they cross the common iliac artery at the junction where it splits into internal and external iliac arteries. The 4th lumbar artery and in fact all lumbar arteries are located medially and posterior to the ureters and therefore are not crossed by the ureters. The inferior mesenteric artery is a midline and unpaired branch of the abdominal aorta. The ureters are more laterally located and do not cross the inferior mesenteric artery.

GAS 331, 358-364; N 314; McM 261

230 C. The gallbladder and its biliary trees are foregut structures. The celiac ganglion contains cell bodies of postganglionic sympathetic fibers from the greater thoracic splanchnic nerve that innervate these structures. A branch of this nerve travels with the cystic artery to supply the gallbladder. The inferior mesenteric plexus contains mostly postganglionic sympathetic fibers to the midgut, mostly from the lesser and then least thoracic splanchnic nerves. The

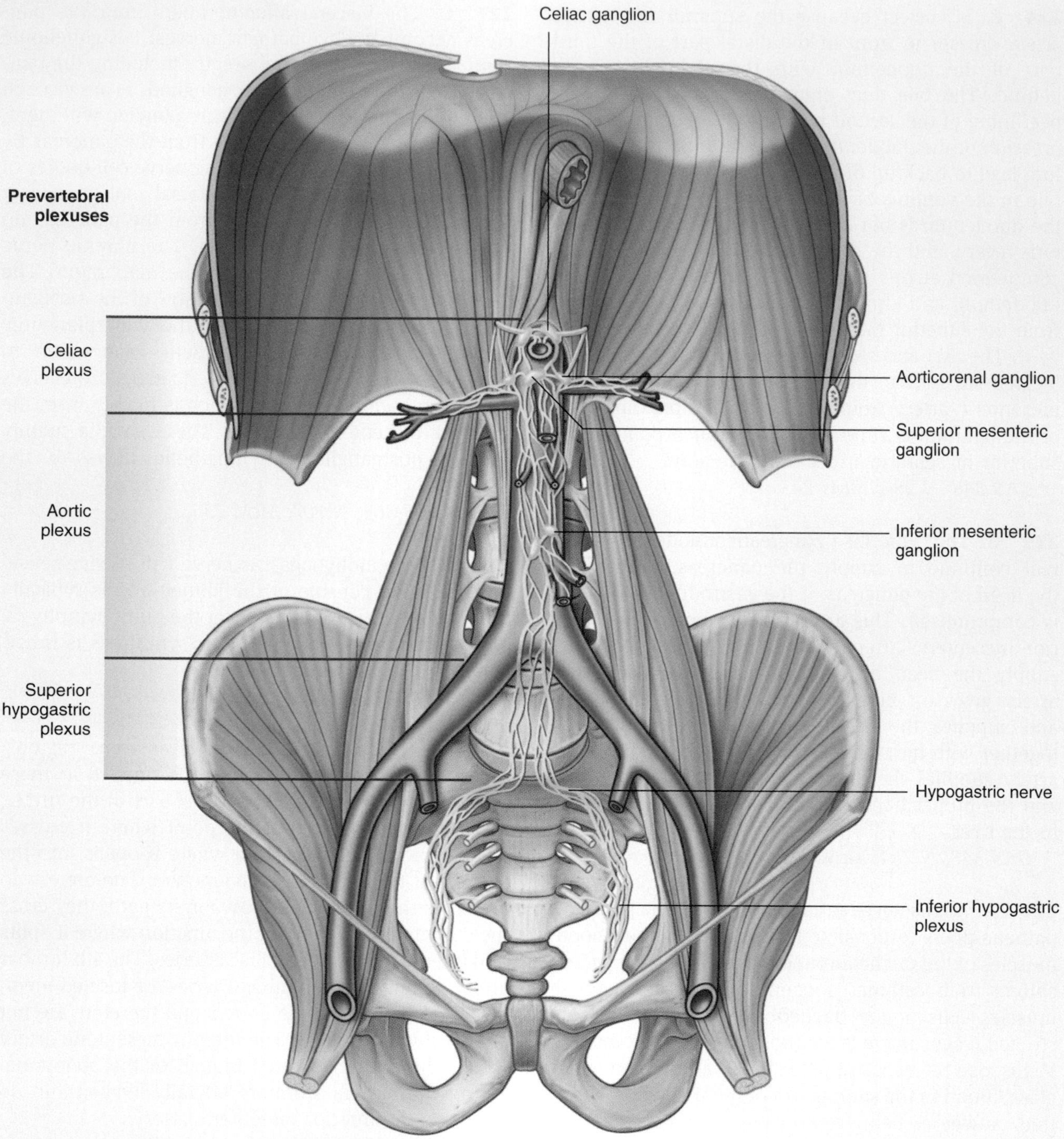

GAS **Fig. 4-126**

superior mesenteric plexus contains postganglionic sympathetic fibers from the lesser thoracic splanchnic nerve to the midgut. The aorticorenal plexus contains postganglionic fibers from the least thoracic splanchnic nerve to the kidney to regulate local blood supply. The superior hypogastric plexus contains postganglionic sympathetic fibers to the pelvic and perineal regions as well as preganglionic parasympathetic fibers to the hindgut (*GAS* Figs. 4-126, 4-127, and 4-157).

GAS 354-364; N 298; McM 246

231 C. Duodenal atresia presents with a distended epigastrium bilious vomiting and double-bubble sign

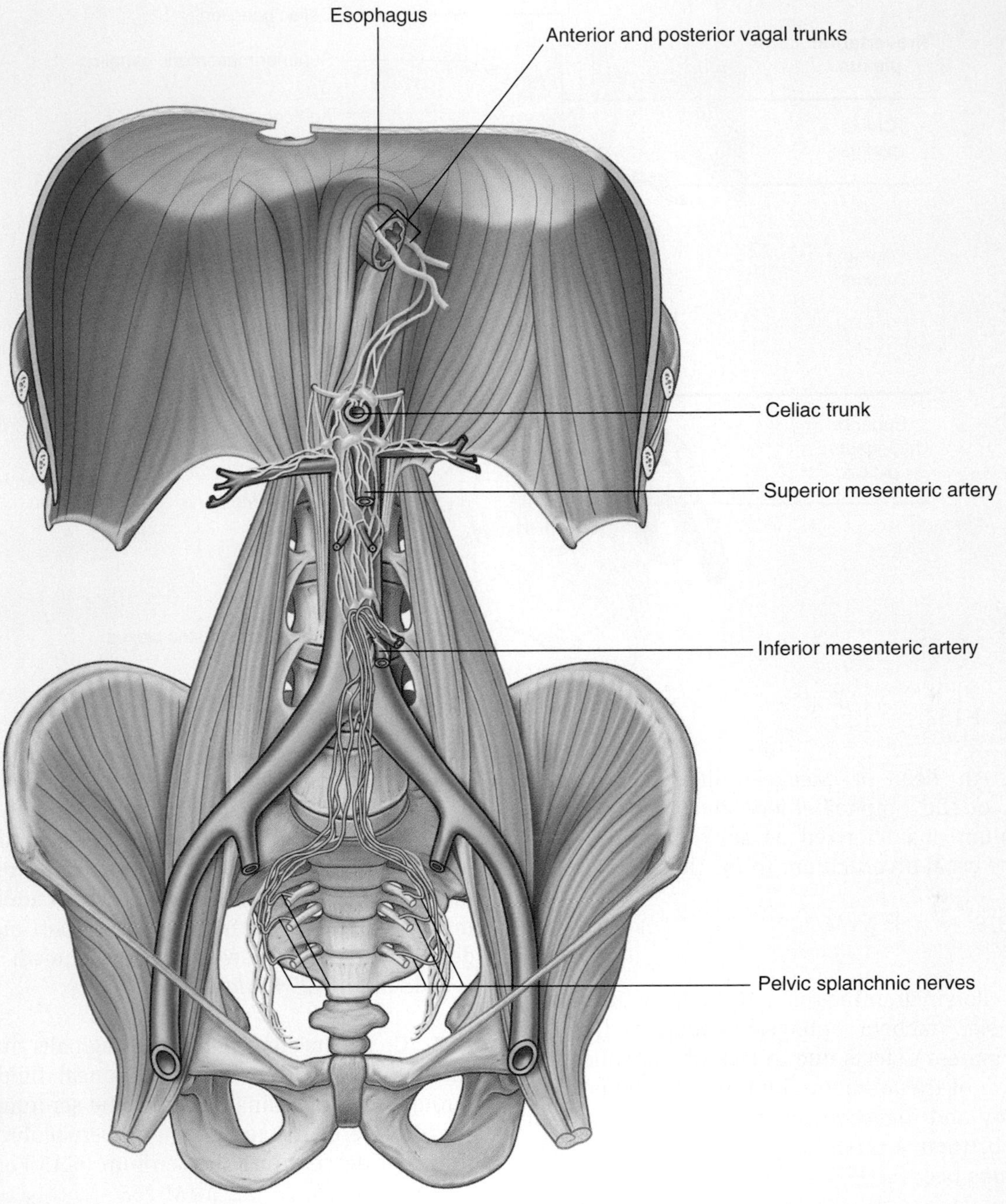

***GAS* Fig. 4-127**

on radiography. Atresia results from failure of recanalization of the duodenum. Defects of the tracheoesophageal septum lead to tracheoesophageal fistulas with nonbilious vomiting. Defects of the pleuroperitoneal folds lead to diaphragmatic hernias whereas malrotation without a concomitant volvulus will not present with bile tainted vomiting or the above radiograph.

GAS 312; N 272; McM 235

232 **E.** Bilateral renal agenesis or obstructive uropathy is associated with oligohydramnios because little or no urine is excreted into the amniotic cavity. Polyhydramnios conversely is associated with esophageal atresia and central nervous system defects. Annular pancreas causes duodenal obstruction. The gonads are not a derivative of the metanephros or its diverticulum.

GAS 373; N 308; McM 257

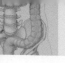

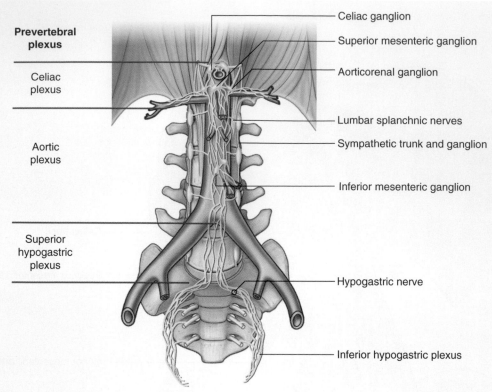

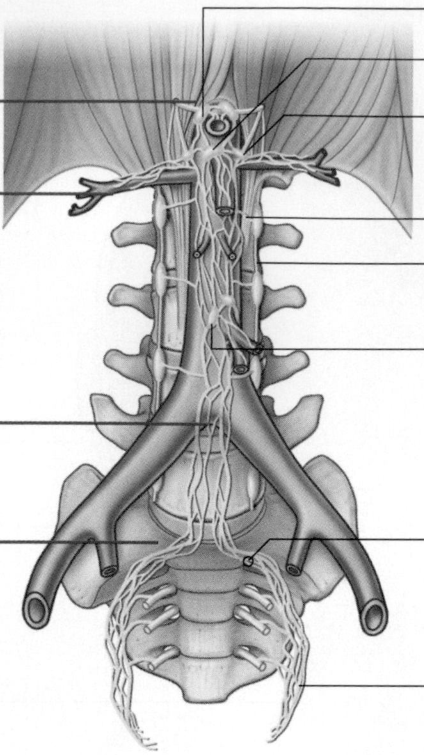

GAS **Fig. 4-157**

233 A. An ileal or Meckel's diverticulum is a remnant of the omphaloenteric duct and is a true diverticulum characterized as above by the rule of twos. The cecal diverticulum forms the appendix and cecum.

GAS 318; N 273; McM 229

234 A. Polyhydramnios is associated with esophageal atresia, tracheoesophageal fistulas and central nervous system defects due to lack of circulation and absorption of the amniotic fluid, which occurs in the respiratory and digestive tracts. Bilateral renal agenesis or obstructive uropathy is associated with oligohydramnios because little or no urine is excreted into the amniotic cavity. Down syndrome not directly related with tracheoesophageal fistulae.

GAS 222; N 231; McM 220

235 C. Omphaloenteric (vitelline) fistula is an abnormal patent connection between the umbilical surface and terminal ileal lumen whereas the omphaloenteric (vitelline) cyst is a cyst connected to the ileum and umbilicus by a fibrous band, which is the remnant of the yolk stalk. An ileal diverticulum is an out pouching of the ileal lumen at the antemesenteric border, which can become ulcerated.

GAS 318; N 321; McM 227

236 C. An annular pancreas, which probably develops from a bifid ventral pancreatic bud, may obstruct the second part of the duodenum either at birth or much later following inflammation or fibrosis. Since the pancreatic buds all develop at the caudal part of the foregut, which forms the second part of the duodenum, the other answer can be excluded.

GAS 336; N 294; McM 235

237 C. A persistent processus vaginalis may be too small for bowel but allow peritoneal fluid passing through the abdominal end into the scrotum forming a hydrocele of the testis. The gubernaculum aids in testicular descent into the scrotum (*GAS* Fig. 4-41).

GAS 294-300; N 321; McM 265

238 C. Cryptorchidism is failure of descent of one or both testes into the scrotum. Testes may be in the abdominal cavity or anywhere along its path to the scrotum. True hermaphroditism is due to presence of both testicular and ovarian tissue whereas pseudohermaphroditism occurs from errors in sexual differentiation leading to contrasting phenotypes. Chordee is congenital ventral or dorsal curvature of the penis.

GAS 294-300; N 321; McM 265

239 D. Gastroschisis is congenital failure of closure of the anterior abdominal wall due to incomplete

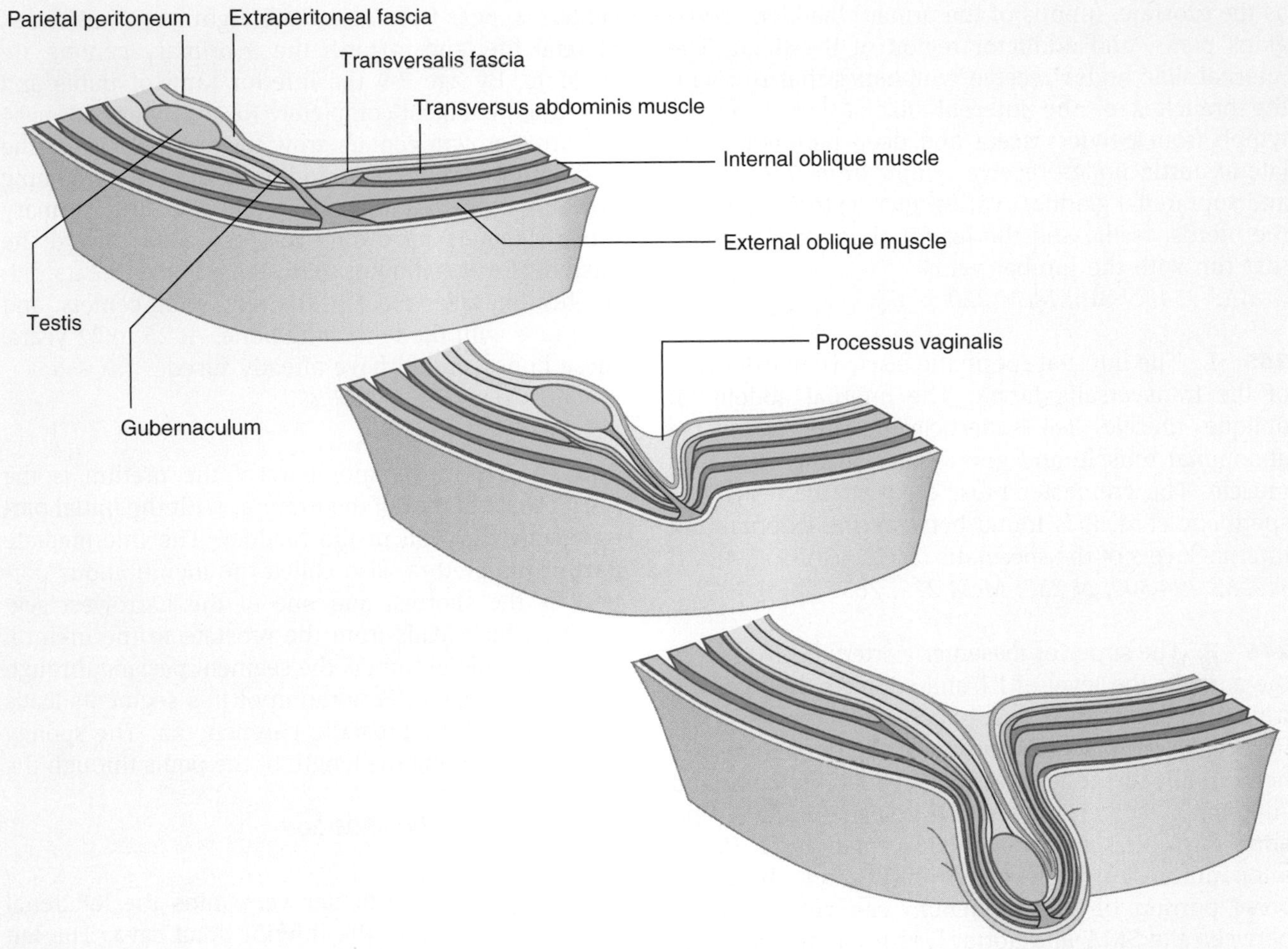

GAS **Fig. 4-41**

closure of lateral folds. Volvulus is twisting around of the bowel and may be a result of a diverticulum. Situs inversus is when all the internal organs are situated in the opposite side of the body.

GAS 265; N 251; McM 227

240 A. Down's syndrome is associated with increased incidence of duodenal atresia but to get bilious vomiting the atresia will have to be distal to the 1st part of the duodenum. All the other conditions occur proximal to the major duodenal papilla.

GAS 312; N 272; McM 231

241 C. Midgut volvulus occurs following failure of the small intestines to enter the abdominal cavity for fixation following rotation of the midgut loop. The resultant twisting of the gut usually occurs and affects the vasculature at the duodenojejunal junction. Congenital megacolon is due to failure of neural crest migration and occurs in the distal colon.

GAS 325; N 321; McM 240

242 A. Congenital (aganglionic) megacolon (Hirschsprung's disease) is due to failure of neural crest migration and occurs in the distal colon. Incomplete separation of the cloaca may be due to defects in the urorectal septum. Rectal atresia is the result of failure of recanalization of the colon.

GAS 322; N 276; McM 240

243 C. The ilioinguinal nerve supplies skin of lower inguinal region, mons pubis, anterior scrotum or labium majus, and adjacent medial thigh; inferior most internal oblique and transversus abdominis.

GAS 398; N 253; McM 220

244 E. The superficial inguinal nodes receive lymph drainage from the abdominal wall below the level of the umbilicus, from the back below the iliac crest, perineum, scrotum, buttock, vulva, and anus. The deep inguinal nodes receive lymph from superficial lymph nodes and lower limbs. The external iliac nodes receive lymphatics from deep structures, such as the prostate, fundus of the urinary bladder, cervix, glans penis, and adductor region of the thigh. The internal iliac nodes receive lymphatics that run with the branches of the internal iliac artery, receiving lymph from pelvic viscera and deep perineum. The lateral aortic nodes receive lymph from the kidneys and suprarenal glands, ovaries, uterine tubes, body of the uterus, testis, and the lateral abdominal muscles that run with the lumbar veins.

GAS 354; N 316; McM 220

245 E. The internal spermatic fascia is an extension of the transversalis fascia. The internal abdominal oblique muscle lies superficial to the transverse abdominal muscle and gives origin to the cremaster muscle. The cremaster muscle covers the testis and spermatic cord. It is found between the external and internal layers of the spermatic fascia. (*GAS* Fig. 4-47).

GAS 294-300; N 257; McM 225, 265

246 E. The superior mesenteric artery (SMA) leaves the aorta at the level of L1 and supplies the intestine from the duodenum and pancreas to the left colic flexure. The transverse portion of the duodenum lies horizontally at the level of L3, between the aorta and superior mesenteric artery. Normally, the SMA and aorta form an approximately 45 degree angle. If this angle diminishes to less than 20 degrees, the transverse portion of the duodenum can get entrapped between the SMA and aorta, leading to symptoms of partial small bowel obstruction. This condition is called superior mesenteric artery, or "nutcracker," syndrome.

GAS 348; N 284; McM 235

247 B. This patient is most likely suffering from gallstone ileus, a condition that occurs in patients with longstanding cholelithiasis (often middle-aged to elderly women). A large (typically 2.5 cm or greater) gallstone causes the formation of a cholecystenteric fistula between the gallbladder and adjoining gut tissue due to persistent pressure on these tissues. The fistula ultimately allows passage of the gallstone into the small bowel, and the resulting communication between the gallbladder and small bowel allows intestinal gas to enter the gallbladder and biliary tree. Often this gas can be observed on abdominal radiographs. Obstruction of the cystic duct or bile duct by a gallstone leads to biliary colic, jaundice, and cholangitis.

GAS 341; N 280; McM 230, 246

248 B. At 16 to 18 years of age the hipbone is ossified from 8 centers, 3 primary and 5 secondary. These centers appear from about the eighth or ninth week of fetal life, and at birth the 3 primary centers are separate. By age 7-9 the inferior rami of pubis and ischium are almost completely fused. By age 13 or 14 the three growth centers grow toward the base of the acetabulum, and at around puberty the remaining portions ossify. At 13 to 15 years the three primary growth centers have only just extended toward the base of the acetabulum. Between 22 to 24 years old, ossification takes place in the remaining centers, and they fuse with the remaining bone. At 25 to 27 years, these bones should have already fused.

GAS 441; N 243; McM 287

249 A. The intramural part of the urethra is the most proximal part of the urethra, with the initial part traversing the wall of the bladder. The intermediate part of the urethra, also called the membranous portion, is the shortest and one of the narrowest segments, which leads from the prostate to the urethral bulb. Prostatic urethra is the segment passing through the prostate gland. Perforation of this segments leads to damage of the prostatic parenchyma. The spongy urethra runs along the length of the penis through the corpus spongiosum.

GAS 466; N 344; McM 266

250 E. The left testicular vein joins the left renal vein, which leads to the inferior vena cava. The left testicular vein after draining the testis and epididymis joins the left renal vein, which later joins the inferior vena cava. The testicular veins drain ipsilateral structures, so the right testicular vein should not be involved in the drainage of the left testicle. The right testicular vein drains directly into the inferior vena cava. The left testicular vein has no direct connection with the left common iliac vein. The median sacral vein receives blood from the sacral region and drains into the left common iliac vein.

GAS 470, 516; N 310; McM 261

251 E. The pubis is described as the anteroinferior part of the pelvis. The mons pubis is a fatty pad that rests above the pubis and can be palpated as a bony prominence below. The ilium articulates posteriorly with the sacrum and terminates anteriorly as the anterior superior iliac spine, which is located lateral to the pubic symphysis away from the midline. The coccyx is the terminal part of the vertebral column. As such, it is too posterior a structure to be palpated through the anterior abdominal wall. The sacrum is formed by the fusion of 5 sacral vertebrae and similar to the coccyx, it cannot be palpated through the anterior

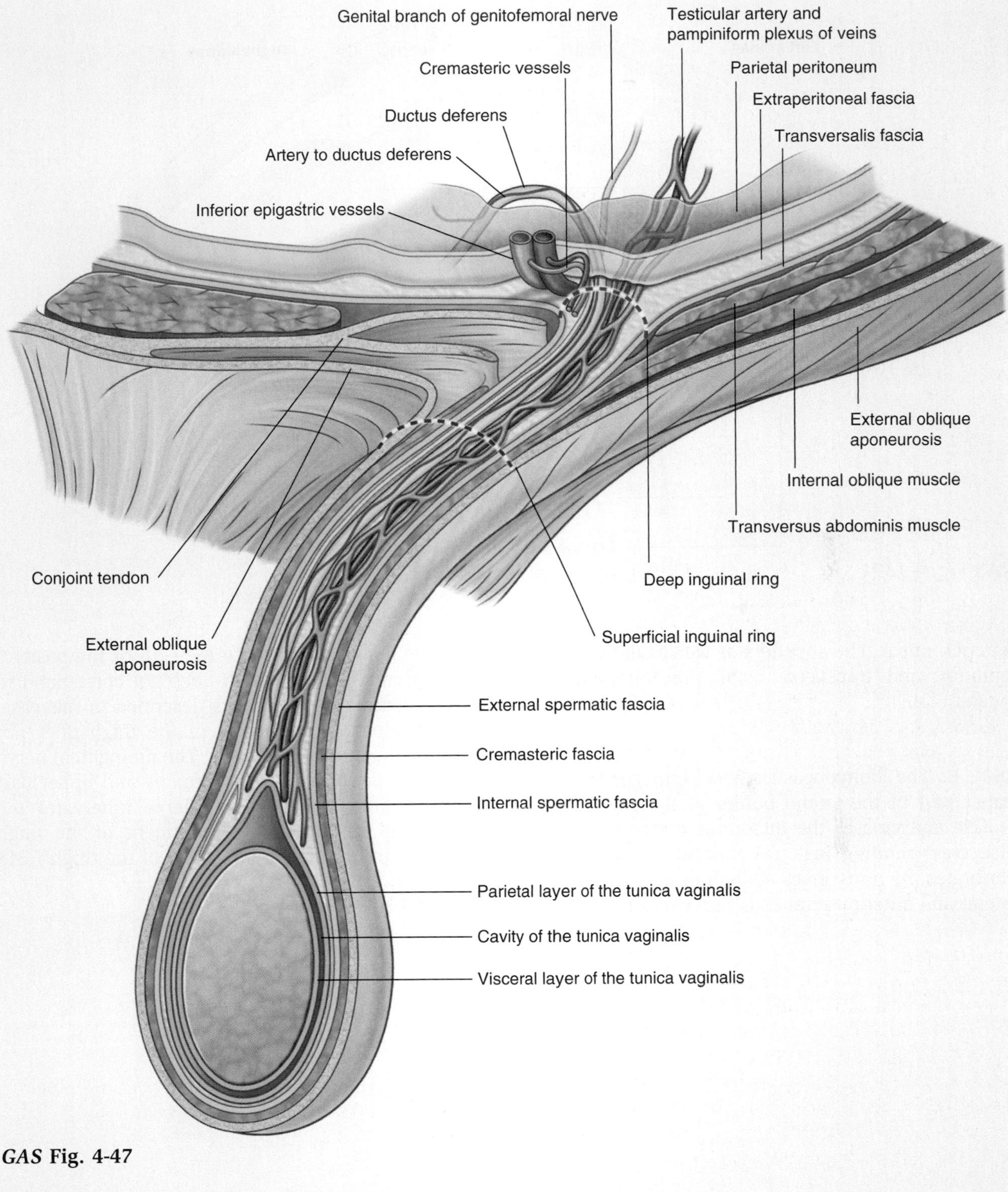

GAS **Fig. 4-47**

abdominal wall. The ischium makes up the posterior inferior part of the pelvic bone. Its most prominent feature is the ischial tuberosity located on the postero-inferior part of the bone, again making palpation as described in this case impossible.

GAS 441; N 243; McM 272

252 A. The descending colon begins at the splenic flexure in the upper left part of the abdomen. It passes downward through the left hypochondrium and lumbar regions, along the lateral border of the left kidney, and ends at the lower left part of the abdomen, where it continues as the sigmoid colon. It is

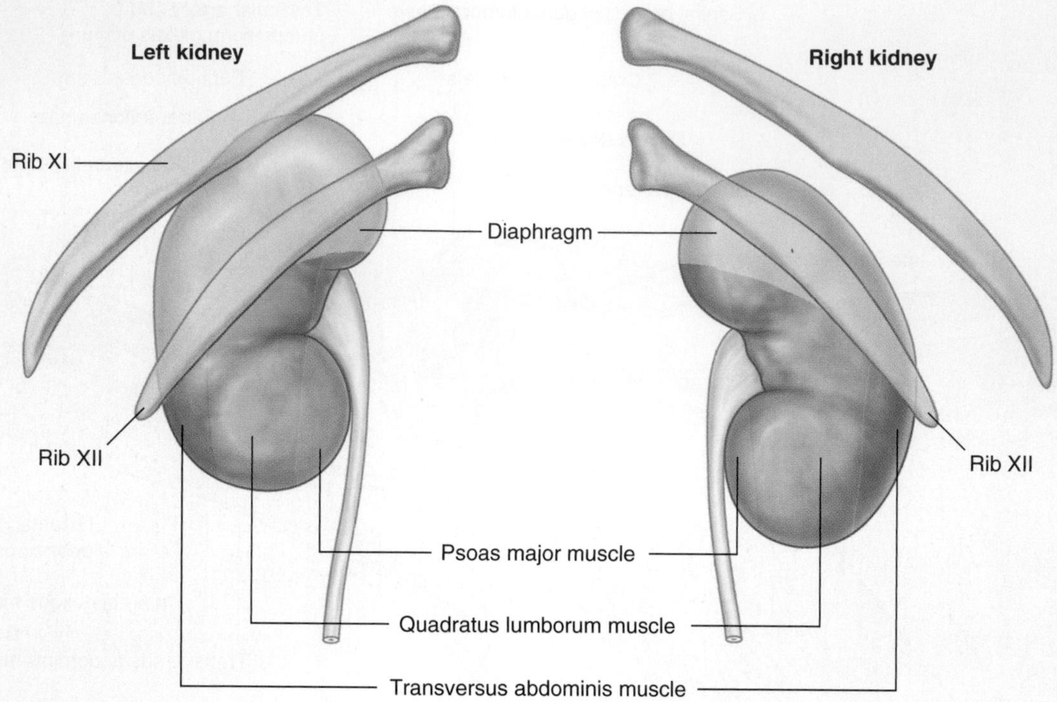

***GAS* Fig. 4-139**

retroperitoneal. The appendix as well as the stomach, jejunum, and transverse colon are intraperitoneal organs.

GAS 319; N 321; McM 228

253 **E.** The iliohypogastric nerve emerges from the upper part of the lateral border of the psoas major muscle and crosses the quadratus lumborum to the iliac crest running just posterior to the kidneys. It perforates the transverses abdominis and divides into lateral and anterior cutaneous branches. The subcostal nerve does not innervate the skin of the posterolateral gluteal region, which does not correspond to the area with sensory deficits described in this case. The lateral cutaneous nerve of the thigh does not relate to quadratus lumborum. The ilioinguinal nerve innervates the skin over the genitals and upper part of the scrotum. The femoral nerve innervates the muscles of the anterior compartment of the thigh and the skin on the medial aspect of the thigh (*GAS* Fig. 4-139).

GAS 398; N 253; McM 253

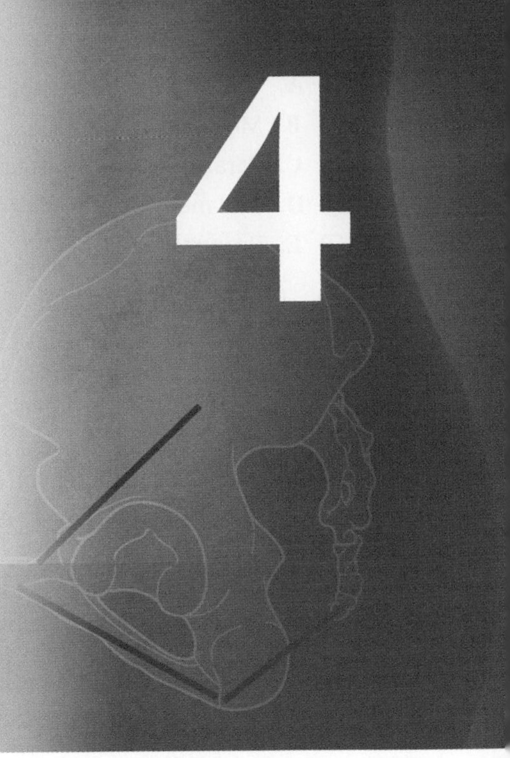

4

PELVIS AND PERINEUM

QUESTIONS

1 A 4-month-old male infant is admitted to the pediatric clinic because he was passing urine near the anus rather than from the tip of his penis. Physical examination reveals that the patient has perineal hypospadias. Which of the following embryologic structures failed to fuse properly?

- ☐ **A.** Labioscrotal folds
- ☐ **B.** Cloacal membrane
- ☐ **C.** Urogenital folds
- ☐ **D.** Genital tubercle
- ☐ **E.** Urogenital membrane

2 A 2-day-old infant girl is diagnosed with tracheoesophageal fistula. In addition, physical examination reveals an imperforate anus. A magnetic resonance imaging (MRI) examination reveals that the rectum, vagina, and colon are joined into a single channel. Which of the following structures is directly involved in this malformation?

- ☐ **A.** Labioscrotal folds
- ☐ **B.** Persistent cloaca
- ☐ **C.** Urogenital folds
- ☐ **D.** Genital tubercle
- ☐ **E.** Urogenital membrane

3 A 6-year-old boy is admitted to the hospital because of a palpable mass located external to the aponeurosis of the external oblique. Radiographic examination reveals that the mass is an ectopic testis, classified as interstitial. Failure of normal development of which of the following embryologic structures is responsible for ectopic testis?

- ☐ **A.** Gubernaculum
- ☐ **B.** Processus vaginalis
- ☐ **C.** Genital tubercle
- ☐ **D.** Seminiferous cords
- ☐ **E.** Labioscrotal swellings

4 A 2-month-old male infant has epispadias and the bladder mucosa is exposed to the outside. Which of the following is the most likely cause of this condition?

- ☐ **A.** Failure of the primitive streak mesoderm to migrate around the cloacal membrane
- ☐ **B.** Failure of urethral folds to fuse
- ☐ **C.** Insufficient androgen stimulation
- ☐ **D.** Klinefelter syndrome
- ☐ **E.** Persistent allantois

5 A bifid ureter or paired unilateral ureters result from partial or complete division of which of the following embryologic structures?

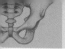

- ☐ **A.** Ureteric bud/metanephric diverticulum
- ☐ **B.** Mesonephric duct
- ☐ **C.** Paramesonephric duct
- ☐ **D.** Metanephric mesoderm
- ☐ **E.** Pronephros

6 A 16-year-old woman is visiting her gynecologist for her first checkup. On ultrasound examination it is noted that the woman has a double uterus. Failure of which of the following processes is responsible for the double uterus?

- ☐ **A.** Fusion of the inferior parts of the paramesonephric ducts
- ☐ **B.** Fusion of the superior parts of the mesonephric ducts
- ☐ **C.** Development of the hymen
- ☐ **D.** Development of the sinovaginal bulbs
- ☐ **E.** Fusion of the inferior parts of the mesonephric ducts

7 A 6-year-old boy has a large intraabdominal mass in the midline just above the pubic symphysis. During surgery a cystic mass is found attached to the umbilicus and to the apex of the bladder. Which of the following is the most likely diagnosis?

- ☐ **A.** Hydrocele
- ☐ **B.** Meckel cyst
- ☐ **C.** Meckel diverticulum
- ☐ **D.** Omphalocele
- ☐ **E.** Urachal cyst

8 A 26-year-old pregnant woman visits her gynecologist for a routine checkup. Ultrasound examination reveals that the patient has a normal pregnancy but that she also has two uteri. What is the most likely embryologic explanation of this condition?

- ☐ **A.** A complete fusion of the paramesonephric ducts
- ☐ **B.** An incomplete fusion of the paramesonephric ducts
- ☐ **C.** Hydronephrosis
- ☐ **D.** Cryptorchidism
- ☐ **E.** Regression of the pronephros

9 A 35-year-old woman is admitted to the emergency department with severe left abdominal and back pain. Radiographic evaluation reveals that the left ureter is blocked with a kidney stone. Because the ureter is completely obstructed, an emergency surgical procedure must be performed. Which of the following landmarks is most reliable for the identification of the ureter?

- ☐ **A.** The left ureter is located anterior to the left common iliac artery.
- ☐ **B.** The left ureter is located medial to the left inferior epigastric artery.
- ☐ **C.** The left ureter is located anterior to the left gonadal artery.
- ☐ **D.** The left ureter is located anterior to the left renal vein.
- ☐ **E.** The left ureter is located anterior to the left inferior epigastric artery.

10 A 1-year-old male infant is admitted to the pediatric clinic because he is passing urine on the underside of the penis as shown in Fig. 4-1. Which embryologic structure failed to fuse?

- ☐ **A.** Spongy urethra
- ☐ **B.** Labioscrotal folds
- ☐ **C.** Urethral folds
- ☐ **D.** Urogenital folds
- ☐ **E.** Genital tubercle

11 A 4-month-old male infant is admitted to the pediatric clinic because urine can be observed passing through an opening on the dorsum of the penis. Which of the following embryologic structures most likely failed to fuse?

- ☐ **A.** Spongy urethra
- ☐ **B.** Labioscrotal folds

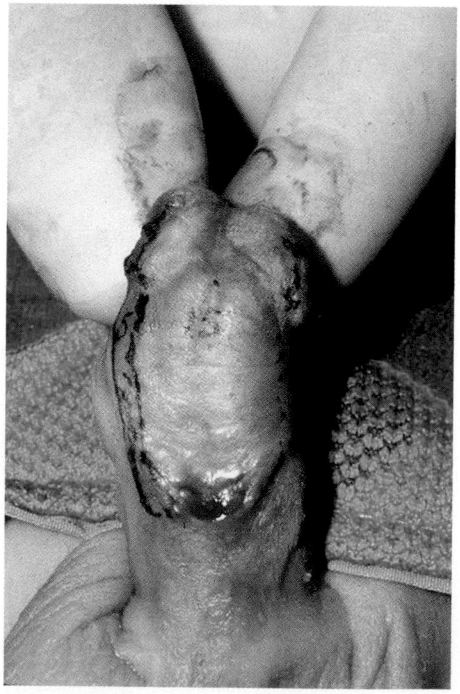

Fig. 4-1

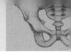

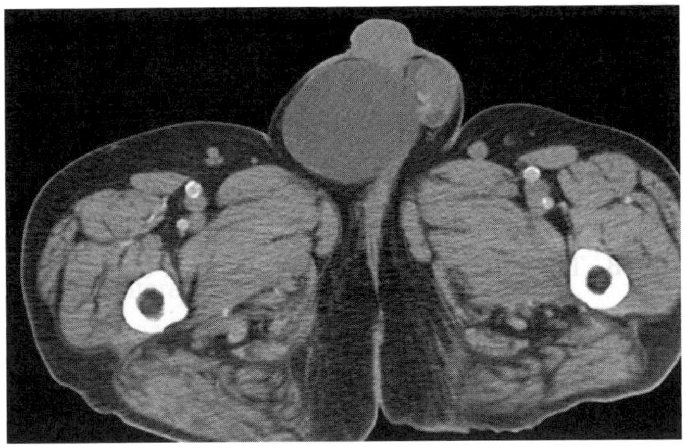

Fig. 4-2

- ▢ **C.** Cloacal membrane
- ▢ **D.** Urogenital folds
- ▢ **E.** Genital tubercle

12 A 25-year-old man is admitted to the hospital with testicular pain. Physical examination reveals a swollen and inflamed right testis. A computed tomography (CT) scan examination reveals abnormal accumulation of fluid in the cavity of the tunica vaginalis (Fig. 4-2). Which of the following is the most likely diagnosis for this patient?

- ▢ **A.** Varicocele
- ▢ **B.** Rectocele
- ▢ **C.** Cystocele
- ▢ **D.** Hydrocele
- ▢ **E.** Hypospadias

13 A 54-year-old man is admitted to the hospital with severe back pain. Radiographic examination suggests carcinoma of the left kidney blocking the drainage of the testicular vein. Which of the following conditions will be most likely associated with these signs?

- ▢ **A.** Varicocele
- ▢ **B.** Rectocele
- ▢ **C.** Cystocele
- ▢ **D.** Hydrocele
- ▢ **E.** Hypospadias

14 A 54-year-old man is admitted to the hospital with severe back pain. Upon radiographic examination (Fig. 4-3) the scrotum resembles a "bag of worms." Which of the following conditions will be most likely associated with this radiographic picture?

- ▢ **A.** Varicocele
- ▢ **B.** Rectocele
- ▢ **C.** Cystocele

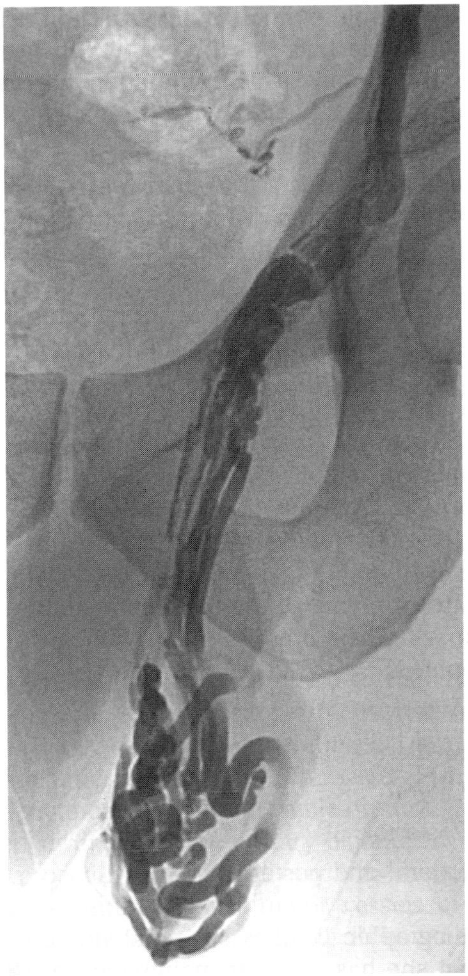

Fig. 4-3

- ▢ **D.** Hydrocele
- ▢ **E.** Hypospadias

15 A 16-year-old woman is brought to the emergency department with severe abdominal pain and fever. Laboratory examination is remarkable for an elevated white blood cell count and a positive test for pregnancy. Colpocentesis is performed to ascertain the presence of blood in the pelvis from a ruptured ectopic pregnancy. Through which of the following structures does the needle need to be inserted to perform colpocentesis?

- ▢ **A.** Through the perineal body into the vesicouterine space
- ▢ **B.** Through the posterior fornix of the vagina into the rectouterine pouch
- ▢ **C.** Through the anterior fornix into the endocervical canal
- ▢ **D.** Through the introitus into the vestibular gland
- ▢ **E.** Through the perineal membrane into the urogenital diaphragm

supplies a small area of skin (over the femoral triangle), just inferior to the midpoint of the inguinal ligament. The femoral nerve (L2 to L4) is motor to the quadriceps and sartorius muscles and sensory to the anterior thigh and the medial thigh and leg. The ilioinguinal supplies the suprapubic region; part of the genitalia and anterior perineum; and the upper, medial thigh. Cutaneous branches of the iliohypogastric nerve innervate skin of the anterolateral gluteal area and suprapubic region.

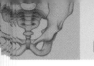

GAS 398; N 391; McM 261

23 **C.** Normally, the uterus is anteflexed at the junction of the cervix and the body and anteverted at the junction of the vagina and the cervical canal.

GAS 477; N 350; McM 273

24 **D.** The cardinal ligament, also known as Mackenrodt's ligament or transverse cervical ligament, is composed of condensations of fibromuscular tissues that accompany the uterine vessels. These bands of pelvic fascia provide direct support to the uterus. The other ligaments listed do not play a direct role in uterine stability.

GAS 481; N 351; McM 274

25 **C.** Ovarian lymph first drains into the para-aortic nodes at the level of the renal vessels. The superficial and deep inguinal nodes drain the body wall below the umbilicus, the lower limbs, and the cutaneous portion of the anal canal and parts of the perineum. The external iliac nodes receive the lymph from the inguinal nodes. The node of Cloquet is located in the femoral ring, adjacent to the external iliac vein and beneath the inguinal ligament. The node of Cloquet drains into the common iliac nodes. The internal iliac nodes accompany the uterine artery and vein, receiving lymph from much of the uterus but not the ovaries.

GAS 501; N 384; McM 362

26 **B.** The external anal sphincter is important for maintaining fecal continence. The external anal sphincter is located immediately posterior to the perineal body (central tendon) and would be susceptible to damage during a median episiotomy. The other structures listed play no role in maintaining fecal continence (*GAS* Fig. 5-17).

GAS 460; N 347; McM 277

27 **C.** The tendinous arch of fascia pelvis is a dense band of connective tissue that joins the fascia of the levator ani to the feltlike pubocervical fascia that covers the anterior wall of the vagina. If this fascial band is torn, the ipsilateral side of the vagina falls, carrying with it the bladder and urethra, often leading

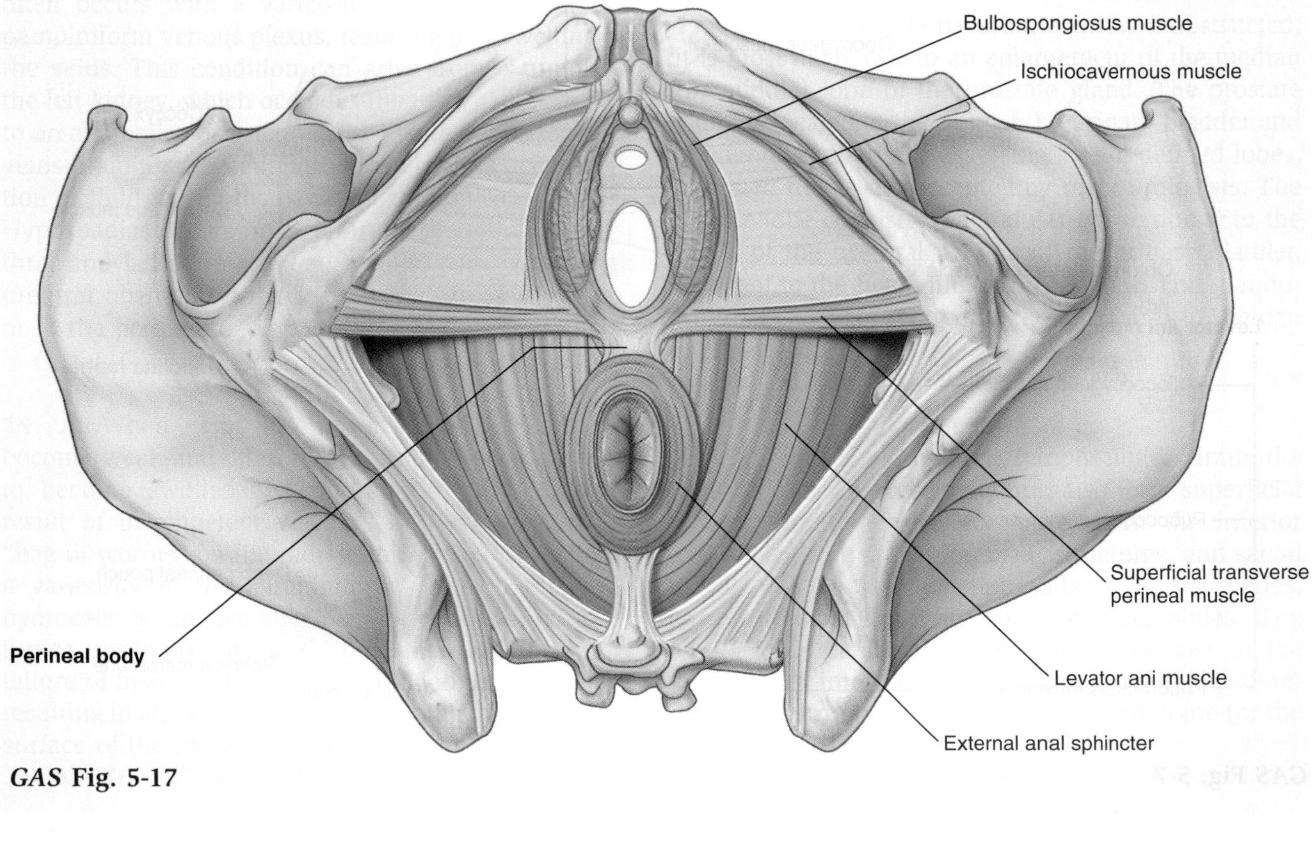

GAS **Fig. 5-17**

to urinary incontinence. The tendinous arch of the levator ani is a thickened portion of the fascia of the obturator internus and provides part of the origin of the levator ani muscle, but it plays no direct role in incontinence. The coccygeus muscle supports and raises the pelvic floor but is not directly associated with urinary incontinence. The obturator internus is involved with lateral rotation of the thigh. If the rectovaginal septum is torn, the patient can be subject to the occurrence of rectocele or enterocele, as the lower portion of the GI tract prolapses into the posterior wall of the vagina (*GAS* Fig. 5-34).

GAS 466, 459; N 356; McM 275

28 A. Lymph from the cutaneous portion of the anal canal (below the pectinate line) drains into the inguinal nodes. Lymph from most parts of the rectum and from the mucosal zone of the anal canal (above the pectinate line) drains into the internal iliac nodes. Lymph from some parts of the rectum also drains into the sacral nodes.

GAS 501; N 384; McM 368

29 C. The retropubic space (of Retzius) is the extraperitoneal space between the pubic symphysis and the bladder. A needle placed over the pubic bone, through the body wall, and into the space of Retzius

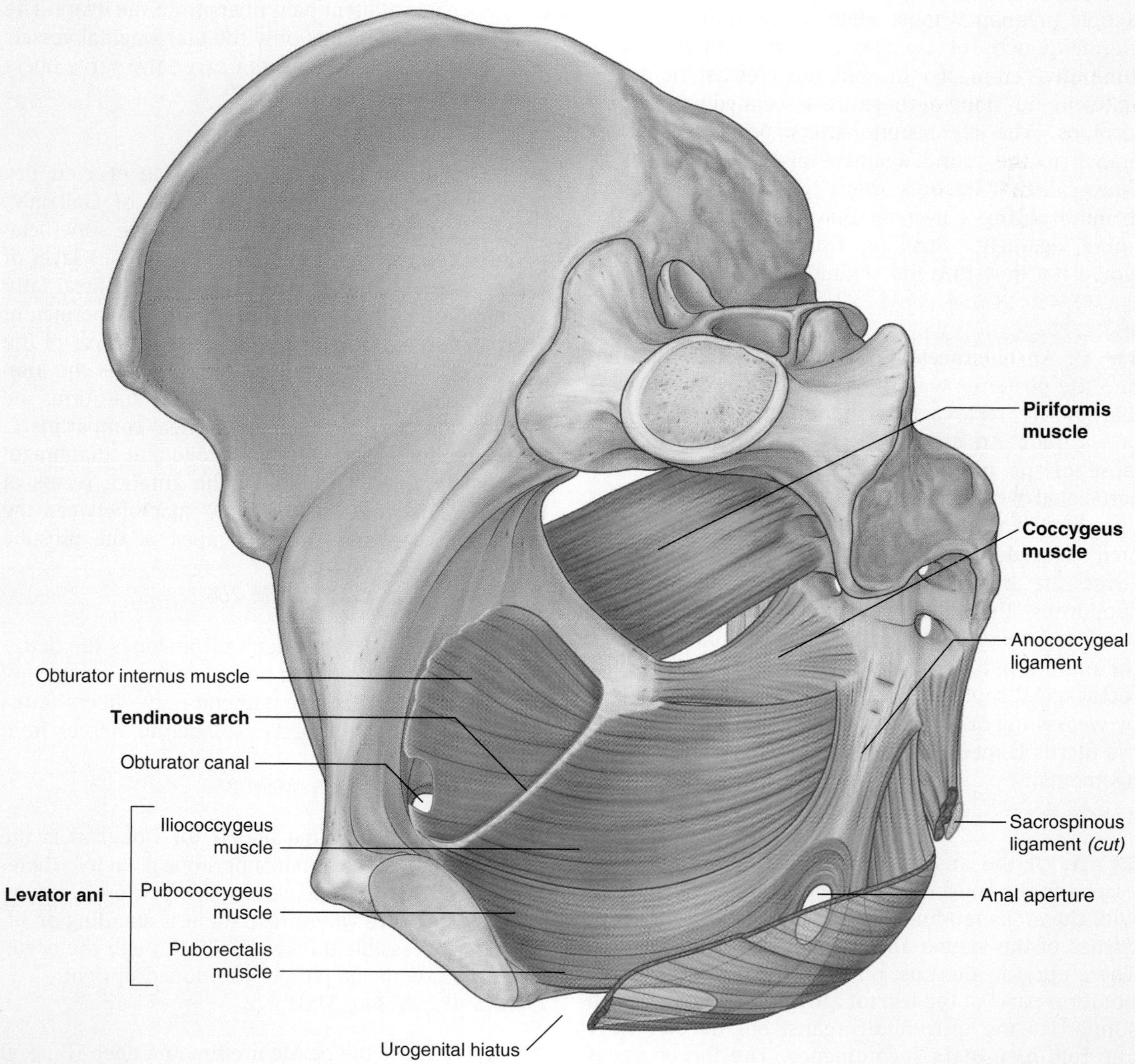

GAS **Fig. 5-34**

will enter the full bladder but avoids entry into the peritoneum and there is little risk of damaging major organs or vessels. Entry through the ischioanal fossa would not provide a direct route to the bladder. With entry through the superficial perineal cleft, perineal body, and deep perineal pouch there is a high risk of damaging important structures.
GAS 463, 466; N 374; McM 266

30 C. Hematocolpos is characterized by filling of the vagina with menstrual blood. This commonly occurs due to the presence of an imperforate hymen. Bartholin's gland ducts open into the vestibule of the vagina; therefore, a cyst in Bartholin's gland would not cause hematocolpos. Blood from a ruptured ectopic pregnancy most often drains into the recto-uterine pouch (of Douglas). Women often have a diminutive cremaster muscle and cremasteric artery and vein, but none of these are associated with hematocolpos. The cremasteric artery provides a small branch to the round ligament of the uterus (sometimes called "Samson's artery"), which must be kept in mind during a hysterectomy, with division of the round ligament. Bleeding from the uterine veins would not flow into the vagina.
GAS 480; N 354; McM 272

31 C. An enterocele (herniation of small intestine into the posterior wall of the vagina) is caused by a tear of the rectovaginal septum that weakens the pelvic floor. An urethrocele is characterized by prolapse of the urethra into the vagina. It is usually associated with a cystocele (prolapse of the bladder into the urethra). Cystocele or urethrocele are associated with defects in the pubocervical fascia that covers the anterior wall of the vagina and assists in supporting the bladder. Urinary incontinence can result from weakening of the muscles that surround the urethra but would not be caused by a tear of the rectovaginal septum. Prolapse of the uterus is caused by weakening or tearing of the ligaments that support the uterus (especially the cardinal and/or uterosacral ligaments).
GAS 480-481; N 343; McM 272

32 A. Of the answer choices listed, the pubococcygeus is the muscle that is most directly associated with the arcus tendineus fascia pelvis and connective tissues of the vagina and the support of the bladder. The obturator internus, piriformis, and coccygeus do not form parts of the levator ani and provide no direct support to the urogenital organs, nor do they have any role in urinary incontinence. The iliococcygeus does form part of the levator ani, but it is located lateral to the pubococcygeus and therefore does not play a direct role in maintaining urinary continence.
GAS 454-456; N 336; McM 264

33 A. The ovarian vessels and nerves lie within the infundibulopelvic ligament (suspensory ligament of the ovary); therefore, cutting this ligament interrupts pain fibers from the ovary. Cutting the sympathetic trunk might help to reduce some of the pain from the ovary, but the results of such a procedure are rather unpredictable, plus locating the lumbar sympathetic trunk is more of a surgical challenge. The clunial nerves are cutaneous nerves that innervate parts of the buttocks. They are not associated with the ovaries. The pudendal nerve innervates the perineum and does not carry afferent pain fibers from the ovary. The broad ligament contains only the uterovaginal vessels and nerve plexus and does not carry any nerve fibers from the ovary (*GAS* Fig. 5-65).
GAS 498; N 342; McM 274

34 C. The superficial perineal space or cleft lies between the external perineal fascia of Gallaudet (fascia of inferior perineal muscles in the superficial perineal compartment) and the membranous layer of Colles' fascia. Camper's fascia is the superficial fatty layer of the anterior abdominal wall and the perineum; Scarpa's fascia is the deep membranous layer of the abdominal wall. The perineal membrane is the inferior fascia of the urogenital diaphragm that forms the inferior boundary of the deep perineal compartment. The superior fascia of the urogenital diaphragm bounds the inferior border of the anterior recess of the ischioanal fossa. There is no space between the urogenital diaphragm and the apex of the prostate gland (*GAS* Fig. 5-69).
GAS 506-512; N 374; McM 266

35 B. The urinary bladder wall includes the detrusor muscle, and it receives both its motor and sensory innervation from parasympathetic nerve fibers transmitted by way of the pelvic splanchnic nerves from S2 to S4.
GAS 492-494; N 395; McM 268

36 A. The rectouterine pouch (of Douglas) is the lowest point of the woman's peritoneal cavity. Therefore, a fluid collection within the peritoneal cavity accumulates here when the patient is standing or sitting. It is accessible transvaginally through the posterior fornix, with the patient positioned upright.
GAS 483; N 340; McM 272

37 E. Because the penile urethra and deep (Buck's) fascia are both located in the superficial perineal

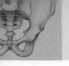

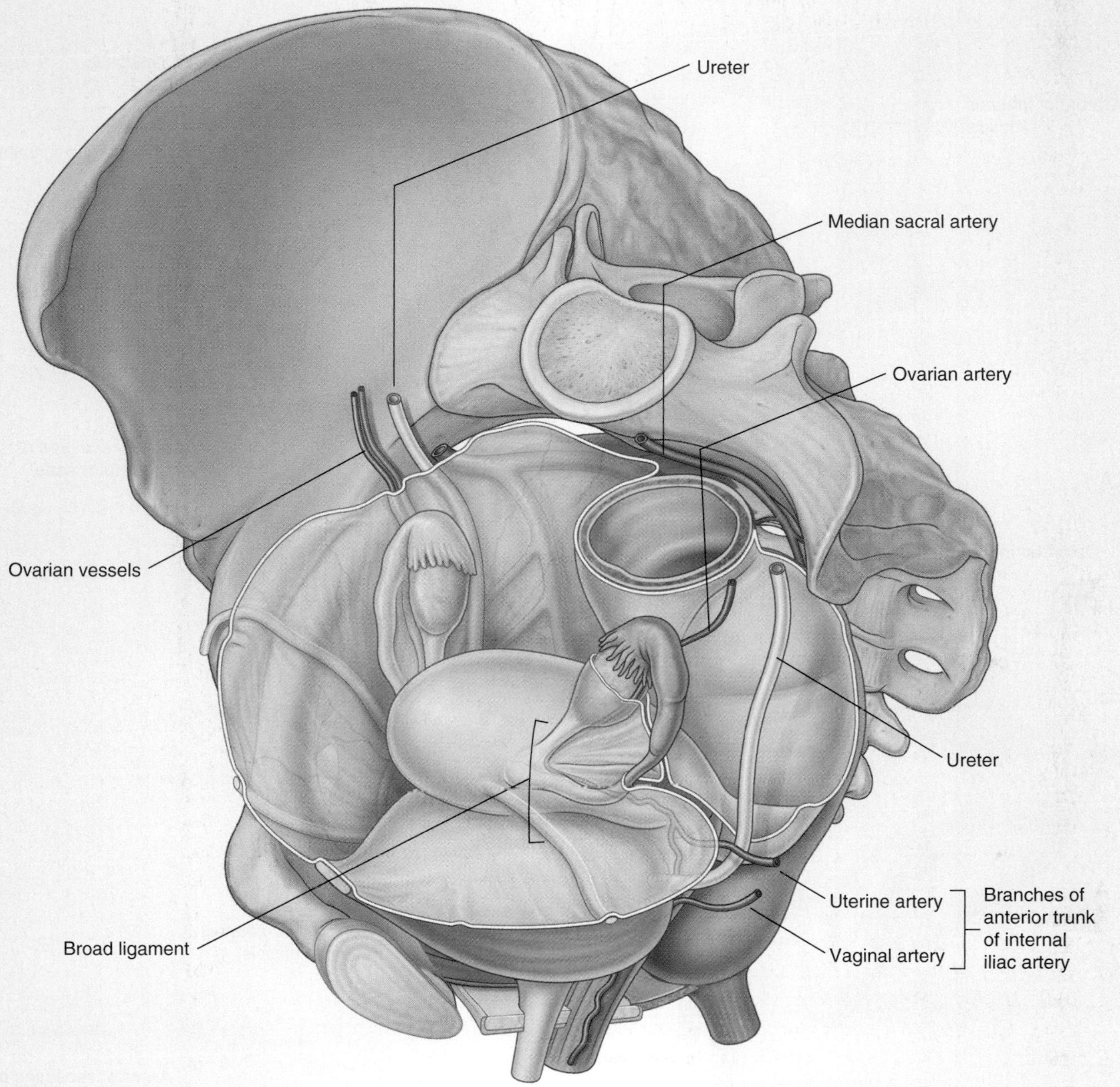

GAS Fig. 5-65

pouch, rupture will occur here, with extravasation of fluids into the superficial perineal cleft. The ischioanal fossa is located posterior to the urogenital triangle, behind the area of injury. The other listed spaces are deep to the superficial compartment or within the pelvis and are not associated with the area of injury.
GAS 466-468, 512; N 374; McM 266

38 **C.** The perineal branch of the pudendal nerve is responsible for the innervation of the external urethral sphincter, and injury to this nerve can result in paralysis of the sphincter and urinary incontinence. Pelvic splanchnic and sacral splanchnic nerves are autonomic nerves that do not supply skeletal muscle. The gluteal nerves innervate gluteal muscles.
GAS 491; N 389; McM 266

39 **D.** The internal pudendal artery gives rise to both the dorsal artery and deep artery of the penis. The deep artery is the main supply for erectile tissue; therefore, significant atherosclerosis of the internal pudendal artery may result in impotence (erectile dysfunction).
GAS 496-497; N 383; McM 267

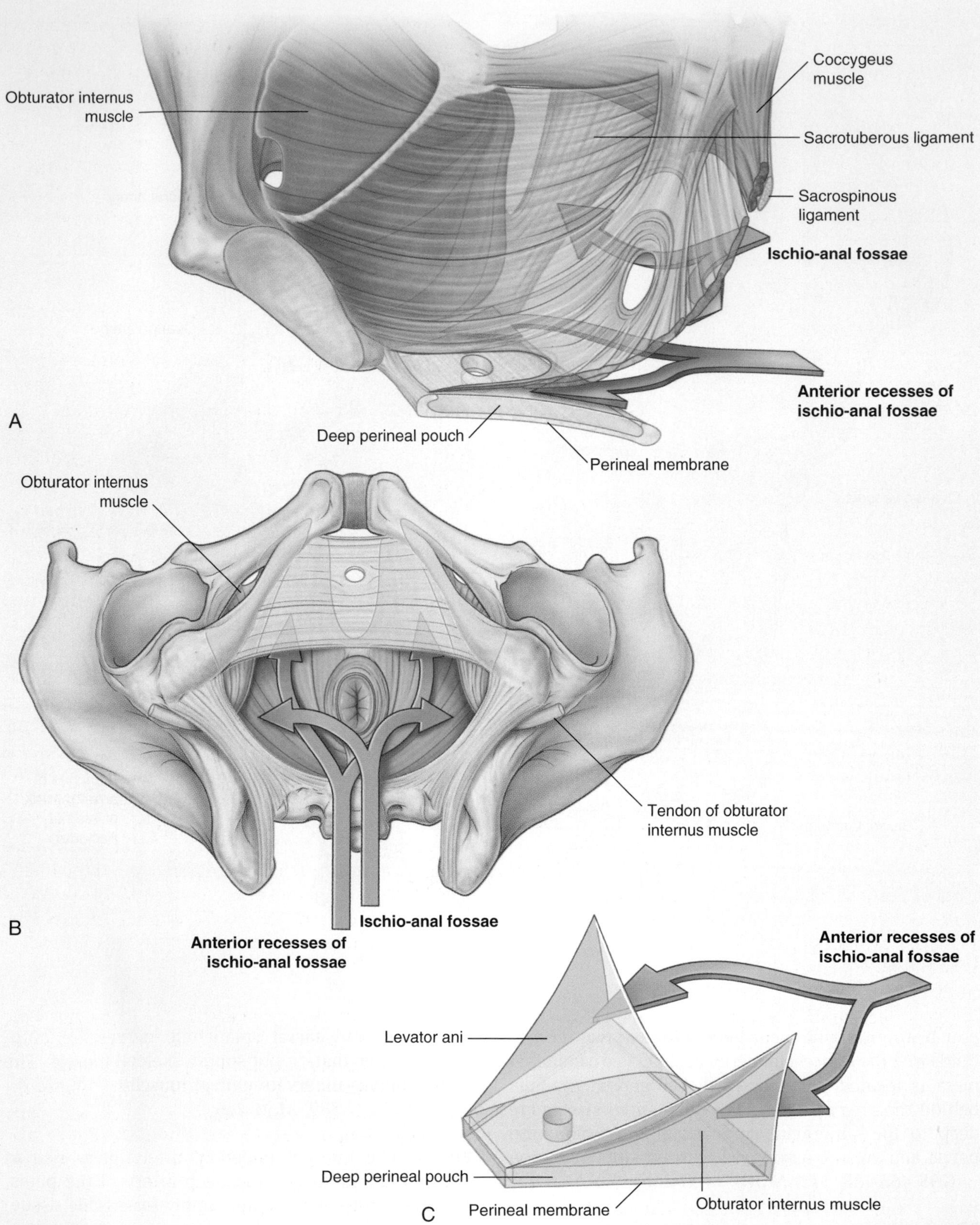
Obturator internus muscle
Coccygeus muscle
Sacrotuberous ligament
Sacrospinous ligament
Ischio-anal fossae
Anterior recesses of ischio-anal fossae
A
Deep perineal pouch
Perineal membrane
Obturator internus muscle
Tendon of obturator internus muscle
B
Ischio-anal fossae
Anterior recesses of ischio-anal fossae
Anterior recesses of ischio-anal fossae
Levator ani
Deep perineal pouch
C
Perineal membrane
Obturator internus muscle

GAS Fig. 5-69

40 A. Cancer present in the inguinal nodes can be indicative of cancer of the uterus at the level of the round ligaments, by which the cancerous cells drain to the inguinal region. Uterine cancer must be especially suspected if the tissues of the lower limb, vulva, and anal canal appear normal. The pectinate line marks the end of the mucosal lining of the anal canal, below which the canal is lined with nonkeratinized, stratified squamous epithelium. The pectinate line is also associated with the distal ends of the anal columns and anal valves. Lymphatic vessels inferior to the pectinate line of the anal canal will drain into the superficial inguinal nodes, but those above the pectinate line flow to internal iliac nodes. Lymph from the ovaries flows to the para-aortic nodes at the level of the kidneys. Lymph from the rectum flows to pelvic lymph nodes.

GAS 501, 519; N 384; McM 274

41 C. The lymphatic vessels of the ovaries join with lymphatics from the uterine tubes and the fundus of the uterus. These ascend to the right and left lumbar (caval/aortic) lymph nodes. These lymph nodes are the first to receive cancerous cells from the ovaries. Superficial inguinal nodes drain the lower limb, the anterior abdominal wall inferior to the umbilicus, and superficial perineal structures. The external iliac nodes drain the deep inguinal nodes that drain the clitoris and superficial inguinal nodes. The internal iliac nodes drain inferior pelvic structures and deep perineal structures.

GAS 501, 519; N 384; McM 362

42 A. The superficial inguinal nodes drain superficial perineal structures, including the superolateral uterine body near attachment of the round ligament, skin of the perineum (including the vulva), and the introitus of the vagina inferior to the hymen. The internal iliac nodes drain the middle and upper vagina, cervix, and body of the uterus. The lumbar/lateral aortic lymph nodes drain the ovaries. The axillary lymph nodes drain the upper limb and chest wall, including the breasts.

GAS 501, 519; N 385; McM 368

43 A. The ischial spine is the correct bony landmark used to administer a pudendal nerve block. The pudendal nerve crosses the sacrospinous ligament, which attaches to the ischial spine. Accessing the ischial spine and thus the pudendal nerve is done most easily using a transvaginal approach. The posterior superior and inferior iliac spines are located on the posterior aspect of the pelvis and articulate with the lateral aspect of the sacrum. They do not relate to the course of the pudendal nerve. The ischial tuberosities are the most inferior aspect of the bony pelvis. The skin and soft tissues around the ischial tuberosities receive sensory supply from the pudendal nerve and perineal branches of the posterior femoral cutaneous nerve. Injections into the area around the tuberosities are less certain, however, than injections at the sacrospinous ligament and often fail to anesthetize the anal triangle well. The coccyx is a poor target for locating and anesthetizing the pudendal nerve.

GAS 441-445; N 391; McM 92

44 D. Hemorrhoids are divided into two categories: internal and external. Pain due to external hemorrhoids is mediated by the pudendal nerve (somatosensory), which serves the majority of the perineum. The sacral splanchnic nerves are postganglionic sympathetic fibers from the sacral sympathetic trunk, and the pelvic splanchnic nerves carry preganglionic parasympathetic fibers and sensory fibers from within the pelvis. Superior hypogastric nerves are mixed nerves located anterior to the sacral promontory and do not mediate pain information from the perineum. The ilioinguinal nerve provides sensory innervation to the skin at the base of the penis; the scrotum; and upper, inner thigh.

GAS 504; N 394; McM 266

45 C. The membranous urethra is shorter in women than in men. Because of its close proximity to the vestibule in women, it commonly leads to infections of the urinary tract. The vagina contains more bacterial flora than the penis. The prostate gland produces a clear, alkaline fluid, but it has not been proved that it protects against bacterial infections. The uterus has no known antibacterial functions. The seminal vesicles produce a fructose-containing fluid that provides nutrients to the sperm for the journey through the female genital tract.

GAS 466-468, 512; N 348; McM 272

46 A. The uterus is stabilized and anchored to the bladder by the pubovesical and vesicocervical fasciae on its anterior surface. During pregnancy and childbirth this connective tissue can be torn, allowing the bladder to herniate into the anterior vaginal wall, with prolapse possible through the vaginal introitus. The transverse cervical (cardinal) ligament is located within the base of the broad ligament and is a major ligament of the uterus but would offer no support if the bladder herniates through the vagina. The uterosacral ligament serves to anchor the uterus to the sacrum for support. Injury to the levator ani would not cause the bladder to herniate through the vagina. The median umbilical ligament contains the urachus and is located on the posterior aspect of the linea alba; the ligament is an embryologic remnant of the allantois.

GAS 477; N 343; McM 275

47 **A.** During a hysterectomy, ligation of or injury to the ureter can happen relatively easily because it is the most susceptible structure due to its location. The ureter is located immediatelly inferior to the uterine vessels ("water passes under the bridge") in the pelvic cavity approximately 1 cm lateral to the supravaginal cervix. The internal iliac artery bifurcates near the pelvic brim but is not in close proximity to the uterine vessels in the vicinity of the cervix. The obturator nerve travels along the pelvic sidewall and is not close to the site of ligation of the uterine vessels. The lumbosacral trunk is located on the lateral side of the sacrum and the pelvic sidewall, not in close proximity to the uterine vessels.

GAS 478; N 378; McM 275

48 **A.** Vaginismus is a painful, psychosomatic gynecologic disorder; it is described as involving distension of the cavernous tissues and the bulbospongiosus and transverse perineal muscles, the stimulation of which triggers the involuntary spasms of the perivaginal and levator ani muscles. This can in turn lead to dyspareunia.

GAS 480; N 350; McM 276

49 **E.** This is a classic example of extravasation of blood and urine from the superficial perineal pouch. This usually is a result of rupture of the spongy urethra. The extravasation of the fluid (urine) will begin to invade the layer between the Buck's fascia and the dartos layer. This extravasation example is evident due to the fluid invading up to the abdomen between the subcutaneous tissues and muscle fascia. If the fluid collects between the other layers of the perineum, the clinical evidence will present differently in the perineum and abdominal area.

GAS 466-468, 502-504; N 374; McM 266

50 **A.** The uterosacral ligaments and the transverse cervical (cardinal) ligaments are the two main ligaments stabilizing the uterus. They help to inhibit the uterus from prolapsing into the vagina. The round ligament of the uterus is related to the descent of the ovaries in embryologic development and continues into the inguinal canal. This ligament is the remnant of the gubernaculum ovary. The broad ligament is the peritoneal covering over the uterine tubes, uterus, and vessels. The arcus tendineus fascia pelvis joins the muscle fascia of the levator ani to the pubocervical fascia on the vagina and is not directly associated with the uterus or its ligaments. The levator ani muscles contribute to the floor of the pelvis and support all of the pelvic viscera indirectly; it does not, however, prevent prolapse of the uterus into the vagina (*GAS* Fig. 5-57).

GAS 481; N 352; McM 275

51 **A.** The internal iliac lymph nodes and sacral nodes would be involved in a pelvic lymphadenectomy, which often would be desired in surgical resection for prostate cancer. Sacral lymphatics can communicate with lymphatics within the vertebral canal and thus metastasize cranially. The external iliac nodes drain all of the anterosuperior pelvic structures, the lower limb and perineum, and the body wall to the level of the umbilicus. The superficial inguinal nodes drain all of the superficial structures below the umbilicus. The deep inguinal nodes drain the glans penis in the male.

GAS 501, 519; N 386; McM 268

52 **E.** The para-aortic and lumbar nodes at the level of the kidneys will most likely be infiltrated by metastasis of testicular cancer because testicular lymphatics run in close association with the testicular vessels and drain the testicles and epididymis. Testicular cancer is a disease that is especially dangerous for young men, as intrabdominal lymph node swelling is often a late clinical presentation. The internal iliac nodes drain the inferior pelvis and deep perineal structures. The external iliac nodes drain all anterosuperior pelvic structures. The superficial inguinal nodes drain all of the superficial structures below the umbilicus. Finally, the deep inguinal nodes receive more superficial vessels and drain the glans penis in males.

GAS 501, 519; N 386; McM 362

53 **C.** Penile erection is a parasympathetic mediated response that is delivered via the pelvic splanchnic nerves that pass through nerve bundles on the posterolateral aspect of the prostate gland. (In prostatectomy, these bundles should be left intact, if at all possible, to avoid erectile dysfunction, also known as impotence.) The pudendal nerve and its terminal branch, the dorsal nerve of the penis, carry the primary skeletal motor and sensory innervation to the external genitalia, and also sympathetic fibers. Sacral splanchnic nerves contain sympathetic fibers.

GAS 492-494, 515; N 394; McM 269

54 **A.** Rupture of the spongy urethra leads to accumulation of fluid (edema) in the superficial perineal cleft. The continuity of Colles' fascia (superficial

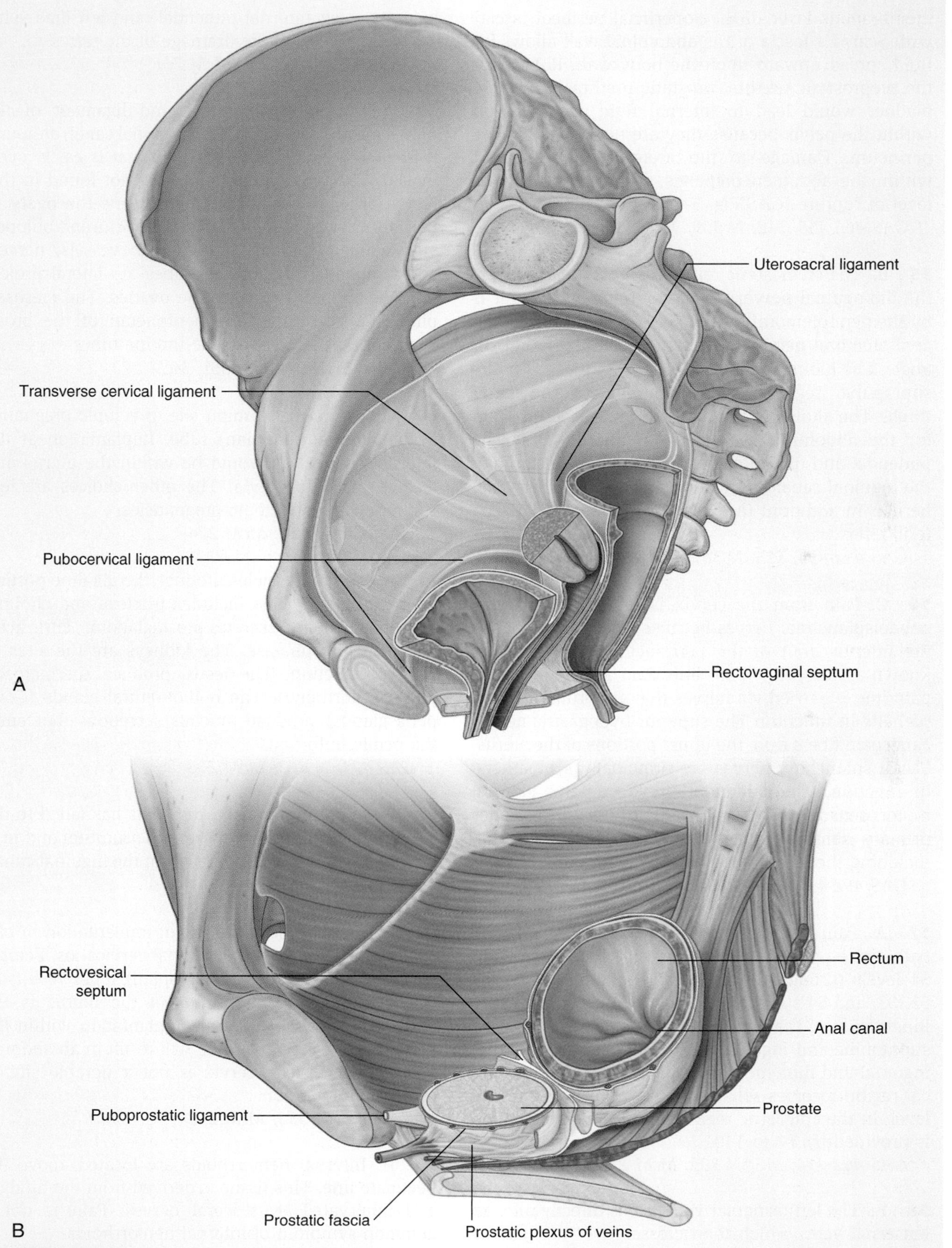
Uterosacral ligament
Transverse cervical ligament
Pubocervical ligament
Rectovaginal septum
A
Rectum
Rectovesical septum
Anal canal
Puboprostatic ligament
Prostate
Prostatic fascia
Prostatic plexus of veins
B

GAS Fig. 5-57

membranous layer of the superficial perineal fascia) with Scarpa's fascia of the abdominal wall allows for fluid spread upward upon the body wall. Rupture of the preprostatic urethra, prostatic urethra, or urinary bladder would lead to internal fluid accumulation within the pelvis because they are not located in the perineum. Damage to the ureter would manifest within the abdomen or pelvis, depending upon the level of rupture (*GAS* Fig. 5-46).

GAS 466-468, 512; N 369; McM 266

55 **B.** The cremasteric reflex afferents are carried by the ilioinguinal nerve; the motor (efferent) output is by the genitofemoral nerve. The sensory fibers of the genitofemoral nerve are to skin over the femoral triangle. The ilioinguinal nerve is sensory to parts of the suprapubic region, anterior perineum, and inner thigh. The iliohypogastric nerve provides sensation for the abdominal wall and suprapubic area. The pudendal and obturator nerves do not travel through the inguinal canal and would not be damaged by the hernia. In addition, they play no role in the cremasteric reflex.

GAS 492-494, 515; N 387; McM 262

56 **C.** Pain from the cervix is transmitted via the pelvic splanchnic nerves because the cervix is below the inferior limit of the peritoneum, which is also known as the pelvic pain line. Pain above the pelvic pain line is carried via nerves that are primarily sympathetic in function. The superior hypogastric nerves carry pain fibers from the upper portions of the uterus. Sacral splanchnic nerves are principally sympathetic in function. The pudendal nerve contains skeletal motor, sensory, and sympathetic fibers and provides primary sensory innervation to external genitalia, including the lower third of the vagina.

GAS 492-494, 515; N 393; McM 269

57 **A.** Pain from this area is mediated via parasympathetic responses and would thus travel to the S2 to S4 levels through the pelvic splanchnic nerves. The S2, S3, and S4 spinal cord levels also provide sensory innervation of the perineum and posterior thigh. The suprapubic and inguinal regions are supplied by ilioinguinal and iliohypogastric nerves (L1). The umbilical region receives sensory innervation from the T10 level. In the epigastric region the sensory innervation is provided by T7 to T10.

GAS 492-494, 515; N 393; McM 272

58 **B.** The left testicular vein drains directly into the left renal vein, which then crosses over the midline to enter the inferior vena cava. The left inferior epigastric, left internal pudendal, and left iliac veins are not involved in the drainage of the testes.

GAS 495-500; N 379; McM 261

59 **A.** During repair, the round ligament of the uterus may be seen within the inguinal canal, although it is often a small, fibrous strand that is easily overlooked. The remaining choices are not found in this region. The ovarian ligament connects the ovary to the uterus, whereas the suspensory (infundibulopelvic) ligament contains the ovarian vessels, nerves, and lymphatic. The uterine tubes are lateral projections of the uterus toward the ovaries. The mesosalpinx is a portion of the peritoneum of the broad ligament that attaches to the uterine tubes.

GAS 476-479; N 350, 351; McM 272

60 **C.** The most common site of ectopic pregnancy is the uterine (fallopian) tube. Implantation at the internal cervical os would be within the uterus and lead to placenta previa. The other choices are less common sites of ectopic pregnancies.

GAS 530; N 352; McM 274

61 **B.** Seminal vesicles produce the alkaline portion of the ejaculate. This includes fructose and choline. The prostate gland secretes prostaglandins, citric acid, and acid phosphatase. The kidneys are the sites of urine production. The testes produce spermatozoa and sex hormones. The bulbourethral glands (Cowper's glands) produce mucous secretions that enter the penile bulb.

GAS 473; N 362; McM 268

62 **C.** In cryptorchidism, the testis has failed to descend into its proper location in the scrotum and may be found within the abdomen or in the inguinal canal.

GAS 470; N 364; McM 266

63 **D.** By definition, the site of implantation in placenta previa overlaps the internal cervical os. Ectopic pregnancy in the uterine (fallopian) tubes results in tubal pregnancy. The fundus of the uterus is the normal site of implantation. Implantation within the mesenteries of the abdomen will result in an abdominal pregnancy. The cervix is not a notable site of ectopic implantation.

GAS 530; N 352; McM 272

64 **D.** Internal hemorrhoids are located above the pectinate line. This tissue is derived from the hindgut and innervated by visceral nerves. Pain is not a common symptom of internal hemorrhoids.

GAS 504; N 377; McM 268

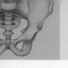

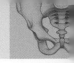

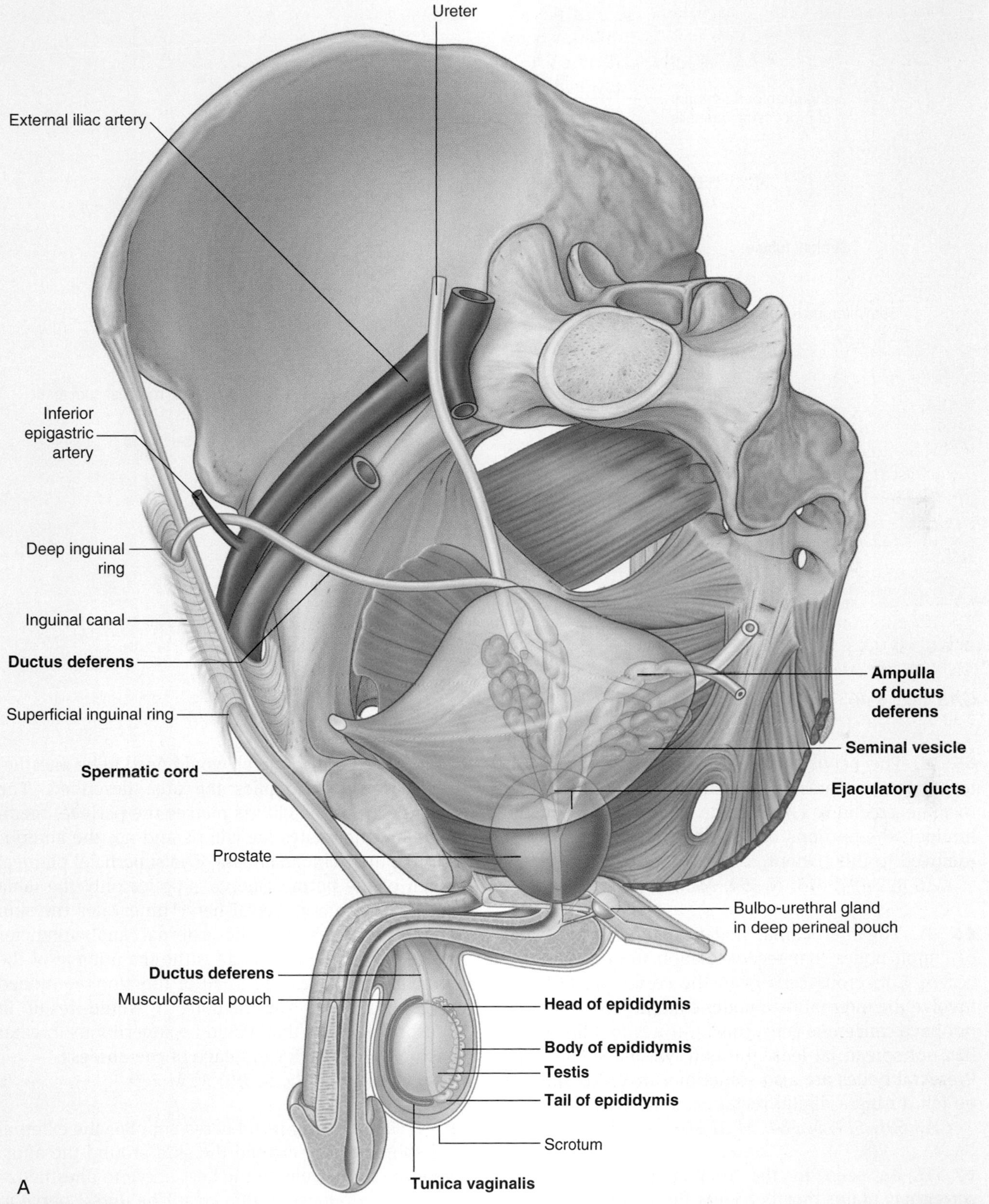
Ureter
External iliac artery
Inferior epigastric artery
Deep inguinal ring
Inguinal canal
Ductus deferens
Superficial inguinal ring
Spermatic cord
Prostate
Ductus deferens
Musculofascial pouch
Ampulla of ductus deferens
Seminal vesicle
Ejaculatory ducts
Bulbo-urethral gland in deep perineal pouch
Head of epididymis
Body of epididymis
Testis
Tail of epididymis
Scrotum
Tunica vaginalis
A

GAS Fig. 5-46

Continued

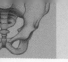

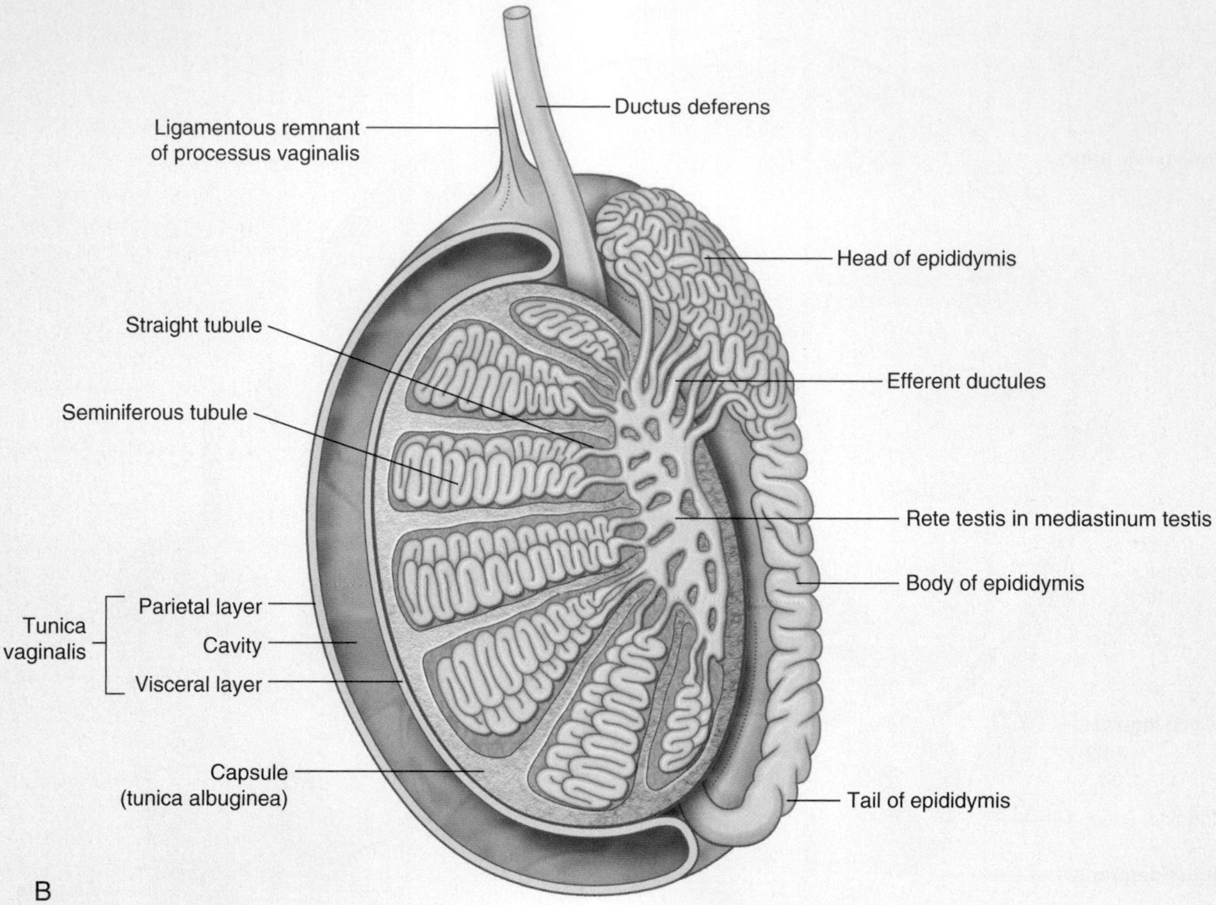

***GAS* Fig. 5-46, cont'd**

65 C. The pelvic splanchnic nerves (nervi erigentes) contain parasympathetic efferent fibers that mediate erection. These same nerves innervate the hindgut, the portions of the large intestine that were removed in this patient.

GAS 492-494, 515; N 394; McM 269

66 A. The internal iliac nodes are the first in a trunk of lymph nodes that receive lymph from the uterine cervix. Cancerous cells from the cervix are likely to involve the internal iliac nodes first. If these nodes do not have cancerous cells, this indicates that the tumor has not spread, at least through lymphatic channels. Presacral nodes are also sometimes involved and can be felt during a digital rectal examination.

GAS 501, 519; N 384; McM 366

67 D. As seen in the photograph, the swollen scrotum contains mostly a clear fluid. Since hydrocele is the accumulation of fluid between the visceral and parietal layers of the tunica vaginalis, this condition best accounts for the findings in this patient.

GAS 470-475; N 365; McM 265

68 C. The perineal nerve would need to be anesthetized because it supplies the area described. The dorsal nerve to the clitoris pierces the perineal membrane and innervates the clitoris and not the anterior recess of the ischioanal fossa. The superficial perineal branch of the perineal nerve supplies only the labia majora. The inferior rectal nerve innervates the skin around the anus and the external anal sphincter muscle. The pudendal nerve is the main nerve of the perineum and gives rise to all of the aforementioned nerves; therefore, anesthetizing it would result in widespread effects that would be superfluous to what is actually needed for drainage of the abscess.

GAS 486-494, 575; N 391; McM 279

69 D. The inferior rectal nerve supplies the external anal sphincter muscle and the skin around the anus. Therefore this would be the best nerve to anesthetize for abscess drainage in this area. The dorsal nerve to the clitoris does not innervate the posterior recess of the perineum. The superficial perineal branch of the perineal nerve supplies the labia majora and would not need to be anesthetized in the event of a horseshoe anal abscess. The perineal nerve supplies all the perineal muscles and the labia majora, but for the area in question it does not have as direct a supply as the inferior rectal nerve. The pudendal nerve gives off all the branches above and thus anesthetizing it would result in additional unwanted side effects (*GAS* Fig. 5-75).

GAS 492-494, 515; N 391; McM 279

70 B. A variant obturator artery arising from the inferior epigastric arteries can be found in 20% to 30% of the population. Patients with this variation are more susceptible to inadvertent damage during certain surgeries if the surgeon is not aware of presence of the aberrant artery. This artery is alternatively called the "corona mortis," which translates as "crown of death," relating to the result of cutting this artery without realizing the seriousness of the error. The other arteries listed would be less likely to be injured because the surgeon would assume they are present and will thus take great care in making sure not to staple them.

GAS 495-500; N 378; McM 272

71 E. The afferents of the testis and most of the ductus accompany sympathetics to enter the trunk at T10 to L2, with cell bodies in the dorsal root ganglia of those spinal nerves. (Which is why a forceful kick to the testes seems to hurt so severely in the periumbilical region of the abdomen.) The more proximal portion of the ductus has sensory fibers in the pelvic splanchnics. The ilioinguinal nerve is somatic and innervates the upper and medial thigh as well as the anterior scrotum and skin at the root of the penis, not the ductus deferens. The iliohypogastric nerve is an anterior abdominal wall nerve that innervates transverse and oblique abdominal muscles, supplies skin above the pubis, and has cutaneous supply to the lateral buttocks. The genital branch of the genitofemoral nerve supplies the cremaster muscle and the scrotum.

GAS 492-494, 515; N 394; McM 265

72 A. The ovarian arteries arise from the abdominal aorta, descend retroperitoneally along the posterior abdominal wall, and cross just anterior to the external iliac vessels. The ovarian arteries are the most likely source of blood from a hematoma following a tubal ligation. The ascending and descending uterine arteries and superior and inferior vesical arteries branch from the internal iliac arteries and are not likely to be the source of blood in this situation.

GAS 495-500; N 378; McM 272

73 C. When an ovariectomy (also called oophorectomy) is performed, the ovarian vessels must be ligated. The ovarian vessels lie anterior to the ureter just proximal to the bifurcation of the aorta. The ureter is the structure that is at the most risk when ligating the ovarian vessels. The vaginal artery is a branch of the uterine artery. The uterine artery does anastomose with the ovarian vessels via the ascending uterine artery; however, it lies too far distally to be at risk during ligation of the ovarian vessels. The internal pudendal artery and pudendal nerve mostly lie in the perineum and are not at risk.

GAS 495-500; N 378; McM 272

74 C. The conjugate diameter of the pelvis (anteroposterior) is not altered by relaxation of the pelvic joints. The transverse diameter is the longest distance extending from the middle of one pelvic brim to the other. The interspinous distance is the distance between the ischial spines and changes dramatically during pregnancy due to relaxation of the joints. The diagonal conjugate and oblique diameters are slightly increased during pregnancy due to the effects of the hormone relaxin.

GAS 446-453; N 332; McM 277

75 D. The obturator nerve runs a course along the lateral pelvic wall and innervates the adductors of the thigh and the skin on the medial aspect of the distal thigh. Damage to the obturator nerve is the most likely cause for the sensory and motor deficit experienced by the patient. The genitofemoral nerve is motor to the cremaster muscle and sensory to the skin over the femoral triangle. The ilioinguinal nerve innervates the skin over the labium majus and upper, inner thigh. The iliohypogastric nerve supplies skin over the anterolateral gluteal region and a strip to the area above the pubis. The lumbosacral trunk contains motor and sensory fibers from L4 and L5 and is the lumbar contribution to the lumbosacral plexus.

GAS 486-494, 515; N 388; McM 272

76 A. The neural cell bodies responsible for erection are located in the sacral parasympathetic nucleus (intermediomedial cell column). The parasympathetic nervous system is responsible for producing an erection. The sacral sympathetic trunk ganglia would not be responsible for the action of erection but rather the action of ejaculation. (Mnemonic: "Point and Shoot": parasympathetics for erection, sympathetics for ejaculation.) The inferior mesenteric ganglion would not contain parasympathetic neural cell bodies responsible for erection because they go to the hindgut. The superior hypogastric plexus contains few if any

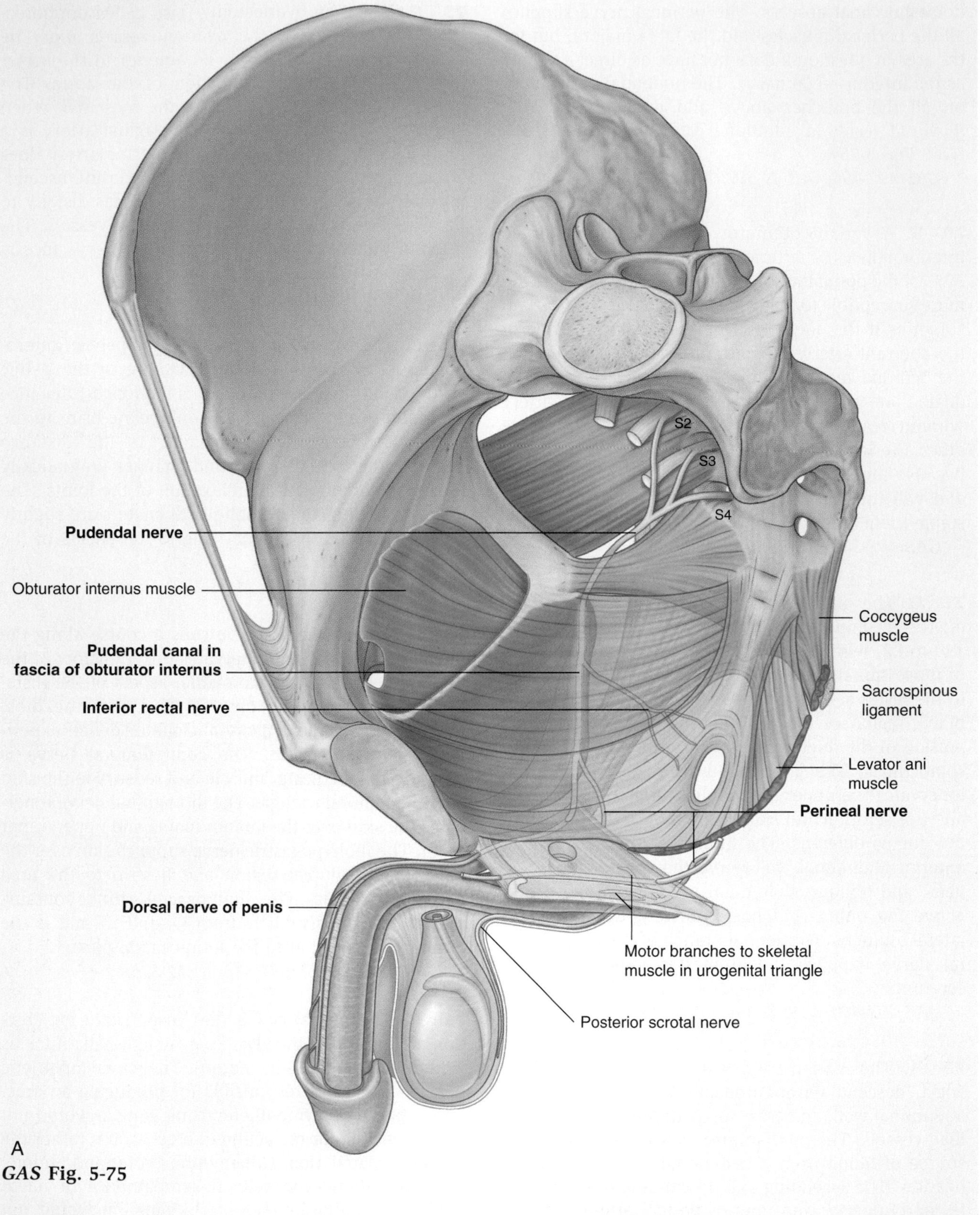
S2
S3
S4
Pudendal nerve
Obturator internus muscle
Coccygeus muscle
Pudendal canal in fascia of obturator internus
Sacrospinous ligament
Inferior rectal nerve
Levator ani muscle
Perineal nerve
Dorsal nerve of penis
Motor branches to skeletal muscle in urogenital triangle
Posterior scrotal nerve

A
GAS **Fig. 5-75**

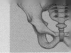

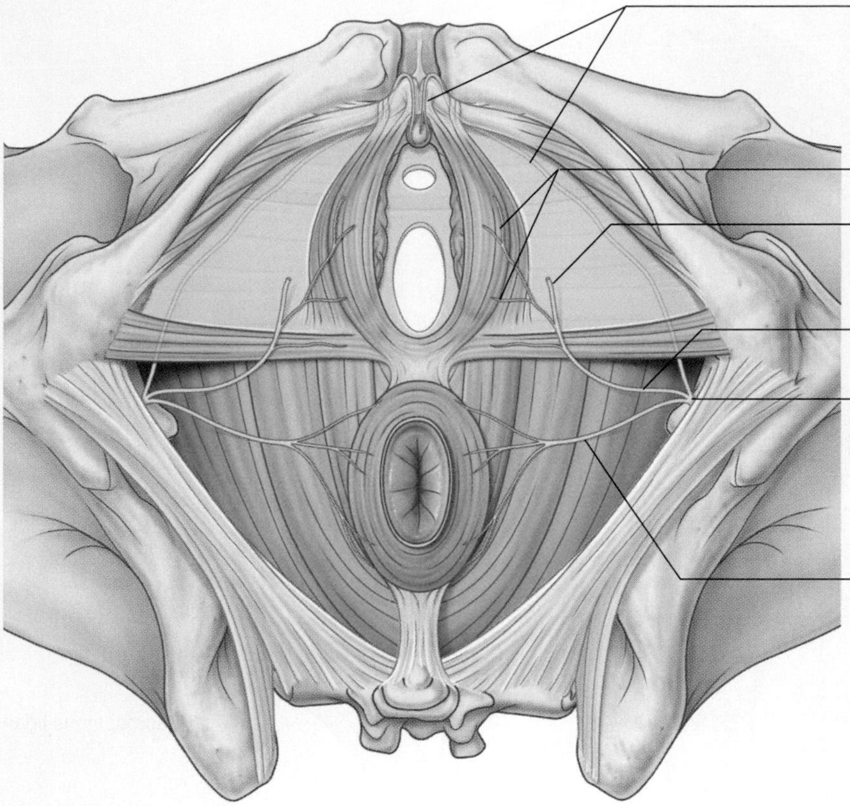

GAS **Fig. 5-75, cont'd**

parasympathetic fibers and is not the primary location for the parasympathetic neural cell bodies. The intermediolateral column of L1 and L2 contains nerve cell bodies of preganglionic sympathetic neurons and therefore would not contribute to producing an erection.

GAS 486-494, 515; N 395; McM 265

77 B. The interspinous distance is the distance between the ischial spines. The interspinous distance is usually the shortest distance, therefore being the minimum dimension along the birth canal. The true conjugate diameter is the anteroposterior distance and does not change. The transverse diameter, oblique diameter, and diagonal conjugate diameter can change slightly during pregnancy, but the interspinous distance changes the most during birth; it is also more easily measured.

GAS 446-453; N 332; McM 276

78 D. Lymph vessels from the testes follow the path of the testicular blood supply (abdominal aorta), and therefore lymph from the testicles drains into the lumbar nodes. The superficial inguinal lymph nodes drain lymph from the lower limb. The deep inguinal nodes drain lymph from the superficial inguinal nodes, the glans of the penis, and spongy urethra. The external iliac nodes drain lymph from anterosuperior pelvic structures and receive lymph from the deep inguinal nodes. Internal iliac nodes drain lymph from inferior pelvic structures and receive lymph from the sacral nodes.

GAS 501, 519; N 386; McM 358

79 C. Uterine artery embolization is performed to starve uterine fibroids of their blood supply resulting in a decrease in size of these benign tumors. Following the procedure, the uterus receives collateral blood supply from the ovarian artery (a direct branch of the abdominal aorta). The external iliac, inferior mesenteric, internal pudendal, and superior mesenteric arteries do not provide adequate collateral blood supply to the uterus.

GAS 459; N 382; McM 270, 275

80 E. The perineal body is a condensed mass of connective tissue to which the muscles of the pelvic floor and the muscles of the perineum attach. In many cases during childbirth, if the fetus' head is arrested, there is a high likelihood of perineal tears. In this situation an episiotomy is performed. This is usually done in an incision 45 degrees away from the midline in

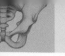

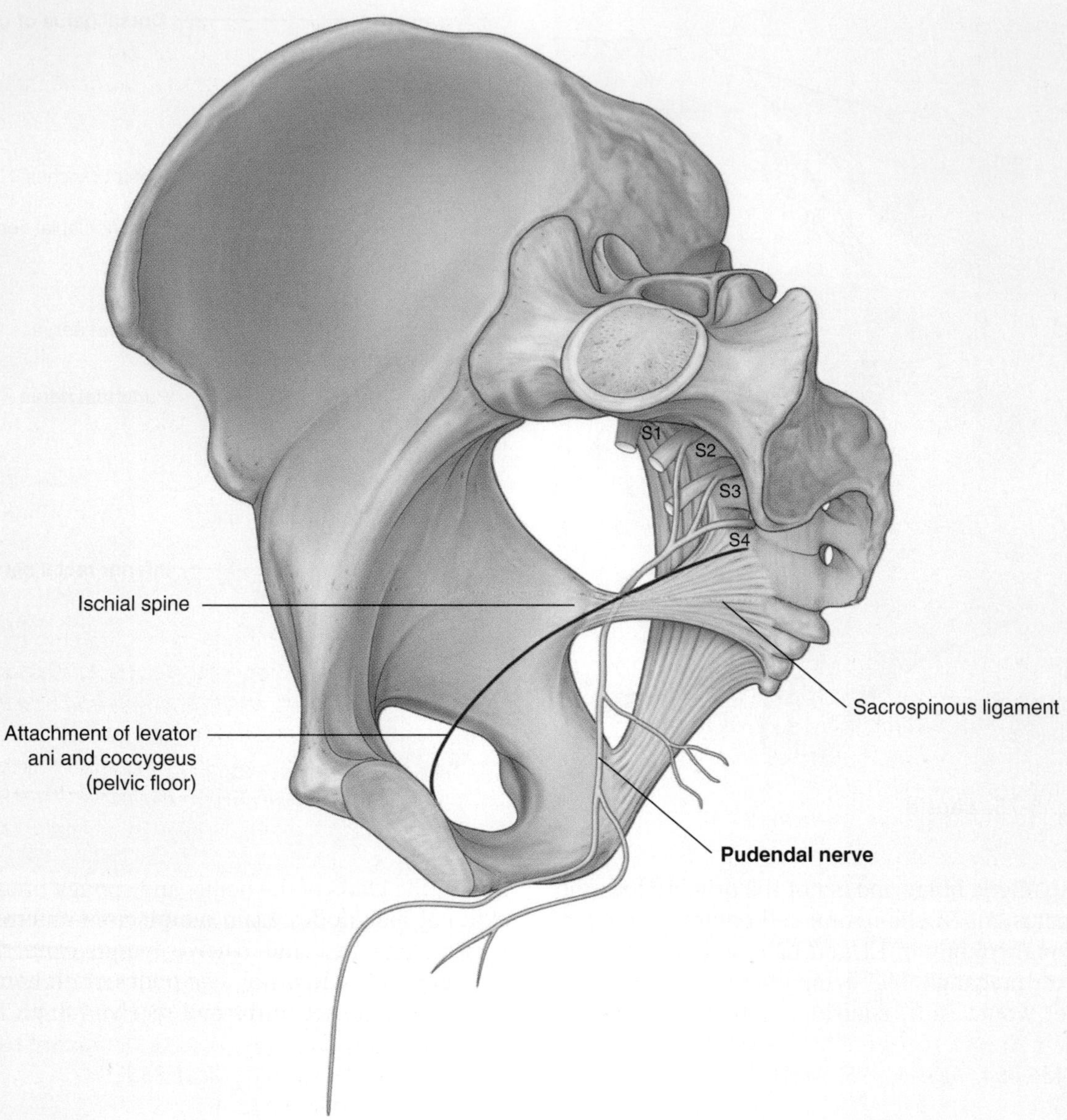

GAS **Fig. 5-15**

order to avoid damaging the perineal body. Damage to this tissue destabilizes the muscles that attach to it and can lead to urinary and fecal incontinence as well as uterine, bladder, and rectal prolapse.

GAS 459; N 356; McM 276

81 **E.** The pudendal nerve is a somatic nerve that innervates the perineum with exception of the anterior part of the labia majora (innervated by the ilio-inguinal and genitofemoral nerves). The pudendal nerve forms from S2 to S4 ventral rami. It leaves the pelvis via the greater sciatic foramen and enters into the perineum via the lesser sciatic foramen by coursing around the sacrospinous ligament where it attaches to the ischial spine. This pudendal nerve block will anesthetize the area of distribution of the pudendal nerve. It will not anesthetize the uterus or cervix as these are visceral organs (*GAS* Fig. 5-15).

GAS 486-494; N 391; McM 271, 276

82 **A.** The prostate is a walnut shaped accessory organ of the reproductive system in men that lies immediately below the bladder and surrounds the exiting urethra. Anatomically, the prostate has four lobes: two lateral lobes, a posterior lobe, and a median lobe that directly surrounds the urethra. A tumor of the posterior lobe does not necessarily obstruct the urethra but it is frequently cancerous. Benign prostatic hyperplasia usually affects the median and lateral lobes. Micturition (urination) will be obstructed and patients present with a variety of symptoms including difficulty in initiating the urinary stream, a slow stream of urine, urinary frequency, and urinary urgency.

GAS 473; N 362; McM 266, 268

83 D. The patient has a tear in the spongy (penile) urethra. This commonly occurs when force is applied to the bulb of the penis. If there is an accompanying tear of the erectile bodies and the Buck's fascia that surrounds it, urine can spill into the superficial perineal pouch. This area is bound by Colles' fascia inferiorly, the perineal body posteriorly, and the perineal membrane superiorly. The attachment of Colles' fascia to the perineal body prevents the urine from spreading posteriorly to the anorectal triangle. The attachment of Colles' fascia to the ischiopubic ramus prevents urine from entering into the thigh.

GAS 466-468; N 374; McM 266, 268

84 C. The rough bony projection at the junction of the inferior end of the body of the ischium and its ramus is the large ischial tuberosity. Much of the upper body's weight rests on these tuberosities when sitting, and it provides the proximal, tendinous attachment of posterior thigh muscles (hamstring muscles and a portion of the adductor magnus). The small pointed posteromedial projection near the junction of the ramus and body is the ischial spine. The inferior pubic ramus is thin and flat and does not bear weight. The pubic tubercle is a prominent forward projecting tubercle on the upper border of the medial portion of the superior ramus of the pubis. The iliac crest extends posteriorly, terminating at the posterior superior iliac spine.

GAS 441-445; N 334; McM 286, 292

85 C. The pelvic inlet or pelvic brim (sagittal inlet) is bounded posteriorly by the sacral promontory, laterally by the iliopectineal lines, and anteriorly by the symphysis pubis. The pelvic outlet (sagittal outlet) is bounded posteriorly by the coccyx, laterally by the ischial tuberosities, and anteriorly by the pubic arc. Bispinous (interspinous) outlet is the distance between the ischial spines. Maximum transverse diameter of inlet extends across the greatest width of the superior aperture, from the middle of the brim on one side to the same point on the opposite side.

GAS 448-453; N 332; McM 92, 223

86 E. Suprapubic (Pfannenstiel) incisions are made 5 cm superior to the pubis symphysis. They are used when access to the pelvic organs is needed. When performing this incision, care must be taken not the perforate the bladder, as the fascia thins around the bladder area. A transverse incision just below the umbilicus is made just inferior and laterally to the umbilicus. This is a commonly used procedure, as it causes least damage to the nerve supply to the abdominal muscles, and heals well. McBurney's incision is performed at McBurney's point (1/3 of the distance between the ASIS and the umbilicus). It is mostly used in appendectomies. Subcostal incisions begin inferior to the xiphoid process, and extend inferior parallel to the costal margin. They are mainly used on the right side to operate on the gallbladder and the liver. Median incisions are made through the linea alba. They can be extended the whole length of the abdomen, by curving around the umbilicus. The linea alba is poorly vascularized, so blood loss is minimal, and major nerves are avoided. However, because it is poorly vascularized it heals slowly.

GAS 466; N 340; McM 266

87 D. The fundiform ligament of the penis is a thickening of the superficial fascia, and is superficial to the suspensory ligament that descends in the midline from the linea alba anterior to the pubic symphysis. The ligament splits to surround the penis and then unites and blends inferiorly with the dartos fascia forming the scrotal septum.

GAS 508; N 344; McM 270

88 A. The ilioinguinal nerve is a branch of the first lumbar nerve (L1). Its fibers are distributed to the skin of the upper and medial part of the thigh, and the skin over the root of the penis and upper part of the scrotum in men and the skin covering the mons pubis and labium majus in women. The iliohypogastric nerve is the superior branch of the ventral ramus of spinal nerve L1, which perforates the transversus abdominis, and divides into lateral and anterior cutaneous branches. The anterior cutaneous branch pierces the internal oblique, becomes cutaneous by perforating the aponeurosis of the external oblique about 2.5 cm above the superficial inguinal ring, and is distributed to the skin of the suprapubic region. The lateral femoral nerve innervates the skin on the lateral upper part of the thigh. The skin of the penis (or clitoris) is mainly supplied by the dorsal nerve (S2), a branch of the pudendal nerve.

GAS 486-494; N 387; McM 218, 220

89 D. Failure of canalization of the vaginal plate results in atresia (blockage) of the vagina. A transverse vaginal septum occurs in approximately 1 in 80,000 females. Usually, the septum is located at the junction of the middle and superior thirds of the vagina. Failure of the inferior end of the vaginal plate to perforate results in an imperforate hymen. Variations in the appearance of the hymen are common. The vaginal orifice varies in diameter from very small to large, and there may be more than one orifice. The most common cause of indirect inguinal hernia is patent processus vaginalis. Most anorectal anomalies result from abnormal development of the urorectal septum, resulting in incomplete separation of the cloaca into urogenital and anorectal parts. Growth of one paramesonephric duct is retarded and does not fuse with the other one, a bicornuate uterus with a rudimentary horn (cornu) will develop.

GAS 480; N 350; McM 272, 273

90 B. The ovaries are supplied by ovarian vessels that originate from the abdominal aorta. Ovarian vessels cross the pelvic brim and descend in the suspensory ligament of ovary to supply the ovaries, fimbrial end of the uterine (fallopian) tube, and portions of the abdominal/pelvic ureter. The ovarian ligament also contains nerves and lymphatics. The remaining ligaments are devoid of major vessels.

GAS 476; N 352; McM 274

91 A. The ureter, which is located retroperitoneally, originates from the renal pelvis and runs inferiorly crossing the pelvic brim close to the bifurcation of the common iliac artery. At this important landmark the ureter is medial to the gonadal vessels as it enters into the pelvis. It is lateral to the internal iliac artery as it descends past the pelvic brim. Although not immediately adjacent, the ureter is medial in relation to the external iliac artery but not close to the inferior vena cava or uterine artery at this location.

GAS 379, 462; N 378; McM 270, 275

92 C. Most anorectal abnormalities including imperforate anus occur from abnormal development of the urorectal septum leading to abnormal or incomplete cloacal separation. This results in abnormal urogenital and anorectal compartments and as such imperforate anus is usually associated with urinary tract defects. VATER syndrome may include tracheoesophageal, vertebral, renal, limb, and cardiac defects but this association is not as common as that between urogenital and anorectal defects. There is no association with ileal atresia.

GAS 460-461; N 372; McM 279

93 A. Pudendal or saddle block is less common than an epidural anesthesia but still used clinically to obtain perineal anesthesia during the final stages of labor or preceding an episiotomy. It is done by locating the pudendal nerve in or as it exits the pudendal canal and anesthetizing either transcutaneously or transvaginally by locating the ischial spine or tuberosity, respectively. The source for the pudendal nerve is S2 to S4 ventral rami.

GAS 486-494; N 391; McM 276, 277

94 E. The superior gluteal artery, which is the largest branch of the posterior division of internal iliac artery, provides spinal branches as it passes between the lumbosacral trunk and ventral ramus of S1 and exits the pelvis via the greater sciatic foramen superior to the piriformis and supplying piriformis, the gluteal muscles, and tensor fasciae latae. Inferior gluteal artery, an anterior division of the internal iliac, runs inferior to the first sacral nerve and it exits the pelvis through the infrapiriform part of the greater sciatic foramen. None of the remaining vessels traverses the greater sciatic foramen.

GAS 495; N 380; McM 268, 276

95 A. Puborectalis, a part of the levator ani group, is crucial to maintaining the anorectal angle and thereby maintaining fecal continence. Relaxation or injury to this muscle decreases the angle between the ampulla of rectum and the upper portion of the anal canal thus aiding defecation or incontinence respectively. None of the remaining muscles functions in maintaining the anorectal angle.

GAS 454-457; N 339; McM 268

96 A. The pudendal nerve passes between the sacrospinous and sacrotuberous ligaments. When performing this block with an internal approach, the ischial spine is used as a landmark as it is easily palpated transvaginally. The ischial tuberosity is used when the procedure is performed externally as it can be easily palpated in the ischioanal fossa. The posterior inferior and the posterior superior iliac spines are posterior; they cannot be palpated transvaginally and are not associated with the pudendal nerve. The coccyx is the most inferior portion of the vertebral column, cannot be palpated transvaginally, and is not near the pudendal nerve.

GAS 486-494; N 389; McM 276, 277

97 D. Nerve supply to the perineum including the anal canal is via the pudendal nerve. The sacral splanchnic nerves carry postganglionic sympathetic nerve fibers to the pelvic organs. The pelvic splanchnic nerves carry preganglionic parasympathetic nerves to the pelvic organs. The superior hypogastric plexus is an autonomic plexus carrying sympathetic and parasympathetic innervation to the lower abdominal

region. The ilioinguinal nerve supplies the skin of the upper medial thigh and anterior perineal area.
GAS 492-494, 515; N 394; McM 276, 277

98 A. The puborectalis muscle is a sling that acts as an internal sphincter around the rectum. The iliococcygeus runs from the obturator fascia to the midline and forms a raphe to which the anal aperture is anchored. The obturator externus and piriformis muscles are located on the lateral walls of the pelvis. The coccygeus muscle runs between the ischial spine and the coccyx and sacrum.
GAS 454-457; N 339; McM 268

99 C. In the perineum lymph drains according to arteries that supply the area, and so the glans penis drains to the deep inguinal nodes. Superficial skin of the penis and scrotum would drain to the superficial inguinal nodes. External iliac nodes receive lymph from the deep inguinal, and the internal iliac from the pelvic organs. The lumbar/lateral aortic nodes receive lymph from the abdominal organs, and the axillary drains the upper limb and external thorax.
GAS 454-457; N 339; McM 268

100 A. Epispadias is the correct option. Epispadias describes the abnormal opening of the urethra on the dorsal side of the penis. During the development of the genital tubercle defective or inadequate interaction between the ectoderm and mesoderm leads to the genital tubercle developing more dorsally. As a consequence, when the more dorsally located urogenital membrane ruptures, the urogenital sinus will open on the dorsal aspect of the penis. Exstrophy of the urinary bladder is a condition in which there is a defect in the anterior abdominal wall with the bladder and part of the urethra are protruding.
GAS 466-468, 512; N 359; McM 365

101 E. Urachal cysts are embryological remnants of the epithelium of the urachus occurring between the umbilicus and bladder. It presents as an extraperitoneal mass in the umbilical region. Urachal cysts are generally asymptomatic; however, if infected, they present with abdominal pain and fever. If fistulation occurs, it may drain through the umbilicus or rupture, leading to peritonitis. Hydroceles are the accumulation of fluids between the two layers of the tunica vaginalis surrounding the testicles. Meckel's cyst and Meckel's diverticulum are formed on the distal ileum and do not have the anatomical relations described in the CT findings. Omphaloceles result from defective development of the muscles of the anterior abdominal wall where abdominal viscera herniate into the umbilical cord where they are outside of the abdomen.
GAS 463; N 341; McM 223, 272

102 B. The sacral components of the craniosacral outflow (parasympathetics) are the pelvic splanchnic nerves. These nerves take their origin from the ventral rami of the S2 to S4 spinal segments and enter the sacral plexus. They carry both preganglionic parasympathetic fibers as well as visceral afferent fibers. The pelvic splanchnics provide innervation to pelvic viscera and genitals regulating the voiding of the bladder, controlling the internal urethral sphincter, rectal motility, as well as sexual functions such as erection. The pelvic splanchnic should not be confused with the lumbar splanchnics or sacral splanchnics which carry preganglionic sympathetics and general visceral afferents.
GAS 492-494, 515; N 394; McM 261, 269

103 A. The rectouterine pouch (or pouch of Douglas) is the extension of the peritoneal cavity situated between the rectum and the posterior uterine wall of the uterus in women. It is the most dependent or lowest part of the abdominopelvic cavity when in the supine position making it a typical site of collection of fluids. Due to its intimacy with the posterior wall of the uterus it can be examined transvaginally or transrectally by digital palpation. Fluids collected there may also be drained through the vagina or rectum without entering the abdominopelvic cavity transabdominally. The pararectal fossa is a feature found only in men. The paravesical space is made up of paired subdivisions of the extraperitoneal space found lateral to the prevesical space. The uterovesical pouch is formed by the peritoneum over the uterus and bladder, continued over the intestinal surface and fundus of the uterus onto its vesical surface. Its more anterior location dictates that when the body is in a supine position, fluid that accumulates there will immediately travel down to deeper parts of the peritoneal cavity (the rectouterine pouch). The superficial perineal pouch can also be ruled out as an option because it is located in the perineum where it is completely enclosed by the deep perineal fascia and the perineal membranes that make up its borders (*GAS* Fig. 5-58).
GAS 483; N 340; McM 272

104 E. The inferior border of the superficial perineal pouch is the deep fascia (Gallaudet's fascia or Buck's fascia). Rupture of the penile urethra leads to extravasation and collection of urine in the superficial perineal pouch. The retrovesical pouch is a peritoneal

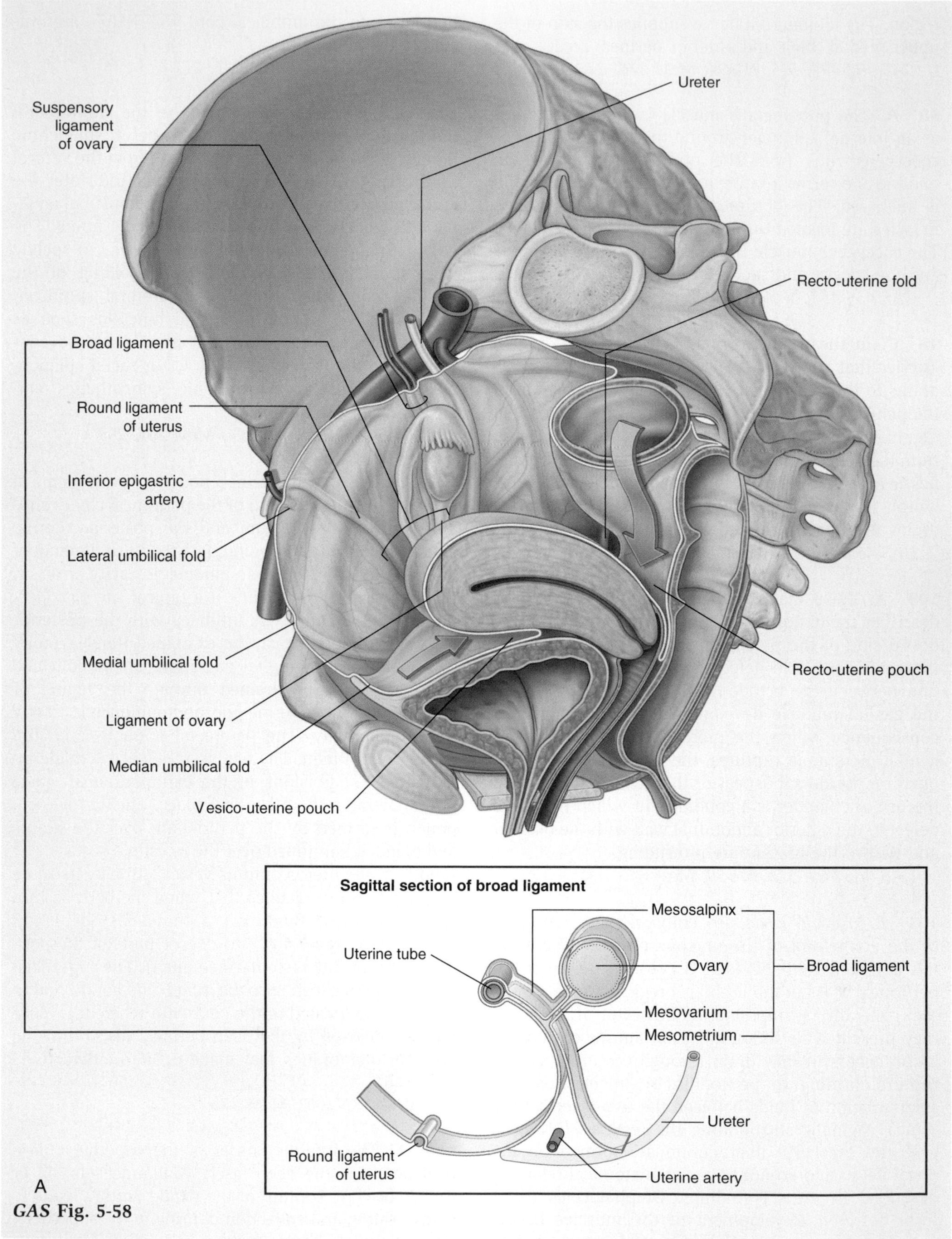
Suspensory ligament of ovary
Ureter
Recto-uterine fold
Broad ligament
Round ligament of uterus
Inferior epigastric artery
Lateral umbilical fold
Medial umbilical fold
Recto-uterine pouch
Ligament of ovary
Median umbilical fold
Vesico-uterine pouch
Sagittal section of broad ligament
Mesosalpinx
Uterine tube
Ovary
Broad ligament
Mesovarium
Mesometrium
Ureter
Round ligament of uterus
Uterine artery
A

GAS Fig. 5-58

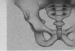

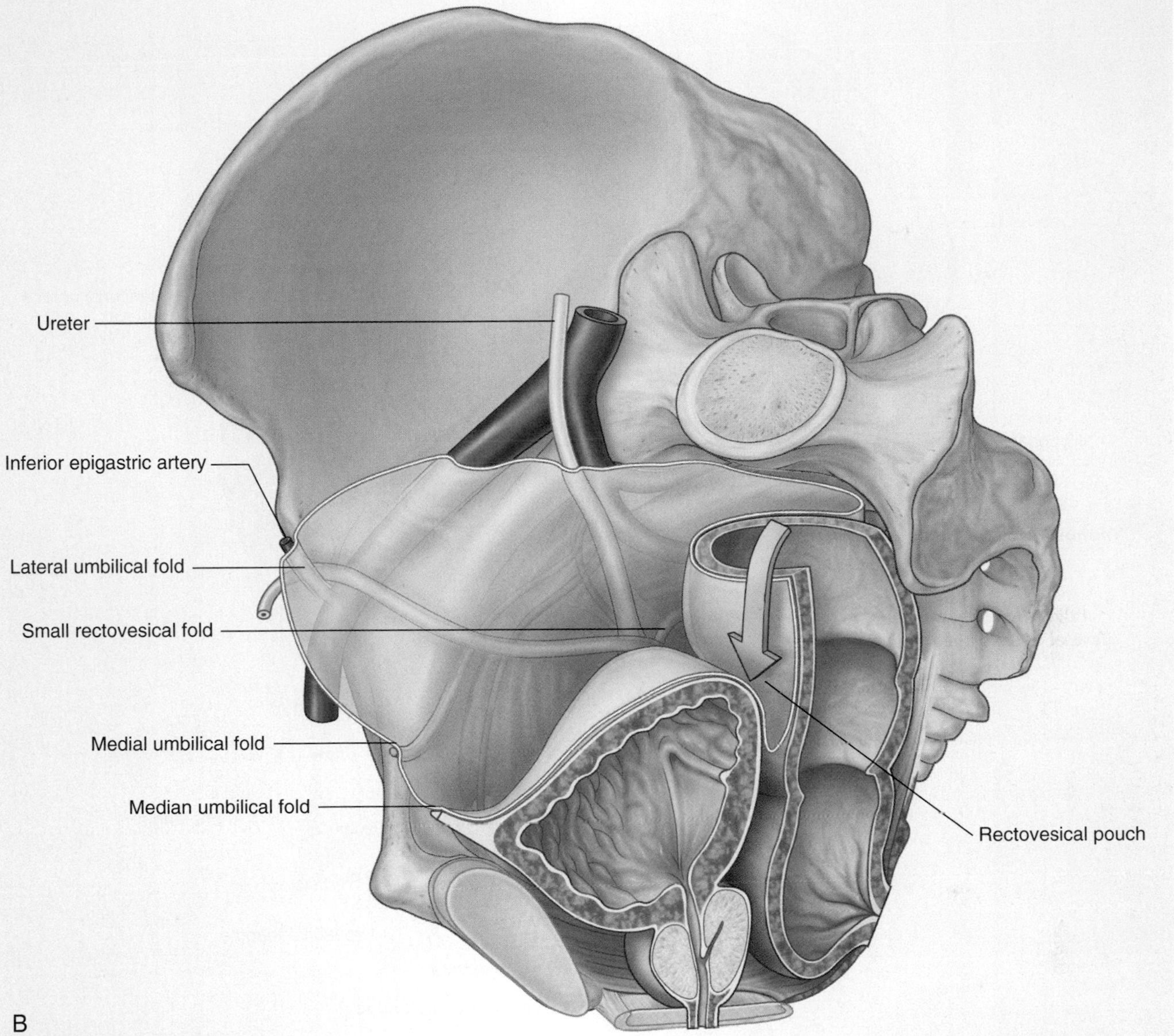

GAS **Fig. 5-58, cont'd**

cavity extension found between the posterior wall of the uterus and the bladder. The deep perineal pouch is the region between the perineal membrane and pelvic diaphragm. The deep perineal pouch is bordered inferiorly by the perineal membrane. It is bordered superiorly by the superior fascia of the urogenital diaphragm. It shares no communication with the deep fascia. The retropubic space, also known as the cave or space of Retzius, is an extraperitoneal space between the pubic symphysis and urinary bladder that bears no relation to the penile urethra.

GAS 506; N 374; McM 365

105 C. The pudendal nerve branches innervate the external urethral sphincter. The pudendal nerve takes its origin from the S2 to S4 spinal segments via the sacral plexus. Its motor branches supply the external urethral sphincter, external anal sphincter, and skeletal muscle of the deep and superficial pouches. Its cutaneous branches supply the skin of the anal triangle and external genitalia. Pelvic and sacral splanchnics carry autonomic fibers, as the external urethral sphincter is a somatic structure. The superior gluteal nerve arises from the dorsal divisions of the fourth and fifth lumbar and the first sacral nerves. Its fibers go on to innervate the gluteus medius, the gluteus minimus, and the tensor fasciae latae, which are unrelated to urinary incontinence. Likewise the inferior gluteal nerve innervates the gluteus maximus muscle.

GAS 486-494; N 389; McM 277

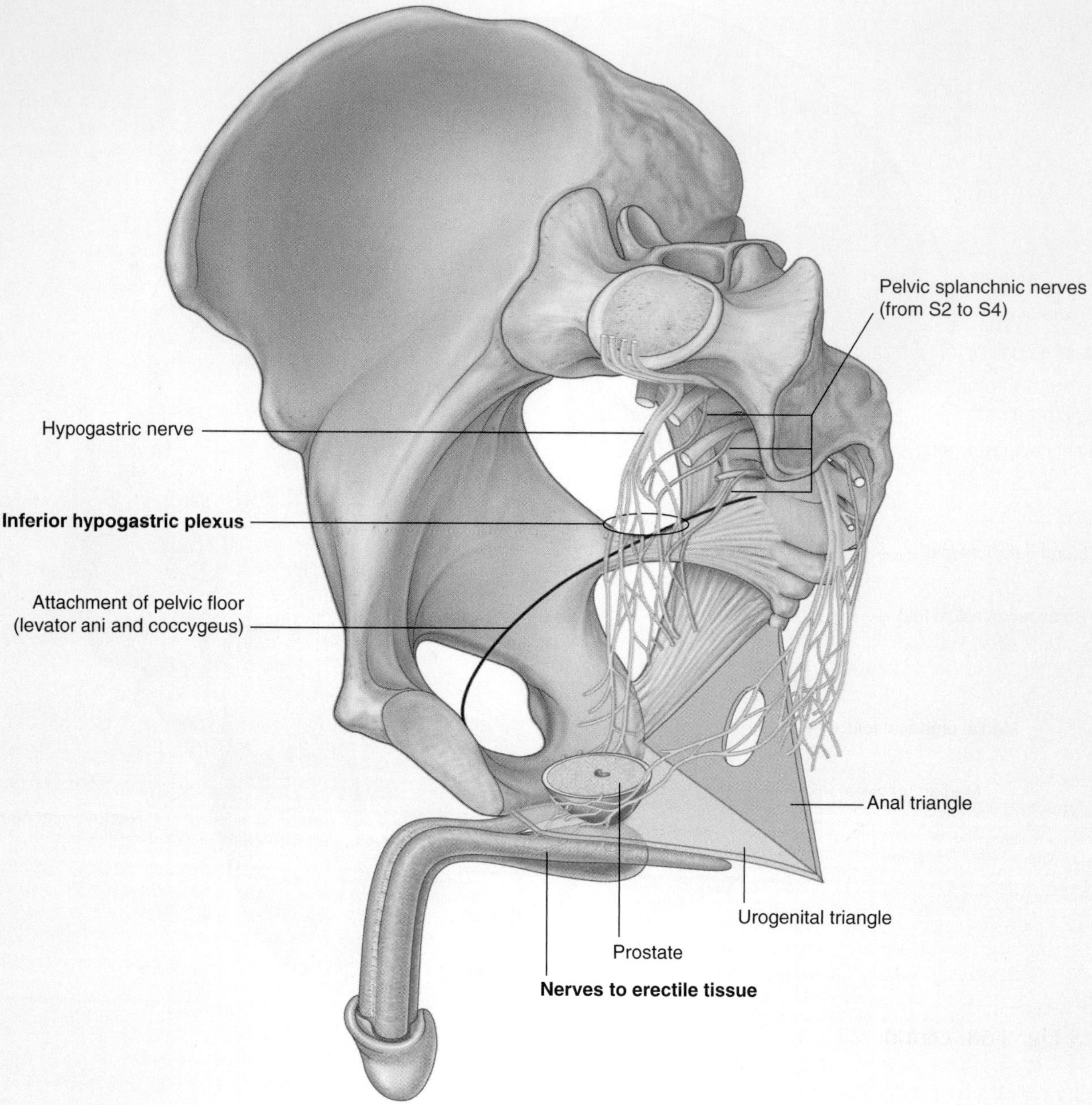

GAS Fig. 5-16

106 A. Cavernous nerves are postganglionic parasympathetic fibers that mediate penile erection. Its preganglionic fibers derive from the pelvic splanchnic nerve (S2 to S4). The glans penis receives its supply from the pudendal nerve. The external urethral sphincter is innervated by a voluntary, somatic nerve called the pudendal nerve. The internal urethral sphincter receives parasympathetic fibers also from the inferior hypogastric plexus, which are very different from the cavernous nerves. The seminal vesicles are innervated by the sympathetic nervous system via the inferior hypogastric plexus (*GAS* Fig. 5-16).

GAS 492-494, 515; N 394; McM 278, 279

107 E. The scrotal skin is drained by superficial lymphatics that will first empty into the horizontal group of superficial inguinal nodes. The external iliac nodes are deep lymph nodes receiving lymphatics from deep abdominal wall structures below the umbilicus, the pelvic viscera as well as from inguinal

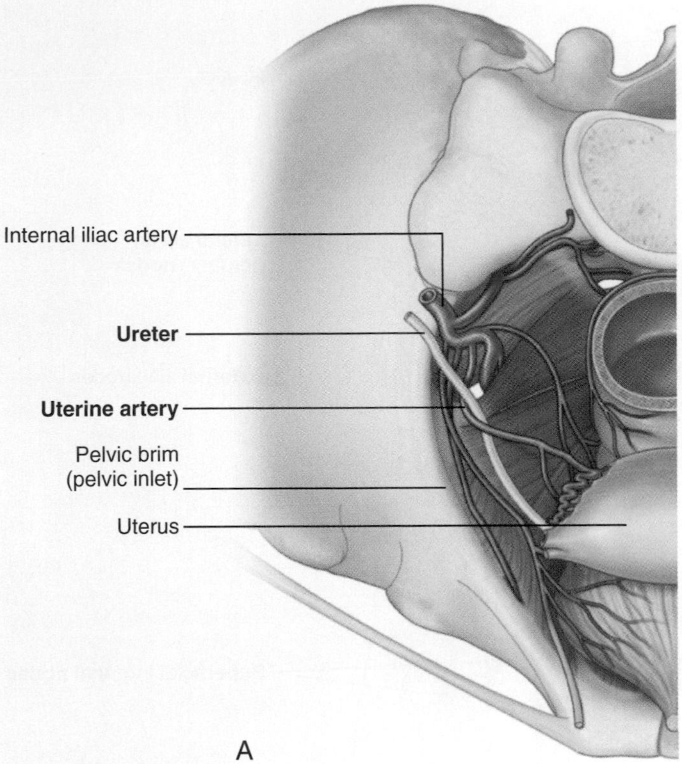

GAS Fig. 5-12A

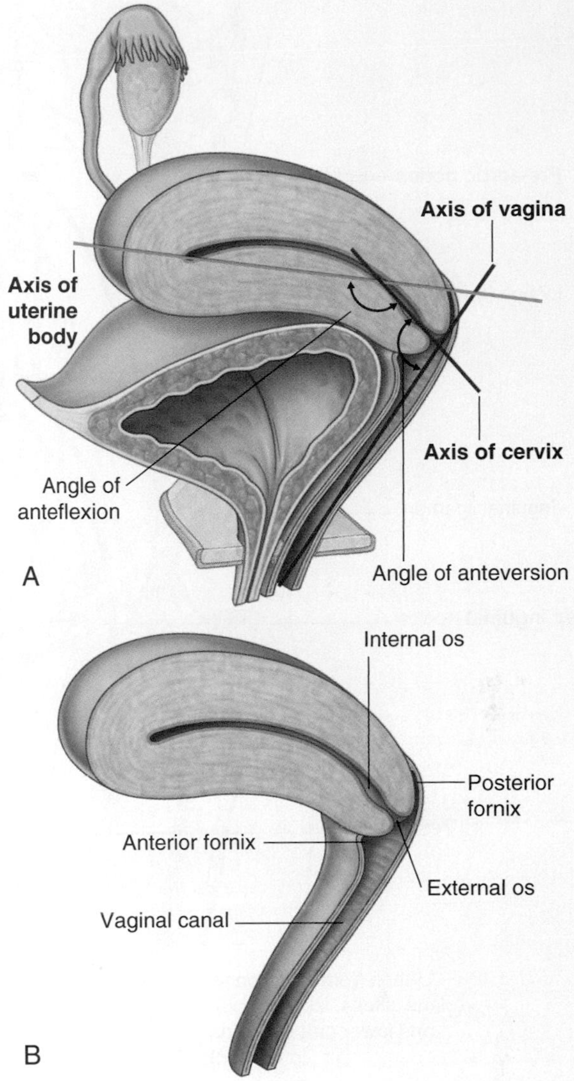

GAS Fig. 5-54

lymph nodes. The internal iliac nodes are also deep nodes that drain pelvic viscera, deeper parts of the perineum, and parts of the urethra. The sacral nodes drain the rectum and posterior pelvic wall.

GAS 501, 519; N 386; McM 368

108 E. During hysterectomy, hemostasis may be ensured by proper ligation of the arteries that supply the uterus. The uterine artery, a branch of the internal iliac artery, is anterior to the ureter in the broad ligament of the uterus. During surgeries, the ureter may be ligated mistakenly in the place of the uterine artery. The ovarian ligament attaches the ovary to the lateral and superior part of the uterus. It is a fibrous cord that is contained in the broad ligament of the uterus and has no direct relationship with the ureters. The mesosalpinx is the part of the broad ligament that stretches from the ovary to the uterine tube above. The round ligament of the uterus is an embryologic remnant of the gubernaculum ovary and has no direct relationship with the ureters (*GAS* Fig. 5-12A).

GAS 478; N 378; McM 274, 275

109 A. The lymph from the inferior part of the anal canal drains to the superficial inguinal nodes. The lymph from the distal rectum drains to the sacral nodes. The lymph from the sigmoid colon drains to the inferior mesenteric nodes and then to the internal iliac nodes. The lymph from the proximal rectum drains to the sacral nodes, and the lymph from the anal canal above the pectinate line drains to the internal iliac nodes.

GAS 501, 519; N 384; McM 368

110 C. Embryologically, the ovaries develop from the posterolateral abdominal wall and descend to their adult location in the pelvis. In doing this, they retain their embryological nerve supply and lymphatic drainage. Therefore, lymphatic drainage from the ovaries drains to the lumbar/lateral aortic nodes. Superficial inguinal nodes receive lymphatics from the lower limb, perineum, anal canal below the pectinate line, and the abdominal wall below the umbilicus. The external iliac nodes drain lymph from deep

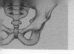

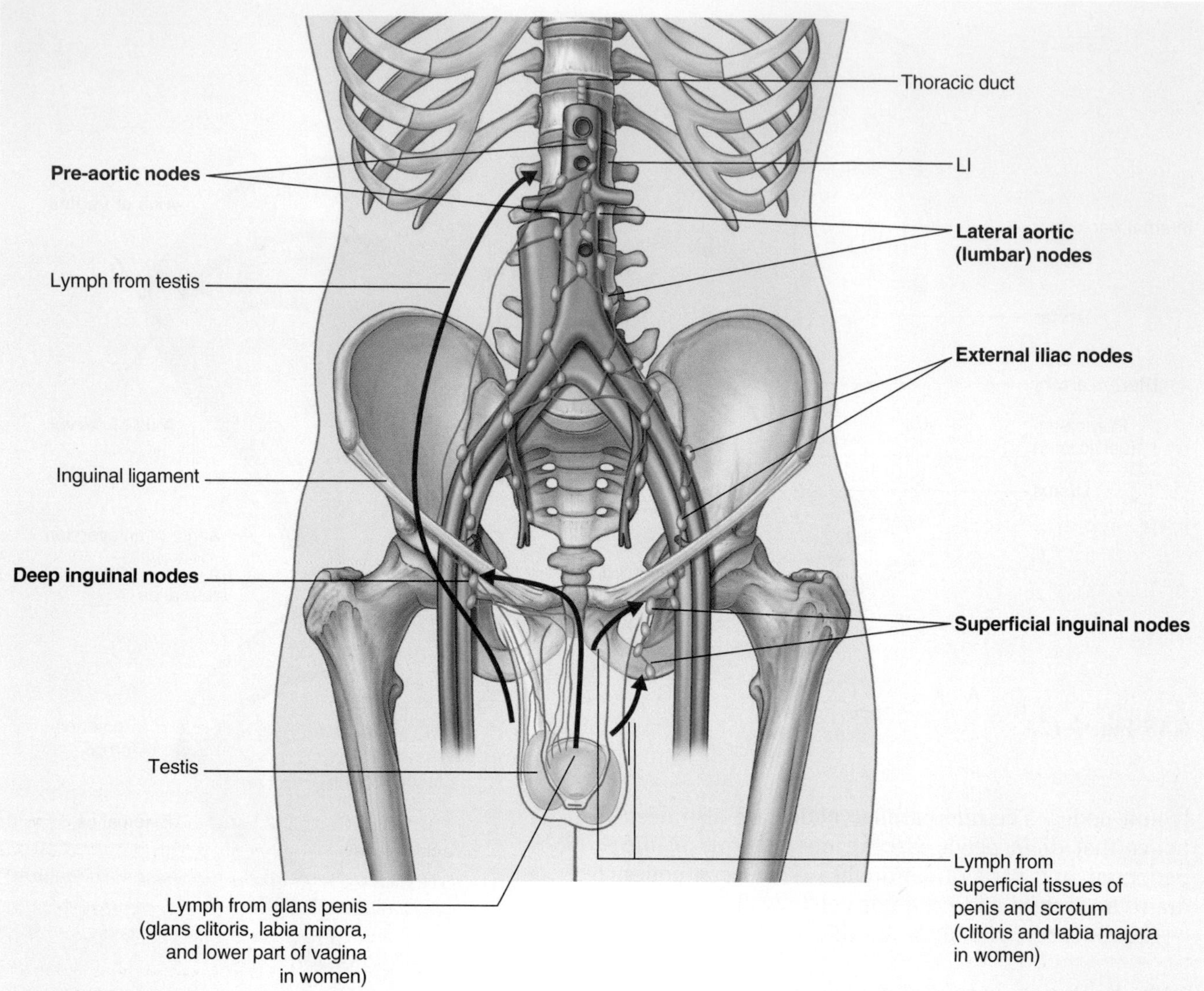

***GAS* Fig. 5-78**

abdominal wall structures below the umbilicus, some pelvic viscera. Deep inguinal nodes are deep lymph nodes that receive lymph from the popliteal nodes, the clitoris in women and the glans penis in men. The internal iliac nodes receive lymph from the pelvic viscera, deep part of the perineum, and the urethra.

GAS 501, 5019; N 367; McM 367

111 C. The normal position of the uterus in most women is anteflexion and anteversion. Anteflexion is the forward bending of the long axis of the uterus in relation to the cervix at the level of the internal os. Anteversion is the forward bending of the long axis of the uterus in relation to the long axis of the vagina (*GAS* Fig. 5-54).

GAS 477-479; N 340; McM 272

112 E. Fig. 4-5 depicts a lymphangiogram showing several lymphatic groups at the pelvic and inguinal region. The lymphatic groups are as follows A=Lumbar, B=Common iliac, C=External iliac, D=Deep iliac, and E=Superficial inguinal. Malignancies involving the lower part of the vagina typically involve the superficial inguinal lymph nodes, so E is the correct answer (*GAS* Fig. 5-78).

GAS 501, 519; N 384; McM 368

5

LOWER LIMB

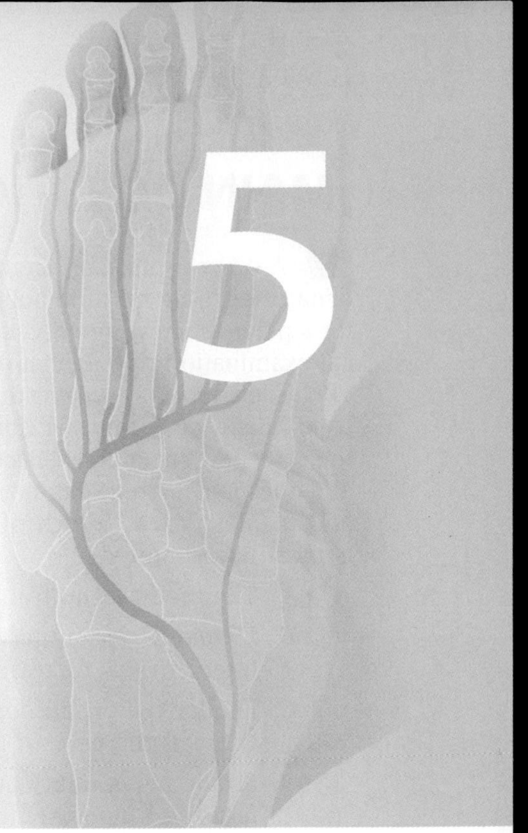

INTRODUCTION

First Order Question

1 The quadriceps femoris muscle group is formed by the rectus femoris, vastus lateralis, vastus medialis, and vastus intermedius. Which of the following nerves innervates this group of muscles?

- ▢ **A.** Sciatic nerve
- ▢ **B.** Femoral nerve
- ▢ **C.** Obturator nerve
- ▢ **D.** Saphenous nerve
- ▢ **E.** Tibial nerve

Explanation

A: Only the femoral nerve innervates the quadriceps femoris. The sciatic nerve, specifically the tibial part, supplies the posterior thigh muscles not the anterior compartment. The obturator nerve supplies the medial compartment and the saphenous nerve does not supply any thigh muscles.

Second Order Question

2 A 24-year-old female motocross racer was involved in a crash that left her right leg pinned under her bike. After the accident, she could no longer extend her right knee. Which of the following nerves was most likely affected?

- ▢ **A.** Sciatic nerve
- ▢ **B.** Femoral nerve
- ▢ **C.** Obturator nerve
- ▢ **D.** Saphenous nerve
- ▢ **E.** Tibial nerve

Explanation

B: Extensors of the knee are the quadriceps femoris muscle, which attaches to the tibia via the patellar ligament. This muscle group is supplied by the femoral nerve. The sciatic nerve supplies the posterior thigh muscles not the anterior compartment. The obturator supplies the medial compartment and the saphenous nerve does not supply motor innervation to any muscles but is a cutaneous branch of the femoral nerve.

Third Order Question

3 A 24-year-old female motocross racer was involved in a crash that left her right leg pinned under her bike. After the accident, she could no longer extend her right knee. The affected nerve gives rise to which of the following cutaneous nerves?

- ▢ **A.** Middle clunial nerve
- ▢ **B.** Lateral femoral cutaneous branch
- ▢ **C.** Superficial fibular (peroneal) nerve
- ▢ **D.** Saphenous nerve
- ▢ **E.** Deep fibular (peroneal)

Explanation

D: The saphenous nerve is a cutaneous branch of the femoral nerve and supplies the skin on the medial leg along the great saphenous vein. Middle clunial is a posterior division of S1 to S3. Lateral femoral cutaneous is from L2 to L3 and the lumbar plexus but is not a femoral nerve branch. Superficial fibular (peroneal) nerve is a branch from the common fibular (peroneal) nerve.

MAIN QUESTIONS

1 A 42-year-old man is admitted to the emergency department after his automobile hit a tree. He is treated for a pelvic fracture and several deep lacerations. Physical examination reveals that dorsiflexion and inversion of the left foot and extension of the big toe are very weak. Sensation from the dorsum of the foot, skin of the sole, and the lateral aspect of the foot has been lost and the patellar reflex is normal. The foot is everted and plantar flexed. Which of the following structures is most likely injured?

- ☐ **A.** The lumbosacral trunk at the linea terminalis
- ☐ **B.** L5 and S1 spinal nerves torn at the intervertebral foramen
- ☐ **C.** Fibular (peroneal) division of the sciatic nerve at the neck of the fibula
- ☐ **D.** Sciatic nerve injury at the greater sciatic foramen ("doorway to the gluteal region")
- ☐ **E.** Tibial nerve in the popliteal fossa

2 A 23-year-old man is admitted to the emergency department with a deep, bleeding stab wound of the pelvis. After the bleeding has been arrested, a magnetic resonance imaging (MRI) examination gives evidence that the right ventral primary ramus of L4 has been transected. Which of the following problems will most likely be seen during physical examination?

- ☐ **A.** Reduction or loss of sensation from the medial aspect of the leg
- ☐ **B.** Loss of the Achilles tendon reflex
- ☐ **C.** Weakness of abduction of the thigh at the hip joint
- ☐ **D.** Inability to evert the foot
- ☐ **E.** Reduction or loss of sensation from the medial aspect of the leg and loss of Achilles tendon reflex

3 A 30-year-old man suffered a superior gluteal nerve injury in a motorcycle crash in which his right lower limb was caught beneath the bike. He is stabilized in the emergency department. Later he is examined and he exhibits a waddling gait and a positive Trendelenburg sign. Which of the following would be the most likely physical finding in this patient?

- ☐ **A.** Difficulty in standing from a sitting position
- ☐ **B.** The left side of the pelvis droops or sags when he attempts to stand with his weight supported just by the right lower limb
- ☐ **C.** The right side of the pelvis droops or sags when he attempts to stand with his weight supported just by the left lower limb
- ☐ **D.** Weakened flexion of the right hip
- ☐ **E.** Difficulty in sitting from a standing position

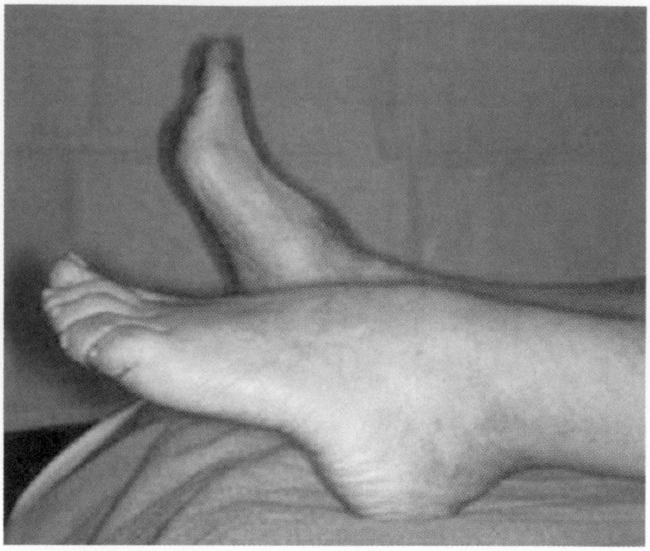

Fig. 5-1

4 A 45-year-old man is treated at the hospital after he fell from his bicycle. Radiologic examination reveals fractures both of the tibia and the fibula. On physical examination the patient has a foot drop, but normal eversion (Fig. 5-1). Which of the following nerves is most likely injured?

- ☐ **A.** Tibial
- ☐ **B.** Common fibular (peroneal)
- ☐ **C.** Superficial fibular (peroneal)
- ☐ **D.** Saphenous
- ☐ **E.** Deep fibular (peroneal)

5 A 49-year-old male construction worker is admitted to the emergency department with a painful lump on the proximal medial aspect of his thigh. Radiologic and physical examinations reveal that the patient has a herniation of abdominal viscera beneath the inguinal ligament into the thigh. Through which of the following openings will a hernia of this type initially pass to extend from the abdomen into the thigh?

- ☐ **A.** Femoral ring
- ☐ **B.** Superficial inguinal ring
- ☐ **C.** Deep inguinal ring
- ☐ **D.** Fossa ovalis
- ☐ **E.** Obturator canal

6 A 37-year-old man is admitted to the hospital after an injury to his foot while playing flag football with friends on a Saturday morning. A series of radiographs demonstrates a fracture involving the talocrural (tibiotalar, ankle) joint. Which movements are the major ones to be affected by this injury?

- ▢ **A.** Plantar flexion and dorsiflexion
- ▢ **B.** Inversion and eversion
- ▢ **C.** Plantar flexion, dorsiflexion, inversion, and eversion
- ▢ **D.** Plantar flexion and inversion
- ▢ **E.** Dorsiflexion and eversion

7 After dividing the overlying superficial tissues and gluteal musculature in a 68-year-old female patient, the orthopedic surgeon carefully identified the underlying structures while performing a total hip arthroplasty. The key landmark in the gluteal region, relied upon in surgical explorations of this area, is provided by which of the following structures?

- ▢ **A.** Gluteus medius
- ▢ **B.** Obturator internus tendon
- ▢ **C.** Sciatic nerve
- ▢ **D.** Piriformis muscle
- ▢ **E.** Spine of the ischium

8 A 16-year-old boy received a superficial cut on the lateral side of his foot while playing football and is admitted to the emergency department where the wound is sutured. Four days later the patient returns to the hospital with high fever and swollen lymph nodes. Which group of nodes will first receive lymph from the infected wound?

- ▢ **A.** Popliteal
- ▢ **B.** Vertical group of superficial inguinal
- ▢ **C.** Deep inguinal
- ▢ **D.** Horizontal group of superficial inguinal
- ▢ **E.** Internal iliac

9 A 45-year-old man presents at the local emergency clinic with the complaint of a painful knee and difficulty in walking. A computed tomography (CT) scan examination reveals a very large cyst in the popliteal fossa compressing the tibial nerve. Which movement will most likely be affected?

- ▢ **A.** Dorsiflexion of the foot
- ▢ **B.** Flexion of the thigh
- ▢ **C.** Extension of the digits
- ▢ **D.** Extension of the leg
- ▢ **E.** Plantar flexion of the foot

10 A 19-year-old football player was hit on the lateral side of his knee just as he put that foot on the ground. Unable to walk without assistance, he is taken to the hospital. An MRI examination reveals a torn medial collateral ligament. Which structure would most likely also be injured due to its attachment to this ligament?

- ▢ **A.** Medial meniscus
- ▢ **B.** Anterior cruciate ligament
- ▢ **C.** Lateral meniscus
- ▢ **D.** Posterior cruciate ligament
- ▢ **E.** Tendon of the semitendinosus

11 A 49-year-old man underwent a coronary bypass graft procedure using the great saphenous vein. Postoperatively, the patient complains of pain and general lack of normal sensation on the medial surface of the leg and foot on the limb from which the graft was harvested. Which nerve was most likely injured during surgery?

- ▢ **A.** Common fibular (peroneal)
- ▢ **B.** Superficial fibular (peroneal)
- ▢ **C.** Lateral sural
- ▢ **D.** Saphenous
- ▢ **E.** Tibial

12 A 22-year-old football player is admitted to the hospital with pain and swelling over the lateral aspect of the ankle. The emergency department doctor diagnoses an inversion sprain. Which ligament was most likely injured?

- ▢ **A.** Plantar calcaneonavicular (spring)
- ▢ **B.** Calcaneofibular
- ▢ **C.** Long plantar
- ▢ **D.** Short plantar
- ▢ **E.** Deltoid

13 A 72-year-old woman is admitted to the hospital with a painful right foot. A CT scan examination reveals a thrombotic occlusion of the femoral artery in the proximal part of the adductor canal. Which artery will most likely provide blood supply to the leg through the genicular anastomosis?

- ▢ **A.** Medial circumflex femoral
- ▢ **B.** Descending branch of the lateral circumflex femoral
- ▢ **C.** First perforating branch of the deep femoral
- ▢ **D.** Inferior gluteal
- ▢ **E.** Descending genicular branch of femoral

14 A 75-year-old woman is admitted to the hospital after falling in her bathroom. Radiologic examination reveals an extracapsular fracture of the femoral neck. Which artery is most likely at risk for injury?

- ▢ **A.** Inferior gluteal
- ▢ **B.** First perforating branch of deep femoral

- ▢ **C.** Medial circumflex femoral
- ▢ **D.** Obturator
- ▢ **E.** Superior gluteal

15 A 56-year-old man with advanced bladder carcinoma suffers from difficulty while walking. Muscle testing reveals weakened adductors of the right thigh. Which nerve is most likely being compressed by the tumor to result in walking difficulty?

- ▢ **A.** Femoral
- ▢ **B.** Obturator
- ▢ **C.** Common fibular (peroneal)
- ▢ **D.** Tibial
- ▢ **E.** Sciatic

16 Upon removal of a knee-high leg cast, a 15-year-old boy complains of numbness of the dorsum of his right foot and inability to dorsiflex and evert his foot. Which is the most probable site of the nerve compression that resulted in these symptoms?

- ▢ **A.** Popliteal fossa
- ▢ **B.** Neck of the fibula
- ▢ **C.** Lateral compartment of the leg
- ▢ **D.** Anterior compartment of the leg
- ▢ **E.** Medial malleolus

17 A 32-year-old patient received a badly placed intramuscular injection to the posterior part of his gluteal region. The needle injured a motor nerve in the area. Later, he had great difficulty rising to a standing position from a seated position. Which muscle was most likely affected by the injury?

- ▢ **A.** Gluteus maximus
- ▢ **B.** Gluteus minimus
- ▢ **C.** Hamstrings
- ▢ **D.** Iliopsoas
- ▢ **E.** Obturator internus

18 During the preparation of an evening meal a female medical student dropped a sharp, slender kitchen knife. The blade pierced the first web space of her foot, resulting in numbness along adjacent sides of the first and second toes. Which nerve was most likely injured?

- ▢ **A.** Saphenous
- ▢ **B.** Deep fibular (peroneal)
- ▢ **C.** Superficial fibular (peroneal)
- ▢ **D.** Sural
- ▢ **E.** Common fibular (peroneal)

19 Following an injury suffered in a soccer match, a 32-year-old woman is examined in a seated position in the orthopedic clinic. Holding the right tibia with both hands, the clinician can press the tibia backward under the distal part of her femur. The left tibia cannot be displaced in this way. Which structure was most likely damaged in the right knee?

- ▢ **A.** Anterior cruciate ligament
- ▢ **B.** Lateral collateral ligament
- ▢ **C.** Medial collateral ligament
- ▢ **D.** Medial meniscus
- ▢ **E.** Posterior cruciate ligament

20 A 22-year-old woman is admitted to the emergency department after another vehicle collided with the passenger side of the convertible in which she was riding. Radiologic examination reveals an avulsion fracture of the greater trochanter. Which of the following muscles would continue to function normally if such an injury was incurred?

- ▢ **A.** Piriformis
- ▢ **B.** Obturator internus
- ▢ **C.** Gluteus medius
- ▢ **D.** Gluteus maximus
- ▢ **E.** Gluteus minimus

21 The news reported that the 58-year-old ambassador received a slashing wound to the medial thigh and died from exsanguination in less than 2 minutes. What was the most likely nature of his injury?

- ▢ **A.** The femoral artery was cut at the inguinal ligament
- ▢ **B.** A vessel or vessels were injured at the apex of the femoral triangle
- ▢ **C.** The femoral vein was transected at its junction with the saphenous vein
- ▢ **D.** The medial circumflex femoral was severed at its origin
- ▢ **E.** The deep femoral artery was divided at its origin

22 A 72-year-old woman suffered a hip dislocation when she fell down the steps to her garage. Which of the following is most significant in resisting hyperextension of the hip joint?

- ▢ **A.** Pubofemoral ligament
- ▢ **B.** Ischiofemoral ligament
- ▢ **C.** Iliofemoral ligament
- ▢ **D.** Negative pressure in the acetabular fossa
- ▢ **E.** Gluteus maximus muscle

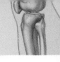

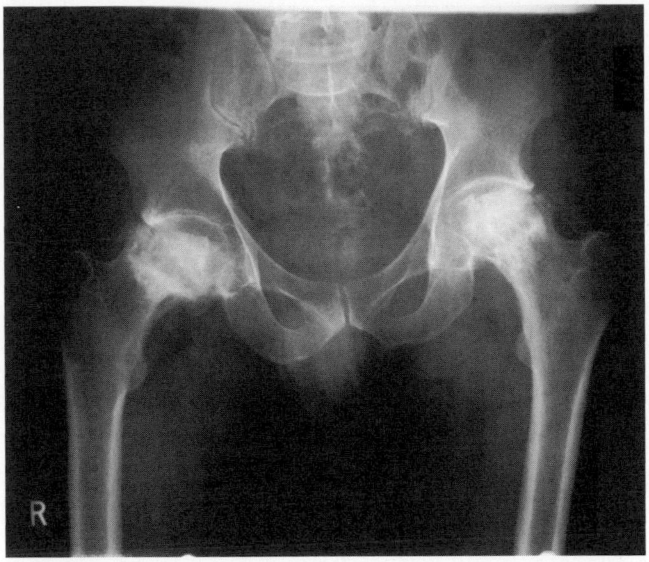

Fig. 5-2

23 A 75-year-old man is transported to the emergency department with severe pain of his right hip and thigh. A radiologic examination reveals avascular necrosis of the femoral head (Fig. 5-2). Which of the following conditions most likely occurred to produce avascular necrosis in this patient?

- ☐ **A.** Dislocation of the hip with tearing of the ligament of the head of the femur
- ☐ **B.** Intertrochanteric fracture of the femur
- ☐ **C.** Intracapsular femoral neck fracture
- ☐ **D.** Thrombosis of the obturator artery
- ☐ **E.** Comminuted fracture of the extracapsular femoral neck

24 A 58-year-old male farmer was accidentally struck with a scythe (a long, curved cutting blade) by another worker while they were cutting wheat. He was admitted to the county hospital with severe bleeding. During physical examination the doctor noted that the patient had a foot drop; sensation was present over the dorsum of the foot and the skin of the posterior calf. Which of the following nerves was injured?

- ☐ **A.** Femoral nerve
- ☐ **B.** Sciatic nerve
- ☐ **C.** Superficial fibular (peroneal) nerve
- ☐ **D.** Deep fibular (peroneal) nerve
- ☐ **E.** Common fibular (peroneal) nerve

25 A 45-year-old man is admitted to the emergency department after experiencing a sharp pain while lifting a box of books. He told the physician that he "felt the pain in my backside, the back of my thigh, my leg, and the side of my foot." During physical examination it is observed that his Achilles tendon jerk is weakened on the affected side. Which is the most likely cause of injury?

- ☐ **A.** Disc lesion at L3-4
- ☐ **B.** Disc lesion at L4-5
- ☐ **C.** Disc lesion at L5-S1
- ☐ **D.** Disc lesion at S1-2
- ☐ **E.** Gluteal crush syndrome of the sciatic nerve or piriformis syndrome

26 A 55-year-old woman is admitted to the emergency department after an automobile crash. Physical examination reveals that the patient's foot is everted and she cannot invert it. A weakness in dorsiflexion and inversion of the foot is noted. Her ipsilateral patellar reflex is reduced in quality, although the Achilles tendon reflex is brisk. Knee extension is almost normal, as are all hip movements and knee flexion. Sensation is greatly reduced on the medial side of the leg. Which of the following nerves is most likely injured?

- ☐ **A.** Femoral nerve
- ☐ **B.** L4 spinal nerve
- ☐ **C.** L4 and L5 spinal nerves
- ☐ **D.** Common fibular (peroneal) nerve
- ☐ **E.** Tibial nerve

27 A 46-year-old woman stepped on a broken wine bottle on the sidewalk and the sharp glass entered the posterior part of her foot. The patient was admitted to the hospital, and a physical examination concluded that her lateral plantar nerve had been transected (cut through). Which of the following conditions will most likely be confirmed by further physical examination?

- ☐ **A.** Loss of sensation over the plantar surface of the third toe
- ☐ **B.** Paralysis of the abductor hallucis
- ☐ **C.** Paralysis of the interossei and adductor hallucis
- ☐ **D.** Flexor hallucis brevis paralysis
- ☐ **E.** Flexor digitorum brevis paralysis

28 A 22-year-old male martial arts competitor was examined by the clinician because of pain and serious disability suffered from a kick to the side of his knee. Physical examination revealed a dark bruise just distal to the head of the fibula. Which of the following muscles will most likely be paralyzed?

- ☐ **A.** Tibialis anterior and extensor digitorum longus
- ☐ **B.** Tibialis posterior
- ☐ **C.** Soleus and gastrocnemius

- ▢ **D.** Plantaris and popliteus
- ▢ **E.** Flexor digitorum longus and flexor hallucis longus

29 A 61-year-old female immigrant had been diagnosed with spinal tuberculosis. The woman had developed a fluctuant, red, tender bulge on one flank, with a similar bulge in the groin on the same side. This presentation is likely due to spread of disease process within the fascia of a muscle with which of the following actions at the hip?

- ▢ **A.** Abduction
- ▢ **B.** Adduction
- ▢ **C.** Extension
- ▢ **D.** Flexion
- ▢ **E.** Internal rotation

30 In an accident during cleanup of an old residential area of the city, the Achilles tendon of a 32-year-old worker was cut through by the blade of a brush cutter. The patient is admitted to the hospital and a laceration of the Achilles tendon is diagnosed. Which of the following bones serves as an insertion for the Achilles tendon?

- ▢ **A.** Calcaneus
- ▢ **B.** Fibula
- ▢ **C.** Cuboid
- ▢ **D.** Talus
- ▢ **E.** Navicular

31 A 27-year-old female tennis pro injured her ankle during the quarterfinal match. A physical examination at the outpatient clinic revealed a severe inversion sprain of the ankle. Which of the following structures is most commonly damaged in such injuries?

- ▢ **A.** Medial plantar nerve
- ▢ **B.** Tibial nerve
- ▢ **C.** Anterior talofibular ligament
- ▢ **D.** Posterior talofibular ligament
- ▢ **E.** Deltoid ligament

32 A 41-year-old man is admitted to the emergency department with a swollen and painful foot. Radiologic examination reveals that the head of the talus has become displaced inferiorly, thereby causing the medial longitudinal arch of the foot to fall. What would be the most likely cause in this case?

- ▢ **A.** Tearing of the plantar calcaneonavicular (spring) ligament
- ▢ **B.** Fracture of the cuboid bone
- ▢ **C.** Interruption of the plantar aponeurosis
- ▢ **D.** Sprain of the anterior talofibular ligament
- ▢ **E.** Sprain of the deltoid ligament

33 During a football game a 21-year-old wide receiver was illegally blocked by a linebacker, who threw himself against the posterolateral aspect of the runner's left knee. As he lay on the ground, the wide receiver grasped his knee in obvious pain. Which of the following structures is frequently subject to injury from this type of force against the knee?

- ▢ **A.** Fibular collateral ligament
- ▢ **B.** Anterior cruciate ligament
- ▢ **C.** Lateral meniscus and posterior cruciate ligament
- ▢ **D.** Fibular collateral and posterior cruciate ligament
- ▢ **E.** All the ligaments of the knee will be affected

34 Lower limb angiography of an 82-year-old woman reveals a possible cause for her limb pain during her workout routines in the health spa. The artery that was occluded is one that should have been demonstrable passing between the proximal part of the space between the tibia and fibula. Which of the following arteries is most likely affected?

- ▢ **A.** Deep femoral
- ▢ **B.** Popliteal
- ▢ **C.** Posterior tibial
- ▢ **D.** Fibular (peroneal)
- ▢ **E.** Anterior tibial

35 A 43-year-old man visits the outpatient clinic with a painful, swollen knee joint. The patient's history reveals chronic gonococcal arthritis. A knee aspiration is ordered for bacterial culture of the synovial fluid. A standard suprapatellar approach is used, and the needle passes from the lateral aspect of the thigh into the region immediately proximal to and deep to the patella. Through which of the following muscles would the needle pass?

- ▢ **A.** Adductor magnus
- ▢ **B.** Short head of biceps femoris
- ▢ **C.** Rectus femoris
- ▢ **D.** Sartorius
- ▢ **E.** Vastus lateralis

36 A 34-year-old male power lifter visits the outpatient clinic because he has difficulty walking. During physical examination it is observed that the patient has a problem unlocking the knee joint to permit flexion of the leg. Which of the following muscles is most likely damaged?

- ▢ **A.** Biceps femoris
- ▢ **B.** Gastrocnemius
- ▢ **C.** Popliteus
- ▢ **D.** Semimembranosus
- ▢ **E.** Rectus femoris

37 A 32-year-old male basketball player comes down hard on his ankle. He is admitted to the outpatient clinic, and radiologic examination reveals a Pott's fracture. What ligament is most likely injured?

- ▢ **A.** Calcaneofibular ligament
- ▢ **B.** Deltoid ligament
- ▢ **C.** Spring ligament
- ▢ **D.** Plantar ligament
- ▢ **E.** Long plantar ligament

38 A 23-year-old man is admitted to the emergency department with pain and cyanosis of his right lower limb. Doppler ultrasound studies reveal deficiency in development of his femoral artery, which appears to terminate midthigh. A thrombotic occlusion is seen in an unusual, rather tortuous, large vessel in the posterior compartment of the thigh, arising in the gluteal area and continuous inferiorly with a normal appearing popliteal artery. It is decided that a vascular graft should be placed from the femoral artery to the popliteal artery. What is the identity of the aberrant artery?

- ▢ **A.** A large, fifth perforating branch of the femoral
- ▢ **B.** An sciatic branch of the inferior gluteal artery
- ▢ **C.** Descending branch of the medial circumflex femoral
- ▢ **D.** Descending branch of the superior gluteal artery
- ▢ **E.** An enlarged descending lateral circumflex femoral artery

39 When he attempted to lift one side of his new electric automobile from the ground to demonstrate his strength, a 51-year-old man felt a sharp pain in his back and quickly dropped the vehicle. Upon examination, it is observed that the patient has deficits in sensation on the dorsum and sole of his foot and marked weakness in abduction and lateral rotation of the lower limb. What was the nature of his injury?

- ▢ **A.** Piriformis syndrome, with entrapment of the sciatic nerve
- ▢ **B.** Disc lesion at L3-4
- ▢ **C.** Disc lesion at L4-5
- ▢ **D.** Disc lesion at L5-S1
- ▢ **E.** Posterior hip dislocation

40 A 43-year-old woman is examined by a neurologist, to whom she complains of pain in her lower limb of 6 months' duration. She has pain in the gluteal area, thigh, and leg. The neurologist observes reduced sensation over the dorsum and lateral side of the involved foot and some weakness in foot dorsiflexion and eversion. A diagnosis of a piriformis entrapment syndrome is made, with compression of the fibular (peroneal) division of the sciatic nerve. Which of the following conditions did the neurologist also most likely find during her physical examination of the patient?

- ▢ **A.** Paralysis of plantar flexion
- ▢ **B.** Instability of the knee, due to paralysis of the quadriceps femoris
- ▢ **C.** Foot drop
- ▢ **D.** Spasm or clonic contractures of the adductor musculature of the thigh
- ▢ **E.** Loss of sensation in the gluteal area, by paralysis of anterior cluneal nerves

41 Three years following a 62-year-old's hip replacement, the man's CT scans indicated that two of his larger hip muscles had been replaced by adipose tissue. The opinion is offered that his superior gluteal nerve could have been injured during the replacement procedure, and the muscles supplied by that nerve had atrophied and been replaced by fat. Which of the following muscles receives its innervation from the superior gluteal nerve?

- ▢ **A.** Tensor fasciae latae
- ▢ **B.** Rectus femoris
- ▢ **C.** Gluteus maximus
- ▢ **D.** Piriformis
- ▢ **E.** Quadratus femoris

42 A popliteal arterial aneurysm can be very fragile, bursting with great loss of blood and the potential loss of the leg if it is not dealt with safely and effectively. In the 18th century, Dr. John Hunter (1728-1793) discovered that if a primary artery of the thigh is temporarily compressed, blood flow in the popliteal artery can be reduced long enough to treat the aneurysm in the popliteal fossa surgically, with safety. What structure is indicated in Fig. 5-3 that is related to his surgical procedure?

- ▢ **A.** Sartorius
- ▢ **B.** Femoral vein
- ▢ **C.** Femoral artery
- ▢ **D.** Gracilis
- ▢ **E.** Adductor brevis

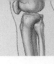

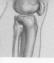

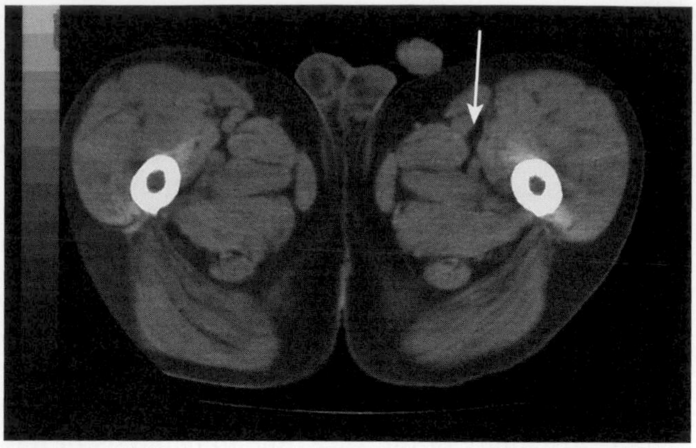

Fig. 5-3

43 A 49-year-old male worker fell from a ladder, with his weight impacting on the heels of his feet. Radiologic examination reveals comminuted calcaneal fractures. After the injury the contraction of which one of the following muscles could most likely increase the pain in the injured foot?

- ☐ **A.** Flexor digitorum profundus
- ☐ **B.** Gastrocnemius
- ☐ **C.** Tibialis posterior
- ☐ **D.** Tibialis anterior
- ☐ **E.** Fibularis (peroneus) longus

44 A 24-year-old woman received a small-caliber bullet wound to the popliteal fossa from a drive-by assailant. The patient was admitted to the emergency department, where the surgeons recognized that the bullet had severed the tibial nerve. Such an injury would most likely result in which of the following?

- ☐ **A.** Inability to extend the leg at the knee
- ☐ **B.** Foot drop
- ☐ **C.** A dorsiflexed and everted foot
- ☐ **D.** A plantar flexed and inverted foot
- ☐ **E.** Total inability to flex the leg at the knee joint

45 An 82-year-old grandmother slipped on the polished floor in her front hall and was transported to the emergency department and admitted for examination with a complaint of great pain in her right lower limb. During physical examination it is observed by the resident that the right lower limb is laterally rotated and noticeably shorter than her left limb. Radiologic examination reveals an intracapsular fracture of the femoral neck. Which of the following arteries supplies the head of the femur in early childhood but no longer in a patient of this age?

- ☐ **A.** Superior gluteal
- ☐ **B.** Lateral circumflex femoral
- ☐ **C.** A branch of the obturator artery
- ☐ **D.** Inferior gluteal
- ☐ **E.** Internal pudendal

46 A 19-year-old patient is admitted to the orthopedic service with a complaint of severe pain in his very swollen and discolored foot. He states that he hurt the foot when jumping from his girlfriend's bedroom window to the concrete driveway below. Plain film radiographic studies reveal that the head of the talus has become displaced inferiorly, thereby causing the medial longitudinal arch of the foot to fall. What would be the most likely, serious problem in such a case?

- ☐ **A.** Tearing of the plantar calcaneonavicular (spring) ligament
- ☐ **B.** Fracture of the cuboid bone
- ☐ **C.** Interruption of the plantar aponeurosis
- ☐ **D.** Sprain of the anterior talofibular ligament
- ☐ **E.** Disruption of the distal tibiofibular ligament

47 A 29-year-old male police officer is examined in a neighborhood clinic, with a complaint of discomfort in the lateral thigh. The physician observes that the policeman is rather overweight and that he is wearing a heavy leather belt, to which numerous objects are attached, including his empty holster. After a thorough physical examination a diagnosis of meralgia paresthetica is confirmed. Which of the following nerves is most likely involved?

- ☐ **A.** Superior gluteal
- ☐ **B.** Femoral
- ☐ **C.** Obturator
- ☐ **D.** Fibular (peroneal) division of sciatic
- ☐ **E.** Lateral femoral cutaneous

48 The swollen and painful left foot of a 23-year-old female long distance runner is examined in the university orthopedic clinic. She states that she stepped on an unseen sharp object while running through the park several days earlier. Emergency surgery is ordered to deal with her tarsal tunnel syndrome. The tarsal tunnel is occupied normally by tendons, vessels, and nerves that pass beneath a very strong band of tissue (flexor retinaculum) on the medial side of the ankle. What is the most anterior of the structures that pass through this tunnel?

- ☐ **A.** Flexor hallucis longus tendon
- ☐ **B.** Plantaris tendon
- ☐ **C.** Tibialis anterior tendon
- ☐ **D.** Tibialis posterior tendon
- ☐ **E.** Tibial nerve

49 A 42-year-old male sign painter is admitted to the emergency department after falling to the sidewalk from his ladder. Radiologic examination reveals a fracture of the proximal femur. Which of the following arteries supplies the proximal part of the femur?

- ☐ **A.** Deep circumflex iliac
- ☐ **B.** Acetabular branch of obturator
- ☐ **C.** Lateral circumflex femoral
- ☐ **D.** A branch of profunda femoris
- ☐ **E.** Medial circumflex femoral

50 A 22-year-old man is admitted to the emergency department after falling from his bicycle. Radiologic examination reveals a fracture of the tibia above the ankle. MRI and physical examination reveal that the tibial nerve is severed on the posterior aspect of the tibia. Which of the following signs will most likely be present during physical examination?

- ☐ **A.** Sensory loss of the dorsum of the foot
- ☐ **B.** Sensory loss on the sole of the foot
- ☐ **C.** Foot drop
- ☐ **D.** Paralysis of the extensor digitorum brevis
- ☐ **E.** Sensory loss of the entire foot

51 A 24-year-old man is admitted to the emergency department after a car collision. Radiologic examination reveals a fracture at the junction of the middle and lower thirds of the femur. An MRI examination provides evidence that the popliteal vessels were injured when the distal fragment of the fracture was pulled posteriorly. Which of the following muscles is most likely to displace the distal fracture fragment?

- ☐ **A.** Soleus
- ☐ **B.** Gastrocnemius
- ☐ **C.** Semitendinosus
- ☐ **D.** Gracilis
- ☐ **E.** Tibialis anterior

52 A 65-year-old man is admitted to the hospital after falling from his roof while cleaning leaves and pine needles from the gutters. Among other injuries suffered in his fall, radiologic examination reveals a fracture of the talus bone in one foot. Much of the blood supply of this bone can be lost in such an injury and can result in osteonecrosis. From what artery does this bone receive its primary vascular supply?

- ☐ **A.** Medial plantar
- ☐ **B.** Lateral plantar
- ☐ **C.** Dorsalis pedis
- ☐ **D.** Anterior tibial
- ☐ **E.** Posterior tibial

53 A 58-year-old female dancer presented to the orthopedic clinic with a complaint of pain during her work because of bilateral bunions. She was referred to a podiatric surgeon who scheduled her for surgery. The protruding bony and soft tissues of the toe were excised, and a muscle was reflected from the lateral side of the proximal phalanx, together with a sesamoid bone, upon which the muscle also inserted. What muscle was this?

- ☐ **A.** Adductor hallucis
- ☐ **B.** Abductor hallucis
- ☐ **C.** First dorsal interosseous
- ☐ **D.** First lumbrical
- ☐ **E.** Quadratus plantae

54 A 34-year-old male long-distance runner complained to the team physician of swelling and pain of his shin. Skin testing in a physical examination showed normal cutaneous sensation of the leg. Muscular strength tests showed marked weakness of dorsiflexion and impaired inversion of the foot. Which nerve serves the muscles involved in the painful swelling?

- ☐ **A.** Common fibular (peroneal)
- ☐ **B.** Deep fibular (peroneal)
- ☐ **C.** Sciatic
- ☐ **D.** Superficial fibular (peroneal)
- ☐ **E.** Tibial

55 A 7-year-old girl accidentally stepped on a sharp snail shell while walking to the beach. She was admitted to the hospital, where she received a tetanus shot, and the wound was cleaned thoroughly and sutured. One week later, during a return visit to her physician, it is seen that she has great difficulty in flexing her big toe, even though there is no inflammation present in the sole of the foot. Which nerve was most likely damaged by the piercing of the shell?

- ☐ **A.** Lateral plantar nerve
- ☐ **B.** Medial plantar nerve
- ☐ **C.** Sural nerve
- ☐ **D.** Superficial fibular (peroneal) nerve
- ☐ **E.** Deep fibular (peroneal) nerve

56 A 49-year-old man is admitted to the emergency department with a cold and pale foot. Physical examination reveals that the patient suffers from peripheral vascular disease; duplex ultrasound studies indicate possible occlusion of his popliteal artery, and the pulse of the posterior tibial artery is absent. What is the most common location for palpation of the pulse of the posterior tibial artery?

- ☐ **A.** Lateral to the muscular belly of the abductor hallucis
- ☐ **B.** Posteroinferior to the medial femoral condyle
- ☐ **C.** Groove midway between the lateral malleolus and the calcaneus
- ☐ **D.** Groove midway between the medial malleolus and the calcaneus
- ☐ **E.** Medially, between the two heads of the gastrocnemius

57 Young parents were concerned that their 14-month-old daughter had not yet begun walking. Their pediatrician reassured them, saying that one of the muscles of the leg, the fibularis (peroneus) tertius, had to complete its central neurologic development before the child could lift the outer corner of the foot and walk without stumbling over her toes. What is the most common nerve supply of this muscle?

- ☐ **A.** Sural
- ☐ **B.** Lateral plantar
- ☐ **C.** Deep fibular (peroneal)
- ☐ **D.** Superficial fibular (peroneal)
- ☐ **E.** Tibial

58 A 22-year-old woman is admitted with high fever and vaginal discharge. Physical and laboratory examinations reveal gonorrheal infection. A series of intramuscular antibiotic injections are ordered. Into which of the following parts of the gluteal region should the antibiotic be injected to avoid nerve injury?

- ☐ **A.** Anterior and superior to a line between the posterior superior iliac spine and the greater trochanter
- ☐ **B.** In the middle of a line between the anterior superior iliac spine and the ischial tuberosity
- ☐ **C.** Inferolateral to a line between the posterior superior iliac spine and the greater trochanter
- ☐ **D.** Inferomedial to a line between the posterior superior iliac spine and the greater trochanter
- ☐ **E.** Halfway between the iliac tuberosity and the greater trochanter

59 A 45-year-old intoxicated man was struck by a tour bus while walking in the middle of the street. The man was admitted to the emergency department and during physical examination was diagnosed with "adductor gait," in which an individual crosses one limb in front of the other, due to powerful hip adduction. Which of the following nerves was most likely involved in this condition?

- ☐ **A.** Tibial
- ☐ **B.** Obturator
- ☐ **C.** Inferior gluteal
- ☐ **D.** Superior gluteal
- ☐ **E.** Femoral

60 The baby was quite large, and the pelvis of the mother-to-be was somewhat narrow, causing her considerable difficulty and pain during the delivery. At her specific request, it was decided to inject local anesthetic into the perineum. The genitofemoral and ilioinguinal nerves were infiltrated anteriorly, and a deep injection was made medial to the ischial tuberosity to anesthetize the pudendal nerve, which supplies much of the perineum in most cases. A few minutes later, it became very obvious to those in attendance that the injection had not been effective enough in the central and posterior parts of the perineum. A separate injection was therefore inserted lateral to the ischial tuberosity. What other nerve(s) can provide much of the sensory supply to the perineum in some individuals?

- ☐ **A.** Posterior femoral cutaneous
- ☐ **B.** Inferior cluneal nerves
- ☐ **C.** Iliohypogastric nerve
- ☐ **D.** Inferior gluteal nerve
- ☐ **E.** Middle cluneal nerves

61 A 55-year-old man is admitted to the hospital for an iliofemoral bypass. The operation is performed successfully and the blood flow between the iliac and femoral arteries is restored. During rehabilitation which of the following arteries should be palpated to monitor good circulation of the lower limb?

- ☐ **A.** Anterior tibial
- ☐ **B.** Deep fibular (peroneal)
- ☐ **C.** Deep plantar
- ☐ **D.** Dorsalis pedis
- ☐ **E.** Dorsal metatarsal

62 A 55-year-old woman is bitten by a dog in the dorsum of the foot and is admitted to the emergency department. The wound is cleaned thoroughly, during which it is seen that no tendons have been cut, but the dorsalis pedis artery and the accompanying nerve have been injured. Which of the following conditions would be expected during physical examination?

- ☐ **A.** Clubfoot
- ☐ **B.** Foot drop
- ☐ **C.** Inability to extend the big toe
- ☐ **D.** Numbness between the first and second toes
- ☐ **E.** Weakness in inversion of the foot

63 A 31-year-old woman presents to the department of surgery with a complaint of facial paralysis (Bell's palsy), which had appeared a year earlier and had resulted in paralysis of muscles of one side of her face. The chief of plastic surgery recommends a nerve graft, taking a cutaneous nerve from the lower limb to replace the defective facial nerve. The surgery is successful. Six months after the procedure, there is restoration of function of previously paralyzed facial muscles. There is an area of skin on the back of the leg laterally and also on the lateral side of the foot that has no sensation. What nerve was used in the grafting procedure?

- ▢ **A.** Superficial fibular (peroneal)
- ▢ **B.** Tibial
- ▢ **C.** Common fibular (peroneal)
- ▢ **D.** Sural
- ▢ **E.** Saphenous

64 A 10-year-old girl is admitted to the emergency department after falling from a tree in which she was playing with her friends. Radiologic and physical examinations reveal Osgood-Schlatter disease (Fig. 5-4). Which of the following bony structures is chiefly affected?

- ▢ **A.** Medial condyle of tibia
- ▢ **B.** Posterior intercondylar area
- ▢ **C.** Intercondylar eminence
- ▢ **D.** Tibial tuberosity
- ▢ **E.** Anterolateral tibial tubercle (Gerdy's tubercle)

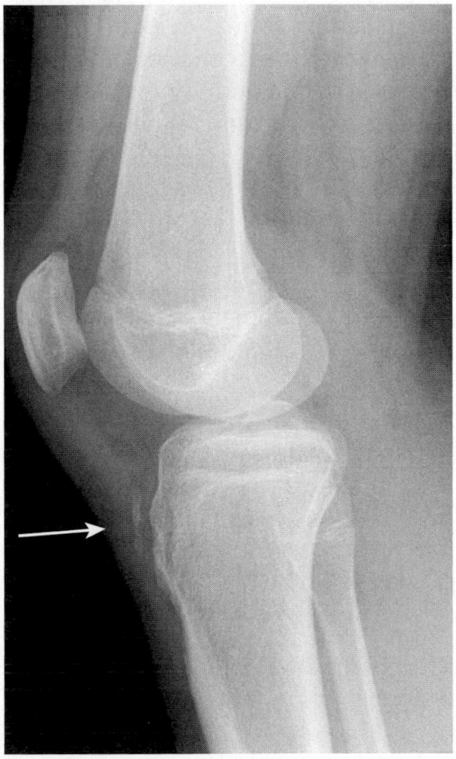

Fig. 5-4

65 An 81-year-old man is admitted to the emergency department with severe pain in his knees. The patient has a long history of osteoarthritis. Radiologic examination reveals degeneration of the joints of his lower limbs. The degeneration is more severe on the medial side of the knees, which causes his knees to be bowed outward when he stands upright. Which of the following terms best describes the condition of his knees?

- ▢ **A.** Genu varus
- ▢ **B.** Genu valgus
- ▢ **C.** Coxa varus
- ▢ **D.** Coxa valgus
- ▢ **E.** Hallux valgus

66 The patellar reflex appears to be markedly reduced in a 33-year-old diabetic female patient, due to deficient vascular supply of the nerves of her lower limb. The tendon of which of the following muscles is stretched during the patellar reflex?

- ▢ **A.** Quadriceps femoris
- ▢ **B.** Quadratus femoris
- ▢ **C.** Sartorius
- ▢ **D.** Pectineus
- ▢ **E.** Biceps femoris

67 A 52-year-old woman is admitted to the emergency department after severely injuring her right lower limb when she fell from a trampoline. Radiologic examination reveals a trimalleolar fracture of the ankle involving the lateral malleolus, medial malleolus, and the posterior process of the tibia. Which of the following bones will also most likely be affected?

- ▢ **A.** Navicular
- ▢ **B.** Calcaneus
- ▢ **C.** Cuneiform
- ▢ **D.** Cuboid
- ▢ **E.** Talus

68 A 72-year-old man visits the outpatient clinic with a complaint of severe pain when walking. Physical examination reveals the problems in his feet as shown in Fig. 5-5. What is the most likely diagnosis?

- ▢ **A.** Coxa varus
- ▢ **B.** Coxa valgus
- ▢ **C.** Genu valgus
- ▢ **D.** Genu vara
- ▢ **E.** Hallux valgus

69 A 63-year-old woman visits the outpatient orthopedic clinic with the complaint of pain in her foot for more than a year. Radiologic and physical

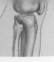

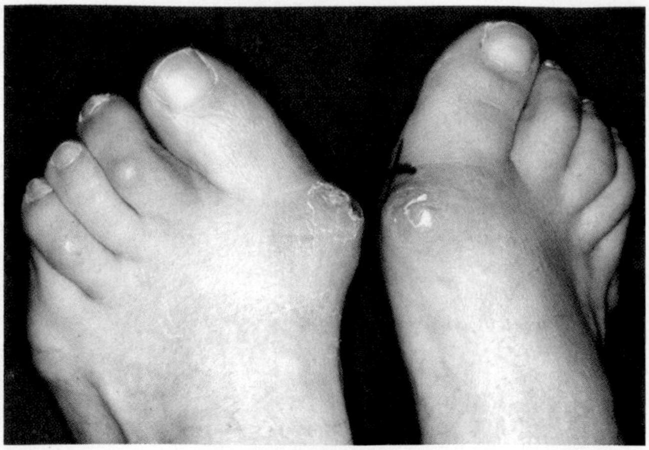

Fig. 5-5

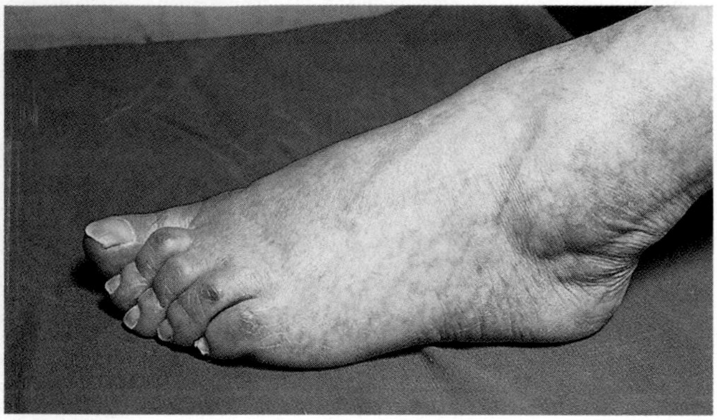

Fig. 5-6

examinations give evidence of constant extension at the metatarsophalangeal joints, hyperflexion at the proximal interphalangeal joints, and extension of distal interphalangeal joints (Fig. 5-6). Which of the following terms is most accurate to describe the signs of physical examination?

- ☐ **A.** Pes planus
- ☐ **B.** Pes cavus
- ☐ **C.** Hammertoes
- ☐ **D.** Claw toes
- ☐ **E.** Hallux valgus

70 A 58-year-old man is admitted to the hospital with pain in his lower limb for the past 2 months. Physical examination reveals point tenderness in the region of his greater sciatic foramen, with pain radiating down the posterior aspect of his thigh. An MRI examination reveals that the patient suffers from piriformis entrapment syndrome. He is directed to treatment by a physical therapist for stretching and relaxation of the muscle. Entrapment of which of the following nerves can mimic piriformis entrapment syndrome?

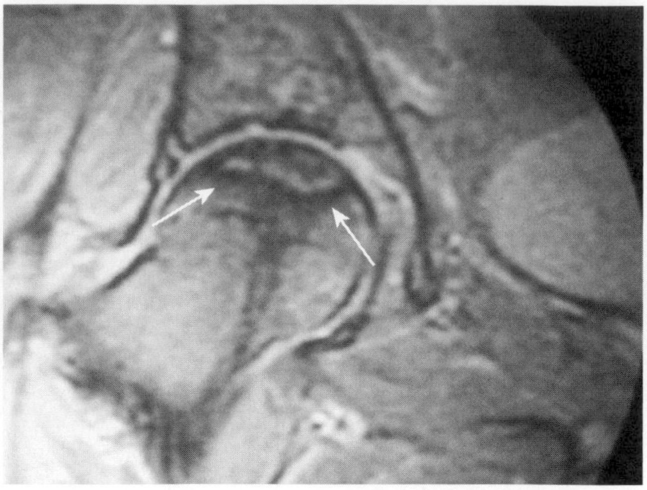

Fig. 5-7

- ☐ **A.** L4
- ☐ **B.** L5
- ☐ **C.** S1
- ☐ **D.** S2
- ☐ **E.** S3

71 A 22-year-old woman is found in a comatose condition, having lain for an unknown length of time on the tile floor of the courtyard. She is found in possession of cocaine. The patient is transported to the hospital while EMT personnel receive instructions for treatment of drug overdose. During the physical examination the patient's gluteal region shows signs of ischemia. After regaining consciousness, she exhibits paralysis of knee flexion and dorsal and plantar flexion and sensory loss in the limb. What is the most likely diagnosis?

- ☐ **A.** Tibial nerve loss
- ☐ **B.** S1-2 nerve compression
- ☐ **C.** Gluteal crush injury
- ☐ **D.** Piriformis entrapment syndrome
- ☐ **E.** Femoral nerve entrapment

72 A 75-year-old man is admitted to the emergency department with severe pain at his right hip and thigh. An MRI examination reveals avascular necrosis of the femoral head (Fig. 5-7). Which of the following arteries is most likely injured, resulting in avascular necrosis?

- ☐ **A.** Deep circumflex iliac
- ☐ **B.** Acetabular branch of obturator
- ☐ **C.** Descending branch of lateral circumflex femoral
- ☐ **D.** First perforating branch of profunda femoris
- ☐ **E.** Ascending branch of medial circumflex femoral

73 A 27-year-old woman had suffered a penetrating injury in the popliteal region by an object thrown from a riding lawnmower. She was admitted to the emergency department for removal of the foreign object. After making a midline incision in the skin of the popliteal fossa, the surgical resident observed a vein of moderate size in the superficial tissues. What vein would be expected at this location?

- ▢ **A.** Popliteal vein
- ▢ **B.** Perforating tributary to the deep femoral vein
- ▢ **C.** Great saphenous vein
- ▢ **D.** Lesser (short) saphenous vein
- ▢ **E.** Superior medial genicular vein

74 A 58-year-old diabetic patient is admitted to the hospital with a painful foot. Physical examination reveals that the patient suffers from peripheral vascular disease. There is no detectable dorsalis pedis arterial pulse, but the posterior tibial pulse is strong. Which of the following arteries will most likely provide adequate collateral supply from the plantar surface to the toes and dorsum of the foot?

- ▢ **A.** Anterior tibial
- ▢ **B.** Fibular (peroneal)
- ▢ **C.** Arcuate
- ▢ **D.** Medial plantar
- ▢ **E.** Lateral plantar

75 A 32-year-old man is admitted to the emergency department after an injury to his foot while playing football with his college friends. An MRI examination reveals multiple tendinous tears (Fig. 5-8). Which of the following bones is associated with the muscle tears?

- ▢ **A.** Navicular
- ▢ **B.** Cuboid
- ▢ **C.** Calcaneus
- ▢ **D.** Sustentaculum tali
- ▢ **E.** Talus

76 An 18-year-old professional tennis player fell when she leaped for an overhead shot and landed with her foot inverted. Radiologic examination in the hospital revealed an avulsion fracture of the tuberosity of the fifth metatarsal. Part of the tuberosity is pulled off, producing pain and edema. Which of the following muscles is pulling on the fractured fragment?

- ▢ **A.** Fibularis (peroneus) longus
- ▢ **B.** Tibialis posterior
- ▢ **C.** Fibularis (peroneus) brevis
- ▢ **D.** Extensor digitorum brevis
- ▢ **E.** Adductor hallucis

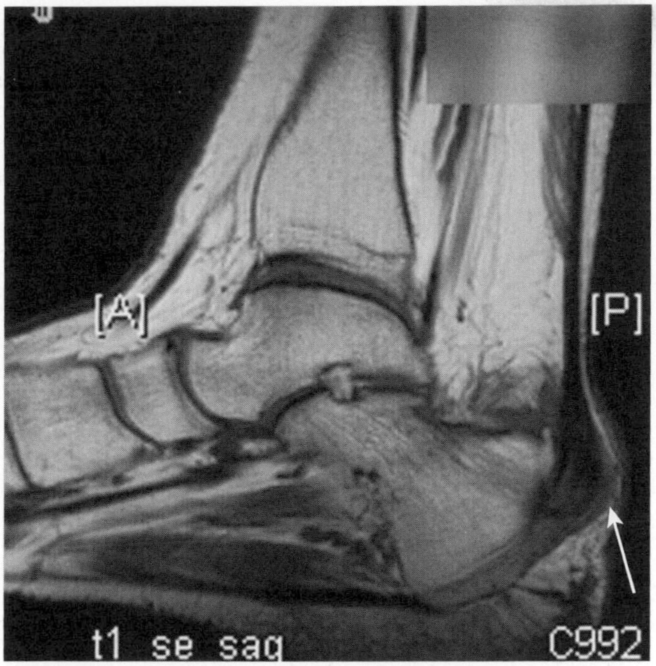

Fig. 5-8

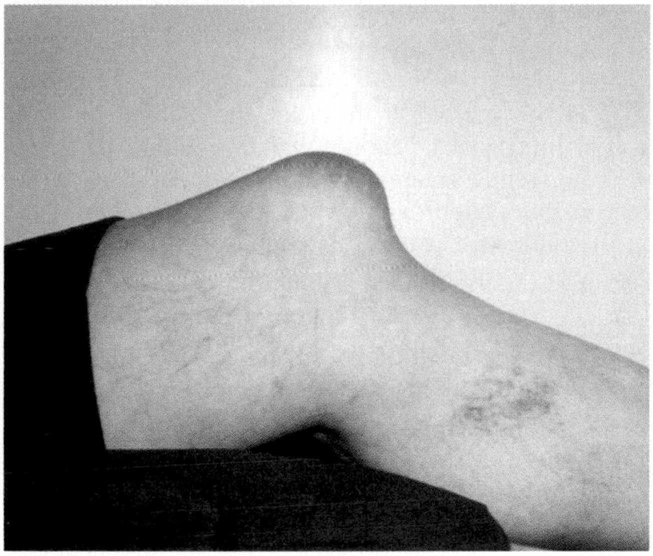

Fig. 5-9

77 A 58-year-old female employee of a housecleaning business visits the outpatient clinic with a complaint of a constant burning pain in her knees. Clinical examinations reveal a "housemaid's knee" condition (Fig. 5-9). Which of the following structures is most likely affected?

- ▢ **A.** Prepatellar bursa
- ▢ **B.** Infrapatellar bursa
- ▢ **C.** Posterior cruciate ligament
- ▢ **D.** Patellar retinacula
- ▢ **E.** Lateral meniscus

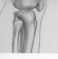

78 A 42-year-old mother of three children visits the outpatient clinic complaining that her youngest son cannot walk yet even though he is 4 years old. Radiologic and physical examinations reveal an unstable hip joint. Which of the following ligaments is responsible for stabilization of the hip joint in childhood?

- ☐ **A.** Iliofemoral
- ☐ **B.** Pubofemoral
- ☐ **C.** Ischiofemoral
- ☐ **D.** Ligament of the head of the femur
- ☐ **E.** Transverse acetabular ligament

79 A 45-year-old is admitted to the hospital after his left leg impacted a fence post when he was thrown from a powerful four-wheel all-terrain vehicle. Radiologic examination reveals posterior displacement of the tibia upon the femur. Which of the following structures was most likely injured?

- ☐ **A.** Anterior cruciate ligament
- ☐ **B.** Posterior cruciate ligament
- ☐ **C.** Lateral collateral ligament
- ☐ **D.** Lateral meniscus ligament
- ☐ **E.** Patellar ligament

80 A 55-year-old man visits the outpatient clinic complaining that he cannot walk more than 5 minutes without feeling severe pain in his feet. An image of the feet of this patient is shown in Fig. 5-10. What is the most common cause of this condition?

- ☐ **A.** Collapse of medial longitudinal arch, with eversion and abduction of the forefoot
- ☐ **B.** Exaggerated height of the medial longitudinal arch of the foot
- ☐ **C.** Collapse of long plantar ligament
- ☐ **D.** Collapse of deltoid ligament
- ☐ **E.** Collapse of plantar calcaneonavicular ligament

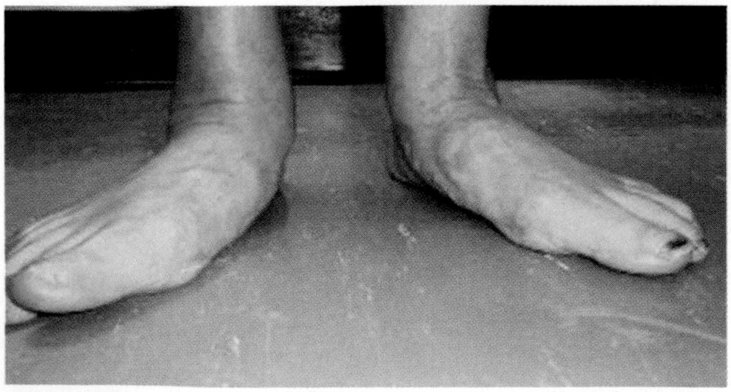

Pes planus

Fig. 5-10

81 A 55-year-old cowboy is admitted to the emergency department after he was knocked from his feet by a young longhorn steer. MRI examination reveals a large hematoma in the knee joint. Physical examination reveals that the patient suffers from the "unhappy triad" (of O'Donoghue). Which of the following structures are involved in such an injury?

- ☐ **A.** Medial collateral ligament, medial meniscus, and anterior cruciate ligament
- ☐ **B.** Lateral collateral ligament, lateral meniscus, and posterior cruciate ligament
- ☐ **C.** Medial collateral ligament, lateral meniscus, and anterior cruciate ligament
- ☐ **D.** Lateral collateral ligament, medial meniscus, and anterior cruciate ligament
- ☐ **E.** Medial collateral ligament, medial meniscus, and posterior cruciate ligament

82 A 32-year-old man is admitted to the emergency department after a car collision. Radiologic examination reveals a distal fracture of the femur. The patient is in severe pain, and a femoral nerve block is administered. What landmark is accurate for localizing the nerve for injection of anesthetics?

- ☐ **A.** 1.5 cm superolateral to the pubic tubercle
- ☐ **B.** 1.5 cm medial to the anterior superior iliac spine
- ☐ **C.** 1.5 cm lateral to the femoral pulse
- ☐ **D.** 1.5 cm medial to the femoral pulse
- ☐ **E.** Midway between the anterior superior iliac spine and pubic symphysis

83 A 39-year-old woman is admitted to the emergency department with a painful foot. Radiologic examination reveals a Morton's neuroma. What is the most typical location of this neuroma?

- ☐ **A.** Between the third and fourth metatarsophalangeal joints
- ☐ **B.** Between the second and third metatarsophalangeal joints
- ☐ **C.** Between the first and second metatarsophalangeal joints
- ☐ **D.** Between the fourth and fifth metatarsophalangeal joints
- ☐ **E.** In the region of the second, third, and fourth metatarsophalangeal joints

84 A 34-year-old male distance runner visits the outpatient clinic with a complaint of pain he has suffered in his foot for the past week. The clinical examination indicates that the patient has an inflammation of the tough band of tissue stretching from the calcaneus to the ball of the foot. Which of the following conditions is most characteristic of these symptoms?

- ▢ **A.** Morton's neuroma
- ▢ **B.** Ankle eversion sprain
- ▢ **C.** Tarsal tunnel syndrome
- ▢ **D.** Plantar fasciitis
- ▢ **E.** Inversion sprain of the ankle

85 A 5-month-old baby boy is admitted to the pediatric orthopedic clinic. During physical examination it is noted that the baby has inversion and adduction of the forefoot relative to the hindfoot and plantar flexion. Which of the following terms is diagnostic for the signs observed on physical examination?

- ▢ **A.** Coxa vara
- ▢ **B.** Talipes equinovarus
- ▢ **C.** Hallux valgus
- ▢ **D.** Hallux varus
- ▢ **E.** Plantar fasciitis

86 A 71-year-old man is admitted to the orthopedic clinic with difficulties walking. The patient has a past history of polio. Physical and radiologic examinations reveal extension at the metatarsophalangeal joints with flexion of both the proximal and distal interphalangeal joints. Which of the following descriptions is most appropriate for this patient's condition?

- ▢ **A.** Hallux valgus
- ▢ **B.** Pes planus
- ▢ **C.** Hammertoes
- ▢ **D.** Claw toes
- ▢ **E.** Pes cavus

87 A 62-year-old man is admitted to the emergency department. Radiologic examination and the available data indicate the likelihood of a transient ischemic attack. During physical examination the ankle jerk reflex is absent. Which of the following nerves is most likely responsible for the reflex arc?

- ▢ **A.** Common fibular (peroneal)
- ▢ **B.** Superficial fibular (peroneal)
- ▢ **C.** Deep fibular (peroneal)
- ▢ **D.** Tibial
- ▢ **E.** Superficial and deep fibular (peroneal)

88 Following the insertion of a prosthetic hip joint in a 72-year-old man, it was observed that the patient had greatly diminished sensation in the region of distribution of the posterior femoral cutaneous nerve. Which of the following is characteristic of this nerve?

- ▢ **A.** Cutaneous supply of the superior aspect of the gluteal region
- ▢ **B.** Arises from sacral spinal nerve levels S1, S2, S3
- ▢ **C.** Motor innervation of the obturator internus and gemelli muscles
- ▢ **D.** Injury results in meralgia paresthetica
- ▢ **E.** Provides origin of the sural nerve

89 A 34-year-old woman has a direct blow to the patella by the dashboard of the vehicle during an automobile crash. The woman is admitted to the emergency department and radiologic examination reveals patellofemoral syndrome. This type of syndrome is characterized by lateral dislocation of the patella. Which of the following muscles requires strengthening by physical rehabilitation to prevent future dislocation of the patella?

- ▢ **A.** Vastus lateralis
- ▢ **B.** Vastus medialis
- ▢ **C.** Vastus intermedius
- ▢ **D.** Rectus femoris
- ▢ **E.** Patellar ligament

90 A 34-year-old man visits the outpatient clinic for an annual checkup. A radiographic examination of his knees is shown in Fig. 5-11. Physical examination reveals no pathology or pain to his knees. The patient has no past history of any knee problems. What is the most likely diagnosis?

- ▢ **A.** Enlarged prepatellar bursa
- ▢ **B.** Osgood-Schlatter disease
- ▢ **C.** Normal intercondylar eminence
- ▢ **D.** Bipartite patella
- ▢ **E.** Injury to lateral meniscus

91 A 48-year-old woman is admitted to the hospital with severe abdominal pain. Several imaging methods reveal that the patient suffers from intestinal ischemia. An abdominopelvic catheterization is ordered for antegrade angiography. A femoral puncture is performed. What is the landmark for femoral artery puncture?

- ▢ **A.** Halfway between anterior superior iliac spine and pubic symphysis
- ▢ **B.** 4.5 cm lateral to the pubic tubercle
- ▢ **C.** Midpoint of the inguinal skin crease
- ▢ **D.** Medial aspect of femoral head
- ▢ **E.** Lateral to the fossa ovalis

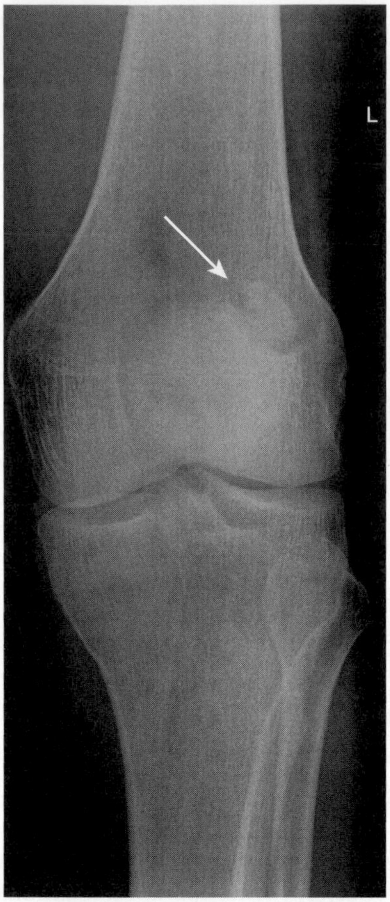

Fig. 5-11

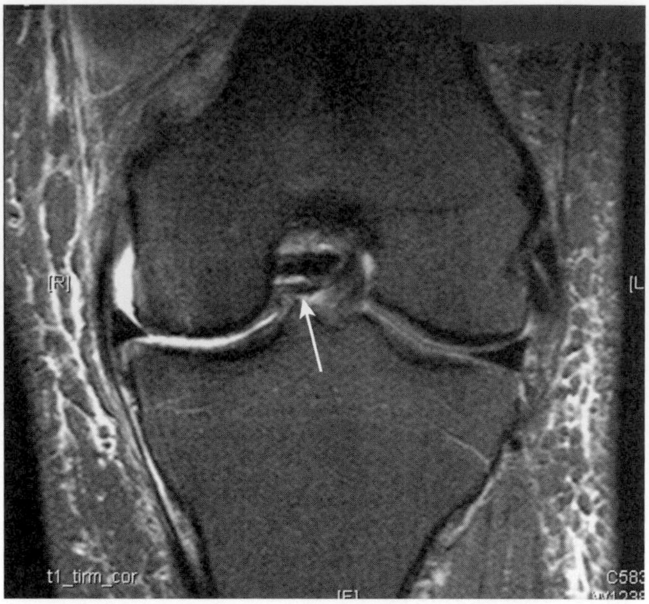

Fig. 5-12

92 A 23-year-old man is admitted to the emergency department after injuring his knee while playing football. During physical examination there is pain and swelling of the knee, in addition to locking of the knee in full extension. Radiologic examination reveals a bucket handle meniscal tear (Fig. 5-12). Which of the following ligaments is most likely injured?

- ☐ **A.** Posterior cruciate
- ☐ **B.** Medial collateral
- ☐ **C.** Lateral collateral
- ☐ **D.** Anterior cruciate
- ☐ **E.** Coronary

93 A 27-year-old male triathlon competitor complained that he frequently experienced deep pains in one calf that almost caused him to drop out of a regional track-and-field event. Doppler ultrasound studies indicated, and surgical exposure confirmed, the existence of an accessory portion of the medial head of the gastrocnemius that was constricting the popliteal artery. Above the medial head of the gastrocnemius, the superior medial border of the popliteal fossa could be seen. Which of the following structures forms this border?

- ☐ **A.** Tendon of biceps femoris
- ☐ **B.** Tendons of semitendinosus and semimembranosus
- ☐ **C.** Tendon of plantaris
- ☐ **D.** Adductor hiatus
- ☐ **E.** Popliteus

94 The neurosurgeon had removed a portion of the dense tissue (dura mater) covering the brain of the patient when she removed the tumor that had invaded the skull. To replace this important tissue covering of the brain, she took a band of the aponeurotic tissue of the lateral aspect of the thigh, covering the vastus lateralis muscle. What muscle, supplied by the inferior gluteal nerve, inserts into this band of dense tissue as part of its insertion?

- ☐ **A.** Gluteus medius
- ☐ **B.** Gluteus minimus
- ☐ **C.** Gluteus maximus
- ☐ **D.** Tensor fasciae latae
- ☐ **E.** Rectus femoris

95 In the radiographs of the knee of a male 28-year-old basketball player, who had apparently suffered a tear in a medial ligament of the knee, the tubercle on the superior aspect of the medial femoral condyle could be seen more clearly than in most individuals. What muscle attaches to this tubercle?

- ☐ **A.** Semimembranosus
- ☐ **B.** Gracilis
- ☐ **C.** Popliteus

- ▢ **D.** Adductor magnus
- ▢ **E.** Vastus medialis

96 In preparing to isolate the proximal portion of the femoral artery, the vascular surgeon gently separated it from surrounding tissues. Posterior to the femoral sheath, what muscle forms the lateral portion of the floor of the femoral triangle?

- ▢ **A.** Adductor longus
- ▢ **B.** Iliopsoas
- ▢ **C.** Sartorius
- ▢ **D.** Pectineus
- ▢ **E.** Rectus femoris

97 A 37-year-old woman had been suffering for months from piriformis entrapment syndrome, which was not relieved by physical therapy. Part of the sciatic nerve passed through the piriformis, and a decision was made for surgical resection of the muscle. When the area of entrapment was identified and cleared, a tendon could be seen emerging through the lesser sciatic foramen, at first hidden by two smaller muscles and several nerves and vessels destined for the region of the perineum. The tendons of which of the following muscles pass through this opening?

- ▢ **A.** Obturator internus
- ▢ **B.** Obturator externus
- ▢ **C.** Quadratus femoris
- ▢ **D.** Gluteus minimus
- ▢ **E.** Gluteus medius

98 A 67-year-old woman has been suffering from osteoporosis for the past year. During her annual checkup, radiologic examination reveals an angle of 160 degrees made by the axis of the femoral neck to the axis of the femoral shaft. Which of the following conditions is associated with these examination findings?

- ▢ **A.** Coxa vara
- ▢ **B.** Coxa valga
- ▢ **C.** Genu valgum
- ▢ **D.** Genu varum
- ▢ **E.** Hallux valgus

99 A 34-year-old male runner visits the outpatient clinic complaining of pain in his foot for the past week. Physical examination reveals inflammation of the tough band of tissue stretching from the calcaneus to the ball of the foot. Which of the following conditions is characteristic of these symptoms?

- ▢ **A.** Pott's fracture
- ▢ **B.** Dupuytren fracture
- ▢ **C.** Tarsal tunnel
- ▢ **D.** Plantar fasciitis
- ▢ **E.** Rupture of spring ligament

100 A 50-year-old man is admitted to the emergency department after a car crash. An MRI examination reveals an injured anterior cruciate ligament. Physical examination reveals a positive drawer sign. Which of the following signs is expected to be present during physical examination?

- ▢ **A.** The tibia can be slightly displaced anteriorly
- ▢ **B.** The tibia can be slightly displaced posteriorly
- ▢ **C.** The fibula can be slightly displaced posteriorly
- ▢ **D.** The fibula can be slightly displaced anteriorly
- ▢ **E.** The tibia and fibula can be slightly displaced anteriorly

101 A 23-year-old male basketball player injured his foot during training and is admitted to the emergency department. An MRI examination reveals a hematoma around the medial malleolus. Upon physical examination the patient shows excessive eversion of his foot. Which of the following ligaments most likely has a tear?

- ▢ **A.** Plantar calcaneonavicular (spring)
- ▢ **B.** Calcaneofibular
- ▢ **C.** Long plantar
- ▢ **D.** Short plantar
- ▢ **E.** Deltoid

102 A 5-year-old boy is admitted to the emergency department after a car collision. Radiologic examination reveals a fracture of the head of the femur. An MRI examination reveals a large hematoma. Which of the following arteries is most likely injured?

- ▢ **A.** Deep circumflex iliac
- ▢ **B.** Acetabular branch of obturator
- ▢ **C.** Descending branch of lateral circumflex femoral
- ▢ **D.** Medial circumflex femoral
- ▢ **E.** Radicular branches of circumflex artery

103 A 72-year-old woman is admitted to the emergency department after an episode of stroke. During neurologic examination the patient shows no response to the ankle reflex test. Which of the following nerve roots is responsible for this reflex?

- ▢ **A.** L2
- ▢ **B.** L3
- ▢ **C.** L4

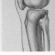

- D. L5
- E. S1

104 A 20-year-old man visits the family physician complaining of difficulty to flex and medially rotate his thigh while running and climbing. Which of the following muscles is most likely damaged in this individual?

- A. Rectus femoris
- B. Tensor fasciae latae
- C. Vastus intermedius
- D. Semimembranosus
- E. Sartorius

105 A 49-year-old man is admitted to the emergency department with a cold and pale foot. Physical examination reveals that the patient suffers from peripheral vascular disease; his popliteal artery is occluded and no pulse is felt upon palpation. What is the landmark to feel the pulse of the femoral artery?

- A. Adductor canal
- B. Femoral triangle
- C. Popliteal fossa
- D. Inguinal canal
- E. Pubic symphysis

106 A 49-year-old man is admitted to the emergency department complaining that he has difficulties walking. Physical examination reveals that the patient suffers from peripheral vascular disease. An ultrasound examination reveals an occlusion of his femoral artery at the proximal portion of the adductor canal. Which of the following arteries will most likely provide collateral circulation to the thigh?

- A. Descending branch of the lateral circumflex femoral
- B. Descending genicular
- C. Medial circumflex femoral
- D. First perforating branch of deep femoral
- E. Obturator artery

107 A 34-year-old man is lifting heavy weights while doing squats. Unfortunately, while making a maximal effort, he drops the weight and immediately grabs at his upper thigh, writhing in pain. The man is admitted to the emergency department and during physical examination is diagnosed with a femoral hernia. What reference structure would be found immediately lateral to the herniated structures?

- A. Femoral vein
- B. Femoral artery
- C. Pectineus muscle
- D. Femoral nerve
- E. Adductor longus muscle

108 A 25-year-old man, an intravenous drug abuser, had been injecting himself with temazepam (a powerful intermediate acting drug in the same group as diazepam (Valium) and heroin for 5 years, leaving much residual scar tissue over points of vascular access. The patient is admitted to the emergency department for a detoxification program requiring an intravenous infusion. The femoral veins in his groin are the only accessible and patent veins for intravenous use. Which of the following landmarks is the most reliable to identify the femoral veins?

- A. The femoral vein lies medial to the femoral artery.
- B. The femoral vein lies within the femoral canal.
- C. The femoral vein lies lateral to the femoral artery.
- D. The femoral vein lies directly medial to the femoral nerve.
- E. The femoral vein lies lateral to the femoral nerve.

109 A 42-year-old man is bitten on his posterior thigh by a dog. The superficial wound is sutured in the emergency department. Four days later the patient returns to the hospital with high fever and swollen lymph nodes. Which group of nodes first receives lymph from the infected wound?

- A. External iliac
- B. Vertical group of superficial inguinal
- C. Deep inguinal
- D. Horizontal group of superficial inguinal
- E. Internal iliac

110 During a battle, a 19-year-old soldier is shot in the lateral aspect of the right foot by a bullet that ricocheted off a building. The soldier is taken to a field hospital. A radiograph of the foot reveals that the base of the fifth metatarsal was completely obliterated. Which of the following muscles is most likely affected by this injury?

- A. Tibialis anterior
- B. Fibularis (peroneus) longus
- C. Gastrocnemius
- D. Fibularis (peroneus) brevis
- E. Extensor hallucis longus

111 A 29-year-old woman is involved in a car crash and is taken to the emergency department. Radiographs reveal a fracture of her pelvis. During healing of the pelvic fracture, a nerve becomes entrapped in the bone callus. Musculoskeletal examination reveals an inability to adduct the thigh. Which of the following nerves is most likely affected?

- ☐ **A.** Obturator
- ☐ **B.** Femoral
- ☐ **C.** Inferior gluteal
- ☐ **D.** Superior gluteal
- ☐ **E.** Tibial

112 A 29-year-old man is brought to the physician for removal of a cast from his left leg. He had sustained a fracture of the left lower extremity 6 weeks prior which was immobilized in a cast that extended from just below the knee to the foot. At the time of injury, there was severe pain but normal strength in the extremity. When the cast was removed, physical examination showed a pronounced left foot drop with paresthesia and sensory loss over the dorsum of the left foot and lateral leg. Injury to which nerve is the most likely cause?

- ☐ **A.** Common fibular (peroneal)
- ☐ **B.** Superficial fibular (peroneal)
- ☐ **C.** Deep fibular (peroneal)
- ☐ **D.** Sciatic
- ☐ **E.** Tibial

113 A 12-year-old boy is brought to the physician by his father because of redness and swelling of his left foot for 24 hours. Three days earlier he had scraped his foot while wading in a drainage ditch. Examination of the foot shows a purulent abrasion with edema, erythema, and tenderness on the lateral side. Infection will most likely spread from the lateral side of the foot to the regional lymph nodes in which area?

- ☐ **A.** Lateral surface of the thigh
- ☐ **B.** Medial malleolus, posteriorly
- ☐ **C.** Popliteal fossa
- ☐ **D.** Sole of the foot
- ☐ **E.** Superficial inguinal area

114 A 22-year-old soccer player collides with one of her teammates. During examination on the field, the posterior drawer test was performed and the tibia moved backward in relation to her femur. Injury to which structure is confirmed by performing this test?

- ☐ **A.** Anterior cruciate ligament
- ☐ **B.** Lateral collateral ligament
- ☐ **C.** Medial collateral ligament
- ☐ **D.** Medial meniscus
- ☐ **E.** Posterior cruciate ligament

115 A 16-year-old boy presents to the emergency department with a fracture of the first and second toes of his right foot. He received an anesthetic injection in the first web space of his foot, to permit easy manipulation and correction. Which nerve was blocked by the anesthesia?

- ☐ **A.** Saphenous
- ☐ **B.** Cutaneous branch of deep fibular (peroneal)
- ☐ **C.** Cutaneous branch of superficial fibular (peroneal)
- ☐ **D.** Sural
- ☐ **E.** Common fibular (peroneal)

116 During an interview, a 30-year-old man who is a psychiatric patient suddenly becomes aggressive. In order to calm him down, the patient is given an intramuscular injection in the upper lateral quadrant of the buttock. The injection is given at this specific location to prevent damage to which of the following nerves?

- ☐ **A.** Lateral femoral cutaneous
- ☐ **B.** Sciatic
- ☐ **C.** Superior gluteal
- ☐ **D.** Obturator
- ☐ **E.** Inferior gluteal

117 A lateral blow to the knee during a tackle in a football game injures a 24-year-old woman. Field examination reveals an "anterior drawer sign." An MRI demonstrates injury to several structures of the knee, including her medial meniscus. Which structure might also have been injured by the tackle?

- ☐ **A.** Medial collateral ligament
- ☐ **B.** Lateral collateral ligament
- ☐ **C.** Lateral meniscus
- ☐ **D.** Posterior cruciate ligament
- ☐ **E.** Tendon of the semitendinosus

118 A 58-year-old woman presents to the outpatient surgery clinic for removal of varicose veins on the medial aspect of her foot. The operation was successful however, one month later she reports loss of sensation over the medial aspect of her leg and foot. Which of the following nerves was most likely injured during the procedure?

- ☐ **A.** Saphenous
- ☐ **B.** Obturator

- ☐ **C.** Lateral femoral cutaneous
- ☐ **D.** Tibial
- ☐ **E.** Femoral

119 A 16-year-old teenage girl suffered an inversion sprain of her ankle during dance class. Physical examination in the clinic most likely reveals severe tenderness over which ligament?

- ☐ **A.** Calcaneonavicular (spring)
- ☐ **B.** Calcaneofibular
- ☐ **C.** Long plantar
- ☐ **D.** Short plantar
- ☐ **E.** Deltoid

120 A 58-year-old man visited his physician for his annual check-up. Physical examination reveals a hyper reflexive patellar reflex. Which muscle(s) contribute(s) to the tendon that is struck when testing this reflex?

- ☐ **A.** Quadriceps femoris
- ☐ **B.** Quadratus femoris
- ☐ **C.** Sartorius
- ☐ **D.** Pectineus
- ☐ **E.** Biceps femoris

121 A 37-year-old unconscious man is rushed to the emergency department after being retrieved from a motor vehicle crash. On physical examination bruising and obvious deformity is seen over his left knee joint. Radiological studies showed a posteriorly dislocated supracondylar fracture with severe compression of the popliteal artery. Which of the following arteries would ensure adequate blood supply to the leg and foot in this patient?

- ☐ **A.** Medial femoral circumflex
- ☐ **B.** Lateral femoral circumflex
- ☐ **C.** Anterior tibial artery
- ☐ **D.** Posterior tibial artery
- ☐ **E.** Fibular (peroneal) artery

122 After a revascularization procedure involving the common iliac artery, a 68-year-old man has difficulty walking. Nerve conduction studies reveal decreased activity in the nerve that innervates the adductors of the thigh. Which nerve is this?

- ☐ **A.** Femoral
- ☐ **B.** Obturator
- ☐ **C.** Common fibular (peroneal)
- ☐ **D.** Tibial
- ☐ **E.** Sciatic

123 A 23-year-old woman was taken to the emergency department after being involved in a head-on collision with a truck. On physical examination a hematoma was seen in the medial thigh. A CT scan revealed a fracture of the femur with a ruptured femoral artery. She was taken to the operating room for repair of the damaged structures. Two days postoperatively during physical examination the patient has loss of sensation to the anterior medial thigh and medial side of her leg and foot. Branches of which of the following nerves were most likely injured in the repair of the fracture?

- ☐ **A.** Femoral
- ☐ **B.** Saphenous
- ☐ **C.** Obturator
- ☐ **D.** Tibial
- ☐ **E.** Fibular (peroneal)

124 A 27-year-old man has had increasing difficulty walking and complained of an area of numbness on the dorsum of his right foot. Examination reveals a hard mass at the anterolateral aspect of his right leg just below the knee. Imaging studies reveal a large bone tumor between the fibula and tibia that is compressing a nerve, accounting for his neurological symptoms. Which of the following is the most likely description of abnormalities on neurological examination?

- ☐ **A.** Decreased/absent knee jerk reflex and decreased sensation on the medial aspect of the leg
- ☐ **B.** Weakness of flexion at the knee and decreased sensation of the plantar aspect of the foot
- ☐ **C.** Weakness of eversion at the ankle and decreased sensation between the first and second toes
- ☐ **D.** Weakness of inversion, dorsiflexion at the ankle, and decreased sensation between the first and second toes
- ☐ **E.** Weakness of plantar flexion at the ankle, weakness of toe flexion, decreased sensation of the plantar aspect of the foot

125 A 60-year-old retired male marathon runner complains to his primary care physician that during his daily morning jog he experiences bouts of numbness and tingling on the medial aspect of his heel. Upon further examination the doctor discovers the patient has trouble tiptoeing and shows a positive Tinel's sign. Which of the following conditions is most characteristic of these symptoms?

- ☐ **A.** Plantar fasciitis
- ☐ **B.** Ankle inversion sprain

- ▢ **C.** Morton's neuroma
- ▢ **D.** Lateral ligament
- ▢ **E.** Tarsal tunnel syndrome

126 A 50-year-old diabetic man presents for a routine wellness checkup. During physical examination it is noted that he has paraesthesia in a classic glove and stocking distribution. The physician decides on a complete peripheral vascular system examination, which includes palpating the pulse of the dorsalis pedis. Where can the dorsalis pedis pulse be palpated?

- ▢ **A.** Between the tendons of extensor hallucis and extensor digitorum longus on the dorsum of the foot
- ▢ **B.** Superior to flexor hallucis longus just distal to the tarsal tunnel
- ▢ **C.** Inferolateral to the pubic symphysis and medial to the deep dorsal vein of the penis
- ▢ **D.** 2 cm anterior to the medial malleolus
- ▢ **E.** 2 cm posterior to the medial malleolus

127 A 43-year-old victim of a drunk driving car crash is undergoing reconstructive arm surgery. The surgeon performs an autograft using a weak adductor of the leg located superficially on the medial side of the thigh. Which muscle is most likely being harvested to perform this reconstruction?

- ▢ **A.** Gracilis
- ▢ **B.** Sartorius
- ▢ **C.** Rectus femoris
- ▢ **D.** Vastus lateralis
- ▢ **E.** Vastus medialis

128 A 39-year-old woman who is a school teacher unwittingly sits on a thumbtack a student placed on her chair. Her left buttock becomes painful and inflamed. Which group of nodes will first receive lymph from the infected wound?

- ▢ **A.** Superficial horizontal group
- ▢ **B.** Superficial vertical group
- ▢ **C.** Superior and inferior gluteal nodes
- ▢ **D.** External iliac
- ▢ **E.** Deep inguinal

129 During a 100-meter sprint a 25-year-old male Olympic athlete suddenly pulls up in discomfort and is seen to be clutching the back of his left thigh in agony. Upon further examination the athlete describes the pain as a "tearing" sensation and is unable to flex his knee. Based on these symptoms which of the following actions are affected due to this injury?

- ▢ **A.** Flexion of the hip and extension of the knee
- ▢ **B.** Extension of the hip and dorsiflexion
- ▢ **C.** Medial rotation of the hip
- ▢ **D.** Lateral rotation of the hip
- ▢ **E.** Hip extension and knee flexion

130 During a gymnastic session, a 24-year-old woman suddenly developed pain and swelling on the right buttock. This happened following a forceful thigh movement. There is severe weakness of right hip extension and knee flexion. Adduction of the thigh is also slightly weak. An avulsion fracture of the ischial tuberosity is found on a radiograph. Which of the following group of muscles has most likely involved in this process?

- ▢ **A.** Adductor brevis, adductor longus, adductor magnus, pectineus, and gracilis
- ▢ **B.** Biceps femoris, semimembranosus, semitendinosus, and adductor magnus
- ▢ **C.** Iliacus and psoas major
- ▢ **D.** Gluteus medius and gluteus minimus
- ▢ **E.** Gluteus maximus and adductor magnus
- ▢ **F.** Iliacus, psoas major, rectus femoris and sartorius

131 A 6-year-old boy with a family history of muscular disease leading to wheelchair dependency in his maternal uncles presents with difficulty in standing from the seated position. He bends forward, uses his hands to help him push up from the floor, and then straightens his knees to stand. Which of the following muscles is most likely involved by this disease process?

- ▢ **A.** Tibialis posterior and gastrocnemius
- ▢ **B.** Quadratus femoris
- ▢ **C.** Gluteus medius and gluteus minimus
- ▢ **D.** Gluteus maximus
- ▢ **E.** Hamstrings
- ▢ **F.** Iliopsoas

132 A 43-year-old woman receives deep intramuscular injections for the past week for treatment of a sexually transmitted disease. She complains to her doctor that she has difficulty walking. During physical examination her right hip drops every time she raises her right foot. Which of the following injection locations will most likely correspond with the clinical presentation of this patient?

- ▢ **A.** Superomedial quadrant of the buttock
- ▢ **B.** Superolateral quadrant of the buttock
- ▢ **C.** Inferomedial quadrant of the buttock

- ▢ **D.** Inferolateral quadrant of the buttock
- ▢ **E.** Posterior thigh

133 A 22-year-old male professional football player is admitted to the emergency department with acute right knee pain after sustaining a kick injury to an extended leg. A radiograph and a subsequent MRI revealed that the trauma caused anterior displacement of the tibia with respect to her femur. Which of the following ligaments was most likely injured?

- ▢ **A.** Fibular (lateral) collateral
- ▢ **B.** Tibial (medial) collateral
- ▢ **C.** Patellar
- ▢ **D.** Anterior cruciate
- ▢ **E.** Posterior cruciate
- ▢ **F.** Oblique popliteal

134 A 51-year-old immigrant with tuberculosis is found to have large flocculent masses over the lateral lumbar spine. There is a similar mass located in the ipsilateral groin. Physical examination reveals increased tenderness just medial to the ipsilateral anterior superior iliac spine on palpation. This pattern of involvement most likely suggests an abscess tracking along which of the following muscles?

- ▢ **A.** Piriformis
- ▢ **B.** Psoas major
- ▢ **C.** Adductor longus
- ▢ **D.** Gluteus maximus
- ▢ **E.** Obturator internus

135 A 23-year-old man is taken to the emergency department because of anorexia, nausea, vomiting, and severe abdominal pain in the right lower quadrant. On examination, he has tenderness in the right lower quadrant with rebound tenderness. The physician suspects appendicitis. To confirm this diagnosis, the physician attempts to straighten the patient's flexed thigh. This causes the patient to wince with pain. Which of the following muscles most likely caused this symptom?

- ▢ **A.** Adductor magnus
- ▢ **B.** Psoas major
- ▢ **C.** Biceps femoris
- ▢ **D.** Obturator internus
- ▢ **E.** Gluteus maximus

136 A 60-year-old man presents with pain on the medial aspect of his thigh. During physical examination he describes the pain to be constant, nonradiating and he also complains of numbness on the medial aspect of his leg and medial plantar arch. The nerve involved in this patient's numbness is closely associated with a structure with which of the following characteristics?

- ▢ **A.** Empties into the popliteal vein
- ▢ **B.** In its ascent in the medial aspect of the leg, it travels posterior to the medial condyle of the femur
- ▢ **C.** In its ascent in the medial aspect of the leg, it travels anterior to the medial condyle of the femur
- ▢ **D.** Arches posterior to the medial malleolus
- ▢ **E.** Is associated with nodes that drain to the horizontal group of inguinal nodes

137 A 56-year-old diabetic man complains of repeated injury and ulcers to his right big toe. He also complains that he finds it difficult maintaining his shoes because the tips of the shoes around the toe area easily wear down. He also complains that for a while now, his first two toes "feel funny." He used to enjoy playing soccer on weekends but has found it difficult to be involved. Which of the following nerves is most likely affected?

- ▢ **A.** Superior gluteal nerve injury
- ▢ **B.** Inferior gluteal nerve injury
- ▢ **C.** Deep fibular (peroneal) nerve injury
- ▢ **D.** Superficial fibular (peroneal) nerve injury
- ▢ **E.** Common fibular (peroneal) nerve injury

138 A 30-year-old man who is a bodybuilder presents to the physician's office complaining of pain and tingling sensation radiating down the inside of his thigh that was exacerbated upon thigh movement. A hernia through which opening would most likely cause this presentation?

- ▢ **A.** Femoral ring
- ▢ **B.** Superficial inguinal ring
- ▢ **C.** Deep inguinal ring
- ▢ **D.** Fossa ovalis
- ▢ **E.** Obturator canal

139 After suffering a deep stab wound to her posterior thigh, a 22-year-old woman presents to the emergency department. The wound is closed but the patient develops a subsequent wound infection. Which group of lymph nodes first receives drainage from this deep wound area, and would most likely be enlarged in this patient?

- ▢ **A.** External iliac
- ▢ **B.** Superficial inguinal
- ▢ **C.** Deep inguinal
- ▢ **D.** Common iliac
- ▢ **E.** Internal iliac

140 A 29-year-old construction worker falls onto some rusty wire mesh and suffers a deep laceration to his right buttock. When the ambulance arrives to transport him to the emergency department and it is noted that he has difficulty stepping up into the ambulance with his right leg. Which nerve has probably been damaged?

- ☐ **A.** Superior gluteal
- ☐ **B.** Tibial
- ☐ **C.** Common fibular (peroneal)
- ☐ **D.** Inferior gluteal
- ☐ **E.** Nerve to piriformis

141 A 69-year-old woman, who fell down the stairs, presents to the emergency department. Radiologic imaging reveals a fracture of the talocrural (tibiotalar) joint. Which movements take place at this joint?

- ☐ **A.** Plantar flexion and dorsiflexion
- ☐ **B.** Inversion and eversion
- ☐ **C.** Plantar flexion, dorsiflexion, inversion, and eversion
- ☐ **D.** Plantar flexion and inversion
- ☐ **E.** Dorsiflexion and eversion

142 After being struck from behind by a motor vehicle, a 55-year-old man presents to the hospital with a swelling of his right knee. Imaging reveals a large hematoma of the popliteal artery compressing his tibial nerve. Upon neurologic examination which movement would likely be diminished in strength?

- ☐ **A.** Dorsiflexion of the foot
- ☐ **B.** Flexion of the thigh
- ☐ **C.** Extension of the digits
- ☐ **D.** Extension of the leg
- ☐ **E.** Plantar flexion of the foot

143 A lateral blow to the knee during a tackle in a football game injures a 24-year-old woman. Field examination reveals an "anterior drawer sign." An MRI demonstrates injury to several structures of the knee, including her medial meniscus. Which structure might also have been injured by the tackle?

- ☐ **A.** Medial collateral ligament
- ☐ **B.** Lateral collateral ligament
- ☐ **C.** Lateral meniscus
- ☐ **D.** Posterior cruciate ligament
- ☐ **E.** Tendon of the semitendinosus

144 A 50-year-old woman is admitted to the emergency department complaining of painful swelling to the left leg, fever, and malaise for 2 days. The patient has a history of type 2 diabetes mellitus, and she was bitten on the left leg by an insect a week before presentation. She scratched the pruritic area and applied alcohol to the site when the swelling increased; a purulent fluid began to drain from it 2 days later. During physical examination, the patient was febrile (40° C) with 5 × 5 cm tender, fluctuant swelling over the anterolateral aspect of the middle third of the left leg, which drained copious amounts of purulent fluid. Which of the following findings is most likely to be also present during physical examination of this patient?

- ☐ **A.** Tender vertical group of superficial inguinal lymph nodes
- ☐ **B.** Enlarged horizontal group of superficial inguinal lymph nodes
- ☐ **C.** Enlarged group of deep inguinal lymph nodes
- ☐ **D.** Enlarged popliteal lymph nodes
- ☐ **E.** Enlarged iliac nodes

145 A 30-year-old woman was admitted to the emergency department after being involved in a motor vehicle crash. The patient complained of pain to the right hip and knee. During physical examination, there is no deformity of the lower limb, but there is tenderness over the right ischiopubic ramus. Pelvic radiographs revealed an inferiorly displaced fracture of the right superior and inferior pubic rami with dislocation of the right sacroiliac joint and pubic symphysis. The patient was referred to the orthopedics team, which had a high suspicion of rupture of the right obturator membrane. What clinical findings are most likely to be present in this patient?

- ☐ **A.** Urinary and fecal incontinence and diminished sensation over the perineum
- ☐ **B.** Weak adduction of the hip and diminished sensation over the upper medial thigh
- ☐ **C.** Weak abduction of the hip and positive Trendelenburg sign
- ☐ **D.** Weak flexion of the hip and diminished sensation over the anterior thigh and medial leg
- ☐ **E.** Weak extension of the hip and diminished sensation over the posterior thigh

146 A 32-year-old man is brought to the emergency department with complaints of pain to the left ankle and knee. The patient recalls that during a football game, his left foot landed in a hole as he was running on an uneven dirt field. The ankle was externally rotated and everted while the knee twisted medially. He was unable to bear weight subsequently. During physical examination, the right ankle is swollen and there is exquisite tenderness over the right medial malleolus and the proximal lateral leg. Radiologic examination of the right lower limb reveals a displaced fracture of the neck of right fibula and a comminuted fracture of the tibial plafond and medial malleolus. Which of the following describes the most likely consequences of this injury?

- ▢ **A.** Weak "push-off" while walking and numbness over the posteromedial leg
- ▢ **B.** Weak ankle eversion and numbness over the dorsum of the foot
- ▢ **C.** High stepping gait and numbness over the dorsum and first web space of the foot
- ▢ **D.** Waddling gait and inability to feel a pin prick over the anterolateral leg
- ▢ **E.** Swing-out gait and numbness over the medial leg

147 A 40-year-old man was brought to the emergency department after being struck by a car. He complained of pain to the left knee and leg and inability to bear weight on the affected limb. On examination, there was a joint effusion of the left knee, and tenderness over the medial and lateral side of the joint. A valgus stress test was positive while the varus stress test was negative. An MRI of the left knee showed complete disruption of multiple ligament support structures of the knee. What other symptoms are most likely possible in this patient?

- ▢ **A.** Inability to extend the knee
- ▢ **B.** Inability to flex the knee
- ▢ **C.** Instability of the knee when walking down a flight of stairs
- ▢ **D.** Instability of the knee when walking up a flight of stairs
- ▢ **E.** Excessive extension of the knee and difficulty walking down stairs

148 A 19-year-old woman is admitted to the emergency department with complaints of pain and swelling to the right ankle. In a recent volleyball game she jumped to spike the ball then landed on the opponent's shoe with her right foot. She recalls hearing a loud "pop" and felt immediate pain to the ankle. She was unable to bear weight subsequently. On examination, the right ankle was swollen, with maximal tenderness inferior and anterior to the lateral malleolus. Radiographs of the ankle showed no fractures. Which of the following structures were most likely injured?

- ▢ **A.** Posterior talofibular ligament
- ▢ **B.** Interosseous ligament between the tibia and fibula
- ▢ **C.** Tibionavicular ligament
- ▢ **D.** Anterior tibiofibular ligament
- ▢ **E.** Calcaneofibular ligament

149 A 30-year-old woman is admitted to the emergency department with complaints of pain to the anterior left thigh. While participating in a 100-meter race, she felt a sudden onset of pain in the anterior midthigh area and could only limp to the finish line. Physical examination revealed a swollen, tender right thigh anteriorly. Extension of the knee was limited due to pain. Ultrasonography of the area revealed a defect in the fibers of the quadriceps muscle, confirmed by CT scan of the limb. Which of the following is the embryologic origin of the affected structure?

- ▢ **A.** Lateral plate mesoderm
- ▢ **B.** Dorsolateral migration of neural crest cells
- ▢ **C.** Preceded the development of chondrification centers
- ▢ **D.** Intermediate mesoderm
- ▢ **E.** Migration of cells from paraxial mesoderm

150 A 23-year-old woman delivered a live male infant at 37 weeks' gestation after an uneventful pregnancy. Examination of the infant revealed the right second and third toes were fused. Radiographs of the right foot indicated 14 phalanges in their correct position. After review by the pediatric orthopedic surgeon, corrective surgery for the deformity was scheduled. Which of the following embryologic conditions explains the infant's condition?

- ▢ **A.** The digital ray for the third toe did not develop
- ▢ **B.** Excessive neural crest cell migration into the foot
- ▢ **C.** Incomplete apoptosis of tissue between digital rays
- ▢ **D.** Lack of signal from the zone of polarizing activity (ZPA)
- ▢ **E.** Faulty development of chondrification centers

151 A 30-year-old man was brought to the emergency department after his involvement in a motor vehicle crash. He complained of pain in the right knee and an inability to bear weight. On examination, there were minor abrasions about his body, in addition to a deep, 5 cm oblique laceration over the anterior right knee, which exposed the patella. He was unable to extend the right knee. Radiographs revealed a displaced transverse fracture of the inferior pole of the patella. The superior fragment of the patella appeared to be "high riding" over the anterior surface of the femur. Which of the following most likely occurred?

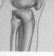

- ▢ **A.** Blood and fat from the injury can enter the popliteus bursa
- ▢ **B.** Blood and fat from the injury can enter the suprapatellar bursa
- ▢ **C.** Joint fluid can enter the subcutaneous infrapatellar bursa
- ▢ **D.** The deep infrapatellar bursa will be affected
- ▢ **E.** The gastrocnemius bursa will not be affected

152 A 53-year-old woman reports difficulty in walking. Physical examination showed a positive Trendelenburg sign when she is asked to stand on her right leg. Which nerve has been compromised to produce the positive sign?

- ▢ **A.** Sciatic
- ▢ **B.** Right superior gluteal
- ▢ **C.** Left inferior gluteal
- ▢ **D.** Left superior gluteal
- ▢ **E.** Right inferior gluteal

153 A 45-year-old man is admitted to the emergency department after a fall and subsequent leg injury. On physical examination the patient has a foot drop but eversion is unaffected. Which nerve is most likely injured?

- ▢ **A.** Tibial
- ▢ **B.** Common fibular (peroneal)
- ▢ **C.** Superficial fibular (peroneal)
- ▢ **D.** Saphenous
- ▢ **E.** Deep fibular (peroneal)

154 A 48-year-old man comes to the physician because of severe back pain for 2 days. The pain radiates down to the buttock, posterior thigh, and posterolateral leg. He also has numbness on the lateral side of his left foot. On physical examination sensation to pain is decreased over the lateral side of the left foot. Deep tendon reflexes are absent at the left ankle, and there is a weakness of dorsiflexion of the left foot. Compression of which of the following nerve roots is the most likely cause of these findings?

- ▢ **A.** T12
- ▢ **B.** L2
- ▢ **C.** L4
- ▢ **D.** S1
- ▢ **E.** S3

155 A 45-year-old man after being diagnosed with a posterior acetabular fracture is taken to the operating room to repair the fracture. During the neurological examination the physician notices loss of sensation to the skin of the inferior half of the buttocks, posterior, and upper medial thigh. The patient had a normal neurovascular examination preoperatively. Which of the following nerves was mostly likely damaged during the operation?

- ▢ **A.** Posterior femoral cutaneous
- ▢ **B.** Obturator nerve
- ▢ **C.** Sciatic
- ▢ **D.** Femoral
- ▢ **E.** Lateral femoral cutaneous

156 A 30-year-old woman is admitted to the emergency department with complaints of pain to the anterior left thigh. While participating in a 100-meter race, she felt a sudden onset of pain in the anterior midthigh area and could only limp to the finish line. Physical examination revealed a swollen, tender right thigh anteriorly. Extension of the knee was limited due to pain. Ultrasonography of the area revealed a defect in the fibers of the quadriceps muscle, confirmed by CT scan of the limb. Which of the following is the embryologic origin of the affected structure?

- ▢ **A.** Lateral plate mesoderm
- ▢ **B.** Dorsolateral migration of neural crest cells
- ▢ **C.** Preceded the development of chondrification centers
- ▢ **D.** Intermediate mesoderm
- ▢ **E.** Migration of cells from paraxial mesoderm

157 A 32-year-old man was brought to the emergency with complaints of pain to the left ankle and leg. During a game of football, his left foot landed in a hole as he was running on an uneven dirt field. He was unable subsequently bear weight on his left limb. On examination, the right ankle was swollen, with exquisite tenderness over the right medial malleolus and over the distal third of the lateral right leg. Radiographs of the right lower limb revealed an inferiorly displaced fracture of the right medial malleolus and a spiral fracture of the distal third of the right fibula. Which of the following describes the most likely mechanism of this injury?

- ▢ **A.** Forceful inversion of the ankle
- ▢ **B.** Direct upward force from the talus into the tibial plafond
- ▢ **C.** Forceful external rotation and eversion of the ankle
- ▢ **D.** Forceful dorsiflexion of the foot
- ▢ **E.** Extreme plantar flexion of the foot

158 A 15-year-old boy falls and injures his ankle while skateboarding. Examination in the emergency department leads to the conclusion that the ankle is mildly sprained, and it is wrapped with an elastic bandage. The boy still complains of pain in his ankle. Which of the following peripheral nerves is involved in carrying pain sensation from the ankle?

- ☐ **A.** Deep fibular (peroneal)
- ☐ **B.** Femoral
- ☐ **C.** Obturator
- ☐ **D.** Posterior femoral cutaneous
- ☐ **E.** Sural

ANSWERS

1 A. The lumbosacral trunk consists of fibers from a portion of the ventral ramus of L4 and all of the ventral ramus of L5 and provides continuity between the lumbar and sacral plexuses. The deep fibular (peroneal) nerve receives supply from segments of L4, L5, and S1. It supplies the extensor hallucis longus and extensor digitorum longus, the main functions of which are extension of the toes and dorsiflexion of the ankle. L5 is responsible for cutaneous innervation of the dorsum of the foot. Injury to L4 would affect foot inversion by the tibialis anterior. Injury to L4 in the lumbosacral trunk would not affect the patellar tendon reflex, for these fibers are delivered by the femoral nerve. Therefore, an injury to the lumbosacral trunk would result in all of the patient's symptoms. Nerve root injury at L5 and S1 would result in loss of sensation of the plantar aspect of the foot and motor loss of plantar flexion, with weakness of hip extension and abduction. The fibularis (peroneus) longus and brevis are supplied by the superficial fibular (peroneal) nerve, which is composed of fibers from segments L5, S1, and S2; these are responsible for eversion of the foot (especially S1). Transection of the fibular (peroneal) division of the sciatic nerve would result in loss of function of all the muscles of the anterior and lateral compartments of the leg. Injury to the sciatic nerve will affect hamstring muscles and all of the muscles below the knee. Injury to the tibial nerve causes loss of plantar flexion and impaired inversion.

GAS 486-487, 563; N 484; McM 271

2 A. The ventral ramus of L4 contains both sensory and motor nerve fibers. Injury from a stab wound could result in loss of sensation from the dermatome supplied by this segment. A dermatome is an area of skin supplied by a single spinal nerve; L4 dermatome supplies the medial aspect of the leg and foot. Loss of the Achilles tendon reflex relates primarily to an S1 deficit. The Achilles tendon reflex is elicited by tapping the calcaneus tendon, which results in plantar flexion. The obturator internus and gluteus medius and minimus are responsible for abduction of the thigh and are innervated by nerves L4, L5, and S1 (with L5 usually dominant). Nerves L5, S1, and S2 are responsible for eversion of the foot (S1 dominant) (*GAS* Fig. 6-16).

GAS 34-35; N 383; McM 285

3 B. Injury to the superior gluteal nerve results in a characteristic motor loss, with paralysis of the gluteus

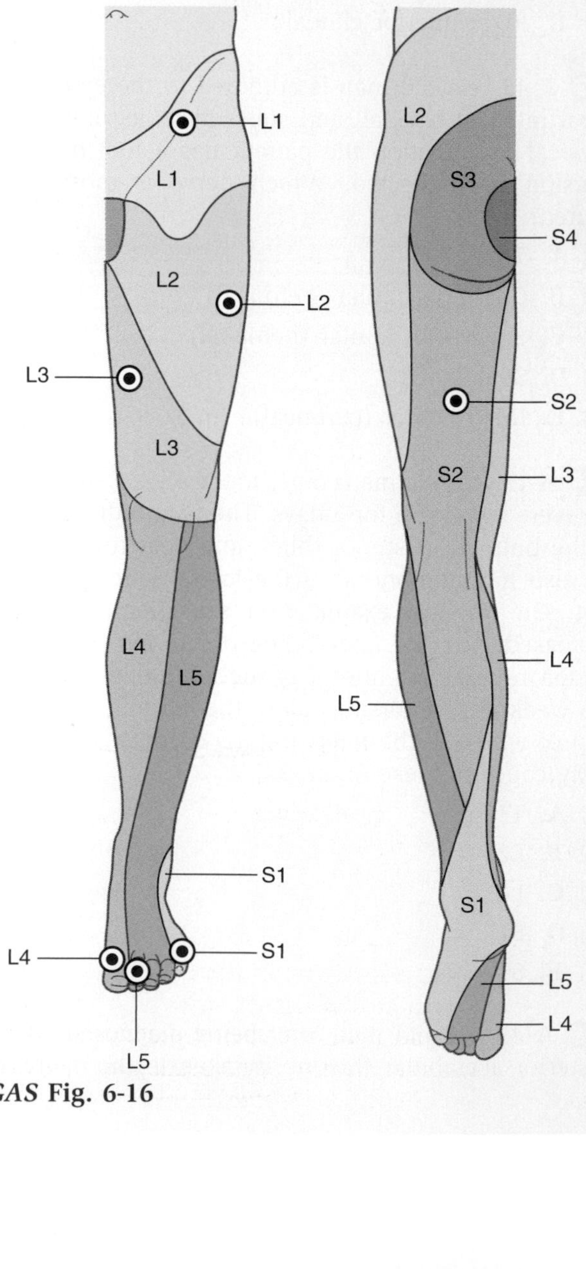

***GAS* Fig. 6-16**

medius and minimus. In addition to their role in abducting the thigh, the gluteus medius and minimus function to stabilize the pelvis. When the patient is asked to stand on the limb of the injured side, the pelvis descends on the opposite side, indicating a positive Trendelenburg test. The gluteal, or lurching, gait that results from this injury is characterized by the pelvis drooping to the unaffected side when the opposite leg is raised. In stepping forward, the affected individual leans over the injured side when lifting the good limb off the ground. The uninjured limb is then swung forward. The gluteus maximus, supplied by the inferior gluteal nerve, is the main muscle responsible for allowing a person to rise to a standing position (extending the flexed hip). Spinal nerve roots L1 and L2 and the femoral nerve are responsible for hip flexion. Injury to the left superior gluteal nerve would result in sagging of the right side of the pelvis when the affected individual stands on the left limb. The hamstring muscles, mainly responsible for flexing the knees to allow a person to sit down from a standing position, are innervated by the tibial branch of the sciatic nerve.

GAS 454, 492, 564, 579; N 489; McM 317

4 E. The deep fibular (peroneal) nerve is responsible for innervating the muscles of the anterior compartment of the leg, which are responsible for toe extension, foot dorsiflexion, and inversion. Injury to this nerve will result in foot drop and also loss of sensation between the first and second toes. Injury to the tibial nerve affects the posterior compartment muscles of the leg, which are responsible for plantar flexion and toe flexion, as well as the intrinsic muscles of the sole of the foot. The common fibular (peroneal) nerve splits into the superficial and deep fibular (peroneal) nerves, and these supply both the lateral and anterior compartments. The superficial fibular (peroneal) nerve innervates the fibularis (peroneus) longus and brevis muscles, which provide eversion of the foot. If the common fibular (peroneal) nerve were injured, eversion of the foot and plantar flexion would be lost in addition to dorsiflexion and inversion. The saphenous nerve, a continuation of the femoral nerve, is a cutaneous nerve that supplies the medial side of the leg and foot and provides no motor innervation.

GAS 627, 660; N 529; McM 337

5 A. The femoral ring is the abdominal opening of the femoral canal. A femoral hernia passes through the femoral ring into the femoral canal deep and inferior to the inguinal ligament. It can appear as a bulging at the saphenous hiatus (fossa ovalis) of the deep fascia of the thigh, the hiatus through which the saphenous vein passes to the femoral vein. The superficial inguinal ring is the triangular opening in the aponeurosis of the external abdominal oblique and lies lateral to the pubic tubercle. The deep inguinal ring lies in the transversalis fascia lateral to the inferior epigastric vessels. Herniation into either of these two openings is associated with an inguinal hernia. The obturator canal, a bony opening between the superior and inferior ramus of the pubic bone, is the site of an obturator hernia.

GAS 301, 545, 573; N 487; McM 225

6 A. The talocrural (tibiotalar, ankle) joint is a hinge-type synovial joint between the tibia and talus. It permits dorsiflexion and plantar flexion, and fracture of this joint would affect these movements.

GAS 635-645; N 514; McM 354

7 D. The piriformis muscle arises from the pelvic surface of the sacrum, passes through the greater sciatic notch, and inserts at the greater trochanter. It is considered the "anatomical key" to gluteal anatomy; the greater sciatic foramen is the "door." The gluteus medius lies posterior to the piriformis. The sciatic nerve emerges from the greater sciatic foramen, normally through the infrapiriformic space. The spine of the ischium separates the greater and lesser sciatic foramina.

GAS 426, 550, 575; N 490; McM 317

8 A. The popliteal lymph nodes are the first to receive lymph from the foot. These nodes will then drain into the deep inguinal nodes and then to the external iliac nodes. The superficial inguinal and internal iliac nodes do not receive lymph from the foot.

GAS 570-571; N 472; McM 340

9 E. The tibial nerve is responsible for innervating the posterior compartment of the leg. These muscles are responsible for knee flexion, plantar flexion, and intrinsic muscle functions of the foot. Compression of this nerve can affect plantar flexion of the foot. Dorsiflexion of the foot would be compromised if the deep fibular (peroneal) nerve were compressed by this Baker's cyst. Flexion of the thigh is a function of muscles supplied by lumbar nerves and the femoral nerve. The deep fibular (peroneal) nerve is also responsible for extension of the digits, whereas the femoral nerve is responsible for extension of the leg.

GAS 492, 545-549, 565; N 503; McM 331

10 A. The medial meniscus is firmly attached to the medial (tibial) collateral ligament. Damage to the medial collateral ligament often causes concomitant damage to the medial meniscus because of this relationship. The anterior cruciate ligament lies inside the knee joint capsule but outside the synovial cavity. It is taut during extension of the knee and may be torn when the knee is hyperextended. If this were damaged along with the medial meniscus and medial cruciate ligament, an "unhappy triad" (of O'Donoghue, or Donahue, both spellings are correct; also called a "blow knee") injury would result. The lateral meniscus is not attached to the medial collateral ligament but receives muscular attachment to the popliteus muscle. The posterior cruciate ligament also lies outside of the synovial cavity and limits hyperflexion of the knee. The tendon of the semitendinosus forms one third of the pes anserinus, with the tendons of the sartorius and gracilis making up the other two thirds. The pes anserinus (goose foot) is located at the medial border of the tibial tuberosity, and a portion can be used for surgical repair of the anterior cruciate ligament.

GAS 607-609; N 495; McM 332

11 D. The great saphenous vein is commonly used in coronary artery bypass grafts. Because branches of the saphenous nerve cross the vein in the distal part of the leg, the nerve can be damaged if the vein is stripped from the ankle to the knee. Stripping the vein in the opposite direction can protect the nerve and lessen the postoperative discomfort of patients. The saphenous nerve is responsible for cutaneous innervations on the medial surface of the leg and the medial side of the foot. Injury to this nerve will result in a loss of sensation and also can create chronic dysesthesias in the area. The common fibular (peroneal) nerve bifurcates at the neck of the fibula into the superficial and deep fibular (peroneal) nerves, which continue on to innervate the lateral and anterior compartments of the leg, respectively. These nerves are lateral and therefore not associated with the great saphenous vein. The lateral sural nerve is a cutaneous nerve that arises from the junction of branches from the common fibular (peroneal) nerve and tibial nerve and innervates the skin on the posterior aspect of the leg and lateral side of the foot. This nerve is often harvested for nerve grafts elsewhere in the body. The tibial nerve is a terminal branch of the sciatic nerve that continues deep in the posterior compartment of the leg.

GAS 550, 568, 603, 659; N 525; McM 338

12 B. The calcaneofibular ligament is a round cord that passes posteroinferiorly from the tip of the lateral malleolus to the lateral surface of the calcaneus. A forced inversion of the foot can result in tearing of the calcaneofibular ligament and sometimes the anterior talofibular ligament as well. Both of these ligaments act to stabilize the foot and prevent an inversion injury. The plantar calcaneonavicular ligament supports the head of the talus. The long plantar ligament passes from the planter surface of the calcaneus to the groove on the cuboid and is important in maintaining the longitudinal arch of the foot. The short plantar ligament is located deep (superior) to the long plantar ligament and extends from the calcaneus to the cuboid and is also involved in maintaining the longitudinal arch of the foot. The deltoid (medial ligament of the ankle) attaches proximally to the medial malleolus and fans out to reinforce the joint capsule of the ankle.

GAS 638; N 514; McM 349

13 B. The lateral circumflex femoral artery arises from the deep femoral (profunda femoris) artery of the thigh and sends a descending branch down the length of the femur to anastomose with the superior medial genicular artery and the superior lateral genicular artery. The medial circumflex femoral artery is responsible for supplying blood to the head and neck of the femur, and it does not anastomose with distal vessels at the knee. The first perforating artery sends an ascending branch that anastomoses with the medial circumflex femoral and the inferior gluteal artery in the buttock. The inferior gluteal artery is a branch of the internal iliac; it has important anastomotic supply to the hip joint. The typically small descending genicular branch of the femoral artery is given off just proximal to the continuation of the femoral artery as the popliteal.

GAS 589-599; N 491; McM 319

14 C. The medial circumflex femoral artery is responsible for supplying blood to the head and neck of the femur by a number of branches that pass under the edge of the ischiofemoral ligament. This artery is most likely at risk for injury in an extracapsular fracture of the femoral neck. The inferior gluteal artery arises from the internal iliac and enters the gluteal region through the greater sciatic foramen, below the piriformis. The first perforating artery sends an ascending branch that anastomoses with the inferior gluteal artery in the buttock. The obturator artery arises from the internal iliac artery and passes through the obturator foramen. It commonly supplies the artery within the ligament of the head of the femur but is not likely to be patent in a person of this age. The superior gluteal artery arises from the internal iliac artery and enters through the greater sciatic foramen above the piriformis.

GAS 589-591; N 491; McM 319

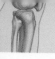

15 B. The obturator nerve arises from the lumbar plexus and enters the thigh through the obturator canal. This nerve is responsible for innervation of the medial compartment of the thigh (adductor compartment). Injury to this nerve can result in weakened adduction and difficulty walking. The femoral nerve innervates muscles of the anterior compartment of the thigh that are responsible for hip flexion and leg extension. The sciatic nerve branches into the common fibular (peroneal) and tibial nerves. The common fibular (peroneal) nerve branches into the deep and superficial branches of the fibular (peroneal) nerve responsible for innervation of the anterior and lateral compartments of the leg, respectively. The tibial nerve innervates the muscles of the posterior compartment of the thigh and leg, which are responsible for extension of the hip, flexion of the leg, and plantar flexion of the foot.

GAS 486, 500, 563-565; N 485; McM 261

16 B. The common fibular (peroneal) nerve winds around the neck of the fibula before dividing into superficial and deep branches that go on to innervate the lateral and anterior compartments of the leg, respectively. These compartments are responsible for dorsiflexion and eversion of the foot, and injury to these nerves would result in deficits in these movements. The tibial nerve lies superficially in the popliteal fossa. This nerve innervates the posterior compartment of the leg, so compression in this area would result in a loss of plantar flexion and weakness of inversion. The lateral compartment of the leg is innervated by the superficial fibular (peroneal) nerve and is mainly involved in eversion of the foot. The cutaneous branches of the superficial fibular (peroneal) nerve emerge through the deep fascia in the anterolateral aspect of the leg and supply the dorsum of the foot. The anterior compartment of the leg is innervated by the deep fibular (peroneal) nerve and is mainly involved in dorsiflexion of the foot. The medial malleolus is an inferiorly directed projection from the medial side of the distal end of the tibia. The tibial nerve runs near the groove behind the medial malleolus, and compression at this location would result in loss of toe flexion, adduction, abduction, and abduction of the great toe.

GAS 486, 550, 563-565, 607; N 529; McM 337

17 A. The gluteus maximus is innervated by the inferior gluteal nerve, and this muscle is responsible for extension and lateral rotation of the thigh. It is the primary muscle that extends the flexed hip and is used to rise from a seated position. The gluteus minimus is innervated by the superior gluteal nerve and is responsible for abduction of the thigh. Hamstring muscles are innervated by the tibial portion of the sciatic nerve, and these are responsible for extension of the thigh and flexion of the leg. The iliopsoas muscle is innervated by L1 and L2 and the femoral nerve, and flexes the thigh. The obturator internus is innervated by the nerve to the obturator internus and is a lateral rotator of the thigh.

GAS 572, 575; N 482; McM 316

18 B. The medial branch of the deep fibular (peroneal) nerve accompanies the dorsalis pedis artery and innervates the skin between the contiguous sides of the first and second toes. The saphenous nerve is responsible for cutaneous innervation of the anteromedial aspect of the leg and foot. The superficial fibular (peroneal) nerve innervates most of the dorsum of the foot, with the exception of the area where sensation was lost (medial branch of deep fibular nerve). The common fibular (peroneal) nerve gives off a cutaneous branch, the sural nerve, which innervates the lateral aspect of the leg and lateral side of the foot.

GAS 630, 659-660; N 508; McM 337

19 E. The posterior cruciate ligament is responsible for preventing the forward sliding of the femur on the tibia. The anterior cruciate ligament prevents posterior displacement of the femur on the tibia. The lateral collateral ligament limits extension and adduction of the leg. The medial meniscus acts as a shock absorber and cushions the articular surfaces of the knee joint.

GAS 584, 606; N 496; McM 332

20 D. The gluteus maximus inserts into the gluteal tuberosity and the iliotibial tract. Although the gluteus maximus would continue to contract at the regions of insertion, their orientation would be displaced by the fracture. The gluteus medius, gluteus minimus, obturator internus, and piriformis all insert on some aspect of the greater trochanter of the femur.

GAS 554-556; N 482; McM 295

21 B. The apex of the femoral triangle occurs at the junction of the adductor longus and sartorius muscles. The subsartorial (Hunter's) canal begins at this location. Immediately deep to this anatomic point lie the femoral artery, femoral vein, deep femoral artery, and deep femoral vein, often overlying one another in that sequence. This has historically been a site of injuries caused by slipping while handling a very sharp butcher's knife. For this reason, injuries at this location are referred to as the "butcher's block" injury. Fatal loss of blood can occur in just a few minutes if pressure, or a tourniquet, is not applied immediately. The common iliac artery becomes the femoral artery at the inguinal ligament. The saphenous vein joins the femoral vein at the saphenous hiatus, or fossa ovalis. The medial circumflex femoral usually arises from the deep femoral artery about 3 to 5 inches inferior to the inguinal ligament, near the origin of the deep femoral artery from the common femoral. Serious blood loss can occur with injury to any of these vessels, although injury to them is not often fatal.

GAS 535-537, 571; N 487; McM 320

22 C. The iliofemoral ligament ("inverted Y ligament of Bigelow") is the most important ligament reinforcing the joint anteriorly that would resist both hyperextension and lateral rotation at the hip joint. The pubofemoral ligament reinforces the joint inferiorly and limits extension and abduction. The ischiofemoral ligament reinforces the joint posteriorly and limits extension and medial rotation. Negative pressure in the acetabular fossa has nothing to do with resisting hyperextension of the hip joint but does help resist dislocation of the head of the femur. The gluteus maximus muscle extends and laterally rotates the thigh and does not particularly resist hyperextension.

GAS 558-561; N 474; McM 324

23 C. An intracapsular femoral neck fracture causes avascular necrosis of the femoral head because the fracture damages the radicular branches of the medial and lateral circumflex arteries that pass beneath the ischiofemoral ligament and pierce the femoral neck. Until an individual reaches about 6 to 10 years of age, blood supply to the head of the femur is provided by a branch of the obturator artery that runs with the ligament of the head of the femur. Thereafter, the artery of the ligament of the head of the femur is insignificant. Intertrochanteric fracture of the femur would not damage the blood supply to the head of the femur but would cause complications because the greater trochanter is an attachment site for several gluteal muscles. During childhood the obturator artery provides the artery of the ligament of the head of the femur. Thrombosis of the obturator artery could result in muscular symptoms, although there are several collateral sources of blood supply in the thigh. Comminuted fracture of the extracapsular femoral neck would not ordinarily imperil the vascular supply.

GAS 558-561, 676; N 491; McM 326

24 D. The farm instrument has injured the deep fibular (peroneal) branch of the common fibular (peroneal) nerve. It is vulnerable to injury as it arises from the common fibular (peroneal) at the neck of the fibula. The muscles denervated are largely dorsiflexors of the foot; hence, foot drop and a high stepping gait can occur. Sensation on the dorsum of the foot is still present; therefore, the superficial branch is mostly or entirely intact, although sensation between the first and second toes would be absent. Femoral nerve injury would result in loss of knee extension. Loss of the sciatic nerve would result in loss of both the tibial and common fibular (peroneal) nerves. Because plantar flexion is still functional, the tibial nerve has not been cut.

GAS 630-632, 660; N 529; McM 337

25 C. The Achilles tendon reflex is a function of the triceps surae muscle, composed of the gastrocnemius and soleus muscles that insert on the calcaneus. The innervation is provided primarily by spinal nerve S1. The S1 root leaves the vertebral column at the S1 foramen of the sacrum, but a herniated disc at the L5-S1 intervertebral space puts the S1 root under tension, resulting in pain and possible weakness or paralysis of S1 supplied muscles, especially the plantar flexors. A disc lesion at L3-4 would affect the L4 spinal nerve (affecting foot inversion and extension); a lesion at L4-5 would cause problems with L5 (hip abduction and knee flexion). A disc lesion at S1-2 in the sacrum is improbable, unless there was lumbarization of the S1 vertebra. The gluteal crush syndrome usually occurs when a patient has been lying unconscious and unmoving on a hard surface for an extended period of time.

GAS 547-548; N 484, 514; McM 345

26 B. An injury to L4 would cause weakness in the patellar reflex and loss of cutaneous innervation to the medial side of the leg. The patellar reflex is used to test L2 to L4 nerve integrity. The motor side of the reflex is primarily derived from spinal nerves L2 and L3, whereas the sensory side of the arc is said to be principally from L4. The L4 spinal nerve supplies the L4 dermatome on the medial side of the leg and foot, by way of the saphenous nerve. It also supplies foot inversion, a function of the tibialis anterior and tibialis posterior muscles; the first is supplied by the deep fibular (peroneal) nerve, and the second supplied by the tibial nerve. Foot dorsiflexion is weakened because of partial denervation of the extensor digitorum longus, but L5 is still contributing to that function. The foot is everted because the S1-supplied (by the superficial fibular nerve) fibularis (peroneus) longus and brevis are unopposed. The Achilles reflex is also primarily supplied by S1. Hip movements are produced primarily by L5- and S1-supplied muscles, as is knee flexion.

GAS 547-548; N 525, 514; McM 328

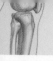

27 C. The lateral plantar nerve innervates the interossei and adductor hallucis. These losses would be obvious when the patient attempts to abduct and adduct the toes. Sensation would be absent over the lateral side of the sole, the fifth and fourth toes, and half of the third toe. The medial plantar nerve provides sensation over the plantar surface of the first and second toes and half of the third toe as well as function of the so-called LAFF muscles: first lumbrical, abductor hallucis, flexor hallucis brevis, and flexor digitorum brevis.
GAS 657-658; N 520, 524, 514; McM 351

28 A. The common fibular (peroneal) nerve passes around the head of the fibula and gives off deep (L4-5) and superficial fibular (peroneal) nerve (L5, S1-2) branches. The two nerves supply the dorsiflexors and evertors of the foot, respectively. In this case, the tibialis anterior and extensor digitorum longus are the only muscles listed that are supplied by either of these nerve branches, and both are innervated by the deep fibular (peroneal) nerve. The fibularis (peroneus) brevis and longus are innervated by the superficial fibular (peroneal) nerve and are evertors of the foot. The tibial nerve supplies each of the other muscles listed.
GAS 486, 550, 563, 607; N 508, 514; McM 337

29 D. Spinal tuberculosis can spread within the sheath of the psoas major to its insertion with the iliacus upon the lesser trochanter, presenting there also with painful symptoms. The iliopsoas muscle is the principal flexor of the hip joint. Abduction of the hips is performed by the gluteus medius and minimus with assistance from short lateral rotator muscles. Extension of the hip is a function of the gluteus maximus, together with the hamstring muscles. Internal rotation is performed by the adductor muscle group.
GAS 368, 589; N 485; McM 326

30 A. The Achilles tendon inserts upon the calcaneus bone. This tendon represents a combination of the tendons of gastrocnemius and soleus muscles. The tendon of the plantaris can insert with this tendon.
GAS 621; N 514; McM 345

31 C. In an inversion injury the most common ligament involvement comes from the anterior talofibular and calcaneofibular ligaments. The medial plantar nerve is medially located within the sole of the foot and might be injured by traction in an eversion injury, not an inversion injury. The posterior talofibular ligament is located posteriorly and is not usually injured in an inversion injury. The deltoid ligament is located medially and would be injured with an eversion injury; it is so strong, however, that eversion is more likely to fracture the medial malleolus rather than tear the deltoid ligament.
GAS 638; N 514; McM 349

32 A. The plantar calcaneonavicular (spring) ligament supports the head of the talus and maintains the longitudinal arch of the foot. A fracture of the cuboid bone would not disrupt the longitudinal arch of the foot. Interruption of the plantar aponeurosis is not the best answer because this aponeurosis provides only passive support, unlike the spring ligament. A sprain of the anterior talofibular ligament would result from an inversion injury of the ankle and would not disrupt the longitudinal arch of the foot. A sprain of the deltoid ligament results from eversion of the ankle joint and would not disrupt the longitudinal arch of the foot.
GAS 638; N 514; McM 349

33 B. This type of injury can result in the "unhappy triad" (of O'Donoghue) injury, with damage to the medial collateral ligament (MCL), anterior cruciate ligament (ACL), and medial meniscus. A blow to the lateral side of the knee stretches and tears the MCL, which is attached to the medial meniscus. The ACL is tensed during knee extension and can tear subsequent to the rupture of the MCL. The remaining answer choices describe structures on the lateral surface of the knee, which are not usually injured by this type of trauma.
GAS 673; N 496; McM 332

34 E. The popliteal artery is the continuation of the femoral artery after it passes through the hiatus of the adductor magnus. The popliteal artery divides into the anterior and posterior tibial arteries. The anterior tibial artery passes between the tibia and fibula proximally in the posterior compartment of the leg, whereas the posterior tibial artery continues in the posterior compartment of the leg, to its division into medial and lateral plantar arteries. The posterior tibial artery provides origin for the fibular (peroneal) artery, which supplies the lateral compartment of the leg. The deep femoral artery provides origin for the three or four perforating branches that supply the posterior compartment of the thigh.
GAS 600, 617; N 509; McM 331

35 E. The vastus lateralis muscle is located on the lateral aspect of the thigh. The distal portion of this muscle lies superficial to the proximal part of the lateral aspect of the joint capsule of the knee. When a needle is inserted superiorly and laterally to the patella, it penetrates the vastus lateralis muscle on its course to the internal capsule. The short head of biceps femoris has its origin on the posterior aspect of the femur, merges with the long head of the biceps femoris, and inserts on the head of the fibula. The rectus femoris passes longitudinally on the medial aspect of the femur and inserts on the tibial tuberosity, via the patellar tendon, or quadriceps tendon. A needle inserted laterally to the patella would not penetrate this muscle. The sartorius originates on the anterior superior iliac spine and forms part of the pes anserinus, which inserts on the medial aspect of the proximal part of the tibia. A needle inserted laterally to the patella would not penetrate this muscle.

GAS 590-593; N 487; McM 320

36 **C.** When the popliteus contracts, it rotates the distal portion of the femur in a lateral direction. It also draws the lateral meniscus posteriorly, thereby protecting this cartilage as the distal femoral condyle glides and rolls backward, as the knee is flexed. This allows the knee to flex and therefore serves in unlocking the knee. The biceps femoris is a strong flexor of the leg and laterally rotates the knee when it is in a position of flexion. The gastrocnemius is a powerful plantar flexor of the foot. The semimembranosus, similar to the biceps femoris, is a component of the hamstring muscles and is involved in extending the thigh and flexing the leg at the knee joint. The rectus femoris is the strongest quadriceps muscle in extending the leg at the knee.

GAS 623-624; N 497; McM 332

37 **B.** Pott's fracture is a rather archaic term for a fracture of the fibula at the ankle. The term is often used to indicate a bimalleolar fracture of fibula and tibia, perhaps with a tear in the medial collateral ligament, allowing the foot to be deviated laterally. (The medial malleolus will often break before the deltoid ligament tears.) This fracture is also known as Dupuytren's fracture. The fracture results from abduction and lateral rotation of the foot in extreme eversion. There can also be fracture of the posterior aspect of the distal tibia. The spring ligament, also known as the plantar calcaneonavicular ligament, extends from the calcaneus to the navicular bone and is a part of the medial longitudinal arch. This ligament would not be affected in eversion or inversion of the ankle. The plantar ligament, which is composed of the long and short plantar ligaments, supports the lateral longitudinal arch of the foot and would therefore not be affected by inversion or eversion of the foot. The calcaneofibular ligament runs from the calcaneus to the fibula. It would be injured during inversion of the foot, not in eversion, as is the case in a Pott's fracture.

GAS 641; N 501; McM 349

38 **B.** The original axial vessel of the lower limb is retained as the (usually tiny) sciatic branch of the inferior gluteal artery. In some cases this vessel is retained as the primary proximal vessel to the limb, wherein there is hypoplastic development of the femoral artery. Aneurysms of the enlarged sciatic artery in the gluteal region are relatively common, as is rupture of the vessel (with profuse bleeding) if they are exposed in the gluteal area. The profunda femoris or deep femoral branch of the femoral artery usually provides three perforating branches to the posterior compartment, but not a branch such as that described. The descending branch of the medial circumflex femoral anastomoses with the first perforator. The superior gluteal artery anastomoses with the inferior gluteal by a descending branch or branches. The descending branch of the lateral circumflex femoral is the descending genicular artery, which anastomoses with the superior lateral genicular branch of the popliteal artery.

GAS 566, 582; N 489; McM 317

39 **C.** Herniation of the intervertebral disc at L4-5 results typically in compression of the L5 spinal nerve. The L4 spinal nerve exits at the L4-5 intervertebral foramen, but the L5 spinal nerve is put under tension as it passes the herniation to reach the L5-1 foramen. Piriformis entrapment of the fibular (peroneal) division of the sciatic nerve is relatively common, but the dermatome affected here appears to be confined to the L5 distribution to the skin of the foot and also includes the superior gluteal nerve, which supplies the large hip abductors. S1 would involve loss of sensation on the lateral side of the foot and potential weakness in hip extension and plantar flexion. A posterior dislocation of the hip would be unlikely in this injury but, even so, would not result in these deficits.

GAS 79; N 528; McM 97

40 **C.** Entrapment compression of all or part of the sciatic nerve by the piriformis can mimic disc herniation, most commonly resembling compression of spinal nerve S1. This results in pain down the posterior aspect of the thigh and leg and the lateral side of the foot. In this case, loss of sensation over the dorsum of the foot and weakness of foot extension, in addition to eversion, indicate that more than S1 is involved. Foot drop would be anticipated with fibular (peroneal) nerve involvement. As noted also in a previous question, compression of the common fibular (peroneal) division of the sciatic nerve by the piriformis gives rise to the clinical condition known as piriformis entrapment. This condition is associated with point pain in the gluteal area, pain in the posterior part of the limb, and possible weakness of muscles in the lateral and anterior compartments of the leg. It can be confused with herniated disc (L5) compression of S1 and sciatica. Paralysis of plantar flexion occurs with a lesion of the tibial division of the sciatic nerve or the tibial nerve. Paralysis of the quadriceps is associated with pathology of the femoral nerve. Clonic contraction of the adductors could result from obturator nerve problems.

GAS 118; N 482, 490; McM 317

41 A. The superior gluteal nerve innervates the gluteus medius, gluteus minimus, and tensor fasciae latae muscles. The tensor fasciae latae arises from the iliac crest, inserts into the iliotibial tract of the lateral aspect of the thigh, and assists in flexion of the hip. The rectus femoris is innervated by the femoral nerve; it flexes the hip and extends the knee, thus acting upon two major joints. It arises in part from the anterior inferior iliac spine and the rim of the acetabulum and inserts into the quadriceps tendon. The gluteus maximus is supplied by the inferior gluteal nerve. The piriformis and quadratus femoris are both short lateral rotators of the hip and are supplied by branches of the sacral plexus.

GAS 565, 575; N 490; McM 320

42 A. The sartorius is indicated by the arrow in Figure 5-3. This muscle forms the roof of the subsartorial canal (Hunter's canal), with the adductor longus and vastus medialis forming other muscular borders. The femoral artery and vein, the saphenous nerve, the nerve to the vastus medialis, and the medial cutaneous nerve of the thigh all pass into this canal. The femoral artery leaves the canal by passing through the hiatus of the adductor magnus. The saphenous nerve emerges from the canal and from beneath the sartorius on the medial side of the lower limb proximally, thereafter providing sensory branches to the medial side of the lower limb and foot. Dr. Hunter mobilized the sartorius, thereby exposing the femoral artery (which continues as the popliteal artery beyond the adductor hiatus), which could be clamped while an aneurysmal popliteal artery was treated surgically.

GAS 590-593; N 487; McM 320

43 B. Contraction of the gastrocnemius on the fractured calcaneus would increase the pain because the gastrocnemius inserts with the soleus upon that bone, via the calcaneal tendon, or tendo Achilles. The flexor digitorum profundus passes the ankle medially to enter the sole of the foot, where it inserts upon the distal phalanges. The tibialis posterior, likewise, passes under the medial malleolus, with complex insertions upon the navicular bone, cuneiform bones, metatarsal bones, and the cuboid bone. The tibialis anterior, a muscle of the anterior leg compartment, inserts upon the navicular bone and, with the tibialis posterior, is a strong invertor of the foot. The fibularis (peroneus) longus is a muscle of the lateral compartment of the leg. It passes under the lateral malleolus, entering the sole of the foot by crossing the lateral surface of the calcaneus, and inserts primarily into the medial cuneiform and base of the first metatarsal bone.

GAS 621, 636; N 503; McM 339

44 C. A severe injury of the tibial nerve in the popliteal fossa would result in a dorsiflexed and everted foot because of the intact muscles of the extensor (anterior) and evertor (lateral) compartments of the leg. It would result also in some weakening of knee flexion because of loss of the gastrocnemius muscle, which flexes the knee and plantar flexes the foot. The hamstrings also flex the knee, so this function would not be lost. Plantar flexion at the ankle would be paralyzed with the loss of the gastrocnemius and soleus, in addition to the flexors of the toes, and inversion by the tibialis posterior. Foot drop results from loss of the anterior compartment, innervated by the deep fibular (peroneal) nerve.

GAS 545; N 514; McM 345

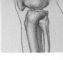

45 C. The obturator artery provides the artery within the ligament of the head of the femur (in about 60% of cases), the artery that supplies the head of the femur, primarily during childhood, later becoming atretic. In the adult this artery supplies only the area of the fovea of the head of the femur. The ligament of the head of the femur arises from the acetabular notch, thereafter receiving the little artery. In some individuals the medial circumflex femoral gives origin to the artery of the head. In the adult the arterial supply of the neck and head is provided by intracapsular branches of the medial circumflex femoral and lateral circumflex femoral arteries that pierce the neck of the femur, with some supply also from the gluteal arteries. The lateral circumflex femoral artery arises from the deep femoral and supplies the vastus lateralis. The pudendal artery arises from the internal iliac and provides blood supply for the structures of the perineum. Quite often, when an older patient with osteoporosis has a hip fracture, the femoral neck may have fractured, precipitating a fall, rather than the fall resulting in the hip fracture.

GAS 558, 568, 676; N 491; McM 326

46 A. With sufficient downward force, the head of the talus can break through the plantar calcaneonavicular (spring) ligament, causing the medial longitudinal arch of the foot to fall, forcing the anterior part of the foot into abduction. The plantar calcaneonavicular ligament is attached between the sustentaculum tali of the calcaneus and the medial surface of the navicular bone, with the head of the talus lying directly upon the inner surface of the ligament. The cuboid bone is located lateral and anterior to the talus bone and would not be fractured. The plantar aponeurosis, a dense, wide band of tissue beneath the fascia of the sole, attaches to the calcaneus and ends distally in longitudinal bands to each of the toes. It stretches very little, even under very heavy loads, and would not rupture in this case. The anterior talofibular ligament is very often injured in "sprained ankle" but would not be directly involved here. The distal tibiofibular joint is a fibrous (and usually nonsynovial) type of joint (called a syndesmosis) between the tibia and fibula, not involved in the displacement of the talus bone (*GAS* Fig. 6-98).

GAS 539-542, 648; N 514; McM 349

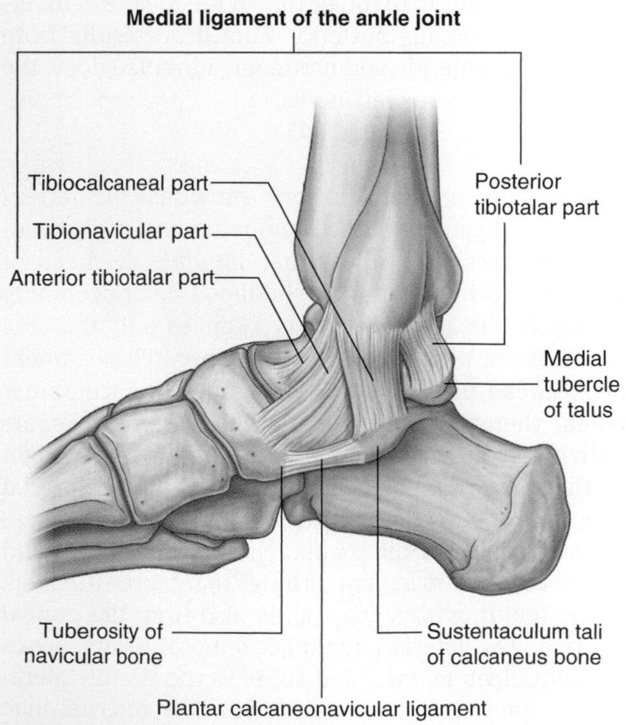

***GAS* Fig. 6-98**

47 E. The lateral femoral cutaneous nerve leaves the pelvis laterally, about 2 cm medial to the anterior superior iliac spine, passing beneath, or through, the inguinal ligament. As a consequence of its site of exit, any tension upon or compression of the inguinal ligament can affect the nerve. If it is thus affected, the individual may feel burning sensations or pain along the lateral aspect of the thigh, which is the region of distribution of the nerve. Obesity, sudden weight loss, wearing a heavy gun belt, wearing trousers that are too tight (Calvin Klein syndrome), or having someone sitting on another's lap for an extended period of time can lead to meralgia paresthetica, the painful lateral thigh. The femoral nerve emerges from beneath the middle of the inguinal ligament and is not usually affected by similar traction or compression. The obturator nerve leaves the pelvis through the obturator canal and enters the thigh deeply in a protected location. It innervates the adductor muscles and supplies sensation on the medial aspect of the thigh. The fibular (peroneal) division of the sciatic nerve supplies the muscles of the anterior and lateral compartments of the leg and provides sensory fibers for the dorsum and lateral side of the foot. The superior gluteal nerve provides motor supply to the gluteus medius and minimus muscles.

GAS 486; N 525; McM 322

48 D. The tibialis posterior tendon is the most anterior of the structures that pass under the laciniate ligament (flexor retinaculum) on the medial side of the ankle to enter the sole of the foot. Increases of pressure within the tissues of the plantar aspect of the foot, usually due to increased fluid from hemorrhage, inflammatory processes, or infections, cause tarsal tunnel syndrome, comparable to carpal tunnel syndrome of the hand. The plantar aponeurosis and other fibrous and osseous tissues of the plantar surface cause this area to be relatively nondistensible; therefore, it takes little increase of fluid content to result in pressures adequate to restrict venous drainage and, thereafter, arterial inflow to the region. Fasciotomy of the medial skin and fascia of the foot and the posterior compartment of the leg can be required to reduce the pressure and allow healing to take place. The structures that pass beneath the flexor retinaculum are, from anterior to posterior: **T**endon of tibialis posterior; tendon of flexor **D**igitorum longus; posterior tibial **V**essels and **N**erve; tendon of flexor **H**allucis longus. (This is the basis of the mnemonic: "Tom, Dick, and a Very Nervous Harry.") Neither the plantaris tendon nor the tibialis anterior tendon pass through this canal (*GAS* Figs. 6-105 and 6-110).

GAS 621-623; N 514; McM 346

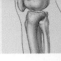

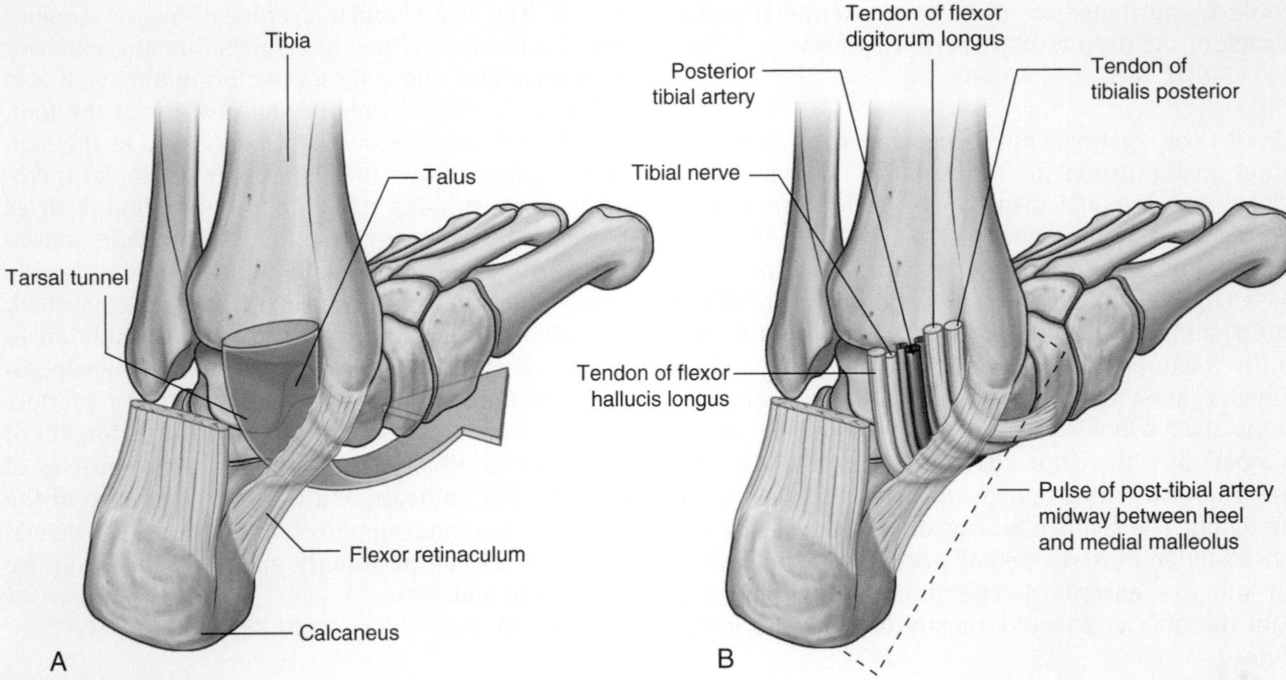

GAS **Fig. 6-105**

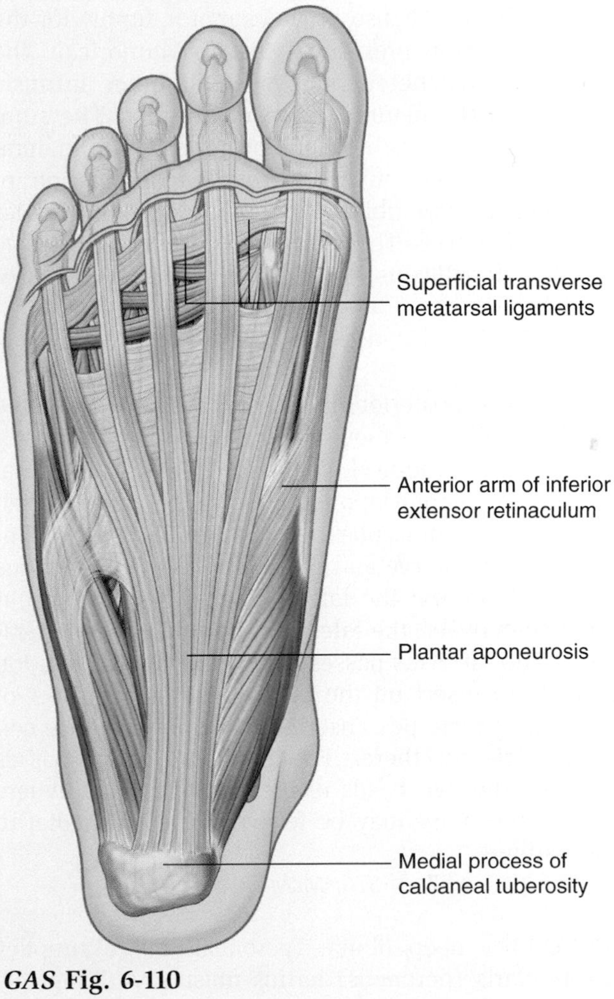

GAS **Fig. 6-110**

49 D. The second perforating branch of the profunda femoris (deep femoral) artery commonly provides the nutrient artery to the femur, a vessel that passes through a rather large foramen to enter the proximal part of the shaft. The deep circumflex branch of the external iliac passes around the medial aspect of the iliac crest, also supplying the lower lateral part of the anterior abdominal wall. The acetabular branch of the obturator artery supplies tissues in the hip socket, usually including a branch to the ligament of the head of the femur. The lateral circumflex femoral branch of the deep femoral artery supplies the vastus lateralis muscle. The medial circumflex femoral branch of the deep femoral artery supplies proximal adductor musculature and the region of the hip joint, including the neck and head of the femur.

GAS 600-602; N 499; McM 322

50 B. The tibial nerve divides into the medial and lateral plantar nerves on the medial side of the ankle. These two nerves provide sensation for the sole of the foot. Sensory supply to the dorsum of the foot is provided mostly by the superficial fibular (peroneal) nerve, with the deep fibular (peroneal) nerve providing sensation for the skin between the first and second toes. Foot drop would be caused by interruption of the common fibular (peroneal) nerve. Sensory loss to the lateral side of the foot results from loss of the sural nerve. Paralysis of the extensor digitorum brevis would be attributed to injury to the terminal motor branch of the deep fibular (peroneal) nerve.

GAS 660; N 528; McM 346

51 **B.** The gastrocnemius muscle arises from the femur just proximal to the femoral condyles. This strong muscle could displace the distal fragment of the fractured femur posteriorly. In addition, the popliteal artery is the deepest structure in the popliteal fossa (right against the popliteal surface of the distal femur) and is susceptible to laceration in this scenario as the fractured end of the distal femoral fragment is pulled against the popliteal artery. Orthopedic surgeons always look for damage to the popliteal artery in a patient with a supracondylar fracture. The soleus arises from the tibia and would have no effect upon the femur. The semitendinosus arises from the ischial tuberosity and inserts medially on the proximal tibia, via the pes anserinus. The tibialis anterior arises from the tibia and inserts mostly onto the navicular bone.

GAS 621-623; N 503; McM 301

52 **E.** The posterior tibial artery provides most of the arterial supply for the neck and body of the talus bone. The fibular (peroneal) artery provides a small amount of vascular supply. The medial plantar and lateral plantar branches of the posterior tibial artery are distributed to tissues in the plantar surface of the foot. The dorsalis pedis is the continuation of the anterior tibial artery on the dorsum of the foot.

GAS 626, 657; N 509; McM 344

53 **A.** The adductor hallucis muscle inserts upon the lateral side of the proximal phalanx of the great toe, and also the lateral sesamoid bone, by way of its oblique and transverse heads. It is supplied by the lateral plantar nerve. The abductor hallucis inserts upon the medial side of the proximal phalanx and the medial sesamoid bone of the great toe. The sesamoid bones are within the tendon of the flexor hallucis brevis and assist it in its function at the first metatarsophalangeal joint. The abductor and flexor hallucis brevis are innervated by the medial plantar nerve. The first dorsal interosseous muscle and the first lumbrical both insert on the medial side of the extensor mechanism of the second toe. The quadratus plantae arises from the calcaneus and inserts on the tendon of the flexor digitorum longus muscle. The first lumbrical is supplied by the medial plantar nerve. The quadratus plantae, the lumbricals 2 to 4, and all interossei are innervated by the lateral plantar nerve.

GAS 660; N 522; McM 351

54 **B.** The deep fibular (peroneal) nerve supplies the dorsiflexors of the foot, including the extensor hallucis longus and extensor digitorum longus. It also supplies the tibialis anterior, an invertor of the foot. This nerve has sensory distribution only to the skin between the first two toes. The common fibular (peroneal) nerve supplies not only the preceding muscles but also the evertors of the foot and provides sensation for most of the dorsum of the foot. The sciatic nerve innervates the muscles of the posterior thigh and all muscles of the leg and foot, in addition to providing sensory supply in those areas. The superficial fibular (peroneal) nerve innervates the evertors of the foot and provides sensation for the dorsum of the foot. The tibial nerve is the nerve for muscles of the posterior compartment of the leg and also of the plantar region and supplies sensation over the medial aspect of the leg posteriorly and the plantar surface of the foot and toes.

GAS 626, 660; N 508; McM 337

55 **B.** The medial plantar nerve innervates the abductor hallucis and both flexor hallucis longus and brevis. This nerve also provides motor supply for the flexor digitorum brevis and the first lumbrical. The lateral plantar nerve innervates all other intrinsic muscles in the plantar region of the foot. The sural nerve is sensory to the lateral posterior leg and lateral side of the foot; it arises from a combination of branches of the tibial nerve and common fibular (peroneal) nerve. The deep fibular (peroneal) nerve supplies dorsiflexors, toe extensors, and invertors of the foot.

GAS 660; N 522; McM 351

56 **D.** The posterior tibial artery passes under the medial malleolus, about halfway between that bony landmark and the heel, or the calcaneus. The medial edge of the plantar aponeurosis can be palpated just medial to the muscular belly of the abductor hallucis. The sural nerve and the short (lesser) saphenous vein pass around the lateral side of the foot, about halfway between the lateral malleolus and the calcaneus. The sartorius passes behind the medial femoral condyle to insert on the proximal, medial aspect of the tibia via the pes anserinus; usually no pulse can be felt clearly there. The popliteal artery passes between the two heads of the gastrocnemius, where the arterial pulse may be felt very deeply, medial to the midline.

GAS 626, 657; N 516; McM 344

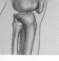

57 **C.** The deep fibular (peroneal) nerve supplies the fibularis (peroneus) tertius muscle. Although its name might lead one to think that this muscle is in the lateral compartment with the other two fibularis (peroneus) muscles, it is in the anterior (extensor) compartment of the leg. It is named for its origin from the fibula. It inserts upon the dorsum of the base of the fifth (or fourth) metatarsal bone and assists in extension and eversion of the foot. The sural nerve is a cutaneous nerve, formed by contributions from the tibial and common fibular (peroneal) nerves; it supplies the posterior lateral leg and the lateral side of the foot. The lateral plantar nerve is a branch of the tibial nerve; it innervates the quadratus plantae, muscles of the little toe, the adductor hallucis, lumbricals 2 to 4, and all of the interossei. It is sensory to the lateral side of the sole and the lateral three and a half digits. The superficial fibular (peroneal) nerve supplies the fibularis (peroneus) longus and brevis and innervates the skin on most of the dorsum of the foot. The tibial nerve supplies the calf muscles and divides into the medial and lateral plantar nerves.

GAS 628-631; N 508; McM 347

58 **A.** Gluteal injections should be given anterior and superior to a line drawn between the posterior superior iliac spine and the greater trochanter to avoid the sciatic nerve and other important nerves and vessels. Occasionally, one can encounter the lateral cutaneous branch of the iliohypogastric nerve, but this usually causes no serious problem. Certainly, one must stay anterior to a vertical line dropped from the highest point of the ilium. If the injected material is too near the sciatic nerve or other motor nerves, it can infiltrate the connective tissue sheath of the nerve, following the nerve, and result in major insult to the neural elements. The needle can cause trauma to this, or other nerves, likewise. Precautions to avoid the sciatic nerve are especially important in injecting the gluteal area in babies. The reduced dimensions are less "forgiving" in babies.

GAS 663; N 468; McM 316

59 **B.** The obturator nerve innervates the adductor muscles, including the gracilis, pectineus, and obturator externus. The tibial nerve supplies the calf muscles and intrinsic muscles in the plantar portion of the foot. The inferior gluteal nerve innervates the gluteus maximus; the superior gluteal nerve supplies the gluteus medius and minimus and tensor fasciae latae. The femoral nerve provides motor supply to the quadriceps femoris, sartorius, and, in some cases, the pectineus. This gait pattern is characteristic of hypertonia in the lower limb. As a result these areas become flexed to various degrees, giving the appearance of crouching, while tight adductors produce extreme adduction.

GAS 468, 500, 563-565; N 488; McM 319

60 **A.** The perineal cutaneous branch of the posterior femoral cutaneous nerve provides a significant portion of the cutaneous innervation of the perineum in some individuals and can require separate anesthetic blockade in childbirth or perineal surgery, if other types of anesthesia are not used. The inferior cluneal branches of the posterior femoral cutaneous nerve supply the lower part of the gluteal skin. The lateral cutaneous branch of the iliohypogastric nerve provides sensation for the anterior superior aspect of the gluteal area. The inferior gluteal nerve innervates the gluteus maximus muscle. The middle cluneal nerves arise from the dorsal primary rami of S1 to S3 and supply skin over the middle of the gluteal region.

GAS 513; N 527; McM 276

61 **D.** The dorsalis pedis is the continuation of the anterior tibial artery into the foot, as it passes the distal end of the tibia and the ankle joint. The pulse of the dorsalis pedis can be felt between the tendon of the extensor hallucis longus and the tendon of the extensor digitorum longus to the second toe. A strong pulse is a positive indicator of circulation through the limb. The fibular (peroneal) artery is a branch of the posterior tibial artery and passes in the calf between the flexor hallucis longus and tibialis posterior, making it difficult to palpate. The deep plantar artery, the extension of the first dorsal interosseous or lateral plantar arteries, passes deep to the aponeurotic tissues and central muscles of the foot, making palpation unlikely. The dorsal metatarsal branches of the dorsalis pedis pass under cover of the extensor digitorum longus and brevis tendons. Palpable pulses of the first or other dorsal metatarsal arteries can therefore be difficult to detect (*GAS* Fig. 6-119).

GAS 658; N 518; McM 344

62 **D.** Injury to the dorsalis pedis artery on the dorsum of the foot can also cause trauma to the terminal portion of the deep fibular (peroneal) nerve. In the proximal part of the foot, this could result in loss of sensation between the first and second toes and paralysis of the extensor digitorum brevis and the extensor hallucis brevis muscles. In the distal part of the foot, only the sensory loss might be apparent. Clubfoot is a congenital malformation observed in pediatric patients. This syndrome combines plantar flexion, inversion, and adduction of the foot. Neither extension of the big toe by the extensor hallucis

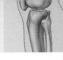

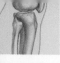

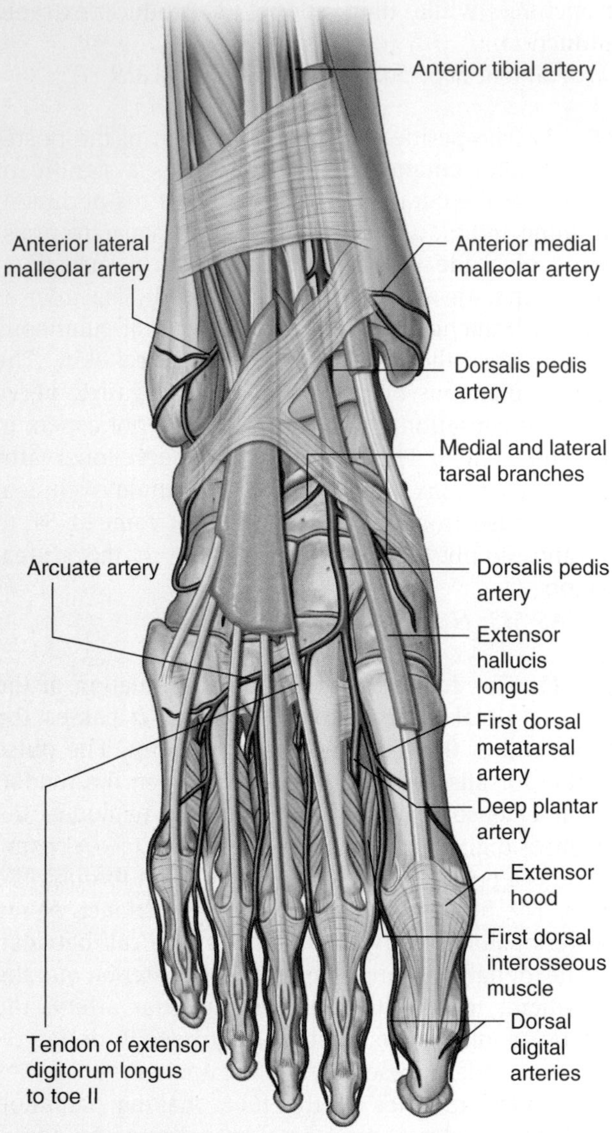

***GAS* Fig. 6-119**

longus nor paralysis of the tibialis anterior (weakness of foot inversion) would occur by this injury because both of these muscles are innervated by the deep fibular (peroneal) nerve much more proximally in the leg.

GAS 658; N 518; McM 348

63 D. The sural nerve is formed by contributions from the tibial nerve and a branch from the common fibular (peroneal) nerve. It provides sensation for the lower lateral portion of the calf and continues beneath the lateral malleolus as the lateral cutaneous nerve of the foot. It is often used for nerve grafting procedures as well as biopsied for diagnostic purposes. When it is grafted to the "living end" of a cut motor or sensory nerve, the severed nerve processes within the "living" nerve grow into the sural nerve sheath, using it as a guide to the distal, surgically anastomosed nerve. Thus, axons from a branch of a functional motor nerve can grow to reinnervate paralyzed muscles. In this case, the surgeon would connect portions of the sural nerve to the functional facial nerve, tunnel it to the opposite side of the face, and join it surgically to the branches of the paralyzed nerve, where it would grow through the now empty nerve sheaths (due to Wallerian degeneration) to the muscles. Growth and reinnervation usually occur at a rate of 1 mm/day (or 1 inch/month) so the time estimated before reinnervation is based on the distance the regenerating fibers need to traverse. The tibial nerve supplies muscles and sensation to the calf and plantar surface of the foot. The common fibular (peroneal) nerve innervates the lateral and anterior compartment muscles and sensation to the dorsum of the foot. The saphenous nerve accompanies the great saphenous vein on the medial side of the leg and foot.

GAS 630, 662; N 529; McM 340

64 D. Osgood-Schlatter disease is also called tibial tuberosity apophysitis and affects the area of the tibial tuberosity. It is not a disease but a problem of overuse, typically in boys of 12 to 14 years or girls 10 to 12 years of age. Very active boys and girls, usually during a growth spurt, are subject to the pain and swelling that occur at the site of attachment of the patellar ligament. The ligament can tear, resulting in a long period of healing following treatment. The medial femoral condyle is the area of attachment of the medial collateral ligament and medial meniscus of the knee joint. The posterior intercondylar eminence is the location of origin of the posterior cruciate ligament. The intercondylar eminence is a bony protuberance on the tibial plateau to which the cruciate ligaments and menisci are attached. The anterolateral tibial tubercle, or Gerdy's tubercle, is the attachment of the iliotibial band or tract; thus it connects the femur and tibia laterally.

GAS 586, 664; N 501; McM 335

65 A. The patient has bowlegs, or genu varus. The opposite of this is genu valgus, or knock knee. The normal angle between the femoral shaft and femoral neck is between 120 and 135 degrees. In coxa vara the angle between the shaft and neck of the femur is less than 120 degrees. This can result from fractures, other injuries, or congenital softness of the bone of the femoral neck. This defect results in limb shortening and limping. In coxa valga there is an increase in femoral shaft neck angulation, which can lead to hip subluxation or dislocation. Coxa valga results from weakness of the adductor musculature. Hallux valgus is commonly known as bunion. In this deformity the big toe points toward the little toe and may override the second toe; the base of the first metatarsal points medially, with a swollen bursal sac at the metatarsophalangeal joint. Excess bony growth of the distal protruding part of the metatarsal bone can also occur. Bunions occur only rarely in people who do not routinely wear shoes.

GAS 554; N 476; McM 332

66 **A.** The patellar ligament is a very heavy ligament that connects the patella to the tibial tuberosity; it provides the insertion of the quadriceps femoris tendon upon the tibia. The patella can be thought of as a bone (a sesamoid bone) that develops within the tendon of the quadriceps femoris muscle. When the reflex hammer strikes the patellar ligament, it stretches the ligament slightly for a brief time, resulting in reflex contraction of the quadriceps femoris muscles. This reflex arc is elicited by the femoral nerve (L4 sensory input component and L2, L3 motor output). The quadriceps femoris includes the rectus femoris and the vastus lateralis, intermedius, and medialis. The patella is the largest sesamoid bone in the body. A sesamoid bone is a bone that develops within a tendon. The quadratus femoris muscle of the gluteal area arises from the ischial tuberosity and inserts on the femur proximally. The sartorius arises from the anterior superior iliac spine and inserts on the proximal, medial aspect of the tibia as one of the three tendinous components of the pes anserinus (goose foot). The biceps femoris of the posterior thigh has a long head that arises from the ischial tuberosity and a short head that arises from the femur; they insert on the head of the fibula.

GAS 586; N 518494 McM 335

67 **E.** The talus can be rotated externally when the ankle sustains a trimalleolar fracture, also called a Henderson fracture. The fracture may be caused by eversion and posterior displacement of the talus. This injury involves the fracture of the distal fibula (lateral malleolus); the medial malleolus of the tibia; and the posterior portion, or lip, of the tibial plafond (the distal articular portion of the tibia, sometimes referred to as the posterior malleolus). The posterior part of the plafond is not truly a malleolus but acts this way in this type of twisting fracture of the ankle. The talus can be forced from its normal position in this fracture, adding to the instability of the ankle. The other bones listed are relatively far from the site of the fractures. The calcaneus resides beneath the talus and articulates distally with the cuboid bone. The head of the talus articulates also with the navicular bone. The navicular bone articulates distally with the three cuneiform bones.

GAS 634-644; N 514; McM 347

68 **E.** Hallux valgus, or lateral displacement of the great toe, usually presents as pain over the prominent metatarsal head, due to rubbing from shoes, and it can be associated with deformity of the second toe, which then tends to override the great toe. Hallux valgus is commonly known as bunion. In this deformity the big toe points toward the little toe; the base of the first metatarsal points medially, with a swollen bursal sac at the metatarsophalangeal joint. Excess bony growth of the distal protruding part of the metatarsal bone can also occur. Bunions occur only rarely in people who do not routinely wear shoes. Genu varus is also referred to as bowlegs, or bandy legs, in which the knees are bowed outward. The opposite of this is genu valgus, or knock knee. The normal angle between the femoral shaft and femoral neck is between 120 and 135 degrees. In coxa vara the angle between the shaft and neck of the femur is less than 120 degrees. This can result from fractures, other injuries, or congenital softness of the bone of the femoral neck. This defect results in limb shortening and limping. In coxa valga there is an increase in femoral shaft neck angulation, which can lead to hip subluxation or dislocation. Coxa valga results from weakness of the adductor musculature.

GAS 631, 634, 644; N 518; McM 350

69 **C.** The patient's complaint is due to her case of hammertoes. Hammer toe can affect any toe but most commonly the second toe, then the third or fourth toes. It results most commonly from wearing shoes that are too short or shoes with heels that are too high. In hammertoe, the metatarsophalangeal joint is extended, the proximal interphalangeal joint is flexed, and the distal phalanx points downward, looking like a hammer. Hammertoe can occur as a result of a bunion. Calluses, or painful corns, can form on the dorsal surface of the joints. In claw toe, both the proximal and distal interphalangeal joints are strongly flexed, the result of muscle imbalance in the foot. Either hammertoe or claw toe can occur from arthritic changes. Pes cavus is the opposite of flat foot. In this case the patient has a high, flexed plantar arch; it occurs as a result of hereditary motor and sensory neural problems. It is painful because of metatarsal compression.

GAS 637-639; N 515; McM 348

70 **C.** In piriformis entrapment, the sciatic nerve can be compressed when the piriformis is contracted, leading to painful sensations in the lower limb. These usually involve pain in the gluteal area, posterior thigh, and leg, most frequently resembling a disc lesion at L5-S1, with compression of the S1 spinal nerve. L4 compression would be rather unusual but would involve the quadriceps femoris knee extension, foot inversion, and sensory loss on the medial side of the leg. L5 compression would be indicated by weakness in hip abduction, knee flexion, and sensory loss on dorsal and plantar surfaces of the foot. S1 compression would weaken plantar flexion and foot eversion. Pudendal nerve entrapment would affect the perineal region. The fibular (peroneal) division of the sciatic nerve passes through the piriformis in some individuals, leading to L5, S1-S3 nerve compression.

GAS 118; N 490; McM 317

71 **C.** Incapacitation and unconsciousness from use of cocaine and other powerful narcotics have led to numerous cases of the "gluteal crush syndrome." Compression of the gluteal region while supine for extended periods of time can lead to gluteal crush injury, in which the nerves and vessels of the gluteal area are compressed. This can result in loss of gluteal muscles and other soft tissues and sciatic nerve compression. The nerve compression can cause paralysis of knee flexors and muscles of the anterior and lateral compartments of the leg, with sensory loss in the posterior thigh and leg and sensory loss in the foot. Tibial nerve loss would not result in loss of dorsiflexion of the foot nor generalized sensory loss. Neither piriformis entrapment nor femoral nerve entrapment is associated with loss of gluteal musculature, nor loss of knee flexion or plantar flexion of the foot, nor do they lead to general sensory loss in the limb.

GAS 535-536, 574; N 489; McM 317

72 **E.** In infants and children until about the age of 8 years, the head of the femur gets its arterial supply by a direct branch of the obturator artery (variably, the medial circumflex femoral). The arterial supply reaches the head of the femur at the fovea capitis by traveling along the ligament of the head of the femur. This source of supply is replaced later by vessels such as branches of the ascending branch of the medial circumflex femoral that pass into foramina of the neck of the femur within the capsule of the hip joint. Similar branches can arise from the lateral circumflex femoral and gluteal arteries. The deep circumflex iliac artery arises from the external iliac artery and supplies branches to the ilium, the iliacus muscle, and lower portions of the abdominal wall. The acetabular branch of the obturator artery often provides the branch to the head of the femur, an artery that normally regresses early in life, so that it supplies only the immediate area of the fovea capitis. The descending branch of the lateral circumflex femoral supplies the vastus lateralis muscle and participates in anastomoses at the knee. The second perforating branch of the deep femoral artery often supplies the nutrient artery of the shaft of the femur (*GAS* Fig. 6-30).

GAS 558-561, 676; N 491; McM 322

73 **D.** The lesser (short) saphenous vein ascends up the middle of the calf from beneath the lateral malleolus, most commonly terminating at the popliteal fossa by piercing the deep fascia and joining the popliteal vein. The popliteal vein is the most superficial of major structures deep to the deep popliteal fascia. The perforating tributaries of the deep femoral vein drain to the deep femoral vein of the posterior compartment of the thigh, thereafter into the femoral vein. The superior medial genicular vein is a tributary to the popliteal vein.

GAS 550, 568, 616, 659; N 503; McM 330

74 **E.** The lateral plantar artery provides origin to the deep plantar arterial arch. Medially, the vascular arch anastomoses with the distal portion of the dorsalis pedis by way of the deep plantar artery. The anterior tibial artery continues as the dorsalis pedis at the ankle joint. The fibular (peroneal) artery, by way of a perforating branch in some individuals, replaces the dorsal pedis. The arcuate artery, a branch of the dorsalis pedis, provides origin for the dorsal metatarsal arteries to the lateral toes.

GAS 657; N 509; McM 351

75 **C.** The bone to which the injured ligament attaches is the calcaneus. The navicular bone, located medially in the foot, articulates posteriorly with the head of the talus and anteriorly with the cuneiform bones. The cuboid bone of the lateral longitudinal arch articulates posteriorly with the calcaneus. The talus articulates with the tibia and fibula in the ankle joint mortise.

GAS 633-644; N 514; McM 345

76 **C.** The fibularis (peroneus) brevis arises from the fibula and inserts upon the tuberosity at the base of the fifth metatarsal bone. Its attachment is often involved in an inversion fracture of the foot. This common fracture can often be overlooked when it is combined with an inversion sprain of the ankle. The fibularis (peroneus) longus arises from the fibula,

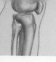

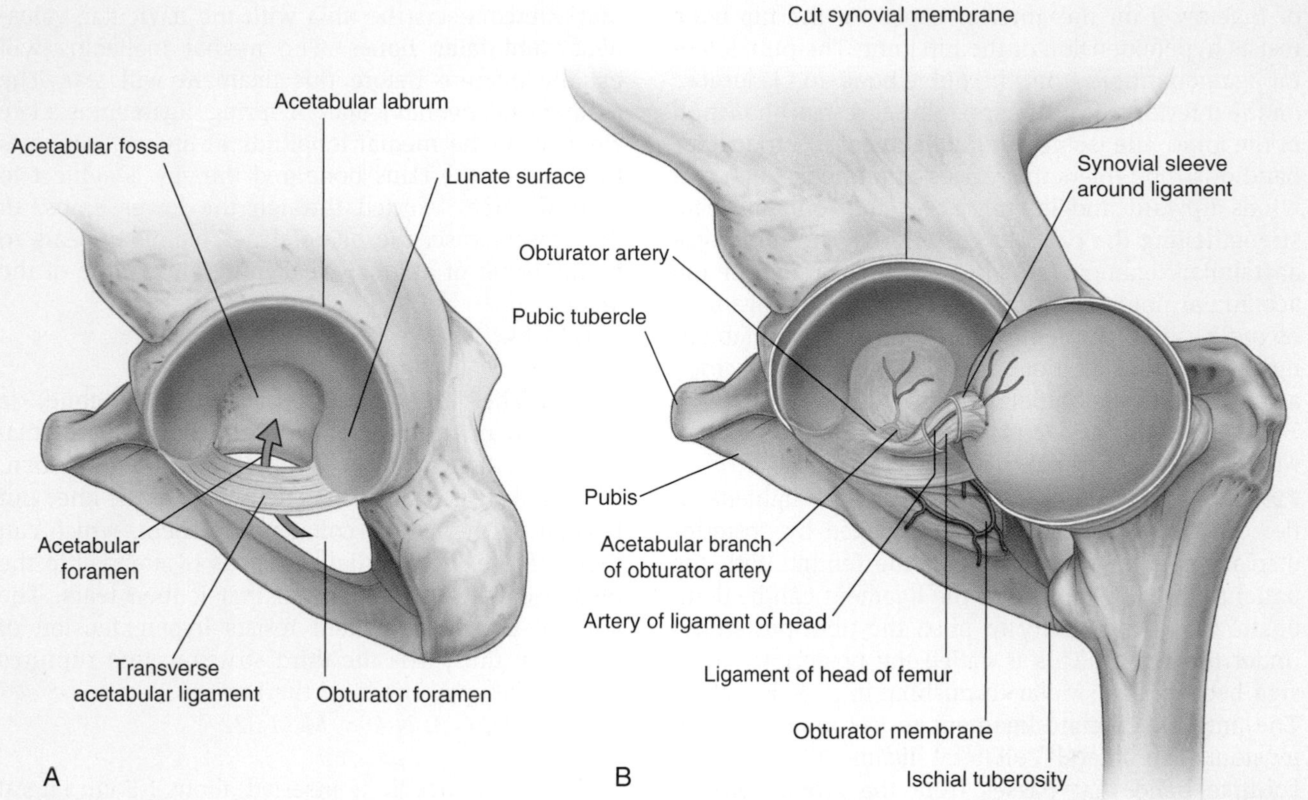

GAS **Fig. 6-30**

passes under the lateral malleolus, and then turns medially into the plantar surface of the foot, where it inserts upon the medial cuneiform and first metatarsal bones. The tibialis posterior arises from the tibia in the posterior compartment of the leg; it passes under the medial malleolus and inserts upon the navicular and metatarsal bones. The extensor digitorum brevis arises dorsally from the calcaneus and inserts upon the proximal phalanges of the lateral toes. The adductor hallucis arises from the lateral metatarsals and transverse tarsal ligament and inserts upon the proximal phalanx and lateral sesamoid bone of the big toe.

GAS 628-629, 646, 668; N 506; McM 353

77 A. Excessive compression of the prepatellar bursa, as in working on bended knees, can result in pain and swelling of the prepatellar bursa, the so called housemaid's knee. Prepatellar bursitis affects plumbers, carpet layers, and other people who spend a lot of time on their knees. The bursa normally enables the patella to move smoothly under the skin. The constant friction of these occupations irritates this small lubricating sac (bursa) located just in front of the patella, resulting in a deformable tense cushion of fluid. Treatment usually requires simple drainage, but this may need to be repeated and occasionally steroids introduced. Excessive irritation of the infrapatellar bursa in kneeling for frequent and long periods of time (as in prayer) can result in "parson's knee." The posterior cruciate ligament of the knee can be injured in sudden, strong flexion of the knee, with posterior displacement of the tibia upon the femur. The patellar retinacula are strong, tendinous bands of tissue that join the quadriceps tendon to the vastus lateralis and medialis muscles. The lateral meniscus is a cartilaginous structure between the lateral condyles of the femur and tibia.

GAS 606-610; N 498; McM 335

78 D. The ligament of the head of the femur conveys a small blood vessel for supply of the head of the femur (primarily in childhood). The ligament is stretched during abduction and lateral rotation of the hip joint and has an important role in stabilizing an infant's hip joint before walking. It has the potential to increase stability of the joint in hip reconstruction in developmental hip dysplasia in the pediatric population. The strength of this ligament is comparable to the anterior cruciate ligament of the knee. The iliofemoral ligament (the inverted "Y-shaped ligament of Bigelow") on the anterior aspect of the hip bone resists hyperextension of the hip joint. The pubofemoral ligament arises from the pubic bone and is located on the inferior side of the hip joint; it resists abduction of the joint. The ischiofemoral ligament is a triangular band of strong fibers that arises from the ischium and winds upward and laterally over the femoral neck, strengthening the capsule posteriorly. The transverse acetabular ligament attaches to the margins of the acetabular notch and provides origin for the ligament of the head of the femur. The transverse acetabular ligament is fibrous, not cartilaginous, but is regarded as part of the acetabular labrum.

GAS 558-561; N 474; McM 325

79 **B.** The posterior cruciate ligament tightens in flexion of the knee. It can be damaged by posterior displacement of the tibia upon the femur. With the patient seated, a rupture of the ligament can be demonstrated by the ability to push the tibia posteriorly under the femur. This is called the posterior drawer sign because it's similar to pushing in a desk drawer. The anterior cruciate ligament resists knee hyperextension. The lateral collateral ligament is a thick, cordlike band that passes from the lateral femoral condyle to the head of the fibula. It is located external to the capsule of the knee joint. The lateral meniscus is a nearly circular band of fibrocartilage that is located laterally within the knee joint. It is less frequently injured than the medial meniscus because it is not attached to the joint capsule or other ligaments. The patellar ligament is the heavy, ligamentous band of insertion of the quadriceps muscle to the tibial tuberosity.

GAS 584-586; N 496; McM 332

80 **A.** Flat foot (pes planus) is due to flattening of the medial longitudinal arch. Often congenital, it may be associated with minor structural anomalies of the tarsal bones. This condition can be seen in wet footprints in which the medial surface of the sole (normally raised in an arch) is visible. Treatment may include intensive foot exercises or arch supports worn in the shoes. Occasionally, surgery is needed in the form of arthrodesis (fusion of the tarsal bones). Pes cavus is a deformity of the foot characterized by a very high medial arch and hyperextension of the toes. The long plantar ligament is a passive ligament of the longitudinal arch. The long plantar ligament connects the calcaneus and cuboid bones. It can be involved with the plantar aponeurosis in plantar fasciitis. The long plantar ligament converts the cuboid groove into a canal for the tendon of the fibularis (peroneus) longus. The deltoid ligament is a very strong ligament that interconnects the tibia with the navicular, calcaneus, and talus bones. The medial malleolus will usually fracture before this ligament will tear. The plantar calcaneonavicular, or spring, ligament is a key element in the medial longitudinal arch; it supports the head of the talus bone and thereby is subject to vertical forces exerted through the lower limbs. In the present case, the bilateral pes planus appears to be the result of gradual weakening and failure of the arches.

GAS 542, 648; N 519; McM 312

81 **A.** The "unhappy triad" (of O'Donoghue) is composed of the medial collateral ligament, medial meniscus, and anterior cruciate ligament. Sudden, forceful thrusts against the lateral side of the knee put tension on the medial collateral ligament, which can then rupture. The medial meniscus is attached to the medial collateral ligament so that it then tears. The anterior cruciate ligament resists hyperextension of the knee; thus, it is the third structure that ruptures in the "unhappy triad" of the knee.

GAS 606, 673; N 496; McM 322

82 **C.** If the needle is inserted about 1.5 cm lateral to the maximal femoral pulse, it will intersect the femoral nerve in most cases. (Fluoroscopic or ultrasound guidance is advisable to avoid iatrogenic errors.) The deep inguinal ring is located about 4 cm superolateral to the pubic tubercle and very close to the origin of the inferior epigastric vessels from the external iliac artery and vein. The approximate site of exit of the lateral femoral cutaneous nerve from the abdomen is 1.5 cm medial to the anterior superior iliac spine. Injections 1.5 cm medial to the femoral artery pulse will enter the femoral vein. Midway between the anterior superior iliac spine and the pubic symphysis can vary approximately 1.5 cm either medial or lateral from the femoral artery.

GAS 566, 664, 671; N 487; McM 320

83 **A.** Morton's neuroma most commonly involves compression (and possible enlargement) of an anastomosing branch that connects the medial and lateral plantar nerves between the third and fourth toes. The pain can be severe. The medial plantar nerve provides sensation for the medial three and a half toes; the lateral plantar nerve supplies the little toe and half of the fourth toe. The neural interconnection can be compressed between the transverse metatarsal ligament and the floor. Women are 10 times more likely than men to be afflicted with this problem, most likely due to wearing shoes that put excessive stress on the forefoot. In about 80% of cases the pain can be eased with different (less confining) shoes or cortisone injections.

GAS 660-661; N 508; McM 351

84 D. Inflammation of the plantar aponeurosis is referred to as plantar fasciitis. Plantar fasciitis is a common clinical condition that results from tearing or inflammation of the tough band of tissue stretching from the calcaneus to the ball of the foot (the plantar aponeurosis). It happens frequently to people who are on their feet all day, such as mail carriers, or engaged in athletics, especially in running and jumping. The pain of plantar fasciitis is usually most significant in the morning, just after you get up from bed and begin to walk. Rest, orthotics, night splints, and antiinflammatory medications are employed in treatment. A Morton's neuroma is a painful lesion of the neural interconnection of the medial and lateral plantar nerves between the third and fourth toes. An eversion sprain of the ankle can break the medial malleolus or tear the deltoid ligament. An inversion sprain commonly injures the fibulocalcaneal ligament or anterior talofibular ligament.

GAS 651; N 519; McM 351

85 B. The child has the problem of talipes equinovarus, or clubfoot. Clubfoot is a congenital malformation observed in about 1 in 1000 pediatric patients and first appears in the first trimester of pregnancy. This syndrome combines plantar flexion, inversion, and adduction of the foot. The heel is drawn upward by the tendo calcaneus and turned inward; the forefoot is also adducted, or turned inward. The foot usually is smaller than normal. In coxa vara, the angle between the femoral shaft and neck is reduced to less than 120 degrees, often due to excessive activity of the adductor musculature. Hallux valgus is also known as bunion, in which the big toe points laterally. Hallux varus involves a medial deviation of the first metatarsal or big toe, sometimes the result of attempted correction of bunions. It can also result from arthritis or muscular problems.

GAS 534-535, 633, 660; N 514; McM 354

86 D. In claw toe, both the proximal and distal interphalangeal joints are strongly flexed, the result of muscle imbalance in the foot. With muscular imbalance, the extensors of the interphalangeal joints are overpowered by the long flexors. The metatarsophalangeal joint is extended, whereas in hammertoe it can be in a neutral position. Either hammer toe or claw toe can occur from arthritic changes. Hammertoe can affect any toe, but it most commonly affects the second toe, then the third or fourth toes. It results most commonly from wearing shoes that are too short or shoes with heels that are too high. In hammertoe, the metatarsophalangeal joint is extended, the proximal interphalangeal joint is flexed, and the distal phalanx may be dorsiflexed, or it may point downward, looking like a hammer. Hammertoe can occur as a result of a bunion. Calluses, or painful corns, can form on the dorsal surface of the joints. Hallux valgus is more commonly referred to as a bunion. The big toe is angulated toward the little toe and may override the second toe. The base of the first metatarsal bone is directed medially and is subject, painfully, to compression. Pes cavus is the opposite of flat foot; the patient has a high, flexed plantar arch. Pes cavus occurs as a result of hereditary motor and sensory neural problems. It is painful because of metatarsal compression.

GAS 542, 642-645; N 515; McM 310

87 D. The ankle jerk reflex, elicited by tapping the tendo Achilles with the reflex hammer, is mediated by the tibial nerve. The superficial fibular (peroneal) nerve supplies the foot evertor muscles of the lateral compartment of the leg and provides sensory supply for the dorsum of the foot. The deep fibular (peroneal) nerve innervates the foot extensor and invertor muscles in the anterior compartment of the leg and supplies skin between the first and second toes. The common fibular (peroneal) nerve combines the functions of the superficial and deep branches. The medial plantar nerve innervates the abductor and flexor muscles of the big toe, the first lumbrical muscle, and flexor digitorum brevis muscle and provides sensation for the medial plantar surface and three and a half toes.

GAS 621-625; N 516; McM 345

88 B. The posterior femoral cutaneous nerve arises from nerves S1 to S3. It provides inferior cluneal branches to the lower portion of the gluteal region and a perineal branch to the perineum and supplies sensation to the posterior thigh to the level of the popliteal fossa. Superior gluteal innervation arises from dorsal rami of L1 to L3. Meralgia paresthetica is the occurrence of pain or burning sensations on the lateral thigh, from compression of the lateral femoral cutaneous nerve. The sural nerve, sensory to the lower calf and lateral foot, arises from contributions from the tibial nerve and common fibular (peroneal) nerve. The posterior femoral cutaneous is a sensory nerve and does not innervate muscles.

GAS 486, 563; N 527; McM 317

89 B. The lower portion of the vastus medialis inserts upon the medial aspect of the patella and draws it medially, especially in the last quarter of extension—during which it is especially palpable in contraction. This lower portion of the muscle is referred to as the vastus medialis obliquus (VMO). Increasing the strength of this muscle can lessen the lateral dislocation of the patella. The rectus femoris arises from the anterior inferior iliac spine and lip of the acetabulum and draws the patella vertically upward, as does the vastus intermedius.

GAS 590; N 494; McM 328

90 D. Bipartite patella is a normal variant of an unfused superolateral secondary ossification center, which can easily be mistaken for a fracture on a radiograph. The subcutaneous prepatellar bursa can become painfully enlarged with acute or chronic compression, as in crawling about on the knees. Osgood-Schlatter disease is painful involvement of the patellar ligament on the tibial tuberosity, commonly in children 10 to 14 years of age. The medial retinaculum is an expanded portion of the vastus medialis tendon toward the patella.

GAS 586; N 494; McM 335

91 D. Femoral artery puncture is one of the most common vascular procedures. The femoral artery can be localized often by simply feeling for the strongest point of the femoral pulse just inferior to the inguinal ligament. The femoral artery can be accessed with fluoroscopic assistance at the medial edge of the upper portion of the head of the femur. It is easily localized by Doppler ultrasound if the pulse is difficult to detect, such as in an obese patient. It is here that catheters are passed into the femoral artery for catheterization of abdominopelvic and thoracic structures and for antegrade angiography. It is also a site where arterial blood can be obtained for gas analysis. The midinguinal point, halfway between the anterior superior iliac spine and the pubic symphysis, can be either medial or lateral to the femoral artery and is not a dependable landmark. A needle inserted at the level of the inguinal crease, or inferior to the femoral head, can enter the femoral artery distal to the origin of the deep femoral artery, presenting more risk for accidental vascular injury. Four centimeters lateral to the pubic tubercle overlies the deep inguinal ring, with potential entry to spermatic cord, femoral vein, or artery. The fossa ovalis is the opening in the deep fascia of the thigh for the termination of the great saphenous vein in the femoral vein.

GAS 664, 671; N 487; McM 320

92 D. Both the medial and lateral menisci are subject to rotational injuries and may be torn. The medial meniscus is much more liable to injury because it is attached to the fused deep layer of the medial collateral ligament and joint capsule. The lateral meniscus is separated from the fibular collateral ligament and is external to the capsule of the knee joint. Commonly seen in football players' knees, meniscal tears are usually diagnosed by MRI or by arthroscopy. The presenting symptoms of tearing may be pain and swelling, or locking of the knee. Locking of the knee suggests a bucket handle tear, in which a partly detached cartilage wedges between the tibia and femur, inhibiting further movement. A bucket handle tear is often associated with rupture of the anterior cruciate ligament. Sometimes a momentary click can be heard in flexion/extension movements of the knee. Meniscectomy is a successful operation, but currently there is greater emphasis on repairing small tears. Meniscal cysts can form secondary to meniscal tears and some of these can also be treated arthroscopically.

GAS 587, 606; N 495; McM 322

93 B. The tendons of the semitendinosus and semimembranosus provide the superior medial border of the popliteal fossa. The semitendinosus inserts with the pes anserinus on the proximal, medial tibia. The semimembranosus inserts on the tibia posteriorly. The biceps femoris forms the superior lateral border of the fossa, as the tendon passes to insertion on the fibula. The plantaris arises from the femur just above the lateral head of the gastrocnemius, passing distally to insert on the calcaneus via the tendo Achilles. The popliteus arises from the tibia and passes superiorly and laterally to insert on the lateral condyle of the femur, with a connection to the lateral meniscus.

GAS 598, 616; N 503; McM 330

94 C. The tensor fasciae latae (which is innervated by the superior gluteal nerve) and the iliotibial tract are dense, wide aponeurosis that receives the insertion of the tensor fasciae latae and about 75% of the gluteus maximus. The gluteus maximus is the only one of the muscles listed that is supplied by the inferior gluteal nerve; in fact, it is the only muscle innervated by the inferior gluteal nerve. Gluteus medius and minimus insert on the greater trochanter and are innervated by the superior gluteal nerve. The rectus femoris, supplied by the femoral nerve, inserts via the quadriceps tendon on the patella and tibial tuberosity.

GAS 571, 664; N 481; McM 320

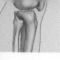

95 D. The tendinous distal portion of the adductor magnus inserts on the adductor tubercle on the upper border of the medial condyle of the femur. The femoral artery passes through the adductor hiatus proximal to this tendinous band, continuing as the popliteal artery. The semimembranosus inserts on the proximal, posterior portion of the tibia. The gracilis inserts with the pes anserinus on the proximal, medial aspect of the tibia. The popliteus inserts on the distal lateral portion of the femur, just above the origin of the lateral head of gastrocnemius. The vastus medialis inserts with other quadriceps muscle components on the patella and then on to the tibial tuberosity.

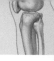

GAS 590-594; N 477; McM 301

96 B. The iliopsoas forms the lateral portion of the troughlike floor of the femoral triangle. The pectineus forms the medial portion of this floor. The adductor longus provides a medial border for the femoral triangle and meets the sartorius, the lateral border of the triangle, at the apex. The rectus femoris is a superficial contributor to the quadriceps femoris, lateral to the femoral triangle (*GAS* Fig. 6-41).

GAS 535, 572; N 487; McM 320

97 A. The tendon of the obturator internus leaves the pelvic cavity by passing through the lesser sciatic foramen, wrapping around the lesser sciatic notch, changing direction by about 90 degrees. It is joined there by the superior and inferior gemelli and inserts with them on the upper portion of the greater trochanter. The obturator externus arises on the external surface of the pubic bone and obturator membrane and inserts on the greater trochanter. The quadratus femoris arises from the ischial tuberosity and inserts on the intertrochanteric line of the femur. The gluteus medius and minimus insert together on the lateral aspect of the greater trochanter.

GAS 426, 448-451; N 486; McM 276

98 B. Generally, the angle of inclination between the neck and shaft of the femur in older age decreases to around 120 degrees. However, in pathologic conditions it can either increase or decrease from the predicted value. When the angle of inclination increases, it is referred to as coxa valga. Coxa vara on the other hand is a condition characterized by a decreased angle of inclination. Genu varum and genu valgum are deformities characterized by a decreased Q-angle and increased Q-angle, respectively. The Q-angle refers to the angle between the femur and tibia. Hallux valgus is a condition that presents with a lateral deviation of the large toe.

GAS 554, 584; N 476; McM 294

99 D. Plantar fasciitis is a common clinical condition that results from tearing or inflammation of the tough band of tissue stretching from the calcaneus to the ball of the foot (the plantar aponeurosis). It usually happens to people who are on their feet frequently or engaged in athletics, especially running and jumping. Plantar fasciitis is usually most painful in the morning, just after getting up from bed and beginning to walk. Rest, orthotics, night splints, and antiinflammatory medications are employed in treatment. A Pott's fracture is a bimalleolar fracture, specifically a fracture of the distal end of the fibula (lateral malleolus) and medial malleolus, with outward displacement of the foot. Dupuytren's fracture involves fracture of the distal fibula with dislocation of the foot. Each of these fractures occurs due to sudden and forceful eversion of the foot.

GAS 649; N 519; McM 349

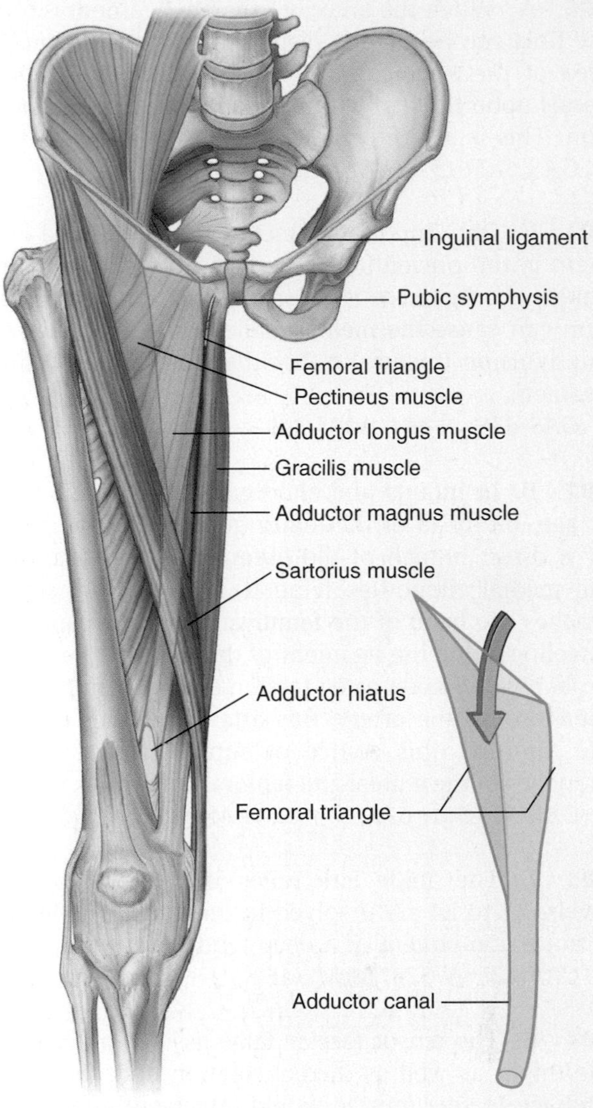

***GAS* Fig. 6-41**

100 **A.** When the anterior cruciate ligament is torn, the tibia can be slightly displaced anteriorly from the area of the knee joint by pulling firmly with both hands upon the leg, with the patient in a seated position. This is a positive anterior drawer sign.
GAS 612-615; N 496; McM 322

101 **E.** One important function of the deltoid ligament is the prevention of excessive extension of the ankle. The ligament is so strong that excessive eversion can cause the medial malleolus to be pulled off (an avulsion fracture) rather than tearing the deltoid ligament.
GAS 638; N 514; McM 349

102 **B.** In infants and children up to about 8 years of age, the head of the femur gets its arterial supply by a direct branch of the obturator artery (variably, the medial circumflex femoral). The arterial supply reaches the head of the femur at the fovea capitis by traveling along the ligament of the head of the femur. Probably due to repeated torsion on the ligament, and therefore on the artery, this artery occludes early in life. In turn, this source of supply is replaced by branches of the gluteal and femoral circumflex vessels.
GAS 558-561, 676; N 491; McM 255

103 **E.** The ankle jerk reflex involves S1 and S2 levels. L2 to L4 are involved in the patellar reflex. L5 is not a component of a deep tendon reflex.
GAS 621; N 527; McM 345

104 **B.** The tensor fasciae latae assists in flexion of the thigh, as well as medial rotation and abduction. Damage to this muscle would adversely affect these motions. The rectus femoris extends the hip. The vastus intermedius extends the knee. The semimembranosus extends the hip and flexes and medially rotates the knee. The sartorius assists in flexion and lateral rotation of the hip, as well as in medial rotation of the knee.
GAS 671; N 481; McM 320

105 **B.** The femoral triangle is the best place to palpate the femoral pulse. It is bounded by the sartorius muscle laterally, adductor longus medially, and the inguinal ligament superiorly. It contains the femoral vein, artery, and nerve (from medial to lateral, respectively). The adductor canal lies deep between the anterior and medial compartments of the thigh and therefore cannot be palpated. The popliteal fossa is the fossa at the back of the knee and contains the popliteal artery and vein, tibial nerve, and common fibular (peroneal) nerve. The femoral pulse cannot be palpated here. The inguinal canal is in the pelvis and is in communication with the anterior abdominal wall. It contains the spermatic cord in males and round ligament of the uterus in females.
GAS 572, 671; N 488; McM 320

106 **A.** If the femoral artery is occluded, the descending branch of the lateral circumflex femoral will provide collateral circulation to the thigh. The descending genicular artery is a branch of the femoral and therefore would also be occluded. The medial circumflex femoral artery is a proximal branch of the deep femoral artery and supplies part of the head of the femur. The first perforating branch of the deep femoral artery supplies a small portion of the muscles of the posterior thigh. Finally, the obturator artery supplies a very small artery and vascularizes only the most proximal part of the head of the femur and usually only during the early years of life.
GAS 561, 566, 582; N 499; McM 322

107 **A.** In a femoral hernia, abdominal contents are forced through the femoral ring, which is just lateral to the lacunar ligament (of Gimbernat) and just medial to the femoral vein. The femoral vein would be found immediately lateral to the femoral hernia. This is correct in most cases because in the majority of people, the femoral vein is found more medial to both the femoral artery and nerve in the femoral triangle. The adductor longus muscle as well as the pectineus muscle would be found deep and medial to the hernia.
GAS 302, 572; N 488; McM 225

108 **A.** The femoral vein lies medial to the femoral artery in the femoral sheath. The femoral sheath is broken into three compartments: lateral, intermediate, and medial. The lateral compartment contains the femoral nerve. The medial compartment encloses the femoral canal and consists of lymphatic tissue and a lymph node, plus areolar tissue. The intermediate contains the femoral vein.
GAS 568, 583; N 488; McM 320

109 **B.** The superficial inguinal nodes are located near the saphenofemoral junction and drain the superior thigh region. The vertical group receives lymph from the superficial thigh, and the horizontal group receives lymph from the gluteal regions and the anterolateral abdominal wall. The deep inguinal lie deep to the fascia lata and receive lymph from deep lymph vessels (popliteal nodes). The external and internal iliac nodes first receive lymph from pelvic and perineal structures (*GAS* Fig. 6-38).
GAS 570; N 472; McM 368

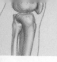

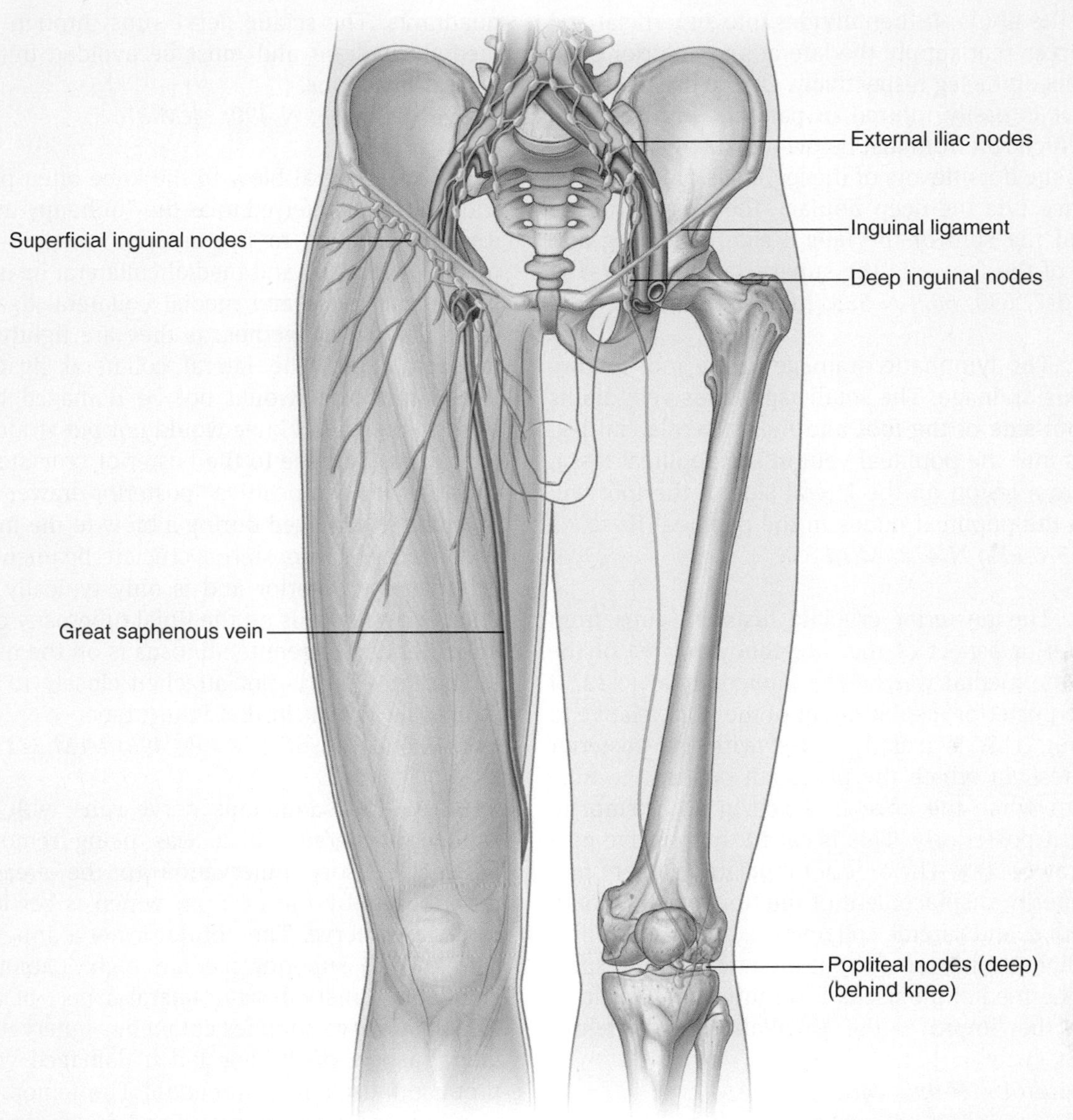

GAS **Fig. 6-38**

110 D. The fibularis (peroneal) brevis muscle originates from the lateral lower two thirds of the shaft of the fibula and inserts on the tubercle at the base of the fifth metatarsal. Any injury to this area will affect this muscle. Patients will present with a weakness in the eversion of the foot. Fibularis (peroneus) longus, extensor hallucis longus and tibialis anterior all insert on the medial side of the foot and will not be affected in this patient. The gastrocnemius inserts via the Achilles tendon to the posterior surface of the calcaneus.

GAS 628-630; N 506; McM 341

111 A. The obturator nerve is a branch of the lumbar plexus that originates from L2 to L4. It descends medial to the psoas on the posterior abdominal wall into the pelvis where it runs along the lateral wall of the lesser pelvis, above and anterior to the obturator vessels. It enters into the medial thigh via the obturator canal (an opening above the obturator membrane) to supply the obturator externus muscle and the adductors of the thigh. The femoral nerve innervates the anterior compartment of the thigh. The inferior gluteal innervates the gluteus maximus muscle, while the superior gluteal innervates the gluteus minimus and medius. The tibial nerve innervates the posterior compartment of the lower limb.

GAS 486, 500, 563-565; N 484; McM 261

112 A. The common fibular (peroneal) nerve is a branch of the sciatic nerve. It descends on the lateral side of the popliteal fossa before winding around the

head of the fibula. It then divides into superficial and deep nerves that supply the lateral and anterior compartments of the leg respectively. Due to its superficial course, it is easily injured in patients with long leg casts (which run from just below the knee). The nerve supplies the dorsiflexors of the leg, the skin of the first web space (via the deep fibular), the evertors of the foot, and the skin of the lateral side of the leg and dorsum of the foot (via the superficial fibular).
GAS 617, 630, 632; N 529; McM 320

113 **C.** The lymphatic drainage of the foot follows its venous drainage. The small saphenous vein drains the lateral side of the foot and the posterolateral leg. It drains into the popliteal vein in the popliteal fossa. Therefore a lesion on the lateral side of the foot will drain to the popliteal nodes in the popliteal fossa.
GAS 570-571; N 472; McM 359

114 **E.** The posterior cruciate ligament runs from the posterior aspect of the intercondylar area of the tibia to the medial wall of the intercondylar fossa. It prevents posterior displacement of the tibia relative to the femur. This is usually tested with the posterior drawer test, in which the physician pushes the tibia backward while the knee is flexed in an attempt to displace it posteriorly. This is called the positive posterior drawer sign. The anterior cruciate ligament prevents anterior displacement of the tibia on the femur. The medial and lateral collateral ligaments stabilize the medial and lateral sides of the knee joint, respectively. The medial meniscus is an intracapsular fibrocartilage that improves the articulation of the femur and tibia.
GAS 612-615; N 496; McM 332

115 **B.** The deep fibular (peroneal) nerve is a branch of the common fibular (peroneal) nerve. It is mainly a motor nerve that innervates the anterior compartment of the leg. Its only cutaneous innervation is to the skin of the first web space. The saphenous nerve innervates the medial side of the leg and foot. The cutaneous branch of superficial fibular (peroneal) nerve innervates the anterior part of the lower leg and the dorsum of the foot. The sural nerve innervates the lateral side of the leg and foot.
GAS 632; N 529; McM 347

116 **B.** The gluteal region can be divided into quadrants by two lines positioned using palpable bony landmarks. One line runs inferiorly from the highest point of the iliac crest. The second line runs horizontally midway between the iliac crests and the ischial tuberosity. This divides the gluteal region into four quadrants. The sciatic nerve runs through the lower medial quadrant and must be avoided during intragluteal injections.
GAS 581, 663; N 490; McM 316

117 **A.** A lateral blow to the knee often produces a trio of injuries referred to as the "unhappy triad." This involves damage to the anterior cruciate ligament, medial meniscus, and medial collateral ligament. The medial meniscus and medial collateral ligament are often damaged together, as they are tightly attached to each other. The lateral collateral ligament and lateral meniscus would not be damaged because a blow to the lateral knee would not put strain on these structures. Damage to the posterior cruciate ligament would produce a positive "posterior drawer sign" and is typically damaged during a blow to the medial side of the knee. The posterior cruciate ligament is stronger than the anterior and is only typically damaged when a person falls on the tibial tuberosity of a flexed knee. Tendon of semitendinosus is on the medial side of the knee but is not attached closely to the other structures or taut in this injury type.
GAS 606-613, 673; N 495, 496; McM 322

118 **A.** The saphenous nerve runs with the great saphenous nerve which was being removed from patient. Sensory innervation to the areas of loss described is by the L4 root, which is carried by the saphenous nerve. The obturator nerve innervates the skin on the superior medial thigh. Lateral femoral cutaneous innervates the lateral aspect of the thigh. The tibial nerve supplies cutaneous innervation to the lateral aspect of the leg and if damaged would also produce muscular dysfunction. The femoral nerve is a motor and sensory nerve and is the origin of the saphenous nerve.
GAS 604; N 525; McM 346

119 **B.** Ligaments act to prevent excessive movement of joints. When a joint is forced into a position, that ligament is stretched and will be tender or rupture if the force is severe enough. Inversion is when the sole of the foot is turned medially and therefore will stretch ligaments that oppose this action. The calcaneofibular ligament is on the lateral side and stretches between the fibula and the calcaneous. It is the only ligament that would be damaged during such an action. The calcaneonavicular and long and short plantar ligaments are located on the plantar surface of the foot and will not be damaged during inversion injuries. The deltoid ligament is located medially and will not be affected.
GAS 638-647; N 514; McM 349

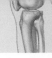

120 A. The patellar reflex causes extension of the knee and is produced by the quadriceps muscle group which consist of; biceps femoris and vastus lateralis, medialis and intermedius. Quadratus femoris is a lateral rotator of the thigh. The sartorius is a flexor of the hip and knee, and the pectineus is an adductor and flexor of the hip.
GAS 586, 606; N 493; McM 323

121 B. The lateral femoral circumflex artery is a branch of the femoral artery close to the hip joint. It gives a branch that runs down the lateral aspect of the thigh and joins the genicular anastomosis via the superior lateral genicular artery. The medial circumflex femoral artery does not provide any branches that descend toward the knee. The anterior and posterior tibial arteries are the terminal branches of the popliteal artery and would not receive any blood if the popliteal is damaged. The fibular (peroneal) artery is a branch of the posterior tibial artery (*GAS* Fig. 6-50).
GAS 566, 582; N 499; McM 220

122 B. The obturator nerve is responsible for innervation of the thigh adductors which form the medial compartment of the thigh. The femoral nerve innervates the anterior compartment and is responsible for extension of the knee. Common fibular (peroneal) nerve supplies the anterior and lateral compartments of the leg while the tibial nerve supplies the posterior compartments of the leg and thigh. The common fibular (peroneal) and tibial nerves are branches of the sciatic nerve.
GAS 486, 500, 563-565; N 488; McM 261

123 A. The skin of the anterior medial thigh and medial leg and foot is supplied by the femoral nerve. The saphenous nerve is a branch of the femoral and only supplies the medial leg and foot. The obturator supplies the medial and medial posterior aspect of the thigh. The tibial nerve supplies the skin of the posterolateral leg, lateral ankle and foot and sole of the foot. The fibular (peroneal) nerve supplies the skin over the lateral aspect of the leg and dorsal aspect of the foot.
GAS 545-549, 604; N 525; McM 320

124 D. The deep fibular (peroneal) nerve is responsible for sensation over the first web space of the foot. Dorsiflexion and inversion of the ankle is produced by the muscles supplied by the deep fibular (peroneal) nerve. The nerves responsible for the knee jerk reflex, knee flexion, eversion, and plantar flexion are all located superior to the location of the tumor and will not be damaged. The nerve located in the space between the tibia and fibula is the deep fibular (peroneal) nerve.
GAS 617, 632; N 529; McM 347

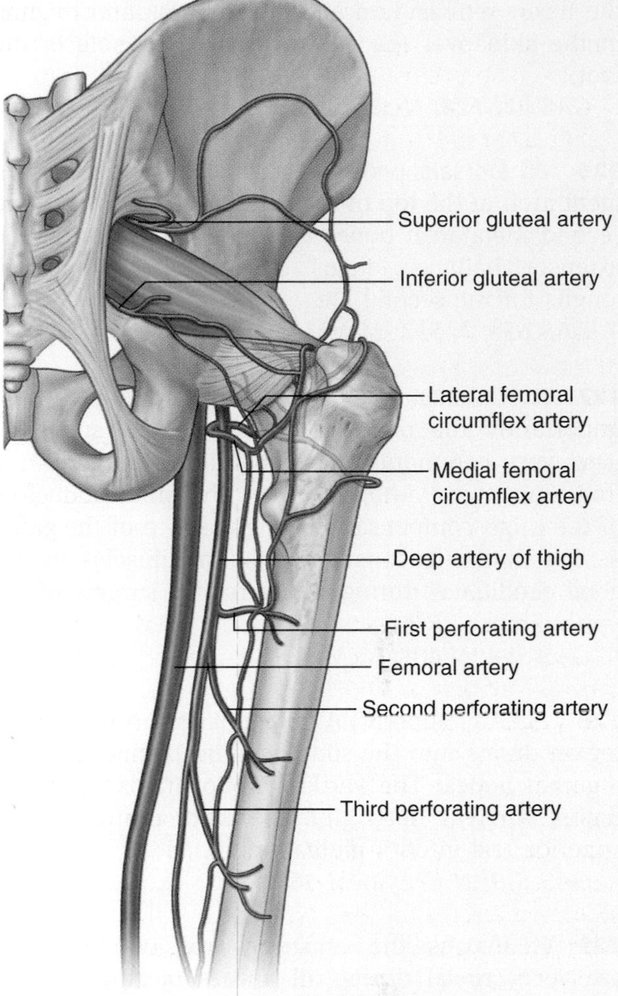

***GAS* Fig. 6-50**

125 E. Tarsal tunnel syndrome is a compression neuropathy resulting from the compression of the tibial nerve in the tarsal tunnel. The tarsal tunnel is located between the medial malleolus, the inferomedial surface of the calcaneus, and the flexor retinaculum. The contents are the tibial nerve and its plantar branches, the tendons of the tibialis posterior, flexor digitorum longus, and the flexor hallucis longus muscles together with the posterior tibial vessels. Any inflammation or swelling in the area will compress on these structures, most significantly the tibial nerve. The posterior tibial vein will be most easily compressed but the nerve is most clinically significant. Clinically, this syndrome is diagnosed with the patient's history and physical examination findings including a positive Tinel's sign (lightly tapping over the flexor retinaculum elicits numbness and tingling in the skin over the calcaneus and the sole of the foot).

GAS 621-628; N 516; McM 345

126 **A.** Dorsalis pedis pulse is palpated at the prominent arch of the top of the foot between the first and second metatarsal bones between the tendon of the extensor hallucis longus and extensor digitorum longus for the second toe.

GAS 658; N 517; McM 348

127 **A.** Gracilis due to its shape, size, and more importantly the nature of neurovascular supply is used very commonly in reconstructive surgery as a free functioning autograft. Also, the other adductors of the thigh compensate for the absence of the gracilis. For similar reasons the remaining muscles are not good candidates during reconstructive surgery of the upper limb.

GAS 594; N 488; McM 323

128 **A.** Any superficial inflammation in the gluteal region drains into the superficial horizontal group of inguinal nodes. The vertical group drains the lower limbs, whereas deep gluteal injuries drain into the superior and inferior gluteal nodes.

GAS 519; N 472; McM 368

129 **E.** Because the hamstrings cross two joints and are very crucial during all phases of running, but especially during the late swing through midstance phase of running, are easily injured. Their normal action includes hip extension and knee flexion. The do not rotate the hip.

GAS 598; N 482; McM 319

130 **B.** The rough bony projection at the junction of the inferior end of the body of the ischium and its ramus is the large ischial tuberosity. Much of the body's weight rests on these tuberosities when sitting, and it provides the proximal, tendinous attachment of the posterior thigh muscles (hamstring muscles and adductor magnus). The hamstring muscles are associated with hip extension and knee flexion. The adduction of the hip joint will be affected slightly because the adductor magnus is affected, although the rest of the adductor muscles are intact.

GAS 551-553, 575, 590, 594; N 478; McM 292

131 **D.** Duchenne muscular dystrophy is a condition that causes muscle weakness. It starts in childhood and may be noticed when a child has difficulty standing up, climbing, or running, which requires extension of the hip. This patient has the classic Gower's sign. The gluteus maximus functions primarily between the flexed and standing (straight) positions of the thigh, as when rising from the sitting position, straightening from the bending position, walking uphill and up stairs, and running.

GAS 575, 590, 594; N 482; McM 318

132 **A.** The gluteal region (buttocks) is a common site for intramuscular injection of drugs, particularly if the volume of the injection is large. To avoid injury to the underlying sciatic nerve, the injection should be given well forward on the upper outer quadrant of the buttock (superolateral quadrant). The patient is showing the Trendelenburg gait pattern (or gluteus medius lurch), which is caused by weakness of the gluteus medius and minimus muscles. These muscles are supplied by the superior gluteal nerve (L4, L5, S1), which emerges from the greater sciatic notch above the upper border of the piriformis and immediately disappears beneath the posterior border of the gluteus medius and runs forward between the gluteus medius and minimus. Intramuscular injection in the upper inner quadrant (superomedially) is most likely to damage this nerve. The sciatic nerve is most likely damaged in the inferomedial quadrant of the buttock.

GAS 581; N 482; McM 316

133 **D.** The anterior cruciate ligament is attached to the anterior intercondylar area and the posterior part of the medial surface of the lateral femoral condyle. Posterior displacement of the femur on the tibia is prevented by the ACL. With the knee joint flexed, the ACL prevents the tibia from being pulled anteriorly. The posterior cruciate ligament is stronger, shorter, and broader, less oblique, and prevents anterior displacement of the femur on the tibia. Lateral collateral ligaments are cordlike and are attached proximally to the lateral side of the head of the fibula overlapped by the tendon of biceps femoris. The medial collateral ligament is a flat band and is attached above to the medial condyle of the femur and below to the medial surface of the shaft of the tibia. It is firmly attached to the edge of the medial meniscus and consequently is more prone to be injured. The oblique popliteal ligament is a tendinous expansion derived from the semimembranosus muscle. It strengthens the posterior aspect of the knee joint capsule. The patellar ligament (tendon) connects the lower border of the patella with the smooth convexity on the tuberosity of the tibia. It represents the continuation of the quadriceps tendon.

GAS 586-588, 612; N 496; McM 332

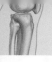

134 B. The psoas muscle arises from the base of the transverse processes, the sides of the vertebral bodies, and the intervertebral discs, from the twelfth thoracic to the fifth lumbar vertebrae and inserted into the lesser trochanter of the femur. The sheath of the psoas retains the pus of a psoas abscess, and spinal tuberculosis may present as a cold abscess in the groin (in the vicinity of the lesser trochanter). The psoas is enclosed in a fibrous sheath that is derived from the lumbar fascia. The sheath is not part of the lumbar fascia, but the lateral edge blends with the anterior layer of that fascia.

GAS 590-591; N 485; McM 263

135 B. The psoas muscle arises from the base of the transverse processes, the sides of the vertebral bodies, and the intervertebral discs, from the twelfth thoracic to the fifth lumbar vertebrae and inserted into the lesser trochanter of the femur. The psoas flexes the thigh at the hip joint on the trunk, or if the thigh is fixed, it flexes the trunk on the thigh, as in sitting up from a lying position. The inflamed appendix is pushed up against the peritoneum from the the contracted psoas. As a result it is in touch with the parietal peritoneum, producing acute pain. In some other cases it may retain the purulence of a psoas abscess, and spinal tuberculosis may present as a cold abscess in the groin. The psoas is enclosed in a fibrous sheath that is derived from the lumbar fascia. The sheath is not part of the lumbar fascia but the lateral edge blends with the anterior layer of that fascia.

GAS 590-591; N 485; McM 264

136 B. The saphenous nerve is the longest and most widely distributed cutaneous branch of the femoral nerve; it is the only branch not from the sciatic nerve to extend beyond the knee. It gives sensory innervations to the medial aspect of the thigh, leg, and the medial planter arch. It accompanies the great saphenous vein over the medial side of the leg. The great saphenous vein is formed by the union of the dorsal vein of the great toe and the dorsal venous arch of the foot. It ascends anterior to the medial malleolus and passes posterior to the medial condyle of the femur and ends when it joins the femoral vein.

GAS 604, 662; N 525; McM 329

137 C. The deep fibular (peroneal) nerve passes deep to the extensor retinaculum and supplies the intrinsic muscles on the dorsum of the foot (extensors digitorum and hallucis longus) and the tarsal and tarsometatarsal joints. When it finally emerges as a cutaneous nerve, it is so far distal in the foot that only a small area of skin remains available for innervation: the web of skin between and contiguous sides of the first and second toes. The superficial fibular (peroneal) nerve supplies the skin on the anterolateral aspect of the leg and divides into the medial and intermediate dorsal cutaneous nerves, which continue across the ankle to supply most of the skin on the dorsum of the foot.

GAS 631-632; N 529; McM 347

138 E. The obturator membrane is a fibrous sheet that almost completely closes the obturator foramen, leaving a small gap, the obturator canal, for the passage of the obturator nerve and vessels as they leave the pelvis to enter the medial thigh. The femoral canal is the small medial compartment for the lymph vessels. It is about 0.5 in (1.3 cm) long, and its upper opening is called the femoral ring. It has following borders: anteriorly the inguinal ligament; posteriorly the superior ramus of the pubis; medially the lacunar ligament; and laterally the femoral vein. A triangular-shaped defect in the external oblique aponeurosis lies immediately above and medial to the pubic tubercle. This is known as the superficial inguinal ring. The deep ring is an oval opening in the transversalis fascia and lies about 0.5 in (1.3 cm) above the inguinal ligament, midway between the anterior superior iliac spine and the pubic symphysis. Fossa ovalis, which refers to an oval opening in the superomedial part of the fascia lata of the thigh, lies 3 to 4 cm inferolateral to the pubic tubercle.

GAS 441, 492, 565, 580; N 488; McM 271

139 C. The deep nodes are located beneath the deep fascia (fascia cribrosa) and lie along the medial side of the femoral vein. The presence of swollen inguinal lymph nodes is an important clinical sign because swelling may indicate an infection in the lower extremities. They then drain superiorly to the external iliac lymph nodes. The superficial nodes lie in the superficial fascia below the inguinal ligament and can be divided into horizontal and vertical groups. External iliac lies along the external iliac vessels; they are arranged in groups of three (anteriorly, medially, and lateral to vessels).

GAS 570-571; N 472; McM 368

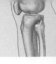

140 D. The inferior gluteal nerve supplies the gluteus maximus muscle, which extends and laterally rotates the hip joint; through the iliotibial tract, it also extends the knee joint. The superior gluteal nerve supplies the gluteus medius and minimus and tensor fasciae latae muscles, which work together as medial rotators of lower limb. The nerve to the piriformis supplies the piriformis muscle, which laterally rotates the femur with hip extension and abducts the femur with hip flexion.

GAS 565, 575, 579; N 490; McM 318

141 A. The talocrural joint is a synovial hinge joint that connects the distal end of the tibia and fibula with the proximal end of the talus. The articulation between the tibia and the talus bears more weight than other joints. Dorsiflexion (toes pointing upward) and plantar flexion (toes pointing downward) are possible. Dorsiflexion is performed by the tibialis anterior, extensor hallucis longus, extensor digitorum longus, and peroneus tertius. Plantar flexion is performed by the gastrocnemius, soleus, plantaris, peroneus longus, peroneus brevis, tibialis posterior, flexor digitorum longus, and flexor hallucis longus. The movements of inversion and eversion take place at the talocalcaneal joint.

GAS 638; N 514; McM 349

142 E. Plantar flexion is mostly due to the gastrocnemius and soleus muscles, which are supplied by the tibial nerve. The tibial nerve leaves the popliteal fossa by passing deep to the gastrocnemius and soleus muscles and lies posterior to the popliteal artery. Therefore a hematoma of the popliteal artery will also compress the nerve. Dorsiflexion of the foot is due to contraction of the muscles in the anterior compartment of the leg.

GAS 621; N 504, 505; McM 330

143 A. A lateral blow to the knee could result in injury to three structures in the knee: anterior cruciate ligament, medial collateral ligament, and the medial meniscus. When all three structures are involved it is collectively called the "unhappy triad." Anterior drawer sign is due to injury to the anterior cruciate ligament and denoted by anterior displacement of the tibia in relation to femur, similar to pulling out a drawer from a desk.

GAS 606, 673; N 496; McM 332

144 C. The lymphatic drainage of the leg is such that superficial lymphatics on the anterolateral side of the foot and leg and all the deep lymphatics in the foot and leg first drain into the popliteal nodes and then to the deep inguinal nodes. This patient has an infected anterolateral midleg injury, which will first drain into the popliteal nodes. The vertical group of superficial inguinal nodes receives superficial lymphatics from the medial side of the foot, leg, and all the superficial lymph from the thigh. The horizontal group of superficial lymphatics receives lymph from the anterior abdominal wall below the umbilicus, perineum (except the glans penis in men and clitoris in women), and lower third of the anal canal. The popliteal nodes eventually drain to the deep inguinal nodes, but are usually not palpable. The iliac nodes are deep structures and are not be palpable during physical examination.

GAS 570-571; N 472; McM 359

145 B. The obturator membrane is a thin membrane that covers the obturator foramen except at its superior part. The obturator nerve exits the pelvis and enters into the medial compartment of the thigh by passing through the obturator canal alongside the obturator vessels. Traumatic injuries to the membrane will most likely lead to obturator nerve damage. The obturator nerve supplies motor innervations to the adductor muscles of the thigh (gracilis, obturator externus, adductor longus, adductor brevis and a portion of the adductor magnus). It also provides sensory innervation to the medial aspect of the thigh. Urinary and fecal incontinence is mediated by autonomic nerves and the pudendal nerve. Both nerves have no relationship with the obturator membrane. The gluteus medius and minimus muscles are the main hip abductors. They also stabilize the hip on the swing-side during motion. These muscles are supplied by the superior gluteal nerve, which leaves the pelvis through the greater sciatic foramen above the piriformis muscle. Flexors of the hip found in the anterior compartment of the thigh are innervated by the femoral nerve, which has no relationship with the obturator membrane. The sciatic nerve supplies the muscles in the posterior compartment of the thigh and also sends cutaneous innervations to the skin of the posterior thigh. It enters the posterior compartment of the thigh from the gluteal region.

GAS 441, 492, 565, 580; N 488; McM 271

146 C. The deep fibular (peroneal) nerve is a branch of the common fibular (peroneal) nerve and begins at about the level of the neck of the fibula, between it and the fibularis (peroneus) longus. This nerve supplies the extensors of the foot (extensor digitorum longus, fibularis [peroneus] tertius, extensor hallucis longus, tibialis anterior, extensor digitorum brevis, and extensor hallucis brevis). It innervates the first web space of the foot. Fracture of the head of the fibula can damage this nerve, resulting in a high stepping gait and numbness over the dorsum and first web space of the foot. Muscles in the posterior compartment of the leg are involved in planter flexion. These muscles are innervated by the tibial nerve, which is a continuation of the sciatic nerve; its medial cutaneous branch supplies sensation to the posteromedial side of the leg. Waddling gait and numbness at the anterolateral side of the leg are associated with the superficial fibular and the lateral sural cutaneous nerves.

GAS 631-632; N 529; McM 337

147 D. A positive valgus stress test indicates injury to the medial collateral ligament. Injuries to this ligament usually involve the anterior cruciate ligament. The femur is usually pushed posteriorly during stair climbing, an action that is opposed by a normal anterior cruciate ligament. Injury to the anterior cruciate ligament results in posterior displacement of the femur in relation to the tibia with difficulty climbing stairs. Extension of the knee is done mainly by the quadriceps femoris muscle. The posterior thigh muscles provide flexion of the knee. Gravity pushes the femur forward while walking down a flight, which is stabilized by the posterior cruciate ligament, which is not damaged in this case. The patient has no difficulty walking down the stairs; the posterior cruciate ligament stabilizes the knee during this action.

GAS 610-615; N 496; McM 332

148 E. The calcaneofibular ligament is located inferior and just anterior to the lateral malleolus and connects the lateral malleolus to the calcaneus. The interosseous ligament between the tibia and the fibula is located medially and superior to the lateral malleolus. The tibionavicular ligaments are located on the medial side of the ankle joint, and the point of injury and tenderness is at the lateral side. The anterior tibiofibular ligament is located anterior to the ankle joint, away from the point of injury (*GAS* Fig. 6-99).

GAS 638-645; N 514; McM 349

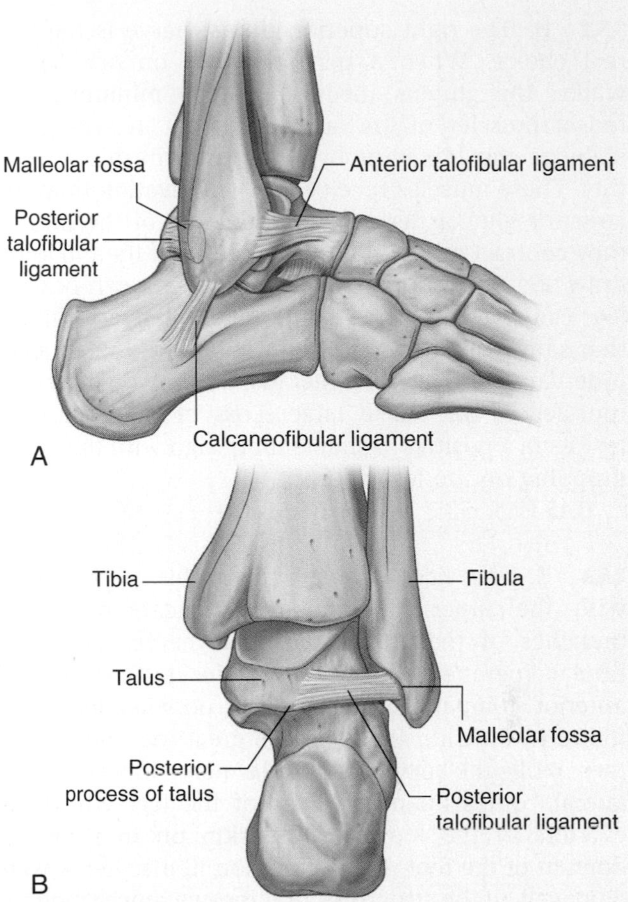

***GAS* Fig. 6-99**

149 E. The paraxial mesoderm develops into somites. Limb muscles develop from the ventral myotome of the somites in response to molecular signals. Embryological derivatives of the lateral plate mesoderm include the circulatory and gut wall, body wall lining, and dermis. Derivative of the neural crest cells does not include the limb muscles. Chondrification is associated with cartilage formation and not muscles. The intermediate mesoderm eventually thins out laterally and becomes the mesoderm, which gives the circulatory and gut walls, plus the lining of the body wall and dermis.

GAS 592; N 479

150 C. Mesenchyme between digital rays undergoes apoptosis for the digits to form. Failure or incomplete apoptosis usually results in fused digits (syndactyly). This may involve the skin and soft tissues alone or may include the bone. Digital rays form from the hand plate. Failure of development of any digital ray results in underdevelopment of a finger or toe. Neural crest cells do not contribute to the formation of the foot. The zone of polarizing activity modulates the patterning of the limb in the anteroposterior diameter. The abnormality described did not involve the phalanges, as shown by radiograph, and thus could not have been caused by faulty chondrification.

GAS 637-638; N 507; McM 335

151 B. The suprapatellar bursa is found in the anterior surface of the inferior part of the femur under the quadriceps femoris muscle. A high-riding superior patellar fragment lead to the exposure of this bursa. In traumatic episodes following this condition, blood and fat from the knee can enter into the suprapatellar bursa. The popliteal bursa is located behind the knee, away from the site of injury. The superficial infrapatellar bursa is located below the patella, between the patella ligament and the skin. The deep infrapatellar bursa is located below the site of the injury, between the upper part of the tibia and the patella ligament. The gastrocnemius bursa is at the back of the knee, as well as below the level of the injury.

GAS 609; N 494; McM 335

152 B. The right superior gluteal nerve is the correct choice. When a person stands on one leg or walks, the gluteus medius, gluteus minimus, and tensor muscles of the fascia latae act in synergy to stabilize the hip joint by abducting the hip (pelvic tilt). These muscles receive their innervation from the superior gluteal nerve. The abductors of the hip, as they contract to maintain the stability of the hip joint, draw the pelvis forcefully toward the weigh-bearing leg, causing the opposite side of the pelvis to tilt in that same direction. The right superior gluteal nerve innervates its ipsilateral medius, minimus, and tensor muscles of the fascia latae. Loss of these muscles results in a positive Trendelenburg sign with the pelvis dropping on the left side.
GAS 565, 575; N 489; McM 318

153 E. The deep fibular (peroneal) nerve along with the superficial fibular (peroneal) nerve are branches of the common fibular nerve. The deep fibular (peroneal) nerve innervates muscles of the anterior compartment of the leg dorsiflexors of the foot and the skin between the great toe and second toes, while the superficial fibular nerve innervates the lateral compartment muscles of the leg, which are evertors of the foot and the skin on most of the dorsum of the foot. If the common fibular nerve were damaged all the structures that receive innervation via this nerve will be compromising dorsiflexion and eversion. Damage to the superficial fibular nerve affects the ability to evert the foot but does not result in foot drop, making the deep fibular nerve, which innervates the dorsiflexors of the foot, the best choice as the injury describes foot drop with the ability to evert the foot conserved. The saphenous nerve is a cutaneous nerve, while the tibial nerve innervates posterior compartment muscles.
GAS 617, 632; N 529; McM 331

154 D. The S1 nerve root provides cutaneous innervation to the lateral aspect of the ankle, the lateral sides of the dorsum and sole of foot, and motor innervation to the gastrocnemius muscle, which plantar flexes the foot and contracts during the ankle jerk reflex. It receives its innervation from the S1, S2 nerve roots via the tibial nerve, making D the correct choice. T12 roots do not reach the foot; L2 roots will reach the hip region and thigh; L4 innervates the invertors of the foot and skin over medial leg, ankle, and side of foot; and S3 innervates the sitting area of the buttocks, posterior scrotum or labia, and the small muscles of the foot.
GAS 545-550; N 528; McM 345

155 A. All the branches of the posterior femoral cutaneous nerve are cutaneous. It arises from the dorsal divisions of the first and second and the ventral divisions of the second and third sacral nerves and travels through the greater sciatic foramen beneath the piriformis muscle to innervate the shin over the lower parts of the gluteus maximus muscle through the inferior clunial nerves and the posterior surface of the thigh and leg and perineum via its perineal branches. The lateral femoral cutaneous nerve, which innervates the lateral surface of the thigh, is an incorrect choice; the obturator, sciatic, and femoral nerves all have both motor and sensory branches and can be eliminated, since no motor deficits were described.
GAS 631-632; N 529; McM 337

156 E. The muscles of the limbs develop from the myotome component of the somites. The somites are condensations of paraxial mesoderm that form after the formation of the trilaminar disc. The lateral plate mesoderm gives rise to the serous membranes, coverings of organs and the heart. The intermediate mesoderm gives rise to the urogenital system and its accessory glands. The chondrification centers precede the formation of the muscles, as it gives the skeletal framework. Neural crest cells give rise to dorsal root ganglia, leptomeninges, Schwann cells, sympathetic ganglia, and the chromaffin cells of the adrenal medulla.
GAS 637-638; N 487

157 C. Forceful external rotation and eversion of the ankle often leads to this type of injury as the bony components are pushed apart forcefully. It is commonly referred to as a Pott fracture (the medial malleolus is pulled forcefully by the strong deltoid ligament as the talus moves laterally, causing a fracture of the lateral malleolus). Inversion, extreme plantar flexion, and forceful dorsiflexion cause a rupture of the ligaments. Direct upward force of the talus is usually due to a fall from great height and will damage the spine and calcaneus.
GAS 641; N 514; McM 349

158 A. Knowledge of Hilton's Law would lead to this correct answer. This law in a modified form, can be remembered as "a joint is innervated by the same nerves that innervate the muscles that move that joint." A complete explanation of this law can be found in an article by Hebert-Blouin et al., *Clinical Anatomy* 27:548-555, 2013. The deep fibular (peroneal) nerve is the only nerve listed that innervates muscles that move the ankle joint.

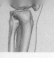

6

UPPER LIMB

INTRODUCTION

First Order Question

1 A 25-year-old man falls on a slippery trail and injures his upper limb. Inspection reveals abrasions over his arm at the area of the triceps muscle. Which of the following nerves innervates the triceps muscle?

- ▢ **A.** Radial
- ▢ **B.** Axillary
- ▢ **C.** Median
- ▢ **D.** Ulnar
- ▢ **E.** Musculocutaneous

Explanation

A: The nerve most likely affected is the radial nerve which innervates the triceps brachii muscle. The axillary, median and ulnar nerves do not innervate any muscles in the arm. The musculocutaneous nerve is innervating the coracobrachialis, biceps brachii, and brachialis muscles in the anterior compartment of the arm.

First Order Question

2 A 25-year-old man falls on a slippery trail and injures his upper limb. Inspection reveals abrasions over his arm. A radiograph shows a fracture at the radial groove of the humerus. Which of the following nerves will most likely be injured?

- ▢ **A.** Radial
- ▢ **B.** Axillary
- ▢ **C.** Median
- ▢ **D.** Ulnar
- ▢ **E.** Musculocutaneous

Explanation

A: The nerve most likely affected is the radial nerve as it travels in the radial groove as it descends along the humerus to the forearm. The axillary nerve runs around the surgical neck of the humerus, the median nerve passes superficial to the muscles of the arm, the ulnar nerve runs at the medial epicondyle, and the musculocutaneous nerve pierces the coracobrachialis muscle and then runs between the brachialis and biceps brachii muscles.

Second Order Question

3 A 25-year-old man falls on a slippery trail and injures his upper limb. Inspection reveals abrasions over his arm. A radiograph shows a fracture at the radial groove of the humerus. Which of the following muscles will most likely be paralyzed?

- ▢ **A.** Triceps brachii
- ▢ **B.** Biceps brachii
- ▢ **C.** Coracobrachialis
- ▢ **D.** Brachialis
- ▢ **E.** Deltoid

Explanation

A: The nerve most likely affected in the radiograph is the radial nerve as it travels in the radial groove along the humerus as it descends to the forearm. The radial nerve innervates the triceps brachii muscle (and extensors in the forearm), whereas the biceps brachii, coracobrachialis, and brachialis muscles are innervated by the musculocutaneous nerve and the deltoid muscle by the axillary nerve.

Third Order Question

4 A 25-year-old man falls on a slippery trail and injures his upper limb. Inspection reveals abrasions over his arm. A radiograph shows a fracture at the radial groove of the humerus. Which of the following will be present during physical examination?

- ▢ **A.** Wrist drop
- ▢ **B.** Inability to flex his hand and loss of pronation
- ▢ **C.** Inability to flex index and middle fingers at the distal interphalangeal (DIP) and proximal interphalangeal (PIP) joints
- ▢ **D.** Inability to flex ring and little fingers at DIP
- ▢ **E.** Paralysis of lumbricals and interosseous muscles

Explanation

A: The nerve likely affected in the radiograph is the radial nerve as it travels in the radial groove as it descends along the humerus to the forearm. The radial nerve innervates the extensor muscles of the forearm. Once these muscles have lost their inability to contract because the radial nerve is injured, the wrist cannot be extended. This is referred to as wrist drop.

B: Inability to flex the hand and loss of pronation is an unlikely choice as flexion of the hand is performed via innervation of muscles by the median and ulnar nerves, pronation of the hand is also performed by muscles innervated by the median nerve.

C: Inability to flex index and middle fingers at the proximal and distal interphalangeal joints is a function of the median nerve.

D: Inability to flex the ring and little fingers at the distal interphalangeal joints describes an ulnar nerve branch deficit.

E: Paralysis of lumbricals and interosseous muscles is an incorrect choice as these muscles are innervated by branches of the median and ulnar nerve which was likely spared during the injury shown on the radiograph (*GAS* Fig. 7-69).

Fourth Order Question

5 A 25-year-old man falls on a slippery trail and injures his upper limb. Inspection reveals abrasions over his arm. The radiograph of his arm is shown in Fig. 6-1. Which deficit will most likely be encountered?

- ▢ **A.** Inability to make a fist
- ▢ **B.** Inability to flex his hand and loss of pronation
- ▢ **C.** Inability to flex index and middle fingers at DIP and PIP joints
- ▢ **D.** Inability to flex ring and little fingers at DIP
- ▢ **E.** Paralysis of lumbricals and interosseous muscles

Explanation

A: The nerve likely affected in the radiograph is the radial nerve as it travels in the radial groove as it descends along the humerus to the forearm. Although the radial nerve does not provide innervations to muscles that close the hand, it does innervate extensor carpi radialis longus and brevis muscles via the posterior interosseous nerve. These muscles act as wrist extensors and are necessary for making a fist, as they contract synergistically with the flexors of the fingers, making it indispensable while performing this action. The "position of function" of the hand is with the wrist extended about 30 degrees.

B: Inability to flex the hand and loss of pronation is an unlikely choice as flexion of the hand is performed via innervation of muscles by the median and ulnar nerves, pronation of the hand is also performed by a muscle innervated by the median nerve.

C: Inability to flex index and middle fingers at the proximal and distal interphalangeal joints is a function of the median nerve.

D: Inability to flex ring and little fingers at the distal interphalangeal describes ulnar nerve branch deficit.

E: Paralysis of lumbricals and interosseous muscles is an incorrect choice as these muscles are innervated by branches of the median and ulnar nerves, which were likely spared during the injury shown on the radiograph (see Fig. 7-22 from GAS 3e).

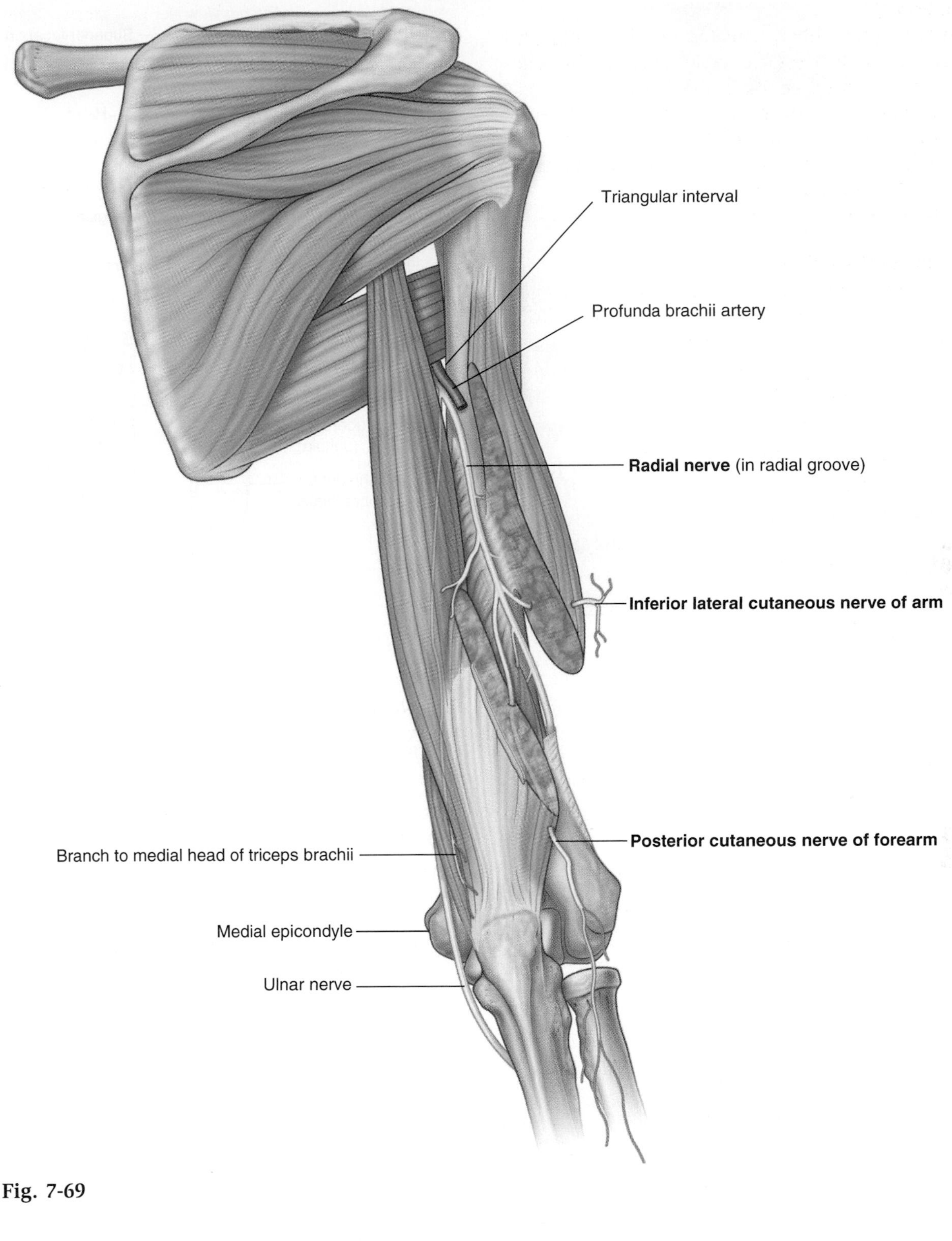

Triangular interval
Profunda brachii artery
Radial nerve (in radial groove)
Inferior lateral cutaneous nerve of arm
Posterior cutaneous nerve of forearm
Branch to medial head of triceps brachii
Medial epicondyle
Ulnar nerve

GAS Fig. 7-69

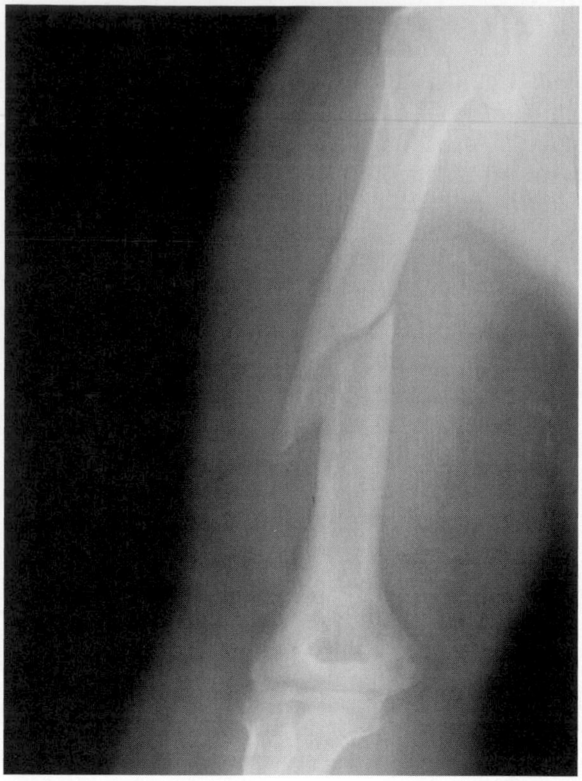

Fig. 6-1

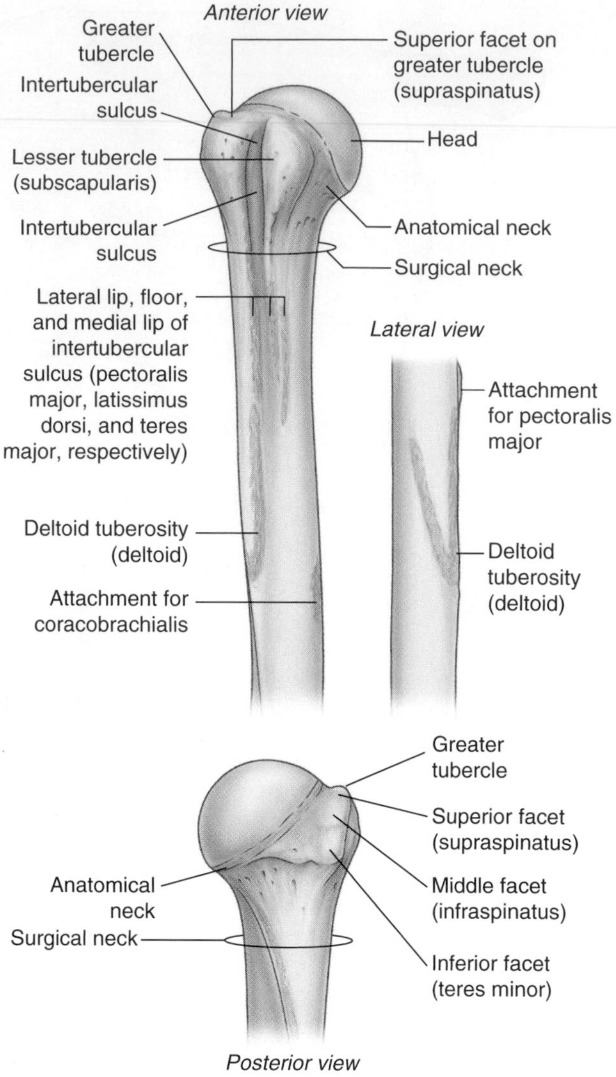
Anterior view
Greater tubercle
Intertubercular sulcus
Lesser tubercle (subscapularis)
Intertubercular sulcus
Lateral lip, floor, and medial lip of intertubercular sulcus (pectoralis major, latissimus dorsi, and teres major, respectively)
Deltoid tuberosity (deltoid)
Attachment for coracobrachialis
Superior facet on greater tubercle (supraspinatus)
Head
Anatomical neck
Surgical neck
Lateral view
Attachment for pectoralis major
Deltoid tuberosity (deltoid)
Greater tubercle
Superior facet (supraspinatus)
Middle facet (infraspinatus)
Inferior facet (teres minor)
Anatomical neck
Surgical neck
Posterior view

GAS Fig. 7-22

MAIN QUESTIONS

1 A 45-year-old woman is being examined as a candidate for cosmetic breast surgery. The surgeon notes that both of her breasts sag considerably. Which structure(s) has most likely become stretched to result in this condition?

- ▢ **A.** Scarpa's fascia
- ▢ **B.** Pectoralis major muscle
- ▢ **C.** Pectoralis minor muscle
- ▢ **D.** Suspensory (Cooper's) ligaments
- ▢ **E.** Serratus anterior muscle

2 A 27-year-old man was admitted to the emergency department after an automobile collision in which he suffered a fracture of the lateral border of the scapula. Six weeks after the accident, physical examination reveals weakness in medial rotation and adduction of the humerus. Which nerve was most likely injured?

- ▢ **A.** Lower subscapular
- ▢ **B.** Axillary
- ▢ **C.** Radial
- ▢ **D.** Spinal accessory
- ▢ **E.** Ulnar

3 A 48-year-old female court stenographer is admitted to the orthopedic clinic with symptoms of carpal tunnel syndrome, with which she has suffered with for almost a year. Which muscles most typically become weakened in this condition?

- ▢ **A.** Dorsal interossei
- ▢ **B.** Lumbricals III and IV
- ▢ **C.** Thenar
- ▢ **D.** Palmar interossei
- ▢ **E.** Hypothenar

4 A 45-year-old man arrived at the emergency department with injuries to his left elbow after he fell in a bicycle race. Plain radiographic and magnetic resonance imaging (MRI) examinations show a fracture of the medial epicondyle and an injured ulnar nerve. Which of the following muscles will most likely be paralyzed?

- ▢ **A.** Flexor digitorum superficialis
- ▢ **B.** Biceps brachii
- ▢ **C.** Brachioradialis
- ▢ **D.** Flexor carpi ulnaris
- ▢ **E.** Supinator

5 While walking to his classroom building, a first-year medical student slipped on the wet pavement and fell against the curb, injuring his right arm. Radiographic images showed a midshaft fracture of the humerus. Which pair of structures was most likely injured at the fracture site?

- ▢ **A.** Median nerve and brachial artery
- ▢ **B.** Axillary nerve and posterior circumflex humeral artery
- ▢ **C.** Radial nerve and deep brachial artery
- ▢ **D.** Suprascapular nerve and artery
- ▢ **E.** Long thoracic nerve and lateral thoracic artery

6 An 18-year-old man is brought to the emergency department after an injury while playing rugby. Imaging reveals a transverse fracture of the humerus about 1 inch proximal to the epicondyles. Which nerve is most frequently injured by the jagged edges of the broken bone at this location?

- ▢ **A.** Axillary
- ▢ **B.** Median
- ▢ **C.** Musculocutaneous
- ▢ **D.** Radial
- ▢ **E.** Ulnar

7 A 52-year-old female band director suffered problems in her right arm several days after strenuous field exercises for a major athletic tournament. Examination in the orthopedic clinic reveals wrist drop and weakness of grasp but normal extension of the elbow joint. There is no loss of sensation in the affected limb. Which nerve was most likely affected?

- ▢ **A.** Ulnar
- ▢ **B.** Anterior interosseous
- ▢ **C.** Posterior interosseous
- ▢ **D.** Median
- ▢ **E.** Superficial radial

8 A 32-year-old woman is admitted to the emergency department after an automobile collision. Radiologic examination reveals multiple fractures of the humerus. Flexion and supination of the forearm are severely weakened. She also has loss of sensation on the lateral surface of the forearm. Which of the following nerves has most likely been injured?

- ▢ **A.** Radial
- ▢ **B.** Musculocutaneous
- ▢ **C.** Median
- ▢ **D.** Lateral cord of brachial plexus
- ▢ **E.** Lateral cutaneous nerve of the forearm

9 A 24-year-old female medical student was bitten at the base of her thumb by her dog. The wound became infected and the infection spread into the radial bursa. The tendon(s) of which muscle will most likely be affected?

- ▢ **A.** Flexor digitorum profundus
- ▢ **B.** Flexor digitorum superficialis
- ▢ **C.** Flexor pollicis longus
- ▢ **D.** Flexor carpi radialis
- ▢ **E.** Flexor pollicis brevis

10 Laboratory studies in the outpatient clinic on a 24-year-old woman included assessment of circulating blood chemistry. Which of the following arteries is most likely at risk during venipuncture at the cubital fossa?

- ▢ **A.** Brachial
- ▢ **B.** Common interosseous
- ▢ **C.** Ulnar
- ▢ **D.** Anterior interosseous
- ▢ **E.** Radial

11 A 22-year-old man is diagnosed with metastatic malignant melanoma of the skin over the xiphoid process. Which lymph nodes receive most of the lymph from this area and are therefore most likely to be involved in metastasis of the tumor?

- ▢ **A.** Deep inguinal
- ▢ **B.** Vertical group of superficial inguinal
- ▢ **C.** Horizontal group of superficial inguinal
- ▢ **D.** Axillary
- ▢ **E.** Deep and superficial inguinal

12 A 49-year-old woman who had suffered a myocardial infarction must undergo a bypass graft procedure using the internal thoracic artery. Which vessels will most likely continue to supply blood to the anterior part of the upper intercostal spaces?

- ▢ **A.** Musculophrenic
- ▢ **B.** Superior epigastric
- ▢ **C.** Posterior intercostal
- ▢ **D.** Lateral thoracic
- ▢ **E.** Thoracodorsal

13 A 22-year-old woman is admitted to the emergency department in an unconscious state. The nurse takes a radial pulse to determine the heart rate of the patient. This pulse is felt lateral to which tendon?

- ▢ **A.** Palmaris longus
- ▢ **B.** Flexor pollicis longus
- ▢ **C.** Flexor digitorum profundus
- ▢ **D.** Flexor carpi radialis
- ▢ **E.** Flexor digitorum superficialis

14 A 45-year-old man is admitted to the hospital after accidentally walking through a plate glass door in a bar while intoxicated. Physical examination shows multiple lacerations to the upper limb, with inability to flex the distal interphalangeal joints of the fourth and fifth digits. Which of the following muscles is most likely affected?

- ▢ **A.** Flexor digitorum profundus
- ▢ **B.** Flexor digitorum superficialis
- ▢ **C.** Lumbricals
- ▢ **D.** Flexor digitorum profundus and flexor digitorum superficialis
- ▢ **E.** Interossei

15 A 24-year-old man is admitted with a wound to the palm of his hand. He cannot touch the pad of his index finger with his thumb but can grip a sheet of paper between all fingers and has no loss of sensation on the skin of his hand. Which of the following nerves has most likely been injured?

- ▢ **A.** Deep branch of ulnar
- ▢ **B.** Anterior interosseous
- ▢ **C.** Median
- ▢ **D.** Recurrent branch of median
- ▢ **E.** Deep branch of radial

16 A 55-year-old man is examined in a neighborhood clinic after receiving blunt trauma to his right axilla in a fall. He has difficulty elevating the right arm above the level of his shoulder. Physical examination shows that the inferior angle of his right scapula protrudes more than the lower part of the left scapula. The right scapula protrudes far more when the patient pushes against the examiner's hand with resistance. Which of the following neural structures has most likely been injured?

- ▢ **A.** The posterior cord of the brachial plexus
- ▢ **B.** The long thoracic nerve
- ▢ **C.** The upper trunk of the brachial plexus
- ▢ **D.** The site of origin of the middle and lower subscapular nerves
- ▢ **E.** Spinal nerve ventral rami C7, C8, and T1

17 A mother tugs violently on her 4-year-old boy's hand to pull him out of the way of an oncoming car and the child screams in pain. Thereafter, it becomes obvious that the child cannot straighten his forearm at the elbow. When the child is seen in the emergency department, radiographic examination reveals a dislocation of the head of the radius. Which of the following ligaments is most likely directly associated with this injury?

- ▢ **A.** Anular
- ▢ **B.** Joint capsular
- ▢ **C.** Interosseous
- ▢ **D.** Radial collateral
- ▢ **E.** Ulnar collateral

18 After a forceps delivery of an infant boy, the baby presents with his left upper limb adducted, internally rotated, and flexed at the wrist. The startle reflex is not seen on the ipsilateral side. Which part of the brachial plexus was most likely injured during this difficult delivery?

- ▢ **A.** Lateral cord
- ▢ **B.** Medial cord
- ▢ **C.** Ventral rami of the lower trunk
- ▢ **D.** Ventral ramus of the middle trunk
- ▢ **E.** Ventral rami of the upper trunk

19 A 35-year-old man has a small but painful tumor under the nail of his little finger. Which of the following nerves would have to be anesthetized for a painless removal of the tumor?

- ▢ **A.** Superficial radial
- ▢ **B.** Common palmar digital of median
- ▢ **C.** Common palmar digital of ulnar
- ▢ **D.** Deep radial
- ▢ **E.** Recurrent branch of median

20 A 25-year-old male athlete is admitted to the emergency department after a bad landing while performing the pole vault. Radiographic examination of his hand reveals a fractured carpal bone in the floor of the anatomic snuffbox (Fig. 6-2). Which bone has most likely been fractured?

- ▢ **A.** Triquetral
- ▢ **B.** Scaphoid
- ▢ **C.** Capitate
- ▢ **D.** Hamate
- ▢ **E.** Trapezoid

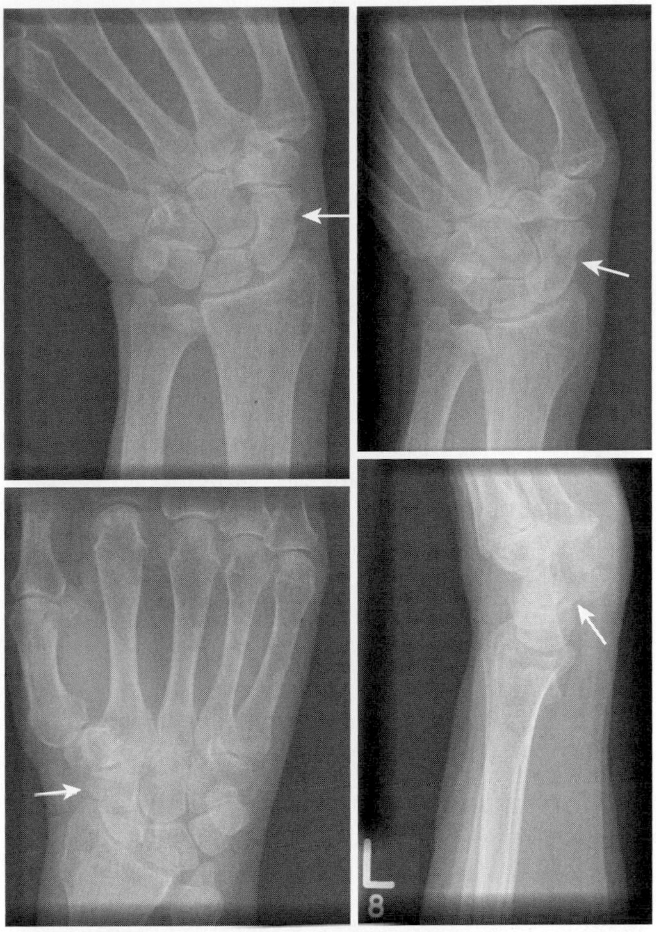

Fig. 6-2

21 A 36-year-old man is brought to the emergency department because of a deep knife wound on the medial side of his distal forearm. He is unable to hold a piece of paper between his fingers and has sensory loss on the medial side of his hand and little finger. Which nerve is most likely injured?

- ▢ **A.** Axillary
- ▢ **B.** Median
- ▢ **C.** Musculocutaneous
- ▢ **D.** Radial
- ▢ **E.** Ulnar

22 A 19-year-old man is brought to the emergency department after dislocating his shoulder while playing soccer. Following reduction of the dislocation, he has pain over the dorsal region of the shoulder and cannot abduct the arm normally. An MRI of the shoulder shows a torn muscle. Which of the following muscles is most likely to have been damaged by this injury?

- ▢ **A.** Coracobrachialis
- ▢ **B.** Long head of the triceps brachii
- ▢ **C.** Pectoralis minor
- ▢ **D.** Supraspinatus
- ▢ **E.** Teres major

23 A 47-year-old female tennis professional is informed by her physician that she has a rotator cuff injury that will require surgery. Her physician explains that over the years of play, a shoulder ligament has gradually caused severe damage to the underlying muscle. To which of the following ligaments is the physician most likely referring?

- ☐ **A.** Acromioclavicular ligament
- ☐ **B.** Coracohumeral ligament
- ☐ **C.** Transverse scapular ligament
- ☐ **D.** Glenohumeral ligament
- ☐ **E.** Coracoacromial ligament

24 A 79-year-old man has numbness in the middle three digits of his right hand and finds it difficult to grasp objects with that hand. He states that he retired 9 years earlier, after working as a carpenter for 50 years. He has atrophy of the thenar eminence (Fig. 6-3). Which of the following conditions is the most likely cause of the problems in his hand?

- ☐ **A.** Compression of the median nerve in the carpal tunnel
- ☐ **B.** Formation of the osteophytes that compress the ulnar nerve at the medial epicondyle
- ☐ **C.** Hypertrophy of the triceps brachii muscle compressing the brachial plexus
- ☐ **D.** Osteoarthritis of the cervical spine
- ☐ **E.** Repeated trauma to the ulnar nerve

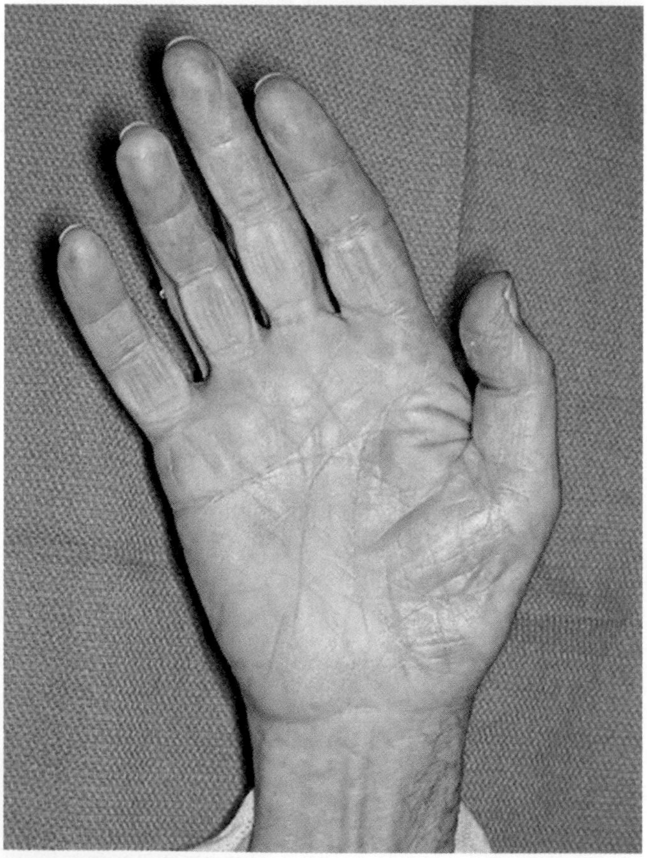

Fig. 6-3

25 A 13-year-old boy is brought to the emergency department after losing control during a motorbike race in which he was hit by several of the other racers. Physical examination reveals several cuts and bruises. He is unable to extend the left wrist, fingers, and thumb, although he can extend the elbow. Sensation is lost in the lateral half of the dorsum of the left hand. Which of the following nerves has most likely been injured to result in these signs, and in what part of the arm is the injury located?

- ☐ **A.** Median nerve, anterior wrist
- ☐ **B.** Median nerve, arm
- ☐ **C.** Radial nerve, midhumerus
- ☐ **D.** Ulnar nerve, midlateral forearm
- ☐ **E.** Ulnar nerve, midpalmar region

26 A 17-year-old boy has weakness of elbow flexion and supination of the left hand after sustaining a knife wound in that arm in a street fight. Examination in the emergency department indicates that a nerve has been severed. Which of the following conditions will also most likely be seen during physical examination?

- ☐ **A.** Inability to adduct and abduct his fingers
- ☐ **B.** Inability to flex his fingers
- ☐ **C.** Inability to flex his thumb
- ☐ **D.** Sensory loss over the lateral surface of his forearm
- ☐ **E.** Sensory loss over the medial surface of his forearm

27 Following several days of 12-hour daily rehearsals of the symphony orchestra for a performance of a Wagnerian opera, the 52-year-old male conductor experienced such excruciating pain in the posterior aspect of his right forearm that he could no longer direct the musicians. When the maestro's forearm was palpated 2 cm distal and posteromedial to the lateral epicondyle, the resulting excruciating pain caused him to grimace. Injections of steroids and rest were recommended to ease the pain. Which of the following injuries is most likely?

- ☐ **A.** Compression of the ulnar nerve by the flexor carpi ulnaris
- ☐ **B.** Compression of the median nerve by the pronator teres
- ☐ **C.** Compression of the median nerve by the flexor digitorum superficialis
- ☐ **D.** Compression of the superficial radial nerve by the brachioradialis
- ☐ **E.** Compression of the deep radial nerve by the supinator

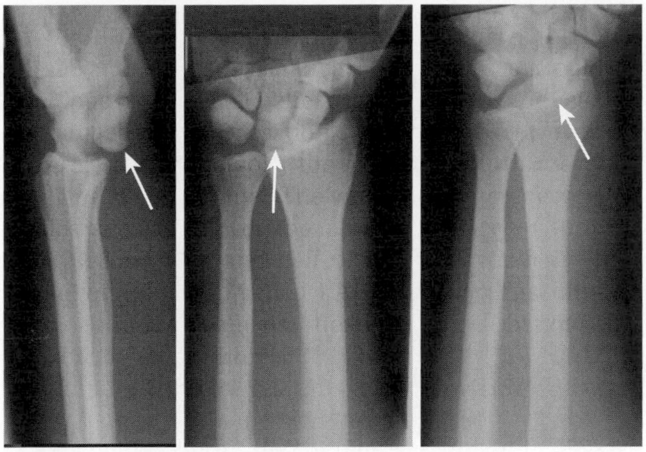

Fig. 6-4

28 A 54-year-old female marathon runner presents with pain in her right wrist that resulted when she fell with force on her outstretched hand. Radiographic studies indicate an anterior dislocation of a carpal bone (Fig. 6-4). Which of the following bones is most likely dislocated?

- ☐ **A.** Capitate
- ☐ **B.** Lunate
- ☐ **C.** Scaphoid
- ☐ **D.** Trapezoid
- ☐ **E.** Triquetrum

29 A 45-year-old man is admitted to the hospital after a car crash. Radiographic examination reveals mild disc herniations of C7, C8, and T1. The patient presents with a sensory deficit of the C8 and T1 spinal nerve dermatomes. The dorsal root ganglia of C8 and T1 would contain cell bodies of sensory fibers carried by which of the following nerves?

- ☐ **A.** Medial antebrachial cutaneous nerve
- ☐ **B.** Long thoracic nerve
- ☐ **C.** Lateral antebrachial cutaneous nerve
- ☐ **D.** Deep branch of ulnar nerve
- ☐ **E.** Anterior interosseous nerve

30 A 23-year-old female maid was making a bed in a hotel bedroom. As she straightened the sheet by running her right hand over the surface with her fingers extended, she caught the end of the index finger in a fold. She experienced a sudden, severe pain over the base of the terminal phalanx. Several hours later when the pain had diminished, she noted that the end of her right index finger was swollen and she could not completely extend the terminal interphalangeal joint. Which one of the following structures within the digit was most likely injured?

- ☐ **A.** The proper palmar digital branch of the median nerve
- ☐ **B.** The vinculum longa
- ☐ **C.** The insertion of the tendon of the extensor digitorum onto the base of the distal phalanx
- ☐ **D.** The insertion of the flexor digitorum profundus tendon
- ☐ **E.** The insertion of the flexor digitorum superficialis tendon

31 A 45-year-old man had fallen on his outstretched hand, resulting in Smith's fracture of the distal end of the radius. The fractured bone displaced a carpal bone in the palmar direction, resulting in nerve compression within the carpal tunnel. Which of the following carpal bones will most likely be dislocated?

- ☐ **A.** Scaphoid
- ☐ **B.** Trapezium
- ☐ **C.** Capitate
- ☐ **D.** Hamate
- ☐ **E.** Lunate

32 A 15-year-old girl was brought to the emergency department with a tear of the tendons in the first dorsal compartment of the wrist from a severe bite by a pit bull dog. The injured tendons in this compartment would include which of the following muscles?

- ☐ **A.** Extensor carpi radialis longus and brevis
- ☐ **B.** Abductor pollicis longus and extensor pollicis brevis
- ☐ **C.** Extensor digitorum
- ☐ **D.** Extensor indicis proprius
- ☐ **E.** Extensor carpi ulnaris

33 As she fell from the uneven parallel bars, a 17-year-old female gymnast grasped the lower bar briefly with one hand but then fell painfully to the floor. An MRI examination reveals an injury to the medial cord of the brachial plexus. Which of the following spinal nerve levels would most likely be affected?

- ☐ **A.** C5, C6
- ☐ **B.** C6, C7
- ☐ **C.** C7, C8
- ☐ **D.** C7, C8, T1
- ☐ **E.** C8, T1

34 A 21-year-old female softball pitcher is examined in the emergency department after she was struck in the arm by a line drive. Plain radiographic and MRI studies show soft tissue injury to the region of the spiral groove, with trauma to the radial nerve. Which of the following muscles would be intact after this injury?

- ▢ **A.** Flexor carpi ulnaris
- ▢ **B.** Extensor indicis
- ▢ **C.** Brachioradialis
- ▢ **D.** Extensor carpi radialis longus
- ▢ **E.** Supinator

35 Examination of a 21-year-old female athlete with an injury of the radial nerve in the spiral groove would typically demonstrate which of the following physical signs?

- ▢ **A.** Weakness of thumb abduction and thumb extension
- ▢ **B.** Weakness of thumb opposition
- ▢ **C.** Inability to extend the elbow
- ▢ **D.** Paralysis of pronation of the hand
- ▢ **E.** Paralysis of abduction and adduction of the arm

36 A 58-year-old convenience store operator had received a superficial bullet wound to the soft tissues on the medial side of the elbow in an attempted robbery. A major nerve was repaired at the site where it passed behind the medial epicondyle. Bleeding was stopped from an artery that accompanied the nerve in its path toward the epicondyle. Vascular repair was performed on this small artery because of its important role in supplying blood to the nerve. Which of the following arteries was most likely repaired?

- ▢ **A.** The profunda brachii artery
- ▢ **B.** The radial collateral artery
- ▢ **C.** The superior ulnar collateral artery
- ▢ **D.** The inferior ulnar collateral artery
- ▢ **E.** The anterior ulnar recurrent artery

37 A 60-year-old male butcher accidentally slashed his wrist with his butcher's knife, partially dividing the ulnar nerve. Which of the following actions would most likely be lost as a result of this injury?

- ▢ **A.** Flexion of the proximal interphalangeal joint of the fifth digit (little finger)
- ▢ **B.** Extension of the thumb
- ▢ **C.** Adduction of the fifth digit
- ▢ **D.** Abduction of the thumb
- ▢ **E.** Opposition of the thumb

38 A 23-year-old male medical student fell asleep in his chair with Netter's *Atlas* wedged into his axilla. When he awoke in the morning, he was unable to extend his wrist or fingers. Movements of the ipsilateral shoulder joint appear to be normal. Which of the following nerves was most likely compressed, producing the symptoms described?

- ▢ **A.** Lateral cord of the brachial plexus
- ▢ **B.** Medial cord of the brachial plexus
- ▢ **C.** Radial nerve
- ▢ **D.** Median nerve
- ▢ **E.** Lateral and medial pectoral nerves

39 The kidneys of a 32-year-old woman were failing, and she needed to be placed on dialysis. However, the search in her upper limb for a suitable vein was unexpectedly difficult. The major vein on the lateral side of the arm was too small; others were too delicate. Finally, a vein was found on the medial side of the arm that passed through the superficial and deep fascia to join veins beside the brachial artery. Which of the following veins was this?

- ▢ **A.** Basilic
- ▢ **B.** Lateral cubital
- ▢ **C.** Cephalic
- ▢ **D.** Medial cubital
- ▢ **E.** Medial antebrachial

40 A 29-year-old woman had sustained a deep laceration in the proximal part of the forearm. After the wound is closed, the following functional deficits are observed by the neurologist on service: the first three digits are in a position of extension and cannot be flexed; digits 4 and 5 are partially flexed at the metacarpophalangeal (MCP) joints and noticeably more flexed at the distal interphalangeal joints; sensation is absent in the lateral side of the palm and the palmar surfaces of digits 1 to 3 and half of digit 4. Which of the following nerve(s) has (have) most likely been injured?

- ▢ **A.** Median nerve
- ▢ **B.** Ulnar and median nerves
- ▢ **C.** Ulnar nerve
- ▢ **D.** Radial and ulnar nerves
- ▢ **E.** Radial nerve

41 A 35-year-old male wrestler is admitted to the emergency department with excruciating pain in his right shoulder and proximal arm. During physical examination, the patient clutches the arm at the elbow with his contralateral hand and is unable to move the injured limb. Radiographic studies show that the patient has a dislocation of the humerus at the glenohumeral joint. Which of the following conditions is the most likely?

- ▢ **A.** The head of the humerus is displaced anteriorly
- ▢ **B.** The head of the humerus is displaced posteriorly
- ▢ **C.** The head of the humerus is displaced inferiorly
- ▢ **D.** The head of the humerus is displaced superiorly
- ▢ **E.** The head of the humerus is displaced medially

42 The 35-year-old woman has a hard breast nodule about 1 cm in diameter slightly above and lateral to the right areola of her right breast. A specific dye is injected into the tissue around the tumor, and an incision is made to expose the lymphatic vessels draining the area, for the lymphatic vessels to take up the dye, which is visible to the eye. The vessels can then be traced to surgically expose the lymph nodes receiving the lymph from the tumor. Which of the following nodes will most likely first encounter the lymph from the tumor?

- ▢ **A.** Anterior axillary (pectoral) nodes
- ▢ **B.** Rotter's interpectoral nodes
- ▢ **C.** Parasternal nodes along the internal thoracic artery and vein
- ▢ **D.** Central axillary nodes
- ▢ **E.** Apical or infraclavicular nodes

43 During a fight in a tavern, a 45-year-old male construction worker received a shallow stab wound from a broken beer bottle at a point near the middle of the left posterior triangle of his neck. Upon physical examination, it is observed that the left shoulder is drooping lower than the right shoulder, and the superior angle of the scapula juts out slightly. Strength in turning the head to the right or left appears to be symmetric. Which of the following nerves is most likely injured?

- ▢ **A.** Suprascapular nerve in the supraspinous fossa
- ▢ **B.** The terminal segment of the dorsal scapular nerve
- ▢ **C.** The upper trunk of the brachial plexus
- ▢ **D.** The spinal accessory nerve in the posterior cervical triangle
- ▢ **E.** The thoracodorsal nerve in the axilla

44 A 44-year-old woman is diagnosed with radial nerve palsy. When muscle function is examined at the metacarpophalangeal (MCP), proximal interphalangeal (PIP), and distal interphalangeal (DIP) joints, what findings are most likely to be present?

- ▢ **A.** Inability to abduct the digits at the MCP joint
- ▢ **B.** Inability to adduct the digits at the MCP joint
- ▢ **C.** Inability to extend the MCP joints only
- ▢ **D.** Inability to extend the MCP, PIP, and DIP joints
- ▢ **E.** Inability to extend the PIP and DIP joints

45 A 27-year-old male painter is admitted to the hospital after falling from a ladder. Physical examination reveals that the patient is unable to abduct his arm more than 15 degrees and he cannot rotate the arm laterally. A radiographic examination reveals an oblique fracture of the humerus. He has associated sensory loss over the shoulder area. Which of the following injuries will most likely correspond to the symptoms of the physical examination?

- ▢ **A.** Fracture of the medial epicondyle
- ▢ **B.** Fracture of the glenoid fossa
- ▢ **C.** Fracture of the surgical neck of the humerus
- ▢ **D.** Fracture of the anatomic neck of the humerus
- ▢ **E.** Fracture of the middle third of the humerus

46 A 47-year-old woman's right breast exhibited characteristics of *peau d'orange*, that is, the skin resembled an orange peel. This condition is primarily a result of which of the following?

- ▢ **A.** Shortening of the suspensory ligaments by cancer in the axillary tail (of Spence) of the breast
- ▢ **B.** Blockage of cutaneous lymphatic vessels
- ▢ **C.** Contraction of the retinacula cutis of the areola and nipple
- ▢ **D.** Invasion of the pectoralis major by the cancer
- ▢ **E.** Ipsilateral (same side) inversion of the periareolar skin from ductular cancer

47 A 29-year-old woman is examined in the emergency department after falling from her balcony. Radiographic examination reveals that she has suffered a broken clavicle, with associated internal bleeding. Which of the following vessels is most likely to be injured in clavicular fractures?

- ▢ **A.** Subclavian artery
- ▢ **B.** Cephalic vein
- ▢ **C.** Lateral thoracic artery
- ▢ **D.** Subclavian vein
- ▢ **E.** Internal thoracic artery

48 A 68-year-old woman is examined by the senior resident in emergency medicine after she fell on a wet bathroom floor in the shopping center. Physical examination reveals a posterior displacement of the left distal wrist and hand. Radiographic examination reveals an oblique fracture of the radius. Which of the following is the most likely fracture involved in this case?

- ▢ **A.** Colles' fracture
- ▢ **B.** Scaphoid fracture
- ▢ **C.** Bennett's fracture
- ▢ **D.** Volkmann's ischemic contracture
- ▢ **E.** Boxer's fracture

49 A 34-year-old female skier was taken by ambulance to the hospital after she struck a tree on the ski slope. Imaging gives evidence of a shoulder separation. Which of the following typically occurs in this kind of injury?

- ▢ **A.** Displacement of the head of the humerus from the glenoid cavity
- ▢ **B.** Partial or complete tearing of the coracoclavicular ligament
- ▢ **C.** Partial or complete tearing of the coracoacromial ligament
- ▢ **D.** Rupture of the transverse scapular ligament
- ▢ **E.** Disruption of the glenoid labrum

50 A 22-year-old male construction worker is admitted to the hospital after he suffers a penetrating injury to his upper limb from a nail gun. Upon physical examination, the patient is unable to flex the distal interphalangeal joints of digits 4 and 5. What is the most likely cause of his injury?

- ▢ **A.** Trauma to the ulnar nerve near the trochlea
- ▢ **B.** Trauma to the ulnar nerve at the wrist
- ▢ **C.** Median nerve damage proximal to the pronator teres
- ▢ **D.** Median nerve damage at the wrist
- ▢ **E.** Trauma to spinal nerve root C8

51 The shoulder of a 44-year-old deer hunter had been penetrated by a bolt released from a crossbow. The bolt had transected the axillary artery just beyond the origin of the subscapular artery. A compress is placed on the wound with deep pressure. After a clamp is placed on the bleeding artery, thought is given to the anatomy of the vessel. What collateral arterial pathways are available to bypass the site of injury?

- ▢ **A.** Suprascapular with circumflex scapular artery
- ▢ **B.** Dorsal scapular with thoracodorsal artery
- ▢ **C.** Posterior circumflex humeral artery with deep brachial artery
- ▢ **D.** Lateral thoracic with brachial artery
- ▢ **E.** Supreme thoracic artery with thoracoacromial artery

52 A 17-year-old boy suffered the most common of fractures of the carpal bones when he fell on his outstretched hand. Which bone would this be?

- ▢ **A.** Trapezium
- ▢ **B.** Lunate
- ▢ **C.** Pisiform
- ▢ **D.** Hamate
- ▢ **E.** Scaphoid

53 A 54-year-old male cotton farmer visits the outpatient clinic because of a penetrating injury to his forearm from a baling hook. After the limb is anesthetized, the site of the wound is opened and flushed thoroughly to remove all debris. The patient is not able to oppose the tip of the thumb to the tip of the index finger, as in making the OK sign. He is able to touch the tips of the ring and little fingers to the pad of his thumb. What nerve has most likely been injured?

- ▢ **A.** Median
- ▢ **B.** Posterior interosseous
- ▢ **C.** Radial
- ▢ **D.** Recurrent median
- ▢ **E.** Anterior interosseous

54 Arthroscopic examination of the shoulder of a 62-year-old woman clearly demonstrated erosion of the tendon within the glenohumeral joint. What tendon was this?

- ▢ **A.** Glenohumeral
- ▢ **B.** Long head of triceps brachii
- ▢ **C.** Long head of biceps brachii
- ▢ **D.** Infraspinatus
- ▢ **E.** Coracobrachialis

55 An orthopedic surgeon exposed a muscle in the supraspinous fossa so that she could move it laterally while repairing an injured rotator cuff. As she reflected the muscle from its bed, an artery was exposed crossing the ligament that bridges the notch in the superior border of the scapula. What artery was this?

- ▢ **A.** Subscapular
- ▢ **B.** Transverse cervical
- ▢ **C.** Dorsal scapular
- ▢ **D.** Posterior circumflex humeral
- ▢ **E.** Suprascapular

56 A 61-year-old man was hit in the midhumeral region of his left arm by a cricket bat. Physical examination reveals an inability to extend the wrist and loss of sensation on a small area of skin on the dorsum of the hand proximal to the first two fingers. What nerve supplies this specific region of the hand?

- ▢ **A.** Radial
- ▢ **B.** Posterior interosseous
- ▢ **C.** Lateral antebrachial cutaneous
- ▢ **D.** Medial antebrachial cutaneous
- ▢ **E.** Dorsal cutaneous of ulnar

57 A 45-year-old woman is admitted to the hospital with neck pain. An MRI examination reveals a herniated disc in the cervical region. Physical examination reveals weakness in wrist extension and paraesthesia on the back of her arm and forearm. Which of the following spinal nerves is most likely injured?

- ▢ **A.** C5
- ▢ **B.** C6
- ▢ **C.** C7
- ▢ **D.** C8
- ▢ **E.** T1

58 A 22-year-old male football player suffered a wrist injury while falling with force on his outstretched hand. When the anatomic snuffbox is exposed in surgery, which artery is visualized crossing the fractured bone that provides a floor for this space?

- ▢ **A.** Ulnar
- ▢ **B.** Radial
- ▢ **C.** Anterior interosseous
- ▢ **D.** Posterior interosseous
- ▢ **E.** Deep palmar arch

59 The right shoulder of a 78-year-old woman had become increasingly painful over the past year. Abduction of the right arm caused her to wince from the discomfort. Palpation of the deltoid muscle by the physician produced exquisite pain. Imaging studies reveal intermuscular inflammation extending over the head of the humerus. Which structure was inflamed?

- ▢ **A.** Subscapular bursa
- ▢ **B.** Infraspinatus muscle
- ▢ **C.** Glenohumeral joint cavity
- ▢ **D.** Subacromial bursa
- ▢ **E.** Teres minor muscle

60 A 55-year-old male metallurgist had been diagnosed with carpal tunnel syndrome. To begin the operation, an anesthetic injection into his axillary sheath was given instead of general anesthesia. From which of the following structures does the axillary sheath take origin?

- ▢ **A.** Superficial fascia of the neck
- ▢ **B.** Superficial cervical investing fascia
- ▢ **C.** Buccopharyngeal fascia
- ▢ **D.** Clavipectoral fascia
- ▢ **E.** Prevertebral fascia

61 A 45-year-old woman is admitted to the hospital with neck pain. A computed tomography (CT) scan reveals a tumor on the left side of her oral cavity. The tumor and related tissues are removed and a radical neck surgical procedure is performed. Two months postoperatively the patient's left shoulder droops quite noticeably. Physical examination reveals distinct weakness in turning her head to the right and impairment of abduction of her left upper limb to the level of the shoulder. Which of the following structures was most likely injured during the radical neck surgery?

- ▢ **A.** Suprascapular nerve
- ▢ **B.** Long thoracic nerve
- ▢ **C.** Spinal accessory nerve
- ▢ **D.** The junction of spinal nerves C5 and C6 of the brachial plexus
- ▢ **E.** Radial nerve

62 A 23-year-old male basketball player is admitted to the hospital after injuring his shoulder during a game. Physical and radiographic examinations reveal total separation of the shoulder (Fig. 6-5). Which of the following structures has most likely been torn?

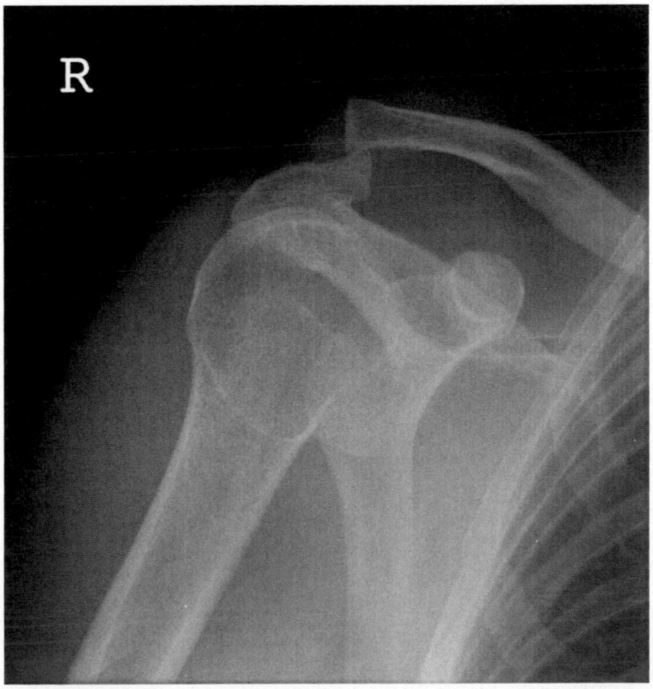

Fig. 6-5

- ▢ **A.** Glenohumeral ligament
- ▢ **B.** Coracoacromial ligament
- ▢ **C.** Tendon of long head of biceps brachii
- ▢ **D.** Acromioclavicular ligament
- ▢ **E.** Transverse scapular ligament

63 A 35-year-old male body builder has enlarged his shoulder muscles to such a degree that the size of the quadrangular space is greatly reduced. Which of the following structures would most likely be compressed in this condition?

- ▢ **A.** Axillary nerve
- ▢ **B.** Anterior circumflex humeral artery
- ▢ **C.** Cephalic vein
- ▢ **D.** Radial nerve
- ▢ **E.** Subscapular artery

64 A 43-year-old woman visits the outpatient clinic with a neurologic problem. Diagnostically, she cannot hold a piece of paper between her thumb and the lateral side of her index finger without flexing the distal joint of her thumb. This is a positive Froment's sign, which is consistent with ulnar neuropathy. Weakness of which specific muscle causes this sign to appear?

- ▢ **A.** Flexor pollicis longus
- ▢ **B.** Adductor pollicis
- ▢ **C.** Flexor digiti minimi
- ▢ **D.** Flexor carpi radialis
- ▢ **E.** Extensor indicis

65 A 48-year-old female piano player visited the outpatient clinic with numbness and tingling in her left hand. A diagnosis was made of nerve compression in the carpal tunnel, and the patient underwent an endoscopic nerve release. Two weeks postoperatively the patient complained of a profound weakness in the thumb, with loss of thumb opposition. The sensation to the hand, however, was unaffected. Which of the following nerves was injured during the operation?

- ▢ **A.** The first common digital branch of the median nerve
- ▢ **B.** The second common digital branch of the median nerve
- ▢ **C.** Recurrent branch of median nerve
- ▢ **D.** Deep branch of the ulnar nerve
- ▢ **E.** Anterior interosseus nerve

66 A 19-year-old man had suffered a deep laceration to an upper limb when he stumbled and fell on a broken bottle. On examination of hand function it is observed that he is able to extend the metacarpophalangeal joints of all his fingers in the affected limb. He cannot extend the interphalangeal (IP) joints of the fourth and fifth digits, and extension of the IP joints of the second and third digits is very weak. There is no apparent sensory deficit in the hand. Which of the following nerves has most likely been injured?

- ▢ **A.** Radial nerve at the elbow
- ▢ **B.** Median nerve at the wrist
- ▢ **C.** Ulnar nerve in midforearm
- ▢ **D.** Deep branch of ulnar nerve
- ▢ **E.** Recurrent branch of the median nerve

67 A 41-year-old woman is scheduled for a latissimus dorsi muscle flap to cosmetically augment the site of her absent left breast after mastectomy. Part of the latissimus dorsi muscle is advanced to the anterior thoracic wall, based upon arterial supply provided in part by the artery that passes through the triangular space of the axilla. Which artery forms the vascular base of this flap?

- ▢ **A.** Circumflex scapular artery
- ▢ **B.** Dorsal scapular artery
- ▢ **C.** Transverse cervical artery
- ▢ **D.** Lateral thoracic artery
- ▢ **E.** Thoracoacromial artery

68 A 31-year-old male hockey player fell on his elbow and is admitted to the emergency department. Radiographic examination reveals a fracture of the surgical neck of the humerus, producing an elevation and adduction of the distal fragment. Which of the following muscles would most likely cause the adduction of the distal fragment?

- ▢ **A.** Brachialis
- ▢ **B.** Teres minor
- ▢ **C.** Pectoralis major
- ▢ **D.** Supraspinatus
- ▢ **E.** Pectoralis minor

69 A 74-year-old woman is admitted to the emergency department after stumbling over her pet dog. Radiographic examination reveals a fracture of the upper third of the right radius, with the distal fragment of the radius and hand pronated. The proximal end of the fractured radius deviates laterally. Which of the following muscles is primarily responsible for the lateral deviation?

- ▢ **A.** Pronator teres
- ▢ **B.** Supinator
- ▢ **C.** Pronator quadratus

- ▢ **D.** Brachioradialis
- ▢ **E.** Brachialis

70 A 12-year-old boy lacerated the palmar surface of the wrist while playing with a sharp knife. The cut ends of a tendon could be seen within the wound in the exact midline of the wrist. Which tendon lies in this position in most people?

- ▢ **A.** Palmaris longus
- ▢ **B.** Flexor carpi radialis
- ▢ **C.** Abductor pollicis longus
- ▢ **D.** Flexor carpi ulnaris
- ▢ **E.** Flexor pollicis longus

71 A 22-year-old male medical student was seen in the emergency department with a complaint of pain in his right hand. He confessed that he had hit a vending machine in the hospital when he did not receive his soft drink after inserting money twice. The medial side of the dorsum of the hand was quite swollen, and one of his knuckles could not be seen when he "made a fist." The physician made a diagnosis of a "boxer's fracture." What was the nature of the impatient student's injury?

- ▢ **A.** Fracture of the styloid process of the ulna
- ▢ **B.** Fracture of the neck of the fifth metacarpal
- ▢ **C.** Colles' fracture of the radius
- ▢ **D.** Smith's fracture of the radius
- ▢ **E.** Bennett's fracture of the thumb

72 Fine motor function in the right hand of a 14-year-old girl with scoliosis since birth appeared to be quite reduced, including opposition of the thumb, abduction and adduction of the digits, and interphalangeal joint extension. Radiography confirmed that her severe scoliosis was causing marked elevation of the right first rib. Long flexor muscles of the hand and long extensors of the wrist appear to be functioning within normal limits. There is notable anesthesia of the skin on the medial side of the forearm; otherwise, sensory function in the limb is intact. Which of the following neural structures is most likely impaired?

- ▢ **A.** Median nerve
- ▢ **B.** Middle trunk of the brachial plexus
- ▢ **C.** Radial nerve
- ▢ **D.** Lower trunk of the brachial plexus
- ▢ **E.** T1 ventral ramus

73 A 23-year-old woman had a painful injury to her hand in a dry ski-slope competition, in which she fell and caught her thumb in the matting. Radiographic and physical examinations reveal rupture of the ulnar collateral ligament of the metacarpophalangeal joint of the thumb. Lidocaine is injected into the area to relieve the pain, and she is scheduled for a surgical repair. From which of the following clinical problems is she suffering?

- ▢ **A.** De Quervain's syndrome
- ▢ **B.** Navicular bone fracture
- ▢ **C.** Boxer's thumb
- ▢ **D.** Gamekeeper's thumb
- ▢ **E.** Bennett's thumb

74 A 26-year-old male power lifter visits the outpatient clinic with a painful shoulder. Radiographic examination reveals tendinopathy of the long head of the biceps brachii muscle. Which of the following conditions will most likely be present during physical examination?

- ▢ **A.** Pain is felt in the anterior shoulder during forced contraction
- ▢ **B.** Pain is felt in the lateral shoulder during forced contraction
- ▢ **C.** Pain is felt during abduction and flexion of the shoulder joint
- ▢ **D.** Pain is felt during extension and adduction of the shoulder joint
- ▢ **E.** Pain is felt in the lateral shoulder during flexion of the shoulder joint

75 A 43-year-old female tennis player visits the outpatient clinic with pain over the right lateral epicondyle of her elbow. Physical examination reveals that the patient has lateral epicondylitis. Which of the following tests should be performed during physical examination to confirm the diagnosis?

- ▢ **A.** Nerve conduction studies
- ▢ **B.** Evaluation of pain experienced during flexion and extension of the elbow joint
- ▢ **C.** Observing the presence of pain when the wrist is extended against resistance
- ▢ **D.** Observing the presence of numbness and tingling in the ring and little fingers when the wrist is flexed against resistance
- ▢ **E.** Evaluation of pain felt over the styloid process of radius during brachioradialis contraction

76 A male skier had a painful fall against a rocky ledge. Radiographic findings revealed a hairline fracture of the surgical neck of the humerus. The third-year medical student assigned to this patient was asked to determine whether there was injury to the nerve associated with the area of injury. Which of the following tests would be best for checking the status of the nerve?

- ▢ **A.** Have the patient abduct the limb while holding a 10 lb weight
- ▢ **B.** Have the patient shrug the shoulders
- ▢ **C.** Test for presence of skin sensation over the lateral side of the shoulder
- ▢ **D.** Test for normal sensation over the medial skin of the axilla
- ▢ **E.** Have the patient push against an immovable object like a wall and assess the position of the scapula

77 A 27-year-old man had lost much of the soft tissue on the dorsum of his left hand in a motorcycle crash. Imaging studies show no other upper limb injuries. Because function of the left extensor carpi radialis longus and brevis tendons was lost, it was decided to replace those tendons with the palmaris longus tendons from both forearms because of their convenient location and relative unimportance. Postoperatively, it is found that sensation is absent in both hands on the lateral palm and palmar surfaces of the first three digits; there is also paralysis of thumb opposition. What is the most likely cause of the sensory deficit and motor loss in both thumbs?

- ▢ **A.** Bilateral loss of spinal nerve T1 with fractures of first rib bilaterally
- ▢ **B.** Lower plexus (lower trunk) trauma
- ▢ **C.** Dupuytren contracture
- ▢ **D.** Left radial nerve injury in the posterior compartment of the forearm
- ▢ **E.** The palmaris longus was absent bilaterally; the nerve normally beneath it looked like a tendon and was cut

78 A 15-year-old boy received a shotgun wound to the ventral surface of the upper limb. Three months after the injury the patient exhibits a complete claw hand but can extend his wrist. What is the nature of this patient's injury?

- ▢ **A.** The ulnar nerve has been severed at the wrist.
- ▢ **B.** The median nerve has been injured in the carpal tunnel.
- ▢ **C.** The median and ulnar nerves are damaged at the wrist.
- ▢ **D.** The median and ulnar nerves have been injured at the elbow region.
- ▢ **E.** The median, ulnar, and radial nerves have been injured at midhumerus.

79 A 68-year-old woman fell when she missed the last step from her motor home. Radiographic examination at the local medical care center reveals a fracture of the distal radius. The distal fragment of the radius is angled forward. What name is commonly applied to this type of injury?

- ▢ **A.** Colles' fracture
- ▢ **B.** Scaphoid fracture
- ▢ **C.** Bennett's fracture
- ▢ **D.** Smith's fracture
- ▢ **E.** Boxer's fracture

80 It was reported by the sports media that the outstanding 27-year-old shortstop for a New York team would miss a number of baseball games. He was hit on a fingertip while attempting to catch a ball barehanded. A tendon had been torn. The team doctor commented that the ballplayer could not straighten the last joint of the long finger of his right hand, and the finger would require surgery. From what injury did the ballplayer suffer?

- ▢ **A.** Claw hand deformity
- ▢ **B.** Boutonnière deformity
- ▢ **C.** Swan-neck deformity
- ▢ **D.** Dupuytren's contracture
- ▢ **E.** Mallet finger

81 A 31-year-old female figure skater is examined in the emergency department following an injury that forced her to withdraw from competition. When her male partner missed catching her properly from an overhead position, he grasped her powerfully, but awkwardly, by the forearm. Clinical examination demonstrated a positive Ochsner test, inability to flex the distal interphalangeal joint of the index finger on clasping the hands. In addition, she is unable to flex the terminal phalanx of the thumb and has loss of sensation over the thenar half of the hand. What is the most likely nature of her injury?

- ▢ **A.** Median nerve injured within the cubital fossa
- ▢ **B.** Anterior interosseous nerve injury at the pronator teres
- ▢ **C.** Radial nerve injury at its entrance into the posterior forearm compartment
- ▢ **D.** Median nerve injury at the proximal skin crease of the wrist
- ▢ **E.** Ulnar nerve trauma halfway along the forearm

82 A 19-year-old man fell from a cliff when he was hiking in the mountains. He broke his fall by grasping a tree branch, but he suffered injury to the C8 to T1 spinal nerve ventral rami. Sensory tests would thereafter confirm the nature of his neurologic injury by the sensory loss in the part of the limb supplied by which of the following?

- ▢ **A.** Lower lateral brachial cutaneous nerve
- ▢ **B.** Musculocutaneous nerve
- ▢ **C.** Intercostobrachial nerve
- ▢ **D.** Medial antebrachial cutaneous nerve
- ▢ **E.** Median nerve

83 The mastectomy procedure on a 52-year-old woman involved excision of the tumor and removal of lymph nodes, including the pectoral, central axillary, and infraclavicular groups. Six months after her mastectomy, the patient complains to her personal physician of an unsightly deep hollow area inferior to the medial half of the clavicle, indicating a significant area of muscle atrophy and loss. She states that the disfigurement has taken place quite gradually since her mastectomy. Physical examination reveals no obvious motor or sensory deficits. What was the most likely cause of the patient's cosmetic problem?

- ▢ **A.** Part of the pectoralis major muscle was cut and removed in the mastectomy
- ▢ **B.** The pectoralis minor muscle was removed entirely in the surgery
- ▢ **C.** A branch of the lateral pectoral nerve was cut
- ▢ **D.** The medial pectoral nerve was cut
- ▢ **E.** The lateral cord of the brachial plexus was injured

84 A 54-year-old woman was found unconscious on the floor, apparently after a fall. She was admitted to the hospital, and during physical examination it was observed that she had unilateral absence of her brachioradialis reflex. Which spinal nerve is primarily responsible for this reflex in the majority of cases?

- ▢ **A.** C5
- ▢ **B.** C6
- ▢ **C.** C7
- ▢ **D.** C8
- ▢ **E.** T1

85 A 43-year-old man is admitted to the hospital, having suffered a whiplash injury when his compact automobile was struck from behind by a sports utility vehicle. MRI examination reveals some herniation of a disc in the cervical region. Physical examination reveals that the patient has lost elbow extension; there is absence of his triceps reflex and loss of extension of the metacarpophalangeal joints on the ipsilateral side. Which of the following spinal nerves is most likely affected?

- ▢ **A.** C5
- ▢ **B.** C6
- ▢ **C.** C7
- ▢ **D.** C8
- ▢ **E.** T1

86 A 29-year-old patient has a dislocated elbow in which the ulna and medial part of the distal humerus have become separated. What classification of joint is normally formed between these two bones?

- ▢ **A.** Trochoid
- ▢ **B.** Ginglymus
- ▢ **C.** Enarthrodial
- ▢ **D.** Synarthrosis
- ▢ **E.** Sellar

87 A 45-year-old female motorcyclist, propelled over the handlebars of her bike by an encounter with a rut in the road, lands on the point of one shoulder. She is taken by ambulance to the emergency department. During physical examination, the arm appears swollen, pale, and cool. Any movement of the arm causes severe pain. Radiographic examination reveals a fracture and a large hematoma, leading to diagnosis of Volkmann's ischemic contracture. At which of the following locations has the fracture most likely occurred?

- ▢ **A.** Surgical neck of humerus
- ▢ **B.** Radial groove of humerus
- ▢ **C.** Supracondylar line of humerus
- ▢ **D.** Olecranon
- ▢ **E.** Lateral epicondyle

88 A 55-year-old female choreographer had been treated in the emergency department after she fell from the stage into the orchestra pit. Radiographs revealed fracture of the styloid process of the ulna. Disruption of the triangular fibrocartilage complex is suspected. With which of the following bones does the ulna normally articulate at the wrist?

- ▢ **A.** Triquetrum
- ▢ **B.** Hamate
- ▢ **C.** Radius and lunate
- ▢ **D.** Radius
- ▢ **E.** Pisiform and triquetrum

89 A 67-year-old woman had a bad fall while walking her dog the evening before. She states that she fell on her outstretched hand. Radiographs do not demonstrate any bony fractures. The clinician observes the following signs of neurologic injury: weakness of flexion of her wrist in a medial direction, a loss of sensation on the medial side of the hand, and clawing of the fingers. Where is the most likely place of nerve trauma?

- ☐ **A.** Behind the medial epicondyle
- ☐ **B.** Between the pisiform bone and the flexor retinaculum
- ☐ **C.** Within the carpal tunnel
- ☐ **D.** At the cubital fossa, between the ulnar and radial heads of origin of flexor digitorum superficialis
- ☐ **E.** At the radial neck, 1 cm distal to the humerocapitellar joint

90 An 18-year-old man suffered a significant laceration through the skin and underlying tissues at the distal crease of the wrist. The medical student rotating through the emergency department suspected (correctly) that the ulnar nerve was cut completely through at this location. Which of the following would most likely occur?

- ☐ **A.** The patient could not touch the tip of the thumb to the tips of the other digits
- ☐ **B.** There would be loss of sensation on the dorsum of the medial side of the hand
- ☐ **C.** The patient would be unable to flex the interphalangeal joints
- ☐ **D.** There would be decreased ability to extend the interphalangeal joints
- ☐ **E.** There would be no serious functional problem at all to the patient

91 A 45-year-old man visits the outpatient clinic after a digit of his left hand was injured when a door was slammed on his hand. A superficial cut on his middle finger has been sutured, but functional deficits are observed in the finger. The proximal interphalangeal joint is pulled into constant flexion, whereas the distal interphalangeal joint is held in a position of hyperextension. What is the most likely diagnosis?

- ☐ **A.** Mallet finger
- ☐ **B.** Boutonnière deformity
- ☐ **C.** Dupuytren's contracture
- ☐ **D.** Swan-neck deformity
- ☐ **E.** Silver fork wrist deformity

92 A 67-year-old housepainter visits the outpatient clinic complaining that his hands are getting progressively worse, becoming more and more painful and losing their function. On physical examination of the hands, there is flexion of the metacarpophalangeal joints, extension of the proximal interphalangeal joints, and slight flexion of the distal interphalangeal joints. What is the most likely diagnosis?

- ☐ **A.** Mallet finger
- ☐ **B.** Boutonnière deformity
- ☐ **C.** Dupuytren's contracture
- ☐ **D.** Swan-neck deformity
- ☐ **E.** Silver fork wrist deformity

93 Several weeks after surgical dissection of her left axilla for the removal of lymph nodes for staging and treatment of her breast cancer, a 32-year-old woman was told by her general physician that she had "winging" of her left scapula when she pushed against resistance during her physical examination. She told the physician that she had also experienced difficulty lately in raising her left arm above her head when she was combing her hair. In a subsequent consult visit with her surgeon, she was told that a nerve was accidentally injured during the diagnostic surgical procedure and that this produced her scapular abnormality and inability to raise her arm normally. What was the origin of this nerve?

- ☐ **A.** The upper trunk of her brachial plexus
- ☐ **B.** The posterior division of the middle trunk
- ☐ **C.** Ventral rami of the brachial plexus
- ☐ **D.** The posterior cord of the brachial plexus
- ☐ **E.** The lateral cord of the brachial plexus

94 A 72-year-old man consulted his physician because he had noticed a thickening of the skin at the base of his left ring finger during the preceding 3 months. As he described it, "There appears to be some hard tissue that is pulling my little and ring fingers into my palm." On examination of the palms of both hands, localized and firm ridges are observed in the palmar skin that extend from the middle part of the palm to the base of the ring and little fingers. What is the medical term for this sign?

- ☐ **A.** Ape hand
- ☐ **B.** Dupuytren's contracture
- ☐ **C.** Claw hand
- ☐ **D.** Wrist drop
- ☐ **E.** Mallet finger

95 A 24-year-old female basketball player is admitted to the emergency department after an injury to her shoulder. Radiographic examination reveals a shoulder dislocation. What is the most commonly injured nerve in shoulder dislocations?

- ☐ **A.** Axillary
- ☐ **B.** Radial

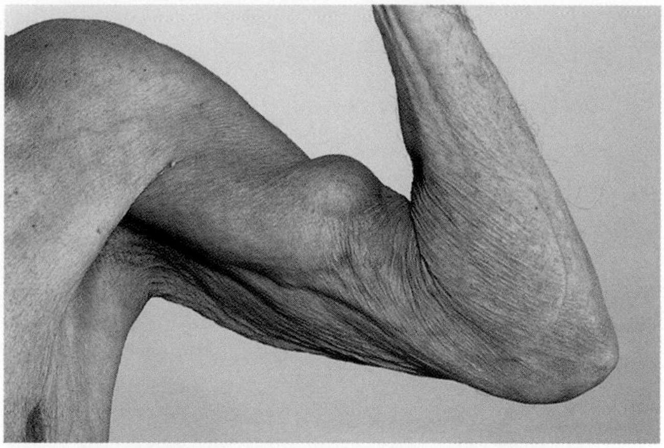

Fig. 6-6

- ☐ **C.** Median
- ☐ **D.** Ulnar
- ☐ **E.** Musculocutaneous

96 An 85-year-old man is admitted to the hospital with a painful arm after lifting a case of wine. Physical examination gives evidence of a rupture of the long tendon of the biceps brachii (Fig. 6-6). Which of the following is the most likely location of the rupture?

- ☐ **A.** Intertubercular groove
- ☐ **B.** Midportion of the biceps brachii muscle
- ☐ **C.** Junction with the short head of the biceps brachii muscle
- ☐ **D.** Proximal end of the combined biceps brachii muscle
- ☐ **E.** Bony insertion of the muscle

97 After an orthopedic surgeon examined the MRI of the shoulder of a 42-year-old woman he informed her that the supraspinatus tendon was injured and needed to be repaired surgically. Which of the following is true of the supraspinatus muscle?

- ☐ **A.** It inserts onto the lesser tubercle of the humerus.
- ☐ **B.** It initiates adduction of the shoulder.
- ☐ **C.** It is innervated chiefly by the C5 spinal nerve.
- ☐ **D.** It is supplied by the upper subscapular nerve.
- ☐ **E.** It originates from the lateral border of the scapula.

98 A 5-year-old boy is admitted to the emergency department after falling from a tree. The parents are informed by the radiologist that their son's fracture is the most common fracture that occurs in children. Which of the following bones was broken?

- ☐ **A.** Humerus
- ☐ **B.** Radius
- ☐ **C.** Ulna
- ☐ **D.** Scaphoid
- ☐ **E.** Clavicle

99 A 22-year-old woman visits the outpatient clinic with pain in her left upper limb. She has a long history of pain in this limb and difficulty with fine motor tasks of the hand. Physical examination reveals paraesthesia along the medial surface of the forearm and palm and weakness and atrophy of gripping muscles ("long flexors") and the intrinsic muscles of the hand. The radial pulse is diminished when her neck is rotated to the ipsilateral side (positive Adson's test). What is the most likely diagnosis?

- ☐ **A.** Erb-Duchenne paralysis
- ☐ **B.** Aneurysm of the brachiocephalic artery, with plexus compression
- ☐ **C.** Thoracic outlet syndrome
- ☐ **D.** Carpal tunnel syndrome
- ☐ **E.** Injury to the medial cord of the brachial plexus

100 Physical examination reveals weakness of medial deviation of the wrist (adduction), loss of sensation on the medial side of the hand, and clawing of the fingers. Where is the most likely place of injury?

- ☐ **A.** Compression of a nerve passing between the humeral and ulnar heads of origin of flexor carpi ulnaris
- ☐ **B.** Compression of a nerve passing at Guyon's canal between the pisiform bone and flexor retinaculum
- ☐ **C.** Compression of a nerve passing through the carpal tunnel
- ☐ **D.** Compression of a nerve passing between the ulnar and radial heads of origin of flexor digitorum superficialis
- ☐ **E.** Compression of a nerve passing deep to brachioradialis muscle

101 A 22-year-old pregnant woman was admitted urgently to the hospital after her baby had begun to appear at the introitus. The baby had presented in the breech position, and it had been necessary to exert considerable traction to complete the delivery. The newborn is shown in Fig. 6-7. Which of the following structures was most likely injured by the trauma of childbirth?

- ☐ **A.** Radial nerve
- ☐ **B.** Upper trunk of the brachial plexus

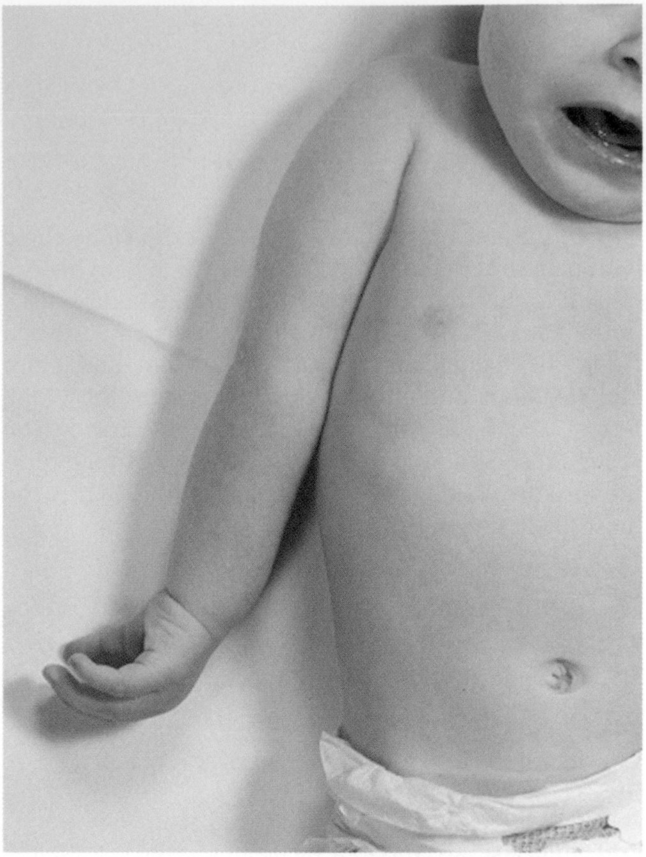

Fig. 6-7

- ▢ **C.** Lower trunk of the brachial plexus
- ▢ **D.** Median, ulnar, and radial nerves
- ▢ **E.** Upper and lower trunks of the brachial plexus

102 A 17-year-old female student of martial arts entered the emergency department with a complaint of pain in her hand. Patient history reveals that she had been breaking concrete blocks with her hand. Examination reveals that the patient has weak abduction and adduction of her fingers but has no difficulty in flexing them. The patient also has decreased sensation over the palmar surfaces of the fourth and fifth digits. Which of the following best describes the nature of her injury?

- ▢ **A.** Compression of the median nerve in the carpal tunnel
- ▢ **B.** Fracture of the triquetrum, with injury to the dorsal ulnar nerve
- ▢ **C.** Dislocation of a bone in the proximal row of the carpus
- ▢ **D.** Fracture of the shaft of the fifth metacarpal
- ▢ **E.** Injury of the ulnar nerve in Guyon's canal

103 A 10-year-old boy suffered a dog bite that entered the common flexor synovial sheath of his forearm. He

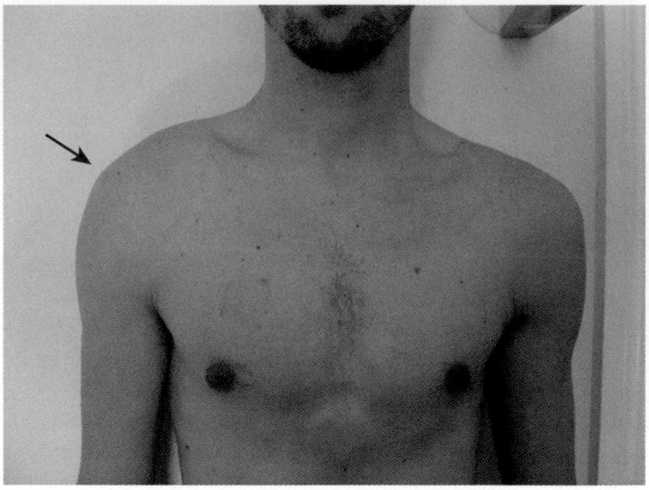

Fig. 6-8

was admitted to the hospital, where the wound was cleaned and dressed and he was treated further with rabies antiserum. Two days later the boy had an elevated temperature and his palm and one digit were obviously swollen, causing him to cry with pain. Into which of the digits could the infection spread most easily, following the anatomy of the typical common flexor sheath?

- ▢ **A.** First
- ▢ **B.** Second
- ▢ **C.** Third
- ▢ **D.** Fourth
- ▢ **E.** Fifth

104 While sharpening his knife, a 23-year-old male soldier accidentally punctured the ventral side of the fifth digit at the base of the distal phalanx. The wound became infected, and within a few days the infection had spread into the palm, within the sheath of the flexor digitorum profundus tendons. If the infection were left untreated, into which of the following spaces could it most likely spread?

- ▢ **A.** Central compartment
- ▢ **B.** Hypothenar compartment
- ▢ **C.** Midpalmar space
- ▢ **D.** Thenar compartment
- ▢ **E.** Thenar space

105 A 36-year-old man is admitted to the emergency department with a dull ache in his shoulder and axilla (Fig. 6-8). During physical examination the pain worsens by activity, and, conversely, rest and elevation relieve the pain. History reveals that the patient was hospitalized 2 days ago and a central venous line was used. What is the most likely diagnosis?

- ▢ **A.** Axillary-subclavian vein thrombosis
- ▢ **B.** Compression of C5 to C8 spinal nerve
- ▢ **C.** Disc herniation of C4 to C8
- ▢ **D.** Impingement syndrome
- ▢ **E.** Injury to radial, ulnar, and median nerves

106 A 22-year-old woman had suffered a severe knife wound to the upper lateral portion of her pectoral region, with entry of the knife at the deltopectoral groove. Pressure applied to the wound had prevented further profuse bleeding. In the emergency department, vascular clamps were applied to the axillary artery, proximal and distal to the site of injury, which had occurred between the second and third parts of the axillary artery. The vascular surgeon knew there was time to repair the wound of the artery because of the rich collateral pathway provided by the anastomoses between which of the following arteries?

- ▢ **A.** Transverse cervical and suprascapular
- ▢ **B.** Posterior circumflex humeral and profunda brachii
- ▢ **C.** Suprascapular and circumflex scapular
- ▢ **D.** Supreme (superior) thoracic and thoracoacromial
- ▢ **E.** Lateral thoracic and suprascapular

107 In a penetrating wound to the forearm of a 24-year-old man, the median nerve is injured at the entrance of the nerve into the forearm. Which of the following would most likely be apparent when the patient's hand is relaxed?

- ▢ **A.** The MCP and IP joints of the second and third digits of the hand will be in a condition of extension.
- ▢ **B.** The third and fourth digits will be held in a slightly flexed position.
- ▢ **C.** The thumb will be flexed and slightly abducted.
- ▢ **D.** The first, second, and third digits will be held in a slightly flexed position.
- ▢ **E.** The MCP and IP joints of the second and third digits of the hand will be in a condition of flexion.

108 A 55-year-old male firefighter is admitted to the hospital after blunt trauma to his right axilla. Examination reveals winging of the scapula and partial paralysis of the right side of the diaphragm. Which of the following parts of the brachial plexus have been injured?

- ▢ **A.** Cords
- ▢ **B.** Divisions
- ▢ **C.** Ventral rami
- ▢ **D.** Terminal branches
- ▢ **E.** Trunks

109 A 69-year-old man has numbness and pain in the middle three digits of his right hand at night. He retired 9 years ago after working as a carpenter for 30 years. He has atrophy of the thenar eminence (see Fig. 6-3). Which of the following conditions will be the most likely cause of this atrophy?

- ▢ **A.** Compression of the median nerve in the carpal tunnel
- ▢ **B.** Formation of the osteophytes that compress the ulnar nerve at the ulnar condyle
- ▢ **C.** Hypertrophy of the triceps brachii muscle compressing the brachial plexus
- ▢ **D.** Osteoarthritis of the cervical spine
- ▢ **E.** Repeated trauma to the ulnar nerve

110 A 54-year-old woman presents with pain in her right wrist that resulted when she fell forcefully on her outstretched hand. Radiographic studies indicate an anterior dislocation of a carpal bone of the proximal row (see Fig. 6-4). Which of the following bones is most commonly dislocated?

- ▢ **A.** Capitate
- ▢ **B.** Lunate
- ▢ **C.** Scaphoid
- ▢ **D.** Pisiform
- ▢ **E.** Triquetrum

111 A 32-year-old man who is an expert target shooter reports pain in his right upper limb and slight tingling and numbness of all digits of the ipsilateral hand. However, the tingling and numbness of the fourth and fifth digits is the most severe. The man states that the problem usually occurs when he is firing his gun with his hand overhead. Radiographic studies reveal the presence of a cervical rib and accessory scalene musculature. Which of the following structures is most likely being compressed?

- ▢ **A.** Axillary artery
- ▢ **B.** Upper trunk of brachial plexus
- ▢ **C.** Subclavian artery
- ▢ **D.** Lower trunk of brachial plexus
- ▢ **E.** Brachiocephalic artery and lower trunk of brachial plexus

112 A 23-year-old woman arrives at the emergency department with a swollen, painful forearm. An MRI examination reveals a compartment syndrome originating at the interosseous membrane between the radius and ulna. Which of the following type of joint will most likely be affected?

- ▢ **A.** Synarthrosis
- ▢ **B.** Symphysis
- ▢ **C.** Synchondrosis
- ▢ **D.** Trochoid
- ▢ **E.** Ginglymus

113 While working out with weights, a 28-year-old woman experiences a severe pain in her chest. The pain is referred to the anterior chest wall, radiating to the mandible and her left arm. The woman felt dizzy and after 10 minutes she collapsed and was unconscious. A physician happened to be near the woman and immediately tried to feel her radial pulse. The radial artery lies between two tendons near the wrist, which are useful landmarks. Which of the following is the correct pair of tendons?

- ▢ **A.** Flexor carpi radialis and palmaris longus
- ▢ **B.** Flexor carpi radialis and brachioradialis
- ▢ **C.** Brachioradialis and flexor pollicis longus
- ▢ **D.** Flexor pollicis longus and flexor digitorum superficialis
- ▢ **E.** Flexor pollicis longus and flexor digitorum profundus

114 A 59-year-old woman is admitted to the hospital in a state of shock. During physical examination, several lacerations are noted in her forearm and her radial pulse is absent. Where is the most typical place to identify the radial artery immediately after crossing the radiocarpal joint?

- ▢ **A.** Between the two heads of the first dorsal interosseous muscle
- ▢ **B.** In the anatomic snuffbox
- ▢ **C.** Below the tendon of the flexor pollicis longus
- ▢ **D.** Between the first and second dorsal interossei muscles
- ▢ **E.** Between the first dorsal interosseous muscle and the adductor pollicis longus

115 A 69-year-old woman visits the outpatient clinic with a complaint of numbness and tingling of her hand for the past 3 months. Physical examination reveals she has numbness and pain in the lateral three digits of her right hand that are relieved by vigorous shaking of the wrist. In addition, the abductor pollicis brevis, opponens pollicis, and the first two lumbrical muscles are weakened. Sensation was decreased over the lateral palm and the volar aspect of the first three digits. Which of the following nerves is most likely compressed?

- ▢ **A.** Ulnar
- ▢ **B.** Radial
- ▢ **C.** Recurrent median
- ▢ **D.** Median
- ▢ **E.** Posterior interosseous

116 A 32-year-old man is admitted to the emergency department after a severe car crash. Radiographic examination reveals multiple fractures of his right upper limb. A surgical procedure is performed and metallic plates are attached to various bony fragments to restore the anatomy. Five months postoperatively the patient visits the outpatient clinic. Upon physical examination the patient can abduct his arm and extend the forearm, and the sensation of the forearm and hand is intact; however, hand grasp is very weak, and he cannot extend his wrist against gravity. Which of the following nerves was most likely injured during the surgical procedure?

- ▢ **A.** Posterior cord of the brachial plexus
- ▢ **B.** Radial nerve at the distal third of the humerus
- ▢ **C.** Radial and ulnar
- ▢ **D.** Radial, ulnar, and median
- ▢ **E.** Radial and musculocutaneous

117 A 52-year-old man is admitted to the emergency department after falling on wet pavement. Radiographic examination reveals fracture of the radius. An MRI study reveals a hematoma between the fractured radius and supinator muscle. Upon physical examination the patient has weakened abduction of the thumb and extension of the metacarpophalangeal joints of the fingers. Which of the following nerves is most likely affected?

- ▢ **A.** Anterior interosseous
- ▢ **B.** Posterior interosseous
- ▢ **C.** Radial nerve
- ▢ **D.** Deep branch of ulnar nerve
- ▢ **E.** Median nerve

118 A 34-year-old woman is admitted to the emergency department after a car crash. Radiographic studies show marked edema and hematoma of the arm, but there are no fractures. During physical examination the patient presents with inability to abduct her arm without first establishing lateral momentum of the limb, and inability to flex the elbow and shoulder. Which of the following portions of the brachial plexus is most likely injured?

- ▢ **A.** Superior trunk
- ▢ **B.** Middle trunk

- ☐ **C.** Inferior trunk
- ☐ **D.** Lateral cord
- ☐ **E.** Medial cord

119 A 22-year-old man is admitted to the hospital after a car collision. Radiographic examination reveals an oblique fracture of his humerus. Upon physical examination the patient is unable to extend his forearm. The damaged nerve was most likely composed of fibers from which of the following spinal levels?

- ☐ **A.** C5, C6
- ☐ **B.** C5, C6, C7
- ☐ **C.** C5, C6, C7, C8, T1
- ☐ **D.** C6, C7, C8, T1
- ☐ **E.** C7, C8, T1

120 A 56-year-old woman is admitted to the hospital after a severe car crash. A large portion of her chest wall needed to be surgically removed and replaced with a musculo-osseous scapular graft involving the medial border of the scapula. Which of the following arteries will most likely recompensate the blood supply to the entire scapula?

- ☐ **A.** Suprascapular
- ☐ **B.** Dorsal scapular artery
- ☐ **C.** Posterior circumflex humeral artery
- ☐ **D.** Lateral thoracic
- ☐ **E.** Supreme thoracic artery

121 A 56-year-old woman visits the emergency department after falling on a wet pavement. Radiographic examination reveals osteoporosis and a Colles' fracture. Which of the following carpal bones are often fractured or dislocated with a Colles' fracture?

- ☐ **A.** Triquetrum and scaphoid
- ☐ **B.** Triquetrum and lunate
- ☐ **C.** Scaphoid and lunate
- ☐ **D.** Triquetrum, lunate, and scaphoid
- ☐ **E.** Triquetrum and pisiform

122 A 3-year-old girl is admitted to the emergency department with severe pain. History taking reveals that the girl was violently lifted by her raised arm by her mother to prevent the girl from walking in front of a moving car. Which of the following is most likely the cause of the pain?

- ☐ **A.** Compression of the median nerve
- ☐ **B.** Separation of the head of the radius from its articulation with the trochlea of the humerus
- ☐ **C.** Separation of the head of the radius from its articulation with the ulna and the capitulum of the humerus
- ☐ **D.** Separation of the ulna from its articulation with the trochlea of the humerus
- ☐ **E.** Stretching of the radial nerve as it passes behind the medial epicondyle of the humerus

123 A 61-year-old man was hit by a cricket bat in the midhumeral region of his left arm. Physical examination reveals normal elbow motion; however, he could not extend his wrist or his metacarpophalangeal joints and he reported a loss of sensation on a small area of skin on the dorsum of the hand proximal to the first two digits. Radiographic examination reveals a hairline fracture of the shaft of the humerus just distal to its midpoint. Which of the following nerves is most likely injured?

- ☐ **A.** Median
- ☐ **B.** Ulnar
- ☐ **C.** Radial
- ☐ **D.** Musculocutaneous
- ☐ **E.** Axillary

124 A 34-year-old man is admitted to the hospital after a car collision. Radiographic examination reveals a fracture at his wrist. Physical examination reveals paralysis of the muscles that act to extend the interphalangeal joints (Fig. 6-9). Which of the following nerves is most likely injured?

- ☐ **A.** Ulnar
- ☐ **B.** Recurrent branch of median
- ☐ **C.** Radial
- ☐ **D.** Musculocutaneous
- ☐ **E.** Anterior interosseous

125 A 45-year-old woman is admitted to the hospital with neck pain. An MRI examination reveals a herniated disc in the cervical region. Physical examination

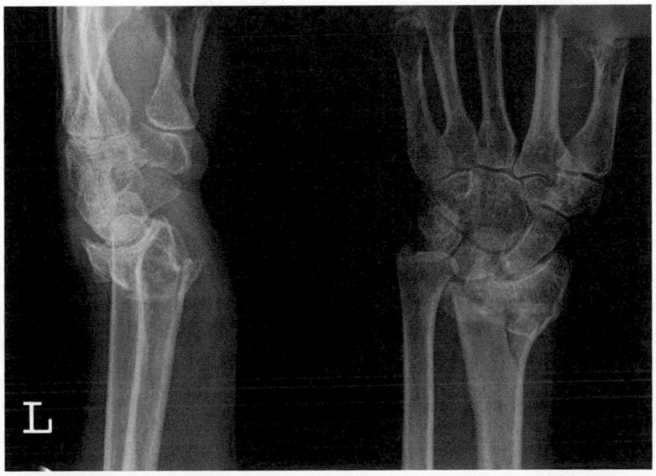

Fig. 6-9

reveals weak triceps brachii muscle. Which of the following spinal nerves is most likely injured?

- ☐ **A.** C5
- ☐ **B.** C6
- ☐ **C.** C7
- ☐ **D.** C8
- ☐ **E.** T1

126 A 34-year-old woman is admitted to the hospital after a car collision. Physical examination reveals a mallet finger. Which of the following conditions is expected to be present during radiographic examination?

- ☐ **A.** A lesion of the ulnar nerve at the distal flexor crease of the wrist
- ☐ **B.** A separation of the extension expansion over the middle interphalangeal joint
- ☐ **C.** Compression of the deep ulnar nerve by dislocation of the lunate bone
- ☐ **D.** Avulsion fracture of the dorsum of the distal phalanx
- ☐ **E.** Fracture of the fourth or fifth metacarpal bone

127 A 42-year-old woman is admitted to the hospital with injury to the upper (superior) trunk of the brachial plexus. The diagnosis is Erb-Duchenne palsy. Which of the following conditions is expected to be present during physical examination?

- ☐ **A.** Winged scapula
- ☐ **B.** Inability to laterally rotate the arm
- ☐ **C.** Paralysis of intrinsic muscles of the hand
- ☐ **D.** Paraesthesia in the medial aspect of the arm
- ☐ **E.** Loss of sensation in the dorsum of the hand

128 A 41-year-old woman is admitted to the hospital after a car crash. Radiographic examination reveals a transverse fracture of the radius proximal to the attachment of the pronator teres muscle. The proximal portion of the radius is deviated laterally. Which of the following muscles will most likely be responsible for this deviation?

- ☐ **A.** Pronator teres
- ☐ **B.** Pronator quadratus
- ☐ **C.** Brachialis
- ☐ **D.** Supinator
- ☐ **E.** Brachioradialis

129 A 45-year-old woman is bitten by a dog on the lateral side of her hand. Two days later the woman develops fever and swollen lymph nodes. Which of the following group of lymphatics will most likely be involved?

- ☐ **A.** Central
- ☐ **B.** Humeral
- ☐ **C.** Pectoral
- ☐ **D.** Subscapular
- ☐ **E.** Parasternal

130 A 25-year-old woman is admitted to the emergency department after a car collision. Radiographic examination reveals a fracture at the spiral groove of the humerus. A cast is placed, and 3 days later she complains of severe pain over the length of her arm. During physical examination the arm appears swollen, pale, and cool. Radial pulse is absent, and any movement of the arm causes severe pain. Which of the following conditions will most likely characterize the findings of the physical examination?

- ☐ **A.** Venous thrombosis
- ☐ **B.** Thoracic outlet syndrome
- ☐ **C.** Compartment syndrome
- ☐ **D.** Raynaud's disease
- ☐ **E.** Injury of the radial nerve

131 A 22-year-old woman is admitted to the hospital after falling from a tree. Radiographic examination reveals fractured pisiform and hamate bones. Which of the following nerves will most likely be injured?

- ☐ **A.** Median
- ☐ **B.** Recurrent median
- ☐ **C.** Radial
- ☐ **D.** Anterior interosseous
- ☐ **E.** Deep ulnar

132 A 43-year-old man visits the outpatient clinic with a painful shoulder. Physical examination reveals a painful arc syndrome due to supraspinatus tendinopathy. Which of the following conditions are expected to be present during physical examination as the patient abducts his arm?

- ☐ **A.** Painful abduction 0 to 15 degrees
- ☐ **B.** Painful abduction 0 to 140 degrees
- ☐ **C.** Painful abduction 70 to 140 degrees
- ☐ **D.** Painful abduction 15 to 140 degrees
- ☐ **E.** Painful abduction 40 to 140 degrees

133 A 54-year-old woman is admitted to the hospital after falling from a tree with an outstretched hand. Radiographic examination reveals a wrist dislocation. Which of the following carpal bones will most likely be involved?

- ▢ **A.** Scaphoid-lunate
- ▢ **B.** Trapezoid-trapezium
- ▢ **C.** Hamate-lunate
- ▢ **D.** Pisiform-triquetrum
- ▢ **E.** Hamate-capitate

134 A 62-year-old man is admitted to the emergency department after falling on wet pavement. Radiographic examination reveals a carpometacarpal fracture at the base of the thumb. What is the term applied to the described fracture?

- ▢ **A.** Colles' fracture
- ▢ **B.** Scaphoid fracture
- ▢ **C.** Bennett's fracture
- ▢ **D.** Smith's fracture
- ▢ **E.** Boxer's fracture

135 A 23-year-old woman is participating in a dry ski-slope competition. The woman is admitted to the emergency department after falling and catching her thumb in the matting. Radiographic and physical examinations reveal rupture of the ulnar collateral ligament of the metacarpophalangeal joint of the thumb. The thumb is extremely painful and an injection of lidocaine is given. What is the most likely diagnosis in this case?

- ▢ **A.** Gamekeeper's thumb
- ▢ **B.** Scaphoid fracture
- ▢ **C.** Bennett's fracture
- ▢ **D.** Smith's fracture
- ▢ **E.** Boxer's fracture

136 A 54-year-old woman is found unconscious in her car. She is admitted to the hospital, and during physical examination her biceps brachii reflex is absent. What is the spinal level of the afferent component of this reflex?

- ▢ **A.** C5
- ▢ **B.** C6
- ▢ **C.** C7
- ▢ **D.** C8
- ▢ **E.** T1

137 A 54-year-old woman is found unconscious in her bed. She is admitted to the hospital, and during physical examination she has absence of her brachioradialis reflex. The ventral ramus of which spinal nerve is responsible for this reflex?

- ▢ **A.** C5
- ▢ **B.** C6
- ▢ **C.** C7
- ▢ **D.** C8
- ▢ **E.** T1

138 A 55-year-old woman is admitted to the emergency department after a car crash. Physical examination reveals severe pain in the flexor muscles of the forearm, fixed flexion position of the finger, and swelling, cyanosis, and anesthesia of the fingers. Which of the following is the most likely diagnosis?

- ▢ **A.** Colles' fracture
- ▢ **B.** Scaphoid fracture
- ▢ **C.** Bennett's fracture
- ▢ **D.** Volkmann's ischemic contracture
- ▢ **E.** Boxer's fracture

139 A 62-year-old man visits the outpatient clinic with pain after falling on his outstretched hand. Radiographic examination reveals a fracture of the pisiform bone and hematoma of the surrounding area. Which of the following nerves will most likely be affected?

- ▢ **A.** Ulnar
- ▢ **B.** Radial
- ▢ **C.** Median
- ▢ **D.** Deep ulnar
- ▢ **E.** Deep radial

140 A 32-year-old woman visits the outpatient clinic after injuring her elbow falling from her bicycle. Physical examination reveals a "benediction attitude" of the hand with the index and long fingers extended and the ring and little fingers flexed. Which of the following is the most likely diagnosis?

- ▢ **A.** Injury to median and radial nerves
- ▢ **B.** Injury to median nerve
- ▢ **C.** Injury to radial and ulnar nerves
- ▢ **D.** Injury to ulnar nerve
- ▢ **E.** Injury to median ulnar and radial nerves

141 A 54-year-old man is admitted to the emergency department with severe chest pain. Electrocardiographic evaluation reveals a myocardial infarction. Due to the severity of the infarction, a coronary artery bypass surgery using a radial artery graft is proposed. Which of the following tests should be performed during physical examination before the bypass graft operation?

- ▢ **A.** Allen test
- ▢ **B.** Triceps reflex
- ▢ **C.** Tinel test
- ▢ **D.** Brachioradialis reflex
- ▢ **E.** Biceps reflex

142 A 34-year-old man visits the outpatient clinic with a painful upper limb after a fall onto a concrete floor. Physical examination reveals that the patient has weak abduction and adduction of his fingers but has no difficulty in flexing them. The patient also has decreased sensation over the palmar surface of the fourth and fifth fingers. Which of the following diagnoses is most likely?

- ☐ **A.** Compression of the median nerve in the carpal tunnel
- ☐ **B.** Injury of the radial nerve from fractured humerus in the radial tuberosity
- ☐ **C.** Compression of the median nerve as it passes between the two heads of the pronator teres
- ☐ **D.** Compression of the radial nerve from the supinator
- ☐ **E.** Injury of the ulnar nerve by a fractured pisiform

143 A 65-year-old man is admitted to the emergency department after falling on his outstretched hand. The patient complains of severe right shoulder pain. Upon physical examination, the patient holds his arm externally rotated and slightly abducted. There is also flattening and sensory loss over the right deltoid muscle. Which of the following is the most likely diagnosis?

- ☐ **A.** Anterior dislocation of the humerus
- ☐ **B.** Acromioclavicular joint subluxation
- ☐ **C.** Clavicular fracture
- ☐ **D.** Spiral fracture of the humeral midshaft
- ☐ **E.** Rotator cuff tear

144 A 4-year-old boy is brought to the emergency department after falling while holding hands and walking with his two parents. The boy cannot move his right upper extremity because any movement produces pain, and he holds it at his side with his elbow extended and forearm pronated. There are no visible hematomas or swelling. Which of the following structures is most likely injured in this patient?

- ☐ **A.** Anular ligament
- ☐ **B.** Biceps brachii tendon
- ☐ **C.** Interosseous membrane
- ☐ **D.** Radial collateral ligament
- ☐ **E.** Ulnar collateral ligament

145 An emergency department physician examines a patient who fell from a motorcycle and injured his shoulder. The clinician notices a loss of the normal contour of the shoulder and an abnormal-appearing depression below the acromion. Which of the following injuries did the patient most likely sustain?

- ☐ **A.** Avulsion of the coronoid process
- ☐ **B.** Dislocated shoulder joint
- ☐ **C.** Fracture of the midshaft of the humerus
- ☐ **D.** Fracture of the surgical neck of the humerus
- ☐ **E.** Laceration of the axillary branch of the posterior cord

146 A 22-year-old woman who is in training to become a phlebotomist is performing venipuncture on another student. She places the needle into the median cubital vein but is unable to withdraw blood. She quickly realizes that she passed the needle completely through the vein. Which of the following structures located deep to the median cubital vein has acted as a barrier and has prevented her from puncturing an artery?

- ☐ **A.** Flexor retinaculum
- ☐ **B.** Pronator teres muscle
- ☐ **C.** Bicipital aponeurosis
- ☐ **D.** Brachioradialis muscle
- ☐ **E.** Biceps brachii tendon

147 A 21-year-old painter sustains a laceration on the anterior surface of his left wrist just distal to the skin fold crease. When he arrives at the emergency department, the physician extends the patient's wrist to determine the depth of the laceration and observes a broad, glistening white structure deep to the superficial fascia. The patient has no numbness or tingling of any of the fingers and is able to discriminate sharp/dull sensation in all of the fingers and palm of the hand. There is no loss of motion in any of the fingers or the hand, and grip strength is normal. Which structure is the physician most likely observing?

- ☐ **A.** Flexor retinaculum
- ☐ **B.** Flexor carpi ulnaris tendon
- ☐ **C.** Palmar skin
- ☐ **D.** Flexor digitorum superficialis tendons
- ☐ **E.** Flexor digitorum profundus tendons

148 While using a wood-carving gouge, a 34-year-old woman lacerates the proximal aspect of her palm from the base of the thumb across to the pisiform bone. Neurological examination reveals pronounced weakness in opposition of the thumb, with intact sensation in the hand. Which of the following injuries best accounts for her findings?

- ☐ **A.** Injury of the median nerve in the carpal tunnel
- ☐ **B.** Injury of the superficial palmar branch of the median nerve
- ☐ **C.** Injury of the recurrent and superficial branch of the median nerve

☐ **D.** Injury of the recurrent median nerve at the wrist

☐ **E.** Injury of the radial and ulnar nerves

149 A 22-year-old football player suffered a wrist injury after falling on his outstretched hand. When the anatomical snuffbox is exposed in surgery, an artery is visualized crossing the fractured bone that provides a floor for this space. Which of the following arteries was most likely visualized?

☐ **A.** Ulnar

☐ **B.** Radial

☐ **C.** Anterior interosseous

☐ **D.** Posterior interosseous

☐ **E.** Deep palmar arch

150 A 36-year-old man is brought to the emergency department because of a deep knife wound on the medial side of his distal forearm. He is unable to hold a piece of paper between his fingers and has lost sensation from the fifth digit and the medial side of the fourth digit. Which of the following nerves is most likely injured?

☐ **A.** Axillary

☐ **B.** Median

☐ **C.** Musculocutaneous

☐ **D.** Radial

☐ **E.** Ulnar

151 A 28-year-old telephone company worker falls off a street pole during a telephone line repair and lands directly on his right shoulder. Plain radiographs reveal a vertical fracture through the entire length of the floor of the intertubercular sulcus of the right humerus. The muscle that is most likely affected by the fracture is innervated by a nerve that is composed of which of the following nerve roots?

☐ **A.** C3 and C4

☐ **B.** C6 to C8

☐ **C.** C4 and C5

☐ **D.** C2 to C4

☐ **E.** C5 to C7

152 A 21-year-old woman who is an athlete dislocated her glenohumeral joint while playing soccer and the shoulder was reduced in the emergency department. However, after 1 week the physician noted that the woman had lost strength when she attempted internal rotation of her arm at the shoulder. This finding was most likely caused by a tear in which of the following muscles?

☐ **A.** Infraspinatus

☐ **B.** Pectoralis minor

☐ **C.** Subscapularis

☐ **D.** Supraspinatus

☐ **E.** Teres minor

153 A 29-year-old man presents with difficulty with fine motor control in his hand. A few weeks ago he fell from a ladder; as he was falling he reached out and grabbed a limb of a tree. Examination reveals a deficit in his ability to abduct and adduct his digits and inability to oppose his thumb on his right hand. Which of the following was most likely injured?

☐ **A.** Lower trunk of the brachial plexus

☐ **B.** Median nerve

☐ **C.** Musculocutaneous nerve

☐ **D.** Ulnar nerve

☐ **E.** Upper trunk of the brachial plexus

154 An emergency department physician evaluates a 28-year-old man who injured his hand in a knife fight. The physician notes that the ring and little fingers cannot be extended at the interphalangeal joints, and the patient cannot spread the fingers of his injured hand. Weakness of which of the following muscles is the major reason for the loss of interphalangeal extension of the medial two fingers?

☐ **A.** Dorsal interosseus muscles

☐ **B.** Extensor digitorum

☐ **C.** Lumbrical muscles

☐ **D.** Palmar interosseus muscles

☐ **E.** Extensor digiti minimi

155 After a fall on her outstretched arm, a 72-year-old woman presents with elbow pain. Physical examination reveals a palpable defect over her biceps brachii tendon. Elbow flexion causes pain but does not limit active movement. Radiographs do not show fractures or dislocations. She is diagnosed with a biceps brachii tendon rupture. Which of the following muscles most likely allow the patient to continue to flex her elbow?

☐ **A.** Brachialis and brachioradialis

☐ **B.** Flexor carpi ulnaris and flexor carpi radialis

☐ **C.** Flexor digitorum superficialis and flexor digitorum profundus

☐ **D.** Pronator teres and supinator

☐ **E.** Triceps brachii and coracobrachialis

156 A 16-year-old girl is brought to the emergency department after attempting suicide by cutting her wrist. The deepest part of the wound is between the tendons of the flexor carpi radialis and the flexor digitorum superficialis. This patient is most likely to have a deficit of which of the following?

- ▢ **A.** Adduction and abduction of the fingers
- ▢ **B.** Extension of the index finger
- ▢ **C.** Flexion of the ring and little finger
- ▢ **D.** Sensation over the base of the little finger
- ▢ **E.** Opposition of the thumb and slightly weakened flexion of the second and third digits

157 A 36-year-old man presents to the emergency department with pain and tenderness in his right wrist after a fall on his outstretched hand two days ago. On examination there is tenderness on the lateral side of the wrist, just proximal to the base of the first metacarpal. What is the most likely diagnosis?

- ▢ **A.** Fracture of the first metacarpal
- ▢ **B.** Fracture of the trapezium
- ▢ **C.** Tenosynovitis of thumb extensors
- ▢ **D.** Fracture of the scaphoid
- ▢ **E.** First carpometacarpal joint arthritis

158 A 55-year-old man is admitted to hospital after blunt trauma at the junction of his neck and shoulder on the right side. Examination reveals winging of the scapula and partial paralysis of the right side of the diaphragm. Which part of the brachial plexus has been injured?

- ▢ **A.** Cords
- ▢ **B.** Divisions
- ▢ **C.** Ventral rami
- ▢ **D.** Terminal branches
- ▢ **E.** Trunks

159 A 55-year-old right-handed woman presents to the clinic with a 1-week history of right elbow pain. The pain started after a long game of competitive tennis. The pain begins in the elbow and at times radiates into the forearm. Splinting of the elbow decreases the intensity of the pain. During physical examination of the elbow mild swelling and tenderness are noted over the lateral epicondyle. Which one of the following wrist movements, if carried out by the patient with a closed fist and against resistance, will most likely exacerbate the pain?

- ▢ **A.** Radial deviation
- ▢ **B.** Ulnar deviation
- ▢ **C.** Flexion
- ▢ **D.** Extension
- ▢ **E.** Flexion and ulnar deviation

160 Following a difficult delivery, a 3-day-old infant girl showed limited movement of the right upper limb, with the arm adducted and internally/medially rotated, the forearm extended at the elbow and pronated, and the wrist slightly flexed. Tearing of fibers in which ventral rami of the brachial plexus best accounts for these symptoms?

- ▢ **A.** C5 and C6
- ▢ **B.** C6 and C7
- ▢ **C.** C7 and C8
- ▢ **D.** C8 and T1
- ▢ **E.** C5 to T1

161 A 48-year-old woman is seen in the orthopedic clinic with symptoms of carpal tunnel syndrome. This could result in weakening of which muscles?

- ▢ **A.** Dorsal and palmar interossei
- ▢ **B.** Lumbricals III and IV
- ▢ **C.** Thenar and lumbricals I and II
- ▢ **D.** Flexor digitorum superficialis and profundus
- ▢ **E.** Hypothenar

162 A 24-year-old man complains of inability to button his shirt. Examination reveals that he can still grip a sheet of paper between his second and third fingers and there is no sensory deficit in the hand. Which nerve has been affected?

- ▢ **A.** Deep branch of ulnar
- ▢ **B.** Anterior interosseous
- ▢ **C.** Median
- ▢ **D.** Recurrent branch of median
- ▢ **E.** Deep branch of radial

163 A 22-year-old man accidentally smashes his hand through a window. He is cut across the entire length of the distal transverse crease on the anterior surface of the wrist. The cut is down to the surface of the flexor retinaculum but not into it. During physical examination which is one of the neuromuscular deficits that will be found?

- ▢ **A.** Weakened pronation of the forearm
- ▢ **B.** Inability to abduct the thumb
- ▢ **C.** Weakened flexion of thumb
- ▢ **D.** Weakened opposition of the thumb
- ▢ **E.** Inability to adduct the thumb

164 A 36-year-old woman is admitted to the emergency department after an athletic injury that has caused weakness in both lateral rotation and the initial 15 to 20 degrees of abduction of the arm. Which nerve was most probably injured?

- ▢ **A.** Lower subscapular
- ▢ **B.** Axillary
- ▢ **C.** Radial
- ▢ **D.** Suprascapular
- ▢ **E.** Upper subscapular

165 A 35-year-old male carpenter suffered a deep cut to the tip of his thumb. Initially the redness, swelling, and pain were limited to the injured part of the thumb, but later the entire thumb and thenar eminence became inflamed. Which group of lymph nodes is the first to receive drainage from this injury?

- ▢ **A.** Posterior axillary
- ▢ **B.** Subclavian
- ▢ **C.** Lateral axillary
- ▢ **D.** Anterior axillary
- ▢ **E.** Central axillary

166 A mother tugs violently on her child's arm to pull him out of the way of an oncoming car and the child screams in pain. The child is admitted to the emergency department and radiographic examination reveals a dislocated head of the radius resulting from the radial head slipping out past which ligament?

- ▢ **A.** Anular
- ▢ **B.** Joint capsule
- ▢ **C.** Interosseous membrane
- ▢ **D.** Radial collateral
- ▢ **E.** Ulnar collateral

167 A 62-year-old woman is seen in the outpatient clinic. A photograph of her hand is shown in Figure 6-10. A radiograph reveals a hairline fracture of the hamate at Guyon's canal. Which of the following will also be present during physical examination?

- ▢ **A.** Numbness and weakness of the little and ring fingers

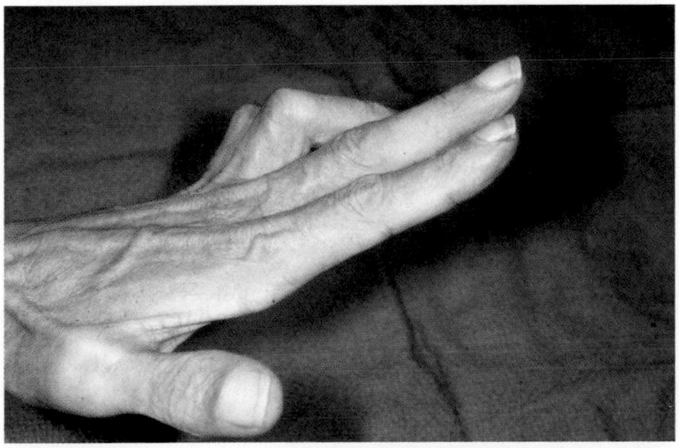

Fig. 6-10

- ▢ **B.** Wrist drop
- ▢ **C.** Atrophy of the thenar muscles
- ▢ **D.** Positive Tinel's test
- ▢ **E.** Trouble turning her forearm outward

168 A 25-year-old woman experiences numbness and tingling in her right arm and hand while carrying a piece of luggage. Physical examination showed no motor or sensory deficits in the upper limb. When asked to abduct her upper limb to 90 degrees and to maintain this position while repeatedly closing and opening her hands, the symptoms are reproduced along the medial border of the limb, from the axilla to the hand. Which nerve structure(s) is/are most likely compressed?

- ▢ **A.** Ulnar nerve at the medial epicondyle
- ▢ **B.** Radial nerve at the neck of the radius
- ▢ **C.** Median nerve in the carpal tunnel
- ▢ **D.** Inferior trunk of the brachial plexus
- ▢ **E.** Divisions of the brachial plexus

169 A 50-year-old woman reports to the physician that she is no longer able to play her viola as she used to because of "locking" of her index finger. During physical examination a snap is heard during passive extension of the finger and the consequent flexion of it. What is the most likely diagnosis of this condition?

- ▢ **A.** Tenovaginitis stenosans (trigger finger)
- ▢ **B.** Dupuytren's contracture
- ▢ **C.** Mallet finger
- ▢ **D.** Boutonniere deformity
- ▢ **E.** Boxer's fracture

170 A 25-year-old woman fashion model has an unsightly lump on her wrist that is causing her great distress. She also reports a tingling sensation on the lateral three and a half digits of the palmar aspect of her hand. Her doctor uses his pen torch to illuminate the lump and then uses a syringe to drain its contents. What is the most likely diagnosis of this condition?

- ▢ **A.** Neurofibroma
- ▢ **B.** Ganglion cyst
- ▢ **C.** Chondroma
- ▢ **D.** Osteoma
- ▢ **E.** Osteophyte

171 An 18-year-old man who is a professional cyclist complains of sensory loss to the medial one and a half fingers on the dorsal aspect of his hand. The orthopedic surgeon diagnoses "Handlebar neuropathy." What other signs may be elicited during physical examination?

- ☐ **A.** Sensory loss of the medial one and a half digits on the palmar aspect of the hand
- ☐ **B.** Weakness in abduction of the thumb
- ☐ **C.** Weakness in extension of the thumb
- ☐ **D.** Thenar muscle atrophy
- ☐ **E.** Tinel's sign at the scaphoid

172 A 20-year-old man who is a racquetball player reports to the physician's office complaining that he is not able to grip his racquet during practice. During physical examination the physician notes that the patient has atrophy of the thenar eminence, inability to oppose the thumb, and difficulty in flexing the middle interphalangeal joints of the digits. What is the most likely diagnosis of this condition?

- ☐ **A.** Hypertrophy of the supinator
- ☐ **B.** Pronator syndrome
- ☐ **C.** Medial supracondylar fracture
- ☐ **D.** Tennis elbow
- ☐ **E.** Golfer's elbow

173 A 54-year-old man presents to his primary care physician complaining of weakness in his fingers. His attempt to make a ring between his thumb and index finger by bringing the tips together is shown in Figure 6-11. He is able to successfully hold a piece of paper between his thumb and index finger. Pronation and wrist flexion are weakened. Which of the following nerves is most likely affected?

- ☐ **A.** Ulnar nerve at Guyon's canal
- ☐ **B.** Median nerve in the carpal tunnel

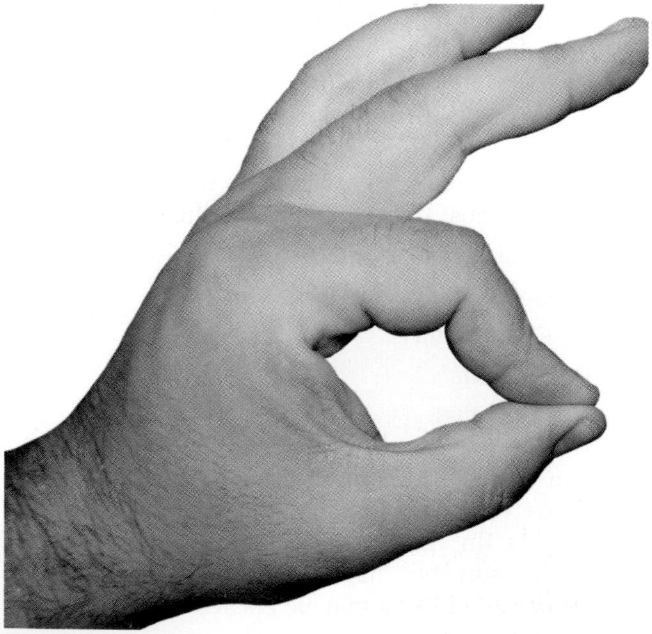

Fig. 6-11

- ☐ **C.** Anterior interosseous nerve beneath the ulnar head of pronator teres
- ☐ **D.** Posterior interosseous nerve beneath the supinator
- ☐ **E.** Median nerve beneath the bicipital aponeurosis

174 A 24-year-old man sustained multiple injuries including complex fractures in the right wrist as the result of a motor vehicle collision. After his injuries were stabilized and surgical repairs planned, neurological testing reveals decreased sensation along the medial border of the hand, as well as the little and ring fingers, and decreased strength of thumb adduction and finger adduction/abduction but with intact flexion of the distal interphalangeal joints of the ring and little fingers. If the nerve injury is not repaired, which of the following will become apparent in the affected hand over the next few weeks to months?

- ☐ **A.** Flattening of the thenar eminence
- ☐ **B.** Wrist drop
- ☐ **C.** Radial deviation at the wrist
- ☐ **D.** Ulnar deviation at the metacarpophalangeal joints
- ☐ **E.** Prominent metacarpal bones with "guttering" between adjacent metacarpals

175 A 30-year-old intoxicated man stumbled while descending stairs and fell on his outstretched and hyperextended hand. Since the fall (2 to 3 hours ago) he has had constant pain in his wrist, but over the past 30 minutes he has developed tingling and burning pain in his hand as well. Radiographs reveal fractures of both the radial and ulnar styloid processes, as well as dislocation of a carpal bone. Which of the following abnormal sensory and motor findings are most likely to be found on examination?

- ☐ **A.** Dysesthesia (tingling in response to light touch) along the medial border of the hand and little finger and weakness in adduction of the thumb
- ☐ **B.** Dysesthesia over the palm and palmar aspect of the thumb, index, and middle fingers and weakness in thumb opposition
- ☐ **C.** Numbness along the medial border of the hand and little finger and weakness in wrist extension
- ☐ **D.** Numbness over the dorsum of the hand laterally including the dorsal aspect of the thumb, index, and middle fingers and weakness in grip strength
- ☐ **E.** Numbness over the palm and palmar aspect of the thumb, index and middle fingers and weakness in adduction of the thumb

176 A 25-year-old man falls on a slippery trail and injures his elbow and hand. Inspection reveals abrasions over the olecranon, medial epicondyle, and palm of the hand. Physical examination reveals decreased sensation with "pins and needles" (paraesthesia) along the ulnar border of the hand and medial one and a half digits. There is also weakness of finger abduction/adduction, thumb adduction, and flexion at the DIP of the ring and little fingers. Which structure was most likely injured?

- ▢ **A.** Ulnar nerve at the medial epicondyle
- ▢ **B.** Ulnar nerve at Guyon's canal
- ▢ **C.** Median nerve in the cubital fossa
- ▢ **D.** Median nerve in the carpal tunnel
- ▢ **E.** Medial cord of brachial plexus in the axillary inlet

177 A 29-year-old woman injures her wrist in a fall on an outstretched hand. Examination reveals pain on movement of the wrist associated with numbness and tingling on the radial side of the palm and palmar aspect of the thumb, index, and middle fingers. A radiograph of the wrist reveals, anterior dislocation of a carpal bone. Which dislocated carpal bone is compressing which structure?

- ▢ **A.** Pisiform compressing ulnar nerve
- ▢ **B.** Hook of hamate compressing ulnar artery
- ▢ **C.** Scaphoid compressing radial artery
- ▢ **D.** Lunate compressing median nerve
- ▢ **E.** Trapezoid bone compressing superficial radial nerve

178 A 54-year-old woman is admitted to the emergency department after a serious motor vehicle accident. Physical examination shows soft tissue edema and bruising around the neck. A radiograph of the humeroscapular region reveals a fracture of the midhumerus. Which of the following areas will most likely have impaired or absent sensation?

- ▢ **A.** Lateral aspect of the forearm
- ▢ **B.** Medial aspect of the arm
- ▢ **C.** Medial aspect of the arm and forearm
- ▢ **D.** Posterior aspect of the forearm
- ▢ **E.** Lateral and posterior aspect of the forearm

179 A 52-year-old man is admitted to the emergency department after a fall. Imaging studies show a fracture at the neck of the radius and a hematoma at the fracture site. Examination reveals weakness of wrist extension, abduction and extension of the thumb, and extension of the metacarpophalangeal and interphalangeal joints of the fingers. However, there was no sensory deficit. Which nerve is most likely affected?

- ▢ **A.** Anterior interosseous
- ▢ **B.** Posterior interosseous
- ▢ **C.** Radial
- ▢ **D.** Ulnar
- ▢ **E.** Superficial radial

180 After falling down concrete steps, a 42-year-old woman complains of tingling and numbness along the medial border of her left hand. Neurological examination reveals several abnormalities including Froment's sign. Weakness of which of the following muscles explains the presence of Froment's sign?

- ▢ **A.** First dorsal interosseous muscle
- ▢ **B.** Opponens pollicis
- ▢ **C.** Adductor pollicis
- ▢ **D.** Flexor pollicis longus
- ▢ **E.** Flexor pollicis brevis

181 A 43-year-old woman visits the outpatient clinic with a painful hand. During physical examination, percussion over the flexor retinaculum causes a sharp pain in the lateral three and a half digits. This sign is indicative of which of the following conditions?

- ▢ **A.** Carpal tunnel syndrome
- ▢ **B.** De Quervain's tenosynovitis
- ▢ **C.** Thoracic outlet syndrome
- ▢ **D.** Mallet finger
- ▢ **E.** Radial nerve damage

182 A 25-year-old woman experiences numbness and tingling in her right arm and hand while carrying a piece of luggage. Physical examination showed no motor or sensory deficits in the upper limb. When asked to abduct her upper limb to 90 degrees and to maintain this position while repeatedly closing and opening her hands, the symptoms are reproduced along the medial border of the limb, from the axilla to the hand. Which nerve structure(s) is/are most likely compressed?

- ▢ **A.** Ulnar nerve at the medial epicondyle
- ▢ **B.** Radial nerve at the neck of the radius
- ▢ **C.** Median nerve in the carpal tunnel
- ▢ **D.** Inferior trunk of the brachial plexus
- ▢ **E.** Divisions of the brachial plexus

183 A 55-year-old woman is admitted to the emergency department after a car crash. Radiographic examination of her hand reveals a fractured carpal bone, which lies in the floor of the anatomical snuffbox. Which bone is fractured?

- ▢ **A.** Triquetrum
- ▢ **B.** Scaphoid

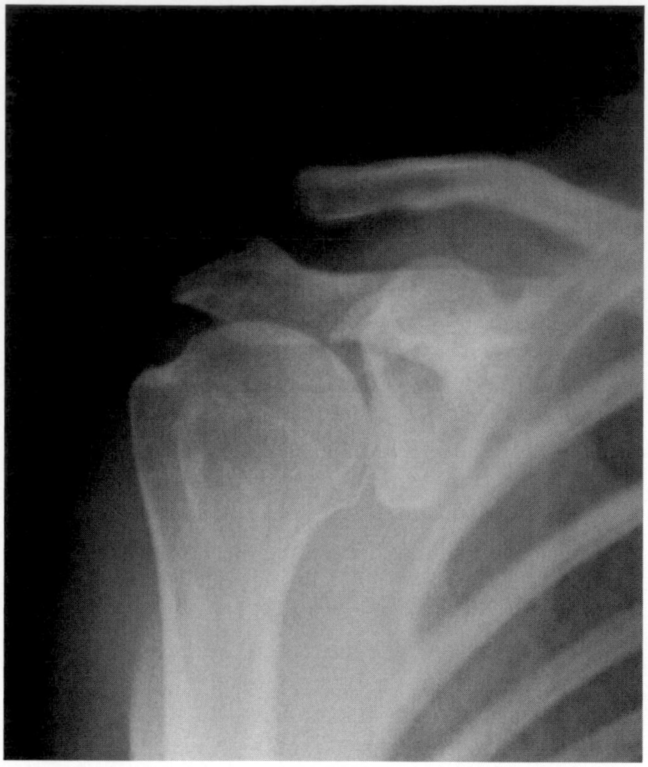

Fig. 6-12

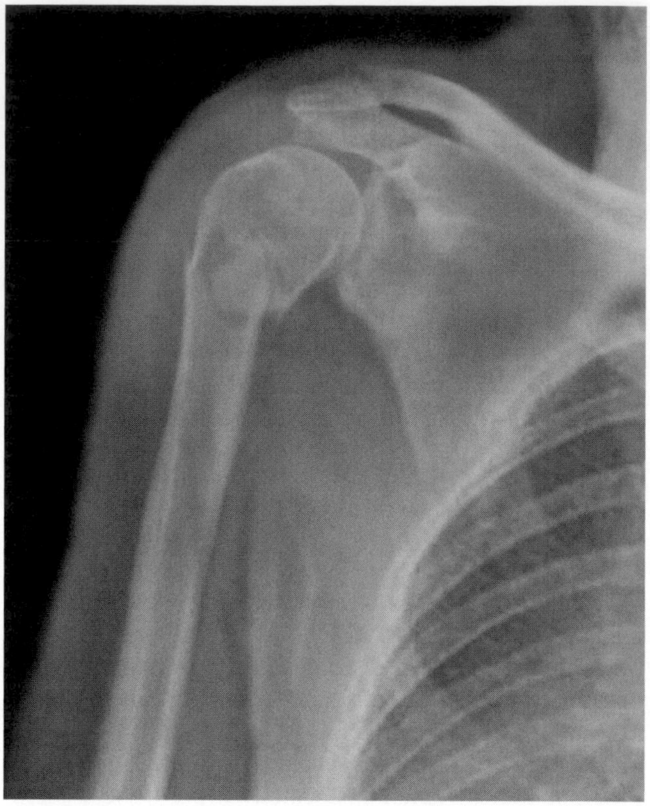

Fig. 6-13

- ▢ **C.** Capitate
- ▢ **D.** Hamate
- ▢ **E.** Trapezoid

184 An 18-year-old man presents to the emergency department with a painful right shoulder after a fall while diving for a soccer ball. A radiograph of the shoulder is shown in Figure 6-12. Examination revealed pain on passive adduction of the right arm across the chest. Which ligamentous structures must have been stretched/torn resulting in this injury?

- ▢ **A.** Acromioclavicular joint capsule and coracoclavicular ligament
- ▢ **B.** Acromioclavicular joint capsule and coracoacromial ligament
- ▢ **C.** Sternoclavicular joint capsule and coracoacromial ligament
- ▢ **D.** Coracoclavicular ligament and transverse scapular ligament
- ▢ **E.** Coracoclavicular ligament and coracoacromial ligament

185 A 67-year-old woman with osteoporosis injured her left shoulder/arm in a fall. Examination reveals bruising and dimpling of the upper part of the arm with exquisite tenderness over the affected area. The shoulder radiograph is shown in Figure 6-13. Which nerve is most likely to be injured?

- ▢ **A.** Radial
- ▢ **B.** Axillary
- ▢ **C.** Ulnar
- ▢ **D.** Median
- ▢ **E.** Musculocutaneous

186 A 14-year-old boy falls on his outstretched hand. Examination reveals point tenderness above the humeral epicondyles and a pulsatile mass just above the cubital fossa. Neurological examination of the upper limb reveals weakness of pronation, wrist flexion, and grip strength. Only flexion at the distal interphalangeal joints of the ring and little fingers is intact. Thumb flexion and opposition are also impaired. A radiograph reveals a supracondylar fracture of the humerus. Which structures injured by the fracture best account for the findings?

- ▢ **A.** Axillary nerve and posterior circumflex humeral artery
- ▢ **B.** Radial nerve and deep brachial artery
- ▢ **C.** Median nerve and brachial artery
- ▢ **D.** Superficial radial nerve and radial artery
- ▢ **E.** Ulnar nerve and ulnar artery

ANSWERS

1 D. The suspensory ligaments of the breast, also known as Cooper's ligaments, are fibrous bands that run from the dermis of the skin to the deep layer of superficial fascia and are primary supports for the breasts against gravity. Ptosis of the breast is usually due to the stretching of these ligaments and can be repaired with plastic surgery. Scarpa's fascia is the deep membranous layer of superficial fascia of the anterior abdominal wall. The pectoralis major and pectoralis minor are muscles that move the upper limb and lie deep to the breast but do not provide any direct support structure to the breast. The serratus anterior muscle is involved in the movements of the scapula.

GAS 131, 139; N 179; McM 179

2 A. The lower subscapular nerve arises from the cervical spinal nerves 5 and 6. It innervates the subscapularis and teres major muscles. The subscapularis and teres major muscles are both responsible for adducting and medially rotating the arm. A lesion of this nerve would result in weakness in these motions. The axillary nerve also arises from cervical spinal nerves 5 and 6 and innervates the deltoid and teres minor muscles. The deltoid muscle is large and covers the entire surface of the shoulder, and contributes to arm movement in any plane. The teres minor muscle is a lateral rotator and a member of the rotator cuff group of muscles. The radial nerve arises from the posterior cord of the brachial plexus. It is the largest branch, and it innervates the triceps brachii and anconeus muscles in the arm. The spinal accessory nerve is cranial nerve XI, and innervates the trapezius muscle, which elevates and depresses the scapula. The ulnar nerve arises from the medial cord of the brachial plexus and runs down the medial aspect of the arm. It innervates muscles of the forearm and hand.

GAS 714-717; N 413; McM 142

3 C. The thenar muscles (and lumbricals I and II) are innervated by the median nerve, which runs through the carpal tunnel. The carpal tunnel is formed anteriorly by the flexor retinaculum and posteriorly by the carpal bones. Carpal tunnel syndrome is caused by a compression of the median nerve, due to reduced space in the carpal tunnel. The carpal tunnel contains the tendons of flexor pollicis longus, flexor digitorum profundus, and flexor digitorum superficialis muscles and their synovial sheaths. The dorsal interossei, lumbricals III and IV, palmar interossei, and hypothenar muscles are all innervated by the ulnar nerve.

GAS 798, 808; N 452; McM 159

4 D. Fracture of the medial epicondyle often causes damage to the ulnar nerve due to its position in the groove behind the epicondyle. The ulnar nerve innervates one and a half muscles in the forearm, the flexor carpi ulnaris and the medial half of the flexor digitorum profundus muscles. The nerve continues on to innervate most of the muscles in the hand. The flexor digitorum superficialis is innervated by the median nerve and the biceps brachii muscle by the musculocutaneous. The radial nerve innervates both the brachioradialis and supinator muscles.

GAS 752, 764-768; N 432; McM 145

5 C. A midshaft humeral fracture can result in injury to the radial nerve and deep brachial artery because they lie in the spiral groove located in the midshaft. Injury to the median nerve and brachial artery can be caused by a supracondylar fracture that occurs by falling on an outstretched hand and partially flexed elbow. A fracture of the surgical neck of the humerus can injure the axillary nerve and posterior circumflex humeral artery. The suprascapular artery and nerve can be injured in a shoulder dislocation. The long thoracic nerve and lateral thoracic artery may be damaged during a mastectomy procedure.

GAS 751, 763; N 418; McM 144

6 B. A supracondylar fracture often results in injury to the median nerve. The course of the median nerve is anterolateral, and at the elbow it lies medial to the brachial artery on the brachialis muscle. The axillary nerve passes posteriorly through the quadrangular space, accompanied by the posterior circumflex humeral artery, and winds around the surgical neck of the humerus. Injury to the surgical neck may damage the axillary nerve. The musculocutaneous nerve pierces the coracobrachialis muscle and descends between the biceps brachii and brachialis muscle. It continues into the forearm as the lateral antebrachial cutaneous nerve. The ulnar nerve descends behind the medial epicondyle in its groove and is easily injured and produces "funny bone" symptoms.

GAS 763, 764; N 434; McM 143

7 C. The radial nerve descends posteriorly between the long and lateral heads of the triceps brachii muscle and passes inferolaterally on the back of the humerus between the medial and lateral heads of the triceps brachii muscle. It eventually enters the anterior compartment and descends to enter the cubital fossa, where it divides into superficial and deep branches. The deep branch of the radial nerve winds laterally around the radius and runs between the two heads of the supinator muscle and continues as the posterior interosseous nerve, innervating extensor muscles of the forearm. Because this injury does not result in loss of sensation over the skin of the upper limb, it is likely that the superficial branch of the radial nerve is not injured. If the radial nerve were injured very proximally, the woman would not be able to extend her elbow. The branches of the radial nerve to the triceps brachii muscle arise proximal to where the nerve runs in the spiral groove. The anterior interosseous nerve arises from the median nerve and supplies the flexor digitorum profundus, flexor pollicis longus, and pronator quadratus muscles, none of which seem to be injured in this example. Injury to the median nerve causes a characteristic flattening (atrophy) of the thenar eminence.

GAS 744-756, 761, 787, 792; N 431; McM 152

8 B. The musculocutaneous nerve supplies the biceps brachii and brachialis muscles, which are the flexors of the forearm at the elbow. The musculocutaneous nerve continues as the lateral antebrachial cutaneous nerve, which supplies sensation to the lateral side of the forearm (with the forearm in the anatomic position). The biceps brachii muscle is the most powerful supinator muscle. Injury to this nerve would result in weakness of supination and forearm flexion and lateral forearm sensory loss. Injury to the radial nerve would result in weakened extension and a characteristic wrist drop. Injury to the median nerve causes paralysis of flexor digitorum superficialis muscle and other flexors in the forearm and results in a characteristic flattening of the thenar eminence. The lateral cord of the brachial plexus gives origin both to the musculocutaneous and lateral pectoral nerves. There is no indication of pectoral paralysis or weakness. Injury to the lateral cord can result in weakened flexion and supination in the forearm, and weakened adduction and medial rotation of the arm. The lateral cutaneous nerve of the forearm is a branch of the musculocutaneous nerve and does not supply any motor innervation. Injury to the musculocutaneous nerve alone is unusual but can follow penetrating injuries.

GAS 760; N 462; McM 139

9 C. Tenosynovitis can be due to an infection of the synovial sheaths of the digits. Tenosynovitis in the thumb may spread through the synovial sheath of the flexor pollicis longus tendon, also known as the radial bursa. The tendons of the flexor digitorum superficialis and profundus muscles are enveloped in the common synovial flexor sheath or ulnar bursa. Neither the flexor carpi radialis nor flexor pollicis brevis tendons are contained in synovial flexor sheaths.

GAS 802; N 448; McM 158

10 A. The three chief contents of the cubital fossa are the biceps brachii tendon, brachial artery, and median nerve (lateral to medial). The common and anterior interosseous arteries arise distal to the cubital fossa; the ulnar and radial arteries are the result of the bifurcation of the brachial artery distal to the cubital fossa.

GAS 768; N 434; McM 151

11 D. Lymph from the skin of the anterior chest wall primarily drains to the axillary lymph nodes.

GAS 748; N 412; McM 179

12 C. The anterior intercostal arteries are twelve small arteries, two in each of the upper six intercostal spaces at the upper and lower borders. The upper artery lying in each space anastomoses with the posterior intercostal arteries, whereas the lower one usually joins the collateral branch of the posterior intercostal artery. The musculophrenic artery is a terminal branch of the internal thoracic artery (also known as the internal mammary artery), and it supplies the pericardium, diaphragm, and muscles of the abdominal wall. It anastomoses with the deep circumflex iliac artery. The superior epigastric artery is the other terminal branch of the internal thoracic artery, and it supplies the diaphragm, peritoneum, and the anterior abdominal wall and anastomoses with the inferior epigastric artery. The lateral thoracic artery runs along the lateral border of the pectoralis minor muscle and supplies the pectoralis major, pectoralis minor, and serratus anterior. The thoracodorsal artery accompanies the thoracodorsal nerve in supplying the latissimus dorsi muscle and lateral thoracic wall.

GAS 155; N 188; McM 183

13 D. The location for palpation of the radial pulse is lateral to the tendon of the flexor carpi radialis, where the radial artery can be compressed against the distal radius. The radial pulse can also be felt in the anatomic snuffbox between the tendons of the extensor pollicis brevis and extensor pollicis longus muscles, where the radial artery can be compressed against the scaphoid.

GAS 782, 827; N 432; McM 150

14 A. The flexor digitorum profundus muscle is dually innervated by the ulnar nerve to the medial two fingers and the median nerve for the long and index fingers. Because of the superficial course of the ulnar nerve, it is vulnerable to laceration. Such an injury would result in an inability to flex the distal interphalangeal joints of the fourth and fifth digits because the flexor digitorum profundus muscle is the only muscle that flexes this joint. The flexor digitorum superficialis muscle is innervated by the median nerve only, and the course of this nerve runs too deep to be usually affected by lacerations. The lumbricals function to flex the MP joints and assist in extending the IP joints. The interossei adduct and abduct the fingers.
GAS 781; N 433; McM 160

15 D. The recurrent branch of the median nerve is motor to the muscles of the thenar eminence, which is an elevation caused by the abductor pollicis brevis, flexor pollicis brevis, and opponens pollicis muscles. If the opponens pollicis is paralyzed, one cannot oppose the pad of the thumb to the pads of the other digits because this is the only muscle that can oppose the thumb by moving the first metacarpal on the trapezium. The recurrent branch does not have a cutaneous distribution. Holding a piece of paper between the fingers is a simple test of adduction of the fingers. These movements are controlled by the deep branch of the ulnar nerve, which is not injured in this patient.
GAS 817; N 460; McM 159

16 B. The condition described in this patient is called "winging" of the scapula. "Winging" of the scapula occurs when the medial border of the scapula lifts off the chest wall when the patient pushes against resistance, such as a vertical wall. The serratus anterior muscle holds the medial border of the scapula against the chest wall and is innervated by the long thoracic nerve. The serratus anterior assists in abduction of the arm above the horizontal plane by rotating the scapula so that the glenoid fossa is directed more superiorly.
GAS 727; N 413; McM 141

17 A. The anular ligament is a fibrous band that encircles the head of the radius, forming a collar that fuses with the radial collateral ligament and articular capsule of the elbow. The anular ligament functions to prevent displacement of the head of the radius from its socket. In a child of this age the head of the radius is almost the same diameter as the shaft of the bone, so the head is relatively easy to dislocate. The joint capsule functions to allow free rotation of the joint and does not function in its stabilization. The interosseous membrane is a fibrous layer between the radius and ulna helping to hold these two bones together. The radial collateral ligament extends from the lateral epicondyle to the margins of the radial notch of the ulnar and the anular ligament of the radius. The ulnar collateral ligament is triangular ligament and extends from the medial epicondyle to the olecranon of the ulna (*GAS* Figs. 7-73A and 7-72).
GAS 764-766; N 424; McM 146

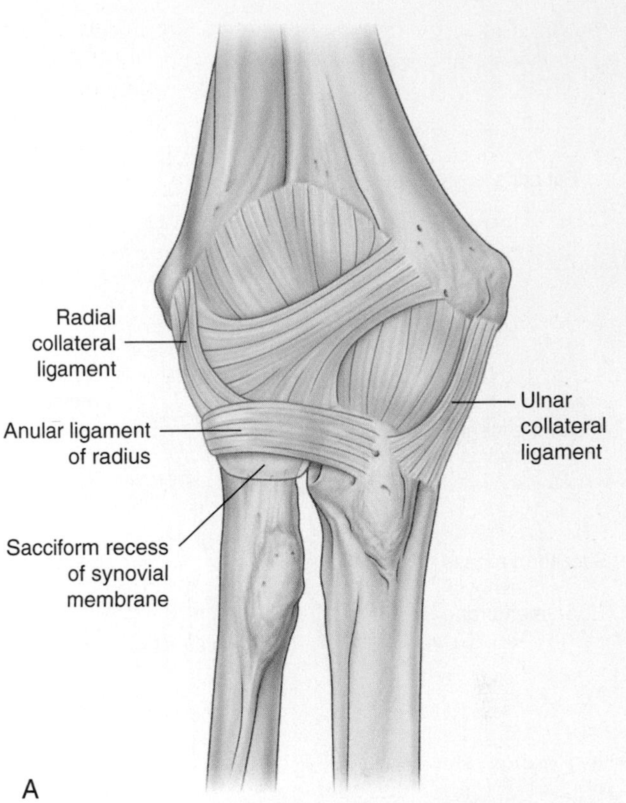

A
***GAS* Fig. 7-73A**

18 E. The injury being described is also known as Erb-Duchenne paralysis or "waiter's tip hand" and is relatively common in children after a difficult delivery. This usually results from an injury to the upper trunk of the brachial plexus, presenting with loss of abduction, flexion, and lateral rotation of the arm. The superior trunk of the brachial plexus consists of spinal nerve ventral rami C5-6.
GAS 738, 747; N 416; McM 139

19 C. The common palmar digital branch comes off the superficial branch of the ulnar nerve and supplies the skin of the little finger and the medial side of the ring finger. The superficial branch of the radial nerve provides cutaneous innervation to the radial (lateral) dorsum of the hand and the radial two and a half

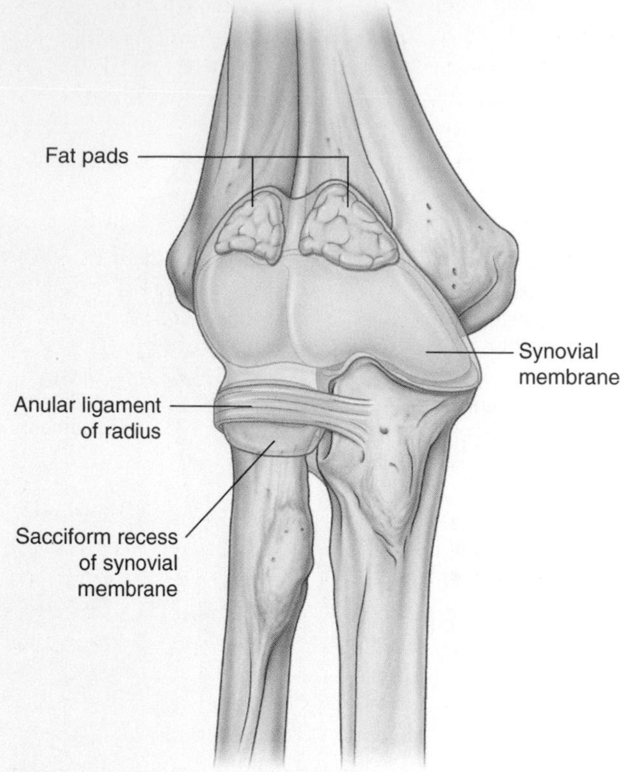

GAS **Fig. 7-72**

digits over the proximal phalanx. The common palmar digital branch of the median nerve innervates most of the lateral aspect of the palmar hand and the dorsal aspect of the second and third finger as well as the lateral part of the fourth digit. The deep radial nerve supplies the extensor carpi radialis brevis and supinator muscles and continues as the posterior interosseous nerve. The recurrent branch of the median nerve supplies the abductor pollicis brevis, flexor pollicis brevis, and opponens pollicis muscles.

GAS 695-699, 814-815; N 460; McM 160

20 B. The anatomic snuffbox is formed by the tendons of the extensor pollicis brevis, the abductor pollicis longus, and the extensor pollicis longus. The floor is formed by the scaphoid bone, and it is here that one can palpate for a possible fractured scaphoid.

GAS 800; N 430; McM 164

21 E. The ulnar nerve innervates the palmar interossei, which adduct the fingers. This is the movement that would maintain the paper between the fingers. The axillary nerve does not innervate muscles of the hand. The median nerve supplies the first and second lumbricals, the opponens pollicis, abductor pollicis brevis, and the flexor pollicis brevis muscles. None of these muscles would affect the ability to hold a piece of paper between the fingers. The musculocutaneous and radial nerves do not supply muscles of the hand.

GAS 808, 814; N 452; McM 162

22 D. The supraspinatus muscle is one of the four rotator cuff muscles—the other three being the infraspinatus, teres minor, and subscapularis muscles. The tendon of the supraspinatus muscle is relatively avascular and is often injured when the shoulder is dislocated. This muscle initiates abduction of the arm, and damage would impair this movement. The coracobrachialis muscle, which runs from the coracoid process to the humerus, functions in adduction and flexion of the arm. The main function of the triceps brachii muscle is to extend the elbow, and damage to its long head would not affect abduction. The pectoralis minor muscle functions as an accessory respiratory muscle and to stabilize the scapula and is not involved in abduction. The teres major muscle functions to adduct and medially rotate the arm.

GAS 717; N 411; McM 137

23 E. The coracoacromial ligament contributes to the coracoacromial arch, preventing superior displacement of the head of the humerus. Because this ligament is very strong, it will rarely be damaged; instead, the ligament can cause inflammation or erosion of the tendon of the supraspinatus muscle as the tendon passes back and forth under the ligament. The acromioclavicular ligament, connecting the acromion with the lateral end of the clavicle, is not in contact with the supraspinatus tendon. The coracohumeral ligament is located too far anteriorly to impinge upon the supraspinatus tendon. The glenohumeral ligament is located deep to the rotator cuff muscles and would not contribute to injury of the supraspinatus muscle. The transverse scapular ligament crosses the scapular notch and is not in contact with the supraspinatus tendon.

GAS 705-706; N 411; McM 136

24 A. The median nerve supplies sensory innervation to the thumb, index, and middle fingers and also to the lateral half of the ring finger. The median nerve also provides motor innervation to muscles of the thenar eminence. Compression of the median nerve in the carpal tunnel explains these deficits in conjunction with normal functioning of the flexor compartment of the forearm because these muscles are innervated by the median nerve proximal to the carpal tunnel. Also, sensory innervation in the proximal palm will be normal because the palmar branch of the radial nerve usually branches off proximal to the flexor retinaculum. The ulnar nerve is not implicated in these symptoms. It does not provide sensation to digits 1 to 3. Compression of the brachial plexus could not be attributed to pressure from the triceps brachii because this muscle is located distal to the plexus. In addition, brachial plexus symptoms would include other upper limb deficits, rather than the focal symptoms described in this case. Osteoarthritis of the cervical spine would also lead to increasing complexity of symptoms.

GAS 798; N 449; McM 160

25 **C.** The radial nerve innervates the extensor compartments of the arm and the forearm. It supplies the triceps brachii proximal to the spiral groove, so elbow extension is intact here. It also provides sensory innervation to much of the posterior arm and forearm as well as the dorsal thumb, index, and middle fingers up to the level of the fingernails. Symptoms are described only in the distal limb due to the mid-humeral location of the lesion. The median nerve innervates flexors of the forearm and thenar muscles and provides sensory innervation to the lateral palmar hand. The ulnar nerve supplies only the flexor carpi ulnaris and the medial half of the flexor digitorum profundus in the forearm. Additionally, its sensory distribution is to both the palmar and dorsal aspects of the medial hand. It does not supply extensor muscles.

GAS 746, 761; N 418; McM 144

26 **D.** The musculocutaneous nerve innervates the brachialis and biceps brachii muscles, which are the main flexors at the elbow. The biceps brachii inserts on the radius and is an important supinator. Because the musculocutaneous nerve is damaged in this case, it leads to loss of sensory perception to the lateral forearm, which is supplied by the distal continuation of the musculocutaneous nerve (known as the lateral antebrachial cutaneous nerve). The name "musculocutaneuous" indicates it is "muscular" in the arm and "cutaneous" in the forearm. Adduction and abduction of the fingers are mediated by the ulnar nerve and would not be affected in this instance. The flexor pollicis brevis muscle flexes the thumb and is mainly innervated by the recurrent branch of the median nerve. Flexion of the fingers is performed by the long flexors of the fingers and lumbrical muscles, innervated by the median and ulnar nerves. Sensory innervation of the medial forearm is provided by the medial antebrachial cutaneous nerve, usually a direct branch of the medial cord of the brachial plexus.

GAS 746, 760; N 417; McM 143

27 **E.** The deep branch of the radial nerve courses between the two heads of the supinator muscle and is located just medial and distal to the lateral epicondyle. After the nerve emerges from the supinator it is called the posterior interosseous nerve. It can be irritated by hypertrophy of the supinator, which compresses the nerve, causing pain and weakness. The ulnar nerve courses laterally behind the medial epicondyle and continues anterior to the flexor carpi ulnaris muscle. The median nerve passes into the forearm flexor compartment; the superficial radial nerve courses down the lateral aspect of the posterior forearm and would not cause pain due to pressure applied to the posterior forearm.

GAS 792; N 466; McM 152

28 **B.** The lunate is the most commonly dislocated carpal bone because of its shape and relatively weak ligaments anteriorly. Dislocations of the scaphoid and triquetrum are relatively rare. The trapezoid and capitate bones are located in the distal row of the carpal bones.

GAS 793; N 439; McM 167

29 **A.** The medial antebrachial cutaneous nerve carries sensory fibers derived from the C8 and T1 levels. The lateral antebrachial cutaneous nerve is the distal continuation of the musculocutaneous nerve, carrying fibers from the C5, C6, and C7 levels. The deep branch of the ulnar nerve and the anterior interosseous nerves carry predominantly motor fibers. The sensory fibers coursing in the radial nerve are derived from the C5 to C8 levels.

GAS 695-699, 742; N 460; McM 148

30 **C.** The contraction of the extensor mechanism produces extension of the distal interphalangeal joint. When it is torn from the distal phalanx, the digit is pulled into flexion by the flexor digitorum profundus muscle. If a piece of the distal phalanx is attached to the torn tendon it is an avulsion fracture. The proper palmar digital branches of the median nerve supply lumbrical muscles and carry sensation from their respective digits. Vincula longa are slender, bandlike connections from the deep flexor tendons to the phalanx that can carry blood supply to the tendons. The insertions of the flexor digitorum superficialis and profundus are on the flexor surface of the middle and distal phalanges, respectively, and act to flex the interphalangeal joints.

GAS 787, 808; N 451; McM 165

31 **E.** In Smith's fracture, the distal fragment of the radius deviates palmarward, often displacing the

lunate bone. The other listed bones are unlikely to be displaced in a palmar direction by Smith's fracture.
GAS 771-774; N 439; McM 167

32 B. The abductor pollicis longus and extensor pollicis brevis muscles are the occupants of the first dorsal compartment of the wrist. The extensor carpi radialis longus and brevis are in the second compartment. The extensor digitorum is in the third compartment, as is the extensor indicis. The extensor carpi ulnaris is located in the sixth dorsal compartment.
GAS 785-790; N 431; McM 165

33 E. The medial cord has been injured by traction on the lower trunk of the brachial plexus. The medial cord is the continuation of the inferior (lower) trunk of the brachial plexus, which is formed by C8 and T1. C5 and C6 are typically associated with the superior (upper) trunk level and thus the lateral cord. C7 forms the middle trunk. An injury to the posterior cord would usually involve the C7 spinal nerve. This is a typical Klumpke paralysis.
GAS 738-747; N 416; McM 139

34 A. The flexor carpi ulnaris muscle is not innervated by the radial nerve but rather by the ulnar nerve. The brachioradialis, extensor carpi radialis longus and brevis, and supinator muscles are all innervated by the radial nerve distal to the spiral groove.
GAS 777, 787; N 418; McM 149

35 A. Injury to the radial nerve in the spiral groove will paralyze the abductor pollicis longus muscle and both extensors of the thumb. This injury will also lead to wrist drop (inability to extend the wrist). Weakness of grip would also occur, although this is not mentioned in the question. If the wrist is flexed, finger flexion and grip strength are weakened because the long flexor tendons are not under tension. Note how much your strength of grip is increased when your wrist is extended versus when it is flexed.
GAS 763, 818; N 427; McM 144

36 C. The superior ulnar collateral branch of the brachial artery accompanies the ulnar nerve in its path posterior to the medial epicondyle and is important in the blood supply of the nerve. The profunda brachii artery passes down the arm with the radial nerve. The radial collateral artery arises from the profunda brachii artery and anastomoses with the radial recurrent branch of the radial artery proximal to the elbow laterally. The inferior ulnar collateral artery arises from the brachial artery and accompanies the median nerve into the forearm. The anterior ulnar recurrent artery arises from the ulnar artery and anastomoses with the inferior ulnar collateral artery anterior to the elbow.
GAS 756; N 435; McM 149

37 C. Adduction of the fifth digit is produced by contraction of the third palmar interosseous muscle. All of the interossei are innervated by the deep branch of the ulnar nerve. Flexion of the proximal interphalangeal joint is a function of the flexor digitorum superficialis, supplied by the median nerve. Opposition of the thumb is a function of the opponens pollicis, supplied by the recurrent branch of the median nerve.
GAS 808; N 452; McM 162

38 C. The radial nerve is the most likely nerve compressed to cause these symptoms. This type of nerve palsy is often called "Saturday night palsy." One reason for this nickname is that people would supposedly fall asleep after being intoxicated on a Saturday night with their arm over the back of a chair or bench, thereby compressing the nerve in the spiral groove. The radial nerve innervates all of the extensors of the elbow, wrist, and fingers. It innervates the triceps brachii muscle but the motor branch typically comes off proximal to the site of compression, so the patient can still extend the elbow. Paralysis of the lateral cord of the brachial plexus would result in loss of the musculocutaneous nerve and the pectoral nerves, which do not mediate extension of the forearm or hand. The medial cord of the brachial plexus branches into the median nerve and ulnar nerve. Neither of these nerves innervates muscles that control extension. The median nerve innervates flexors of the forearm and the thenar muscles. The lateral and median pectoral nerves do not extend into the arm and innervate the pectoralis major and minor muscles.
GAS 761-763; N 415; McM 139

39 A. The basilic vein can be used for dialysis, especially when the cephalic vein is judged to be too small, as in this case. The basilic vein can be elevated from its position as it passes through the fascia on the medial side of the arm (brachium). The cephalic vein passes more laterally up the limb. The lateral cubital vein is a tributary to the cephalic vein, and the medial cubital vein joins the basilic vein, both of which are rather superficial in position. The medial antebrachial vein courses up the midline of the forearm (antebrachium) ventrally.
GAS 700, 759, 769-770; N 401; McM 148

40 A. The patient exhibits the classic "benediction attitude" of the thumb and fingers from injury to the median nerve proximally in the forearm. The thumb is somewhat extended (radial supplied abductor and extensors unopposed); digits 2 and 3 are extended (by intact interossei); digits 4 and 5 are partially flexed (by their intact flexor digitorum profundus). A lesion of the median nerve would result in weakened flexion of the proximal interphalangeal joints of all digits (flexor digitorum superficialis muscle), loss of flexion of the interphalangeal joint of the thumb, the distal interphalangeal joints of digits 2 and 3 (flexor digitorum profundus muscle), and weakened flexion of the metacarpophalangeal joints of the second and third digits (first and second lumbricals). A lesion of both the ulnar and median nerves would cause weakness or paralysis of flexion of all of the digits. A lesion of the ulnar nerve would mostly cause weakness in flexion of the DIP of the fourth and fifth digits and would affect all of the interosseous muscles and the lumbricals of the third and fourth digits. A lesion of the radial nerve would cause weakness in extension of the wrist, thumb, and metacarpophalangeal joints.
GAS 784, 817; N 434; McM 149

41 C. The head of the humerus is displaced inferiorly because in that location it is not supported by rotator cuff muscle tendons or the coracoacromial arch. It is also pulled anteriorly (relative to the tendon of the triceps brachii) beneath the coracoid process by pectoralis and subscapularis muscles. It would not be displaced posteriorly because it is supported by the teres minor and infraspinatus muscle tendons. It would not be displaced superiorly because the coracoacromial ligament and supraspinatus reinforce in that direction. A medial dislocation is blocked by the subscapularis tendon.
GAS 712; N 408; McM 136

42 A. The anterior axillary (or anterior pectoral) nodes are the first lymph nodes to receive most of the lymph from the breast parenchyma, areola, and nipple. From there, lymph flows through central axillary, apical, and supraclavicular nodes in sequence. The interpectoral Rotter's nodes lie between the pectoral muscles and are, unfortunately, an alternate route in some patients, speeding the rate of metastasis. The parasternal nodes receive lymph from the medial part of the breast and lie along the internal thoracic artery and vein.
GAS 748; N 403; McM 179

43 D. The left spinal accessory nerve (CN XI) has been injured distal to the sternocleidomastoid muscle, resulting in paralysis of the trapezius, allowing the shoulder to droop and the superior angle to push out posteriorly. The sternocleidomastoid muscles are intact, as demonstrated by symmetry in strength in turning the head to the right and left. There is no indication of paralysis of the lateral rotators of the shoulder or elbow flexors (suprascapular nerve or upper trunk). Thoracodorsal nerve injury would result in paralysis of the latissimus dorsi muscle, an extensor, and medial rotator of the humerus.
GAS 714; N 413; McM 132

44 C. Inability to extend the metacarpophalangeal (MCP) joints. The tendons of the extensor digitorum and extensor digiti minimi muscles, innervated by the radial nerve, are responsible for extension of the MCP and, to a much lesser degree, the proximal (PIP) and distal (DIP) interphalangeal joints. Abduction and adduction of the MCP joints are functions of the interossei, all of which are innervated by the deep ulnar nerve. Extension of the PIP and DIP joints is performed by the lumbricals and interossei. The first two lumbricals are supplied by the median nerve; the other lumbricals and the interossei, by the deep branch of the ulnar nerve.
GAS 792, 814-818; N 451; McM 155

45 C. Fracture of the surgical neck of the humerus often injures the axillary nerve, which innervates the deltoid and teres minor muscles. Abduction of the humerus between 15 degrees and the horizontal is performed by the deltoid muscle. Lateral rotation of the humerus is mainly performed by the deltoid muscle, teres minor, and the infraspinatus. The deltoid and teres minor are both lost in this case. Fracture of the glenoid fossa would lead to drooping of the shoulder. Fracture of the anatomic neck of the humerus will similarly lead to a drooping of the shoulder but would not necessarily affect abduction of the humerus. It is also quite unusual. Fracture of the middle third of the humerus would most likely injure the radial nerve. The ulnar nerve would be potentially compromised in a fracture of the medial epicondyle of the humerus.
GAS 705; N 405; McM 140

46 B. When cutaneous lymphatics of the breast are blocked by cancer, the skin becomes edematous, except where hair follicles cause small indentations of the skin, giving an overall resemblance to orange peel. Shortening of the suspensory ligaments (of Cooper) or retinacula cutis leads to pitting of the overlying skin, pitting that is intensified if the patient raises her arm above her head. Invasion of the pectoralis major by cancer can result in fixation of the breast, seen upon elevation of the ipsilateral limb. Inversion of areolar skin with involvement of the ducts would also be due to involvement of the retinacula cutis.

GAS 748; N 181; McM 179

47 **D.** The subclavian vein traverses between the clavicle and first rib and is the most superficial structure to be damaged following a fracture of the clavicle. The subclavian artery runs posterior to the subclavian vein, and though it is in the appropriate location, it would likely not be damaged because of its deep anatomic position. The cephalic vein is a tributary to the axillary vein after ascending on the lateral side of the arm. Its location within the body is too superficial and lateral to the site of injury. The lateral thoracic artery is a branch from the axillary artery that runs lateral to the pectoralis minor. It courses inferior and medial from its point of origin from the axillary artery, and it does not maintain a position near the clavicle during its descent. The internal thoracic artery arises from the first part of the subclavian artery before descending deep to the costal cartilages. Its point of origin from the subclavian artery is lateral to clavicular injury. Furthermore, its course behind the costal cartilages is quite medial to the clavicular fracture.

GAS 694, 736-737; N 415; McM 129

48 **A.** A Colles' fracture is a fracture of the distal end of the radius. The proximal portion of the radius is displaced anteriorly, with the distal bone fragment projecting posteriorly. The displacement of the radius from the wrist often gives the appearance of a dinner fork, thus a Colles' fracture is often referred to as a "dinner fork" deformity. A scaphoid fracture results from a fracture of the scaphoid bone and would thus not cause displacement of the radius. This fracture usually occurs at the narrow aspect ("waist") of the scaphoid bone. Bennett's and boxer's fractures both result from fractures of the metacarpals (first and fifth, respectively). Volkmann's ischemic contracture is a muscular deformity that can follow a supracondylar fracture of the humerus, with arterial laceration into the flexor compartment of the forearm. Ischemia and muscle contracture, with extreme pain, accompany this fracture.

GAS 771-774; N 439; McM 124

49 **B.** In shoulder separation, either or both the acromioclavicular and coracoclavicular ligaments can be partially or completely torn through. The acromioclavicular joint can be interrupted and the distal end of the clavicle may deviate upward in a complete separation, while the upper limb droops away inferiorly, causing a "step off" that can be palpated and sometimes observed. Displacement of the head of the humerus is shoulder dislocation, not separation. The coracoacromial ligament is not torn in separation (but it is sometimes used in the repair of the torn coracoclavicular ligament). Disruption of the glenoid labrum often accompanies shoulder dislocation.

GAS 711; N 411; McM 136

50 **A.** The nail was fired explosively from the nail gun and then pierced the ulnar nerve near the coronoid process of the ulna and the trochlea of the humerus. Paralysis of the medial half of the flexor digitorum profundus muscle would result (among other significant deficits), with loss of flexion of the distal interphalangeal joints of digits 4 and 5. Ulnar trauma at the wrist would not affect the interphalangeal joints, although it would cause paralysis of interossei, hypothenar muscles, and so on. Median nerve damage proximal to the pronator teres would affect proximal interphalangeal joint flexion and distal interphalangeal joint flexion of digits 2 and 3 as well as thumb flexion. Median nerve injury at the wrist would cause loss of thenar muscles but not long flexors of the fingers. Trauma to spinal nerve ventral ramus C8 would affect all long finger flexors.

GAS 784, 814; N 434; McM 149

51 **C.** The injury has occurred just beyond the third part of the axillary artery. The only collateral arterial channel between the third part of the axillary artery and the brachial artery is between the posterior circumflex humeral and the ascending branch of the profunda brachii, and this anastomotic path is often inadequate to supply the arterial needs of the limb. The posterior circumflex humeral arises from the third part of the axillary artery. It typically anastomoses with a variably small, ascending branch of the profunda brachii branch of the brachial artery. The suprascapular artery anastomoses with the circumflex scapular deep to the infraspinatus. The dorsal scapular artery (passing beneath the medial border of the scapula) has no anastomosis with thoracodorsal within the scope of the injury. The lateral thoracic artery has no anastomoses with the brachial artery. The supreme thoracic artery (from first part of axillary) has no helpful anastomoses with the thoracoacromial (second part of axillary) (*GAS* Figs. 7-39 and 7-50).

GAS 719-721; N 420; McM 139

52 **E.** The scaphoid (or the older term, navicular) bone is the most commonly fractured carpal bone.

GAS 797; N 439; McM 167

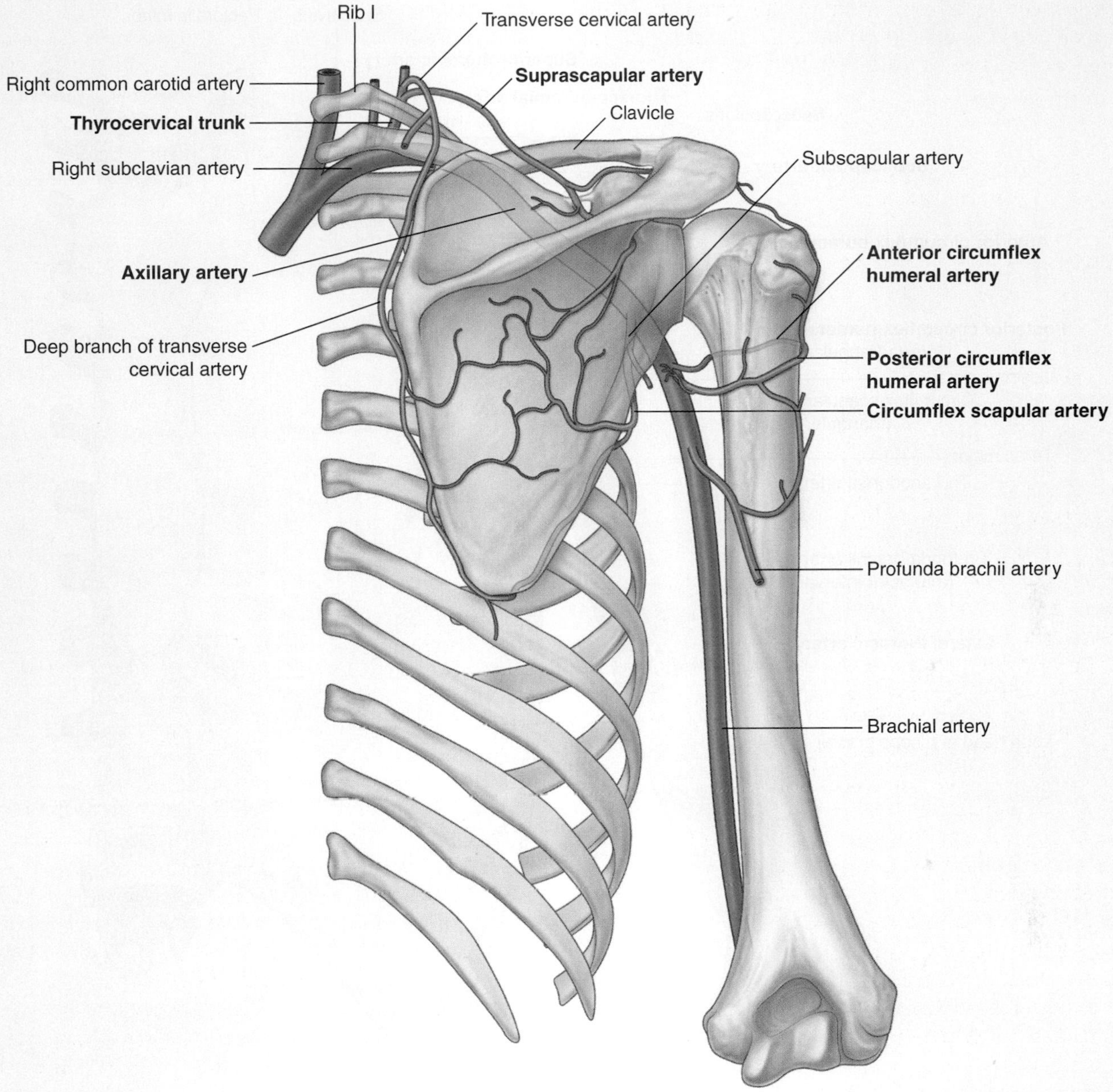

GAS Fig. 7-39

53 E. The anterior interosseous nerve is a branch of the median nerve that supplies the flexor pollicis longus, the lateral half of the flexor digitorum profundus, and the pronator quadratus muscles. If it is injured, flexion of the interphalangeal joint of the thumb will be compromised. The median nerve gives rise to the anterior interosseous nerve but is not a direct enough answer as injury to it would result in more widespread effects. The posterior interosseous nerve supplies extensors in the forearm, not flexors. The radial nerve gives rise to the posterior interosseous nerve and is not associated with the anterior interosseous nerve; therefore, it would not have any effect on the flexors of the forearm. The recurrent median nerve is also a branch of the median nerve but supplies the thenar eminence muscles, and its injury would result in problems with opposable motion of the thumb (*GAS* Fig. 7-87).

GAS 784; N 463; McM 151

54 C. The tendon of the long head of the biceps brachii muscle passes through the glenohumeral joint, surrounded by synovial membrane. The glenohumeral is a ligament that attaches to the glenoid labrum. The long head of the triceps brachii arises from the infraglenoid tubercle, beneath the glenoid fossa. The

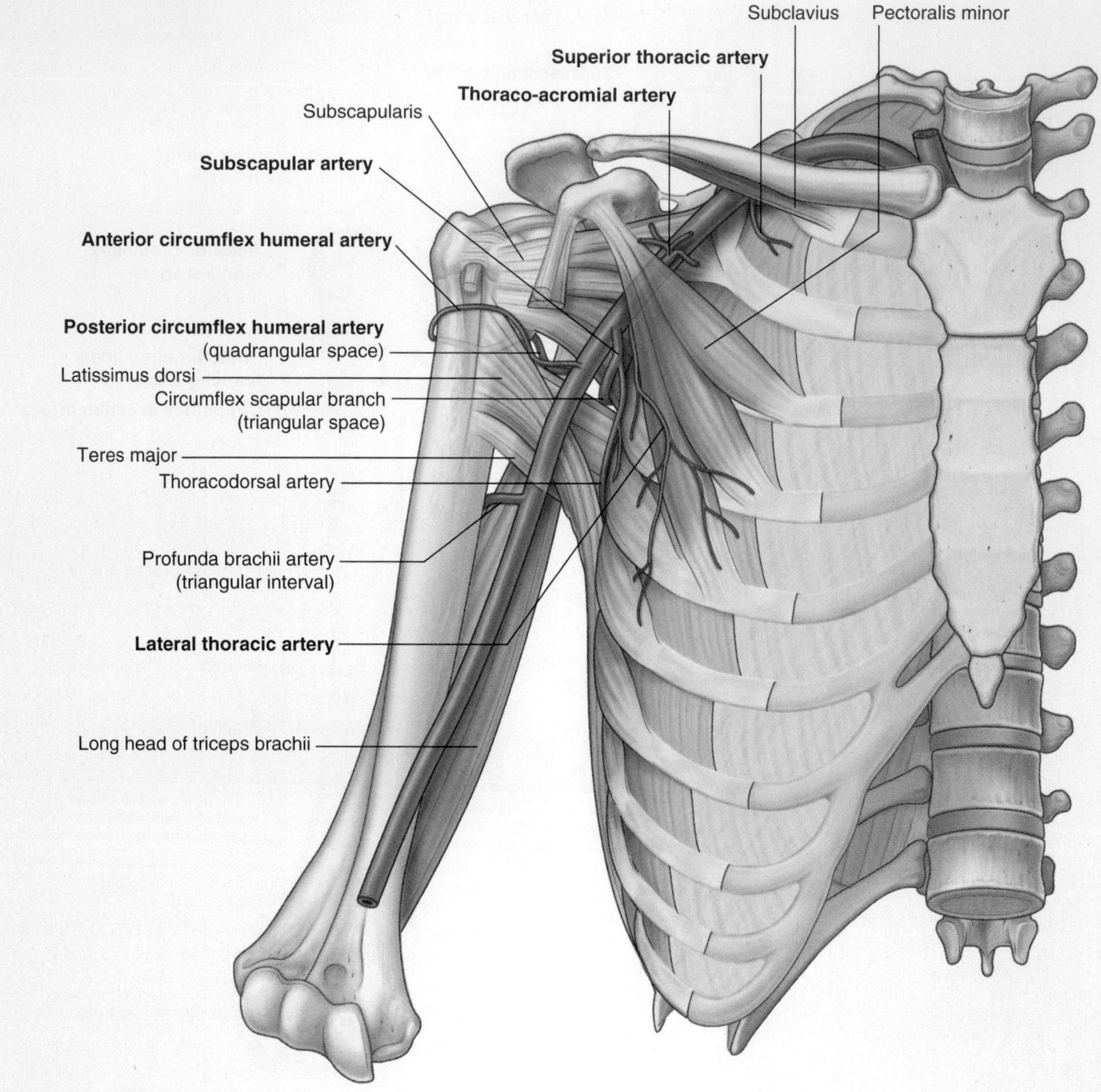

GAS **Fig. 7-50**

infraspinatus tendon passes posterior to the head of the humerus to insert on the greater tubercle. The coracobrachialis arises from the coracoid process and inserts on the humerus.

GAS 707; N 417; McM 137

55 E. The suprascapular artery passes over, and the suprascapular nerve passes under, the superior transverse scapular ligament. This ligament bridges the suprascapular notch in the upper border of the scapula, converting the notch to foramen. The artery and nerve then pass deep to the supraspinatus muscle, thereafter supplying it and then passing through the spinoglenoid notch to supply the infraspinatus. The subscapular artery is a branch of the third part of the axillary artery; it divides into circumflex scapular and thoracodorsal branches. The transverse cervical artery courses anterior to this site. The dorsal scapular artery and nerve pass deep to the medial border of the scapula. The posterior circumflex humeral branch of the axillary artery passes through the quadrangular space with the axillary nerve.

GAS 719-720; N 414; McM 133

56 A. The patient has suffered injury to the radial nerve in the midhumeral region. The nerve that

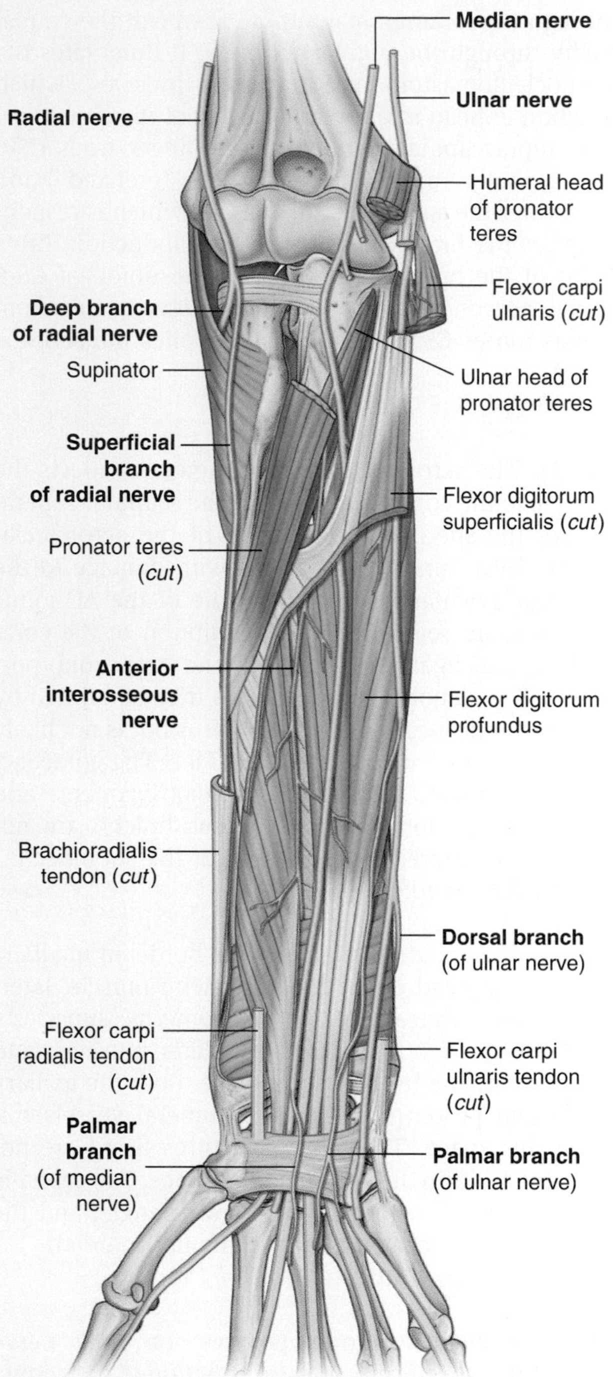

GAS Fig. 7-87

provides sensation to the dorsum of the hand proximal to the thumb and index finger is the superficial branch of the radial nerve. The posterior interosseous nerve supplies a strip of skin on the back of the forearm and wrist extensors. The lateral antebrachial cutaneous nerve is a continuation of the musculocutaneous nerve and supplies the lateral side of the forearm. The medial antebrachial cutaneous is a direct branch of the medial cord and supplies skin of the medial side of the forearm. The dorsal cutaneous branch of the ulnar nerve supplies the medial side of the dorsum of the hand.

GAS 761, 792; N 418; McM 144

57 **C.** The seventh cervical nerve makes a major contribution to the radial nerve, and this nerve is the prime mover in wrist extension. The dermatome of C7 is in the region described.

GAS 745, 787, 790; N 416; McM 153

58 **B.** As the radial artery passes from the ventral surface of the wrist to the dorsum, it crosses through the anatomic snuffbox, passing over the scaphoid bone. The ulnar artery at the wrist is located on the medial side of the wrist, passing from beneath the flexor carpi ulnaris to reach Guyon's canal between the pisiform bone and the flexor retinaculum. Guyon's canal is adjacent to but not in communication with the carpal tunnel. The anterior interosseous and posterior interosseous arteries arise from the common interosseous branch of the ulnar artery and pass proximal to distal in the forearm between the radius and ulna, in the flexor and extensor compartments, respectively. The deep palmar branch of the ulnar artery passes between the two heads of the adductor pollicis to anastomose with the radial artery in the palm (*GAS* Fig. 7-86).

GAS 810-814; N 454; McM 166

59 **D.** The patient is suffering from subacromial or subdeltoid bursitis. (If the pain on palpation is less when the arm has been elevated to the horizontal, the bursitis may be thought of as being more subacromial, that is, associated more with the supraspinatus tendon perhaps, for such a bursa may be drawn back under the acromion when the limb is abducted.) The subscapular bursa, beneath the subscapularis muscle, would not present as superficial pain. It can communicate with the glenohumeral joint cavity. Inflammation or arthritic changes within the glenohumeral joint present as more generalized shoulder pain than that present here. The teres minor muscle and tendon are located inferior to the point of marked discomfort.

GAS 708, 713; N 424; McM 136

60 **E.** The axillary sheath is a fascial continuation of the prevertebral layer of the deep cervical fascia extending into the axilla. It encloses the nerves of the neurovascular bundle of the upper limb. Superficial fascia is loose connective tissue between the dermis and the deep investing fascia and contains fat, cutaneous vessels, nerves, lymphatics, and glands. The

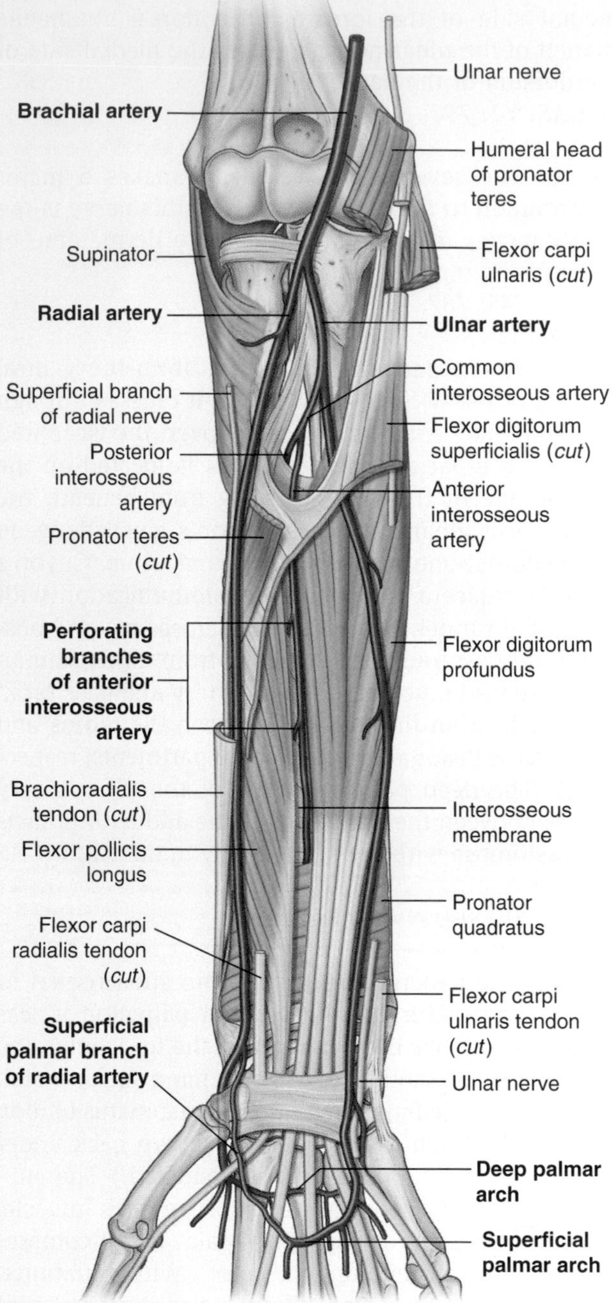

***GAS* Fig. 7-86**

buccopharyngeal fascia covers the buccinator muscles and the pharynx mingles with the pretracheal fascia. The clavipectoral muscle invests the clavicle and pectoralis minor muscle. The axillary fascia is continuous with the pectoral and latissimus dorsi fascia and forms the hollow of the armpit.

GAS 721, 731; N 412; McM 361

61 C. The spinal accessory nerve (CN XI) arises from the ventral rootlets of C1 to C4 that ascend through the foramen magnum to then exit the cranial cavity through the jugular foramen. It innervates the sternocleidomastoid and trapezius muscles, which function in head rotation and raising of the shoulders. The suprascapular nerve receives fibers from C5-6 (occasionally from C4 if the plexus is "prefixed") and innervates the supraspinatus muscle, which is responsible for the first 15 degrees of arm abduction. Erb's point of the brachial plexus is at the union of C5-6 spinal nerves. The long thoracic nerve arises from plexus routes C5, 6, and 7, and supplies the serratus anterior.

GAS 714; N 33; McM 132

62 D. The acromioclavicular ligament connects the clavicle to the coracoid process of the scapula. Separation of the shoulder (dislocation of the acromioclavicular [AC] joint) is associated with damage to the acromioclavicular ligament (capsule of the AC joint) and, in more severe injuries, disruption of the coracoclavicular ligaments (conoid and trapezoid portions). The glenohumeral ligament may be injured by an anterior dislocation of the humerus but is not likely to be injured by a separated shoulder. The coracoacromial ligament, transverse scapular ligament, and tendon of the long head of triceps brachii are not likely to be injured by separation of the shoulder.

GAS 706; N 408; McM 136

63 A. The quadrangular space is bordered medially by the long head of the triceps brachii muscle, laterally by the surgical neck of the humerus, superiorly by the teres minor and subscapularis muscles, and inferiorly by the teres major muscle. Both the axillary nerve and posterior circumflex humeral vessels traverse this space. The other structures listed are not contained within the quadrangular space. The cephalic vein is located in the deltopectoral triangle, and the radial nerve is located in the triangular interval.

GAS 718-720, 730; N 413; McM 139

64 B. Froment's sign is positive for ulnar nerve palsy. More specifically it tests the action of the adductor pollicis muscle. The patient is asked to hold a sheet of paper between the thumb and a flat palm. The flexor pollicis longus is innervated by the anterior interosseous branch of the median nerve. The flexor digiti minimi is innervated by the deep branch of the ulnar nerve and would not be used to hold a sheet of paper between the thumb and palm. The flexor carpi radialis is innervated by the median nerve, and the extensor indicis is innervated by the radial nerve (Fig. 6-14).

GAS 814-816, 826; N 464; McM 157

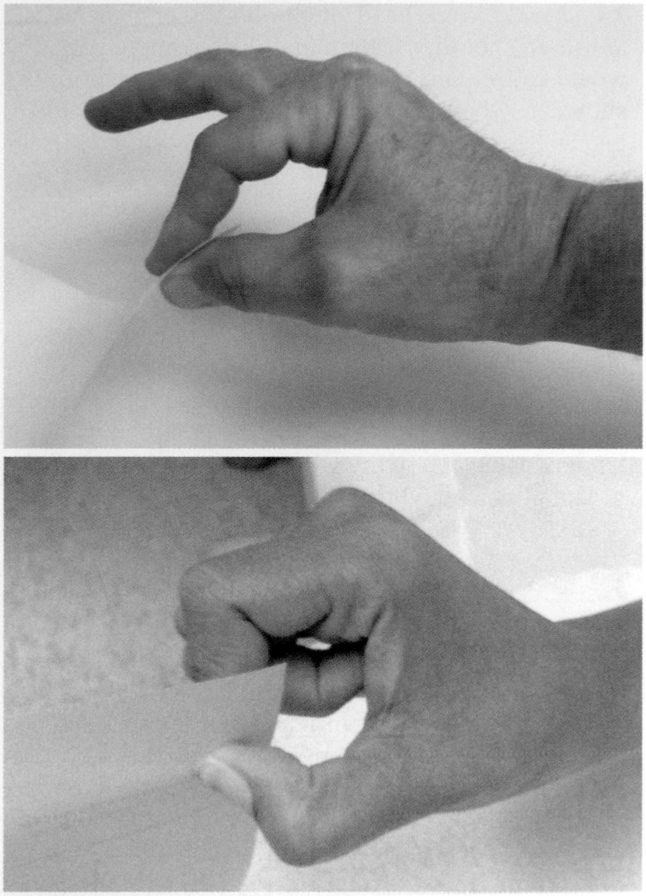

Fig. 6-14

65 C. The recurrent branch of the median nerve innervates the thenar muscles (opponens pollicis, abductor pollicis brevis, and flexor pollicis brevis) and is not responsible for any cutaneous innervation. Damage to the palmar cutaneous branches of the median nerve or to the ulnar nerve would not cause weakness of opposition of the thumb for they are principally sensory in function. The deep branch of the ulnar nerve supplies the hypothenar muscles, adductor and abductor muscles of digits 2–5, and does not innervate the abductor pollicis brevis.

GAS 817; N 463; McM 159

66 D. Injury to the deep branch of the ulnar nerve results in paralysis of all interosseous muscles and the lumbrical muscles of digits 4 and 5. Extension of the metacarpophalangeal joints is intact, a function of the radial nerve. Interphalangeal extension of digits 4 and 5 is absent, due to the loss of all interosseous muscle and the lumbricals of digits 4 and 5. Some weak interphalangeal joint extension is still present in digits 2 and 3 because the lumbricals of these two fingers are innervated by the median nerve. The radial nerve and the median nerve appear to be intact in this case. If the ulnar nerve were injured in the midforearm region, there would be sensory loss in the palm and digits 4 and 5 and on the dorsum of the hand. The recurrent branch of the median nerve supplies the thenar muscles; it does not supply lumbricals. Moreover, paralysis of this nerve would have no effect on the interphalangeal joints.

GAS 814; N 464; McM 159

67 A. The circumflex scapular artery passes through the triangular space after arising from the subscapular artery. It provides superficial branches to the overlying latissimus dorsi, whereas its deep portion passes into the infraspinous fossa to anastomose with the suprascapular artery. The dorsal scapular artery passes between the ventral rami of the brachial plexus and then deep to the medial border of the scapula. The transverse cervical artery arises from the thyrocervical trunk at the root of the neck and can provide origin for a dorsal scapular branch. The lateral thoracic and thoracoacromial arteries are branches of the second part of the axillary artery and provide no supply to the latissimus dorsi.

GAS 721; N 414; McM 141

68 C. The surgical neck of the humerus is a typical site of fractures. The fracture line lies above the insertions of the pectoralis major, teres major, and latissimus dorsi muscles. The supraspinatus muscle abducts the proximal fragment, whereas the distal fragment is elevated and adducted. The elevation results from contraction of the deltoid, biceps brachii, and coracobrachialis muscles. The adduction is due to the action of pectoralis major, teres major, and latissimus dorsi.

GAS 705; N 413; McM 140

69 B. The fracture line of the upper third of the radius lies between the bony attachments of the supinator and the pronator teres muscles. The distal radial fragment and hand are pronated due to unopposed contraction of pronator teres and pronator quadratus muscles. The proximal fragment deviates laterally by the unopposed contraction of the supinator muscle. The brachioradialis inserts distally on the radius. The brachialis inserts on the coronoid process of the ulna and would not be involved in the lateral deviation of the radius.

GAS 772-774; N 431; McM 152

70 A. The palmaris longus passes along the midline of the flexor surface of the forearm. The flexor carpi radialis is seen in the lateral portion of the forearm superficially, passing over the trapezium to insert at the base of the second metacarpal. The abductor pollicis longus tendon is laterally located in the wrist, where it helps form the lateral border of the anatomic snuffbox. The flexor carpi ulnaris tendon can be seen and palpated on the medial side of the wrist ventrally. The flexor pollicis longus tendon passes deep through the carpal tunnel.

GAS 777; N 432; McM 158

71 B. The student had broken the neck of the fifth metacarpal when hitting the machine with his fist. This is the more common type of "boxer's fracture." Neither a fracture of the ulnar styloid nor a Colles' fracture nor Smith's fracture of the distal radius would present with the absence of a knuckle as observed here. Bennett's fracture involves dislocation of the carpometacarpal joint of the thumb. Indications are that the injury is on the medial side of the hand, not the wrist, nor the lateral side of the hand or wrist.

GAS 793-794; N 440; McM 167

72 E. Scoliosis (severe lateral curvature of the spine) in the patient is causing compression or stretching of the T1 spinal nerve ramus by the first rib as the nerve ascends to join C8 and form the lower trunk of the brachial plexus. T1 provides sensation for the medial side of the forearm, via the medial antebrachial cutaneous nerve from the medial cord of the brachial plexus. T1 is the principal source of motor supply to all of the intrinsic muscles in the palm. Its dysfunction affects all fine motor movements of the digits. Long flexors of the fingers are intact; therefore, the median nerve and ulnar nerve are not injured. The extensors of the wrist are functional; therefore, the radial nerve is not paralyzed. The only sensory disturbance is that of the T1 dermatome.

GAS 695-700, 744-745; N 161; McM 94

73 D. Interestingly, "gamekeeper's thumb" was a term coined because this injury was most commonly associated with Scottish gamekeepers who, it is said, killed small animals such as rabbits by breaking their necks between the ground and the gamekeeper's thumb and index finger. The resulting valgus force on the abducted metacarpophalangeal (MCP) joint caused injury to the ulnar collateral ligament. These days this injury is more commonly seen in skiers who land awkwardly with their hand braced on a ski pole, causing the valgus force on the thumb as is seen in this patient. Whereas the term "skier's thumb" is sometimes used, "gamekeeper's thumb" is still in common usage.

GAS 795-796; N 441; McM 163

74 A. The long head of the biceps brachii muscle assists in shoulder flexion and during a tendinopathy would cause pain in the anterior compartment of the shoulder, where it originates at the supraglenoid tubercle. Also, forced contraction would cause a greater tension force on the tendon.

GAS 732; N 419; McM 136

75 C. The common extensor tendon originates from the lateral epicondyle, and inflammation of this tendon is lateral epicondylitis, nicknamed "tennis elbow" because the tendon is often irritated during the backhand stroke in tennis. Because the extensors of the wrist originate as part of the common extensor tendon, extension of the wrist will exacerbate the pain of lateral epicondylitis.

GAS 768, 785; N 427; McM 152

76 C. The axillary nerve passes dorsally around the surgical neck of the humerus (accompanied by the posterior circumflex humeral artery) and can be injured when the humerus is fractured at that location. The axillary nerve provides sensation to the skin over the upper, lateral aspect of the shoulder. Therefore, although the patient might not be able to abduct the arm because of the injury, a simple test of skin sensation can indicate whether there is associated nerve injury of the axillary nerve (CN XI). Shrugging the shoulders can help assess trapezius function, thereby testing the spinal accessory nerve. Intact sensation of the skin on the medial aspect of the axilla and arm is an indication that the radial and intercostobrachial nerves are functional. Pushing against an immovable object tests the serratus anterior muscle and the long thoracic nerve.

GAS 718-720; N 465; McM 139

77 E. The surgeon took the distal segments of the median nerves from both forearms, mistakenly believing them to be palmaris longus tendons. Both of the structures lie in the midline of the ventral surface of the distal forearm and are often of similar appearance in color and diameter. The nerve is located deep to the tendon, when the tendon is present, but when the tendon is absent, the nerve appears to be where the tendon belongs. There is no evidence of rib fractures; even so, a fractured rib would not explain loss of sensation on the lateral portion of the palm. Lower plexus trauma (C8, T1) would result in paralysis of forearm flexor muscles and all intrinsic hand muscles and sensory loss over the medial dorsum of the hand, in addition to palmar sensory loss. Dupuytren's contracture is a flexion contracture of (usually) digits four and five from connective tissue disease in the palm.

Radial nerve injury in the posterior forearm would affect metacarpophalangeal joint extension, thumb extension, and so on, not palmar disturbances.

GAS 784-785; N 432; McM 150

78 C. Trauma both to the median and ulnar nerves at the wrist results in total clawing of the fingers. The metacarpophalangeal joints of all digits are extended by the unopposed extensors because the radial nerve is intact. All interossei and lumbricals are paralyzed because the deep branch of the ulnar nerve supplies all of the interossei; lumbricals I and II are paralyzed, for they are innervated by the median nerve; lumbricals III and IV are paralyzed, for they receive supply from the deep ulnar nerve. The interossei and lumbricals are responsible for extension of the interphalangeal joints. When they are paralyzed, the long flexor tendons pull the fingers into a position of flexion, completing the "claw" appearance. If the median nerve were intact, the clawing would be less noticeable in the index and long fingers because the two lumbricals would still be capable of some degree of extension of those interphalangeal joints. If the median nerve alone is injured in the carpal tunnel, there would be loss of thenar opposition but not clawing. If the median and ulnar nerves are both transected at the elbow, the hand appears totally flat because of the loss of long flexors, in addition to intrinsic paralysis.

GAS 784, 814-818; N 434; McM 157

79 D. Colles' fracture is a fracture of the distal radius with the distal fragment displaced dorsally. Smith's fracture involves the distal fragment displaced in a volar direction. Smith's fracture is sometimes referred to as a reverse Colles' fracture.

GAS 771-774; N 440; McM 153

80 E. The extensor tendons of the fingers insert distally on the distal phalanx of each digit. If the tendon is avulsed, or the proximal part of the distal phalanx is detached, the distal interphalangeal joint (DIP) is pulled into total flexion by the unopposed flexor digitorum profundus muscle. This result gives the digit the appearance of a mallet. In boutonnière deformity, the central portion of the extensor tendon expansion is torn over the proximal interphalangeal (PIP) joint, allowing the tendon to move palmarward, causing the tendon to act as a flexor of the PIP joint. This causes the DIP joint to be hyperextended. Swan-neck deformity involves slight flexion of the metacarpophalangeal (MCP) joints, hyperextension of PIP joints, and slight flexion of DIP joints. This condition results most often from shortening of the tendons of intrinsic muscles, as in rheumatoid arthritis. Dupuytren's contracture results from connective tissue disorder in the palm, usually causing irreversible flexion of digits 4 and 5. Claw hand occurs with lesions to the median and ulnar nerves at the wrist. In this clinical problem all intrinsic muscles are paralyzed, including the extensors of the interphalangeal joints. The MCP joint extensors, supplied by the radial nerve, and the long flexors of the fingers, supplied more proximally in the forearm by the median and ulnar nerves, are intact and are unopposed, pulling the fingers into the "claw" appearance.

GAS 787-790, 802; N 451; McM 153

81 A. Because the median nerve is injured within the cubital fossa, the long flexors are paralyzed, including the flexor pollicis longus muscle. The flexor pollicis longus would not be paralyzed if the median nerve were injured at the wrist. Lateral palm sensory loss confirms median nerve injury. If only the anterior interosseous nerve were damaged, there would be no cutaneous sensory deficit. The radial nerve supplies wrist extensors, long thumb abductor, and metacarpophalangeal joint extensors. The ulnar nerve does not supply sensation to the lateral palm.

GAS 768, 804; N 434; McM 149

82 D. In a lesion of the lower trunk of the brachial plexus, or the C8 and T1 ventral rami, there is sensory loss on the medial forearm and the medial side of hand (dorsal and ventral). The medial cord is an extension of the lower trunk. The medial cord gives origin to the medial antebrachial cutaneous nerve, which supplies the T1 dermatome of the medial side of the antebrachium. The lower lateral brachial cutaneous nerve arises from the radial nerve, C5 and C6. The musculocutaneous nerve arises from the lateral cord, ending in the lateral antebrachial cutaneous nerve, with C5 and C6 dermatome fibers. The intercostobrachial nerve is the lateral cutaneous branch of the T2 ventral primary ramus and supplies skin on the medial side of the arm. The median nerve distributes C6 and C7 sensory fibers to the lateral part of the palm, thumb, index, long finger, and half of the ring finger.

GAS 738-745; N 416; McM 138

83 C. The first branch of the lateral pectoral nerve is typically the only source of motor supply to the clavicular head of the pectoralis major muscle. If it is injured (as in this case of an iatrogenic injury when the infraclavicular nodes were removed), this part of the muscle undergoes atrophy, leaving an infraclavicular cosmetic deficit. The remainder of the lateral

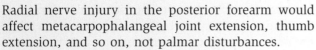

pectoral nerve joins the medial pectoral nerve in a neural arch that provides motor supply to the remaining parts of the pectoralis major and the pectoralis minor. Physical examination reveals no obvious motor or sensory deficits. Loss of the medial pectoral nerve would have no effect on the clavicular head of pectoralis major and might not be discernible. Injury to the lateral cord would lead to loss not only of all of the lateral pectoral nerve but also the musculocutaneous nerve, resulting in biceps brachii and brachialis paralysis and lateral antebrachial sensory loss.
GAS 724, 742; N 415; McM 141

84 **B.** The C6 spinal nerve is primarily responsible for the brachioradialis reflex. C5 and C6 are both involved in the biceps brachii reflex; C5 for motor, C6 for the sensory part of the reflex arc; C7 is the key spinal nerve in the triceps reflex.
GAS 755; N 432; McM 143

85 **C.** C7 is the main spinal nerve that contributes to the radial nerve and innervates the triceps brachii. Absence of the triceps reflex is usually indicative of a C7 radiculopathy or injury.
GAS 745-746, 756; N 416; McM 144

86 **B.** Ginglymus joint is the correct technical term to describe a hinge joint. It allows motion in one axis (flexion and extension in the case of the humeroulnar joint) and is therefore a uniaxial joint. The other types of joints listed allow motion in more than one axis.
GAS 764; N 442; McM 120

87 **C.** A fracture of the humerus just proximal to the epicondyles is called a supracondylar fracture. This is the most common cause of a Volkmann ischemic fracture. The sharp bony fragment often lacerates the brachial (or other) artery, with bleeding into the flexor compartment. Diminution of arterial supply to the compartment results in the ischemia. Bleeding into the compartment causes greatly increased pressure, first blocking venous outflow from the compartment, then reducing the arterial flow into the compartment as the pressure rises to arterial levels. The ischemic muscles then undergo unrelieved contracture. A humeral fracture is sometimes placed in a cast from shoulder to wrist, often concealing the ischemia until major tissue loss occurs. Cold, insensate digits, and great pain are warnings of this compartmental syndrome, demanding that the cast be removed and the compartment opened ("released") for pressure reduction and vascular repair. Fracture of the surgical neck endangers the axillary nerve and posterior circumflex humeral artery, although not ischemic contracture. Fracture of the humerus in the spiral groove can injure the radial nerve and profunda brachii artery. Fracture of the olecranon does not result in Volkmann's contracture, although the triceps brachii can displace the distal fractured fragment of the ulna.
GAS 766; N 420; McM 149

88 **D.** Normally the distal part of the ulna articulates only with the radius at the distal radioulnar joint at the wrist, a joint that participates in pronation and supination. The head of the ulna does not articulate with any of the carpal bones; instead, it is separated from the triquetrum and lunate bones by the triangular fibrocartilage complex between it and the radius. The pisiform articulates with the triquetrum. The carpal articulation of the radius is primarily that of the scaphoid (the old name is navicular) bone.
GAS 764-765; N 439; McM 123

89 **A.** The force of the woman's fall on the outstretched hand was transmitted up through the forearm, in this case resulting in dislocation of the olecranon at the elbow, putting traction on the ulnar nerve as it passes around the medial epicondyle of the humerus. Ulnar trauma at the elbow can cause weakness in medial flexion (adduction) at the wrist, from loss of the flexor carpi ulnaris. Ulnar nerve injury also results in sensory loss in the medial hand and paralysis of the interossei and medial two lumbricals, with clawing especially of digits 4 and 5. Injury of the ulnar nerve at the pisiform bone would not affect the flexor carpi ulnaris, nor would it produce sensory loss on the dorsum of the hand because the dorsal cutaneous branch of the ulnar branches off proximal to the wrist. Carpal tunnel problems affect median nerve function, which is not indicated here. The ulnar nerve passes medial to the cubital fossa between the heads of the flexor carpi ulnaris, not between the heads of the flexor digitorum superficialis. Injuries at the radial neck affect the site of division of the radial nerve, and its paralysis would not result in the clinical problems seen in this patient.
GAS 768, 784; N 464; McM 145

90 **D.** The interossei are the most important muscles in extension of the interphalangeal (IP) joints because of the manner of their insertion into the extensor expansion of the fingers, which passes dorsal to the transverse axes of these joints. The lumbrical muscles assist in IP extension, in addition to flexing the metacarpophalangeal joints. Ulnar nerve injury at the wrist results in paralysis of all the interossei and the medial two lumbricals. Extensors of the metacarpophalangeal

(MCP) joints are innervated by the deep radial nerve. Unopposed extension of the MCP joints causes them to be held in extension whereas unopposed long flexors of the fingers (supplied by median and ulnar nerves proximally in the forearm) cause them to be flexed into the "claw" position. The lumbricals of digits two and three are still intact because they are supplied by the median nerve, so clawing is not seen as much on these digits. Loss of opposition would result from median or recurrent nerve paralysis. If the ulnar nerve is cut at the wrist, its dorsal cutaneous branch to the dorsum of the hand is unaffected.

GAS 808-809; N 451; McM 159

91 B. In boutonnière deformity, the central portion of the extensor tendon expansion is torn over the proximal interphalangeal (PIP) joint, allowing the tendon to move toward the palm, causing the tendon to act as a flexor of the PIP joint. This causes the distal interphalangeal (DIP) joint to be hyperextended. The tear in the extensor tendon is said to resemble a buttonhole (*boutonnière* in French), and the head of the proximal phalanx may stick through the hole.

GAS 795-796; N 451; McM 166

92 D. Swan-neck deformity involves slight flexion of the metacarpophalangeal (MCP) joints, hyperextension of the proximal interphalangeal (PIP) joints, and slight flexion of the distal interphalangeal (DIP) joints. This condition results most often from shortening of the tendons of intrinsic muscles, as in rheumatoid arthritis. When asked to straighten the injured finger, the patient is unable to do so and the curvature of the finger somewhat resembles the neck of a swan.

GAS 795-796; N 451; McM 159

93 C. The long thoracic nerve was injured during the axillary dissection, resulting in paralysis of the serratus anterior muscle. The serratus anterior is important in rotation of the scapula in raising the arm above the level of the shoulder. Its loss results in protrusion of the medial border ("winging" of the scapula), which is more obvious when one pushes against resistance. The long thoracic nerve arises from the ventral rami of C5, C6, and C7. The upper trunk (C5, C6) supplies rotator and abductor muscles of the shoulder and elbow flexors. The posterior division of the middle trunk contains C7 fibers for distribution to extensor muscles; likewise, the posterior cord supplies extensors of the arm, forearm, and hand. The lateral cord (C5, C6, and C7) gives origin to the lateral pectoral nerve, the musculocutaneous nerve, and the lateral root of the median nerve. There is no sensory loss in the limb in this patient; injury to any of the other nerve elements listed here would be associated with specific dermatome losses.

GAS 726-727; N 413; McM 138

94 B. Dupuytren's contracture or deformity is a result of fibromatosis of palmar fascia, resulting in irregular thickening of the fascial attachments to the skin, which causes gradual contraction of the digits, especially digits 4 and 5. In 50% of cases, it is bilateral in occurrence. Ape hand, or flat hand, is a result of loss of the median and ulnar nerves at the elbow, with paralysis of all long flexors of the fingers and all intrinsic hand muscles. The term can also be specific for just median nerve injury and a flattened thenar eminence. Claw hand results from paralysis of interphalangeal joint extension by interossei and lumbricals, innervated primarily by the ulnar nerve. Wrist drop occurs with radial nerve paralysis and loss of the extensors carpi radialis longus and brevis. Mallet finger results from detachment of the extensor mechanism from the distal phalanx of a finger and unopposed flexion of that distal interphalangeal joint.

GAS 800; N 446; McM 157

95 A. The axillary nerve is a direct branch of the posterior cord and wraps around the surgical neck of the humerus to innervate the teres minor and the deltoid muscles. With this anatomic arrangement, the axillary nerve is tightly "tethered" to the proximal humerus. When the head of the humerus is dislocated, it often puts traction on the axillary nerve.

GAS 718-719; N 413; McM 142

96 A. The tendon of the long head of the biceps brachii muscles runs in the intertubercular groove on the proximal humerus as it changes direction and turns medially to attach to the supraglenoid tubercle of the scapula. This change in direction within an osseous structure predisposes the tendon to wear and tear, particularly in people who overuse the biceps brachii muscle. This type of injury presents with a characteristic sign called the "Popeye sign" after the cartoon character.

GAS 731-732; N 417; McM 114

97 C. The supraspinatus muscle inserts on the greater tubercle of the humerus and is said to initiate abduction of the arm at the shoulder. It is supplied principally by spinal nerve C5. The subscapularis muscle is the only muscle that inserts on the lesser tubercle. The subscapularis muscle is innervated by the upper and lower subscapular nerves. The teres minor muscle takes origin from the lateral border of the scapula; the teres major muscle takes origin from

the region of the inferior angle and the lateral border of the scapula.
GAS 717; N 411; McM 115

98 **E.** During a fall on an outstretched upper limb, the forces are conducted through the hand on up through the bones of the limb in succession. Often these bones do not fracture but rather pass the compressive forces proximally. The appendicular skeleton joins with the axial skeleton at the sternoclavicular joint. The forces are not sufficiently transferred to the sternum, causing the clavicle to absorb the force, resulting in common pediatric fracture of this sigmoidal-shaped bone.
GAS 711; N 461; McM 112

99 **C.** The patient is suffering from thoracic outlet syndrome, involving neural and vascular elements. This results from any condition that decreases the dimensions of the superior thoracic aperture (the formal name of the thoracic outlet). It could be a result of a cervical rib, accessory muscles, and/or atypical connective tissue bands at the root of the neck. In this case, symptoms involve the arm, forearm, and hand. Paraesthesia along the medial forearm and hand and atrophy of long flexors and intrinsic muscles point to a possible compression or traction problem of the lower trunk (C8, T1) rather than a lesion of either the median or ulnar nerve. The lateral palm has no sensory problem, which tends to rule out median nerve involvement. Changes in the radial artery pulse point to vascular compression. Erb-Duchenne paralysis of the upper trunk would affect proximal limb functions, such as arm rotation, abduction, and so on. This lesion is on the left side, so the brachiocephalic artery could not be involved because it arises from the right side of the aortic arch; moreover, it would not compress the brachial plexus. Carpal tunnel syndrome would not explain the problems of the forearm and medial hand, or the long flexor atrophy. An isolated medial cord lesion would not explain the atrophy of all long flexors and intrinsic muscles and does not explain the radial pulse characteristics. The ischemic pain in the arm is due to vascular compression.
GAS 150; N 183; McM 138

100 **A.** The ulnar nerve enters the forearm by passing between the two heads of the flexor carpi ulnaris and descends between and innervates the flexor carpi ulnaris (for medial wrist deviation) and flexor digitorum profundus (medial half) muscles. Injuring the ulnar nerve results in claw hand. It enters the hand superficial to the flexor retinaculum and lateral to the pisiform bone, where it is vulnerable to damage. The ulnar nerve also enters Guyon's canal, but damage to it here would not present with the aforementioned symptoms. The median nerve enters the carpal tunnel and the radial nerve passes deep to the brachioradialis.
GAS 777, 784; N 464; McM 145

101 **B.** During a breech delivery as described here, downward traction is applied to the shoulders and upper limbs as the baby is forcibly extracted from the birth canal. This exerts traction on the upper cord of the brachial plexus, often causing a traction injury from which the baby can often recover. If the ventral rami of C5 and C6 are avulsed from the spinal cord, the injury is permanent.
GAS 738, 747; N 416; McM 31

102 **E.** Striking the concrete blocks with the medial side of her hand has injured the ulnar nerve in Guyon's canal. This is the triangular tunnel formed by the pisiform bone medially, the flexor retinaculum dorsally, and the deep fascia of the wrist ventrally. This injury would result in loss of sensation to the medial palm and the palmar surface of the medial one and a half digits and motor loss of the hypothenar muscles, the interossei, and the medial two lumbricals. The median nerve is not involved because the thenar muscles and lateral palmar sensations are intact. The dorsal ulnar nerve arises proximal to the wrist, thus it would not be lost. Carpal bone dislocation is unlikely. If the lunate bone were dislocated, it would not cause compression of the ulnar nerve at the wrist. There is no indication of fifth metacarpal fracture, the so-called boxer's fracture.
GAS 784, 814; N 449; McM 159

103 **E.** The common flexor sheath encloses the long flexor tendons of the fingers in the carpal tunnel and proximal palm. This sheath is usually continuous with the flexor sheath of the little (fifth) finger, which continues within the palm, having no connection with sheaths of the other digits, which do not extend into the digits.
GAS 800-802; N 448; McM 158

104 **C.** The infectious agent was introduced into the synovial sheath of the long tendons of the little (fifth) finger. Proximally, this sheath runs through the midpalmar space, and inflammatory processes typically rupture into this space unless aggressively treated with the appropriate antibiotics.
GAS 800-801; N 448; McM 158

105 **A.** Axillary-subclavian vein thrombosis is becoming much more common in recent years because of the extensive use of catheters in cancer patients and other chronic medical conditions. Effort-induced thrombosis is seen with strenuous use of the dominant arm with hyperabduction and external rotation of the arm or backward and downward rotation of the shoulder as in playing cricket, volleyball, or baseball, or chopping wood. Because the symptoms of subclavian stenosis are fairly dramatic, most patients present promptly, usually within 24 hours. They complain of a dull ache in the shoulder and axilla, the pain worsened by activity. Conversely, rest and elevation often relieve the pain. Patients with catheter-associated axillary-subclavian deep vein thrombosis report similar symptoms at the arm or shoulder on the side with the indwelling catheter.

GAS 759; N 420; McM 206

106 **C.** The injury is at the second part of the axillary artery. The suprascapular artery is a branch of the thyrocervical trunk off the subclavian artery, proximal to the axillary artery. The subscapular artery is the major branch of the third part of the axillary artery, giving off the thoracodorsal and the circumflex scapular arteries. In this case blood would be flowing from the circumflex scapular artery in a retrograde direction into the axillary artery, supplying blood distal to the injury.

GAS 733-735; N 420; McM 134

107 **A.** This proximal injury to the median nerve would paralyze all of the long flexors of the digits, except for the muscle that flexes the distal interphalangeal joints of digits 4 and 5, thereby swinging the "balance of power" to the muscles that extend the digits, all of which are innervated by the radial nerve. The intrinsic hand muscles can aid in flexion of the metacarpophalangeal joints, and are innervated by the ulnar nerve. However, they are of insufficient size to compensate for the extensor forces exerted on fingers.

GAS 742-746; N 463; McM 148

108 **C.** The winged scapula results from a lesion of the long thoracic nerve, which supplies the serratus anterior muscle. This muscle is responsible for rotating the scapula upward, which occurs during abduction of the arm above the horizontal. The long thoracic nerve arises from the ventral rami of C5 to C7 of the brachial plexus. The diaphragm is supplied by the phrenic nerve, which comes from the ventral rami of C3 to C5 (mnemonic: C3, 4 and 5 keep the diaphragm alive).

GAS 727; N 413; McM 129

109 **A.** The median nerve supplies sensory innervation to the thumb, index, and middle fingers as well as to the lateral half of the ring finger. The median nerve also provides motor innervation to muscles of the thenar eminence. Compression of the median nerve in the carpal tunnel explains these deficits in conjunction with normal functioning of the flexor compartment of the forearm. The ulnar nerve is not implicated in these symptoms. Compression of the brachial plexus could not be attributed to pressure from hypertrophy of the triceps brachii muscle, it is located distal to the plexus. In addition, symptoms would include several upper limb deficits rather than the focal symptoms described in this instance. Osteoarthritis of the cervical spine would also lead to increasing complexity of symptoms.

GAS 745, 817; N 463; McM 159

110 **B.** The lunate bone is the most commonly dislocated carpal bone. Displacement is almost always anteriorly. Dislocation of the lunate bone can precipitate the signs associated typically with carpal tunnel syndrome.

GAS 793-795; N 443; McM 122

111 **D.** A cervical rib (usually found at C7) may cause thoracic outlet syndrome, which is a condition characterized by weak muscle tone in the hand and loss of radial pulse when the upper limb is abducted above the shoulder. The mechanism of injury with the gun being fired overhead suggests a lower trunk injury to the brachial plexus. The axillary artery supplies the shoulder muscles, and there is no loss of function to these muscles. The upper trunk of the brachial plexus also supplies innervation to the shoulder muscles, which are unaffected based on the patient's presenting abnormalities. The subclavian artery is located anterior to the brachial plexus until the plexus separates into cords as it passes under the clavicle. The brachiocephalic artery and lower trunk of the brachial plexus is only partially correct; the brachiocephalic artery is not directly associated with the brachial plexus due to its location at the midline of the body behind the sternum.

GAS 150; N 183, 416; McM 129

112 **A.** A synarthrosis joint is a fibrous connection that allows minimal to no movement. In this case, virtually no movement is allowed by the interosseous membrane joint between the radius and ulna. Symphysis joints are permanent fibrocartilaginous fusions between two bones; pubic symphysis is an example. Synchondrosis is a temporary joint made of cartilage that transitions to bone typically after growth completes (i.e., epiphyseal plate). Trochoid joints are pivot joints, and the humeral-radial portion of the elbow joint is an example. Ginglymus joints are hinge joints located at the interphalangeal junctions in the hand and foot (PIPs and DIPs).

GAS 18-20, 774-775; N 425; McM 146

113 B. The radial pulse is best located on the forearm (antebrachium) just proximal to the wrist joint. At this point the radial artery travels on the distal radius between the flexor carpi radialis and brachioradialis tendons. The palmaris longus tendon travels more medially to the radial artery and above the flexor retinaculum. The flexor pollicis longus tendon is a deeper structure in the antebrachium and is also located medially to the radial artery.

GAS 827; N 432; McM 161

114 B. The radial artery enters the palm through the anatomic snuffbox. The artery then moves on to pierce through the two heads of the first dorsal interosseous muscle and enter the deep aspect of the palm. The flexor pollicis longus tendon runs on the palmar aspect of the hand and the radial artery runs on the dorsal aspect of the hand before entering the deep aspect of the palm, and therefore the radial artery does not run below this tendon. The radial artery does not run between the first and second interosseous muscle and therefore cannot be used as a landmark to identify the artery. Finally, the artery does not run between the first dorsal interosseous muscle and the adductor pollicis longus.

GAS 800, 812; N 454; McM 161

115 D. The median nerve provides innervation to most of the muscles in the flexor compartment of the forearm; cutaneous innervation of the second, third, and fourth digits and palmar and dorsum aspects of the hand; and innervation of four intrinsic hand muscles: first and second lumbricals, abductor pollicis brevis, opponens pollicis, and flexor pollicis brevis. The thenar compartment contains the abductor pollicis brevis, opponens pollicis, and flexor pollicis brevis muscles, and these muscles are innervated by the recurrent branch of the median nerve. The patient has weakening of the first two lumbricals and not simply the thenar muscles, so the median nerve is most likely to be compressed. Another indication that the median nerve is compressed is the vigorous shaking of the wrist. Because the median nerve traverses the carpal tunnel, carpal tunnel compression could lead to this action on part of the patient. The ulnar nerve provides innervation for part of the flexor digitorum profundus and flexor carpi ulnaris muscles. These muscles are not weakened in this patient. The radial nerve provides cutaneous supply to the dorsum of the hand and forearm as well as extensor muscles of the forearm. The posterior interosseous nerve is a branch of the radial nerve and provides innervation of the extensor muscles in the forearm.

GAS 745, 784; N 463; McM 157

116 B. The patient can extend his forearm, which suggests that the triceps brachii muscle is not weakened. Supination appears to be weak along with hand grasp and wrist drop. This would indicate that part of the radial nerve has been lost below the innervation of the triceps brachii and above the branches to the supinator and extensors in the forearm. However, sensation on the forearm and hand is intact, indicating that the superficial branch of the radial nerve is intact. The superficial branch of the radial nerve separates from the deep radial nerve at the distal third of the humerus. The posterior cord of the brachial plexus is responsible for providing innervation of the axially and radial nerves. This patient does have some radial nerve innervation and no loss of axillary nerve function. The patient does not have weakened adduction of the wrist, indicating that the ulnar nerve is not injured. If both the radial and musculocutaneous nerves are injured, supination would not be possible as the supinator and biceps brachii muscles provide supination of the forearm.

GAS 761-763, 785; N 465; McM 143

117 B. The posterior interosseous nerve is an extension of the deep branch of the radial nerve after it emerges distal to the supinator. It is responsible for innervation of several muscles in the extensor compartment of the posterior aspect of the forearm, including extension of the metacarpophalangeal joints. The deep radial nerve courses laterally around the radius and passes between the two heads of the supinator muscle and is thus likely to be compressed by a hematoma between the fractured radius and the supinator muscle. Though the radial nerve gives rise to the posterior interosseous nerve, this answer choice is too general and would not indicate the precise injured branch of the radial nerve. Both the deep branch of the ulnar nerve and the median nerve traverse the medial and anteromedial aspect of the arm, respectively. These nerves primarily supply the flexor compartment of the arm. The anterior interosseous nerve is a branch of the median nerve and supplies the flexor digitorum profundus, flexor pollicis longus, and the pronator quadratus muscles (*GAS* Fig. 7-90).

GAS 785, 792; N 466; McM 152

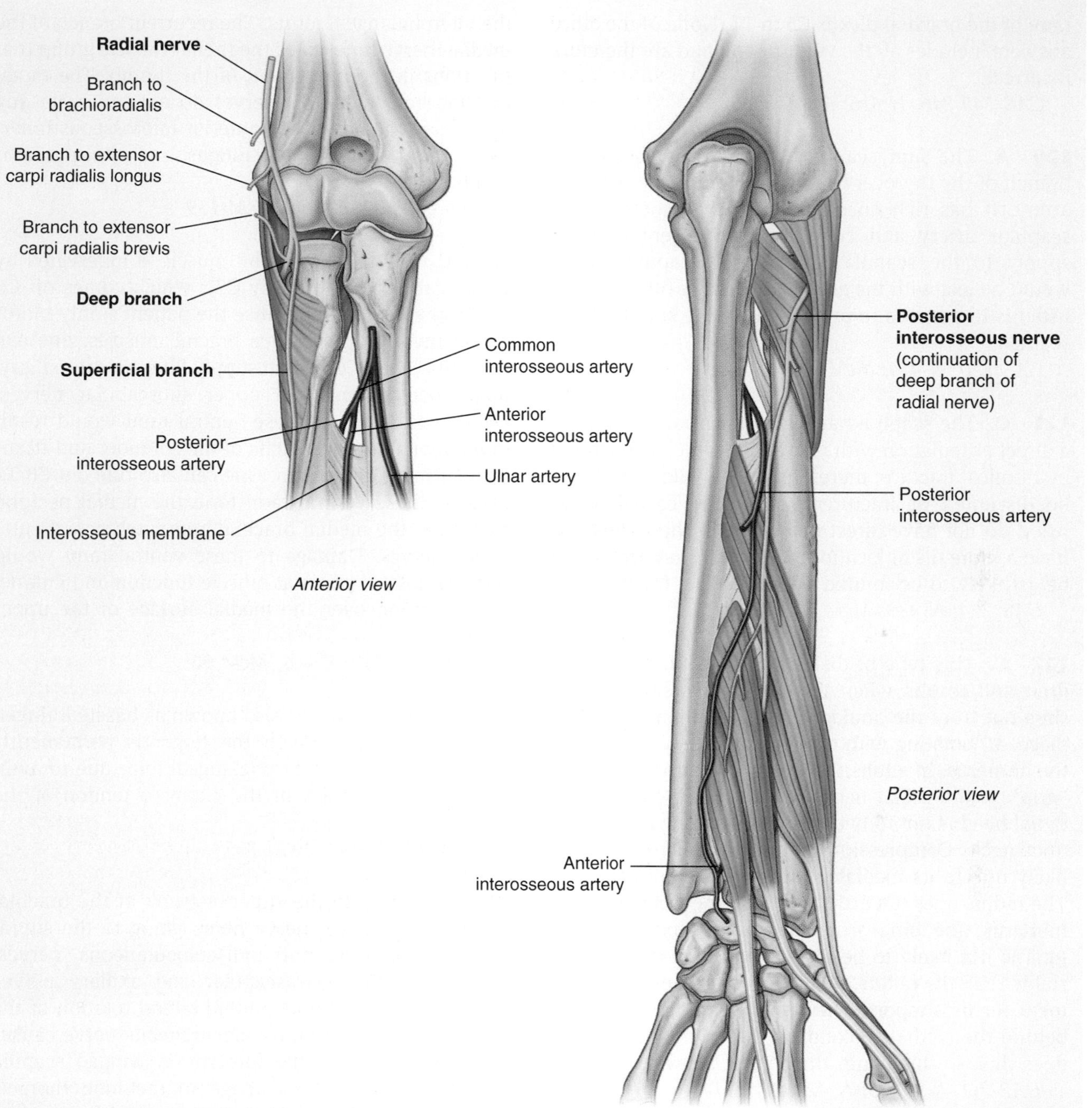

GAS Fig. 7-90

118 **A.** The superior trunk of the brachial plexus includes C5 and C6, which give rise to the suprascapular nerve, which innervates the supraspinatus muscle. The supraspinatus muscle is the primary muscle involved in abduction of the arm from 0 to 15 degrees. The deltoid muscle, supplied primarily by C5, abducts the arm from 15 to 90 degrees. The middle trunk is just C7 and has nothing to do with the muscle involved in initial abduction of the arm. The inferior trunk is C8-T1 and does not supply the supraspinatus muscle; therefore, it is not the right answer. The cords are distal to the branching of the supraspinatus muscle; therefore, neither lateral cord nor medial cord is the correct answer.

GAS 738, 747; N 416; McM 28

119 **C.** The radial nerve acts to extend the forearm at the elbow. This nerve is derived from all the ventral

rami of the brachial plexus C5 to T1. None of the other answers includes all the ventral rami and are therefore incorrect.
GAS 745-746; N 416; McM 96

120 **A.** The suprascapular artery arises as a major branch of the thyrocervical trunk from the subclavian artery. It has rich anastomoses with the circumflex scapular artery and could provide essential blood supply to the scapula. The dorsal scapular artery would be lost with the graft. None of the other vessels listed is in position to provide adequate supply to the scapula.
GAS 720; N 414; McM 31

121 **C.** The scaphoid and lunate carpal bones have a direct articulation with the radius, which is fractured in a Colles' fracture; therefore, they would most likely be disrupted or fractured. The other carpal bones listed do not have direct contact with the radius and have a more distal location; therefore, they would not be as likely to be injured with a Colles' fracture.
GAS 774; N 439; McM 123

122 **C.** This type of dislocation is common in children and results when the radius is dislocated and slips out from the anular ligament, which holds it in place, articulating with the ulna and the capitulum of the humerus. In adults the anular ligament has a good "grip" at the radial neck, but in young children the radial head is not fully developed, leading to an indistinct neck. Compression of the median nerve is not likely due to its medial position in the cubital fossa. The radius does not articulate with the trochlea of the humerus; the ulna articulates at this position. The ulna is not likely to be dislocated because it is more stable than the radius, which has only the anular ligament for its support. The radial nerve does not pass behind the medial epicondyle; rather, the ulnar nerve does this, so this is not the correct answer.
GAS 766-768, 775; N 424; McM 146

123 **C.** Injury to the radial nerve can be caused by a blow to the midhumeral region because the nerve winds around the shaft of the humerus. The symptoms described include the loss of wrist and finger extension and a loss of sensation in an area of skin supplied by the radial nerve.
GAS 763; N 465; McM 144

124 **A.** The ulnar nerve innervates the dorsal and palmar interossei, which act to abduct and adduct the fingers and assist the lumbricals in their actions of flexing the metacarpophalangeal joints and extending the interphalangeal joints. The recurrent branch of the median nerve innervates the thenar muscle group that functions in the movement of the thumb. The radial and musculocutaneous nerves do not innervate any muscles in the hand. The anterior interosseous innervates the flexor pollicis longus and the pronator quadratus.
GAS 808-809; N 464; McM 159

125 **C.** The triceps brachii muscle is innervated by the radial nerve (primarily C7), which comes off C5 to T1 spinal nerves. Because the patient's only motor deficit involves the triceps brachii muscles, one can rule out C5 and C6, which supply fibers to the axillary, musculocutaneous, and upper subscapular nerves. Damage to either of these ventral rami would result in additional motor deficits of the shoulder and flexor compartment of the arm. One can also rule out C8-T1 because these ventral rami form the medial pectoral nerve and the medial brachial and antebrachial cutaneous nerves. Damage to these ventral rami would result in loss of pectoral muscle function and cutaneous sensation over the medial surface of the upper limb.
GAS 745, 761; N 416; McM 96

126 **D.** Mallet finger, also known as baseball finger, is a deformity in which the finger is permanently flexed at the distal interphalangeal joint due to avulsion of the insertion of the extensor tendon at the distal phalanx.
GAS 802; N 443; McM 165

127 **B.** Injury to the superior trunk of the brachial plexus can damage nerve fibers going to the suprascapular, axillary, and musculocutaneous nerves. Damage to the suprascapular and axillary nerves causes impaired abduction and lateral rotation of the arm. Damage to the musculocutaneous nerve causes impaired flexion of the forearm. A winged scapula would be caused by damage to the long thoracic nerve. The long thoracic nerve is formed from spinal cord levels C5, C6, and C7, so the serratus anterior muscle would be weakened from the damage to C5 and C6, but the muscle would not be completely paralyzed. The intrinsic muscles of the hand are innervated by the ulnar nerve, which would most likely remain intact. Paraesthesia in the medial aspect of the arm would be caused by damage to the medial brachial cutaneous nerve (C8-T1; inferior trunk). Loss of sensation on the dorsum of the hand would be caused by damage to either the ulnar or radial nerves (C6 to T1).
GAS 738, 747; N 416; McM 31

128 **D.** The supinator muscle attaches to the radius proximally and when fractured would cause a lateral deviation. The pronator teres muscle originates on the medial epicondyle and coronoid process of the ulna and inserts onto the middle of the lateral side of the radius, pulling the radius medially below the fracture. The pronator quadratus muscle originates on the anterior surface of the distal ulna and inserts on the anterior surface of the distal radius, pulling the radius medially. The brachioradialis muscle originates on the lateral supracondylar ridge of the humerus and inserts at the base of the radial styloid process, far below the fracture. The brachialis muscle originates in the lower anterior surface of the humerus and inserts in the coronoid process and ulnar tuberosity, hence not causing an action on the radius.

GAS 777, 787-788; N 426; McM 121

129 **A.** Lymph from the lateral side of the hand drains directly into humeral (epitrochlear) nodes then to the central (axillary) nodes. Pectoral nodes receive lymph mainly from the anterior thoracic wall, including most of the breast. Subscapular nodes receive lymph from the posterior aspect of the thoracic wall and scapular region. Parasternal nodes receive lymph from the lower medial quadrant of the breast (*GAS* Fig. 7-57).

GAS 748; N 403; McM 364

130 **C.** Compartment syndrome is characterized by increased pressure within a confined space by a fascial compartment, which impairs blood supply, resulting in paleness and loss of pulses distal to the compartment. Venous thrombosis would not cause pain but could cause death from a pulmonary embolism if a thrombus (clot) broke free and became lodged in the pulmonary trunk. Thoracic outlet syndrome affects nerves in the brachial plexus and the subclavian artery and blood vessels between the neck and the axilla, far above the cast. Raynaud's disease affects blood flow to the limbs when they are exposed to temperature changes or stress. The fracture at the radial groove probably resulted in a radial nerve injury but would not be responsible for these symptoms.

GAS 590, 763; N 432; McM 143

131 **E.** The deep branch of the ulnar nerve arises at the level of the pisiform bone and passes between the pisiform and the hook of the hamate; hence the deep branch of the ulnar nerve is most likely to be injured in this patient. The median nerve enters the forearm between the humeral and ulnar heads of the pronator teres muscle then becomes superficial near the wrist. The recurrent branch of the median nerve branches off after the median nerve enters the palm through the carpal tunnel. The radial nerve divides into superficial and deep branches when it enters the cubital fossa.

GAS 814; N 452; McM 162

132 **A.** The supraspinatus initiates abduction of the arm during the first 15 degrees of abduction; palpation of the tendon during this phase would result in pain from a tendinopathy of the supraspinatus.

GAS 717; N 411; McM 132

133 **A.** The hallmark fracture caused by a fall on an outstretched hand is a scaphoid-lunate fracture; the scaphoid and lunate are the two wrist bones most proximal to the styloid process of the radius. All the other wrist bones are less likely to be affected by this injury.

GAS 793-794, 797; N 439; McM 122

134 **C.** Bennett's fracture is a carpometacarpal fracture at the base of the thumb. Smith's fracture is also called a reverse Colles' fracture and is caused when the distal fragment of the radius angles forward. Colles' fracture is also called "silver fork deformity" because the distal fragment is displaced posteriorly. Boxer's fractures of the necks of metacarpal bones are fractures to the fingers. A scaphoid fracture would be indicated by pain in the anatomical snuffbox.

GAS 793-796; N 439; McM 122

135 **A.** Interestingly, "gamekeeper's thumb" was a term coined to describe an injury common among Scottish gamekeepers who, it is said, killed small animals such as rabbits by breaking their necks between the ground and the gamekeeper's thumb and index finger. The resulting valgus force on the abducted metacarpophalangeal (MCP) joint caused injury to the ulnar collateral ligament. Today this injury is more commonly seen in skiers who land awkwardly with their hand braced on a ski pole, causing the valgus force on the thumb, as seen in this patient. Whereas the term "skier's thumb" is sometimes used, "gamekeeper's thumb" is still in common usage. Bennett's fracture is a fracture at the base of the metacarpal of the thumb. Scaphoid fracture occurs after a fall on an outstretched hand, involving the scaphoid and lunate bone. Colles' fracture is also called silver fork deformity because the distal fragment of the radius is displaced posteriorly. Boxer's fracture is a fracture of the necks of the second and third (and sometimes the fifth) metacarpals. Smith's fracture is also called a reverse Colles' fracture and is caused when the distal

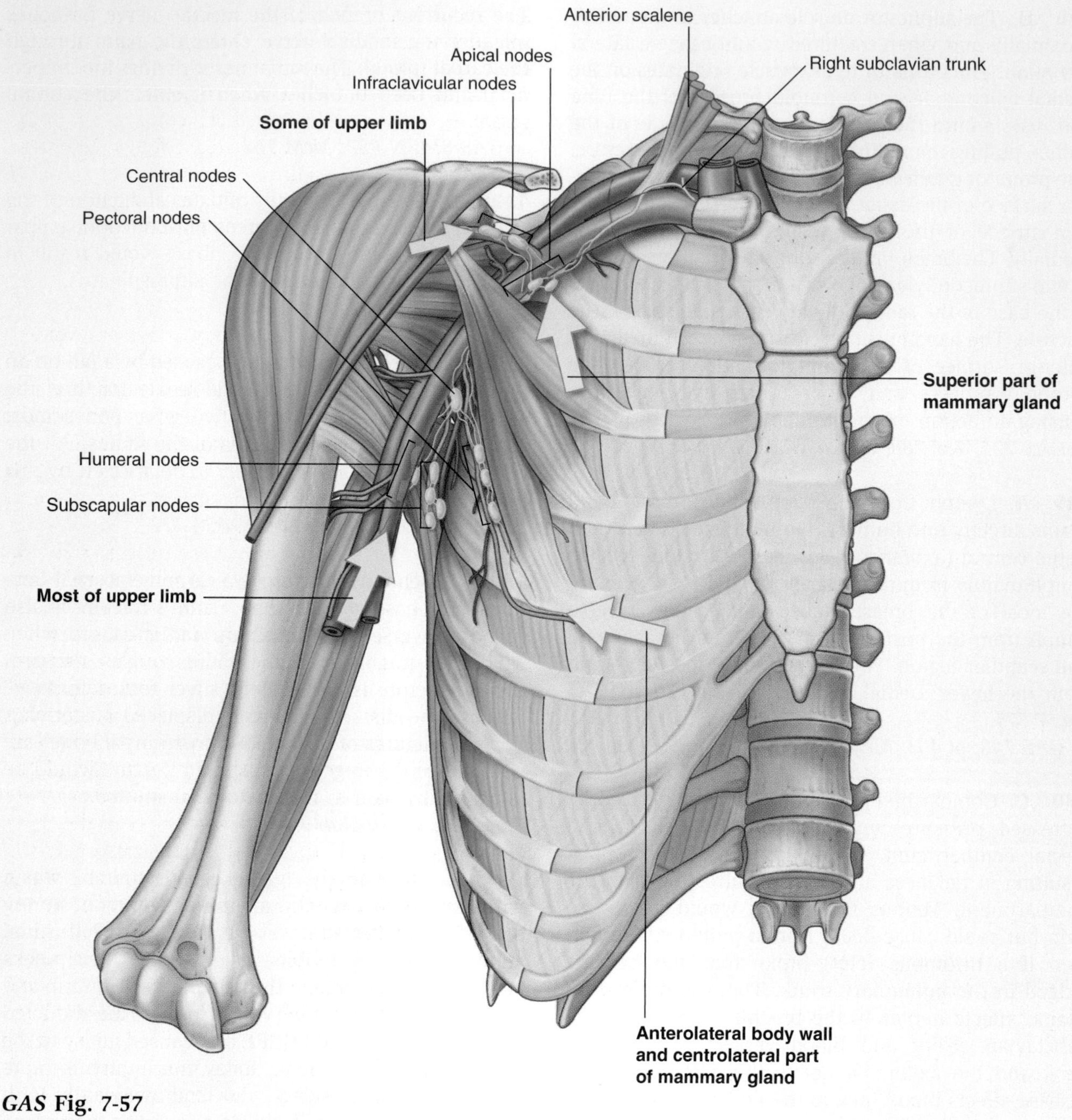

GAS **Fig. 7-57**

radius is fractured and the distal radial fragment is angled forward.

GAS 793-796; N 442; McM 163

136 B. The biceps brachii reflex is elicited by tapping on the tendon of the biceps near its insertion on the radius. The biceps brachii reflex involves C5 and C6 spinal nerves. C5 provides the motor component; C6 the afferent side of the reflex arc.

GAS 731-732; N 417; McM 148

137 B. The brachioradialis reflex is elicited by tapping the tendon of the brachioradialis muscle. The reflex involves spinal nerves C5, C6, and C7. The major contribution is from C6.

GAS 785-787; N 432; McM 150

138 D. Volkmann's contracture is a flexion deformity of the fingers and sometimes the wrist from an ischemic necrosis of the forearm flexor muscles. Bennett's fracture is a fracture at the base of the metacarpal of the thumb. Scaphoid fracture occurs after a fall on an outstretched hand and involves the scaphoid and lunate bones. Colles' fracture is also called silver fork deformity because the distal fragment of the radius is displaced posteriorly. Boxer's fracture is a fracture of the necks of the second and third (and sometimes the fifth) metacarpals. Smith's fracture is also called a reverse Colles' fracture and is caused when the distal radius is fractured, with the radial fragment angled forward.

GAS 774; N 432; McM 150

139 D. The ulnar nerve enters the forearm by passing between the two heads of the flexor carpi ulnaris and descends between and innervates the flexor carpi ulnaris and flexor digitorum profundus (medial half) muscles. It enters the hand superficial to the flexor retinaculum and lateral to the pisiform bone, where it is vulnerable to damage and provides the deep ulnar branch. The deep branch of the radial nerve arises proximally in the forearm.

GAS 784; N 464; McM 149

140 B. "Benediction attitude" of the hand with the index and long fingers straight and the ring and little fingers flexed is caused by an injury to the median nerve. The long flexors of the digits are supplied by the median nerve; the unopposed radial nerve and deep ulnar nerve supply the extensors of the digits 1–3, causing them to be in the extended position. Digits 4 and 5 are slightly flexed because the flexors of the proximal interphalangeal joints are supplied by the ulnar nerve.

GAS 784, 417; N 463; McM 157

141 A. The Allen test involves compression of the radial and ulnar arteries at the wrist with the fingers flexed tightly to move the blood out the palm. Pressure is then released on the radial and ulnar arteries successively to determine the degree of supply to the hand by either vessel and the patency of the anastomoses between them. The usefulness of the radial artery for bypass can thereby be assessed. If the the palm does not flush with blood when the radial artery is released, then the ulnar artery is not sufficient to supply the hand if the radial artery is harvested for a graft. The other tests have nothing to do with the patency of the radial artery.

GAS 814; N 435; McM 160

142 E. The ulnar nerve enters the hand superficial to the flexor retinaculum and lateral to the pisiform bone and innervates all the interossei via the deep branch. These muscles are responsible for adduction and abduction of the fingers. Flexion of the fingers is spared because the flexor digitorum superficialis and most of the flexor digitorum profundus are innervated by the median nerve, which is unaffected by this injury. Had the median nerve been compressed in the carpal tunnel, one would have difficulty with motion of the thumb as a result of a lack of innervation of the thenar muscles. An injury of the radial nerve in the arm results in extension deficit in the forearm and hand.

GAS 814; N 452; McM 158

143 A. The glenohumeral joint is an extremely mobile joint with a wide range of movement. Anterior dislocation is the most common. Anterior dislocations of the humerus usually follow injuries where abnormal force is applied to the shoulder while the arm is extended, abducted, and externally rotated. When the head of the humerus is displaced anteriorly and inferiorly, there is flattening of the deltoid prominence (due to the increased weight of the humerus pulling on the muscle), protrusion of the acromion, and anterior axillary fullness (due to the movement of the humeral head into this location). The most commonly injured nerve is the axillary nerve, which innervates the teres minor and deltoid and also provides cutaneous supply to the posterior arm and the skin overlying the deltoid muscle. Acromioclavicular joint subluxation typically results from a blow to the tip of the shoulder when the arm is at the side and slightly adducted. It produces swelling and superior displacement of the clavicle. It is not associated with specific major nerve injuries or sensory deficits. The clavicle is a commonly fractured bone typically after direct trauma. Most fractures occur in the middle third of the clavicle. There is local swelling and tenderness but rarely any neurovascular damage. A spiral humerus midshaft fracture may result from a fall on an outstretched hand. The radial nerve is commonly fractured as it runs in the radial groove. Rotator cuff tears usually occur when there is some degenerative injury to the tendons. The rotator cuff is made up of the subscapularis, supraspinatus, infraspinatus, and teres minor and tendons.

GAS 707; N 422, 424; McM 136

144 A. The patient is experiencing radial head subluxation ("nursemaid's elbow"), the most common elbow injury in children. The injury often results from a sharp pull on the hand while the forearm is pronated and the elbow is extended. The underdevelopment of the radial head and the laxity of the anular ligament allows for the radial head to sublux (partially dislocate) from this cuff of tissue. This condition is extremely painful but can be easily treated with supination and compression of the elbow joint. Although it is uncommon for muscle tendons to rupture, the most common is the tendon of the long head of the biceps brachii. It produces a characteristic deformity when flexing the elbow: an extremely prominent bulge of unattached muscle belly called the "Popeye sign." The interosseous membrane is an expansive sheet of connective tissue that connects the radius and ulna at their midsection. It serves as an attachment site for the muscles of the forearm. The radial collateral ligament lies on the lateral side of the elbow joint reinforcing the radiohumeral joint. The ulnar collateral ligament lies on the medial side of the elbow joint reinforcing the ulnohumeral joint.

GAS 764, 766; N 424; McM 146

145 **B.** The glenohumeral joint is an extremely mobile joint with a wide range of motion. Anterior dislocation of the humerus is most common and usually associated with an isolated traumatic incident. When the head of the humerus is displaced anteriorly and inferiorly, flattening of the deltoid prominence occurs, leading to loss of the normal contour of the humerus. There is protrusion of the acromion, and the slope of the shoulder lateral to the acromion is depressed and has a "dented" appearance. Avulsion of the coronoid process of the ulna usually occurs with elbow hyperextension, which affects the shoulder joint. A fracture of the midshaft of the humerus damages the radial nerve. Although a fracture to the surgical neck of the humerus and a laceration to the axillary part of the posterior cord affect the axillary nerve, which innervates the deltoid muscle, there will not be any depression beneath the acromion in either case.

GAS 707; N 422, 424; McM 136

146 **C.** The median cubital vein is a superficial vein that lies on the biceps brachii aponeurosis. The biceps brachii aponeurosis, also known as lacertus fibrosus, is a flat sheet of connective tissue that fans out from the medial side of the biceps brachii tendon to blend with the deep fascia of the biceps brachii muscle. It reinforces the cubital fossa and protects the brachial artery, which runs beneath it.

GAS 768-769; N 403; McM 148

147 **A.** The flexor retinaculum is a thick connective tissue ligament that spans the space between the medial and lateral sides of the base of the carpal tunnel. It protects and stabilizes the tendons that run beneath it. Damage to the flexor carpi ulnaris tendon, flexor digitorum superficialis tendons, and flexor digitorum profundus tendons result in functional losses in the hand. The palmar skin is loose connective tissue and does not have a shiny, glistening appearance (*GAS* Fig. 7-103).

GAS 798; N 449; McM 158

148 **D.** The recurrent branch of the median nerve usually originates from the lateral side of the median nerve at the distal margin of the flexor retinaculum. It innervates the three thenar muscles: the opponens pollicis, flexor pollicis brevis, and abductor pollicis brevis muscles. Injury of the median nerve in the carpal tunnel, as well as injury of the recurrent and superficial branch of the median nerve, causes both sensory and motor deficits. Injury of the superficial palmar branch of the median nerve results in loss of sensation only of the palm. Injury to the radial and ulnar nerves results in a greater number of sensory and motor deficits in the distribution of theses nerves (*GAS* Fig. 7-103).

GAS 817; N 463; McM 157

149 **B.** The radial artery enters the anatomical snuffbox as it passes to the posterior aspect of the hand to pass between the two heads of the 1st dorsal interosseous muscle. The ulnar artery continues anteriorly and enters the hand on the palmar surface. The anterior and posterior interosseous arteries are found anteriorly and posteriorly, respectively, on the interosseous membrane, which is located between the radius and ulna. The deep palmar arch is an anastomosis on the palmar surface of the hand that is formed by the radial artery and the deep branch of the ulna artery and lies on the anterior surface of the hand.

GAS 782, 800, 810-815; N 454; McM 161

150 **E.** The ulnar nerve is responsible for cutaneous innervation to the medial one and a half digits and motor innervation to most of the intrinsic muscles of the hand including the interossei. The interossei muscles are responsible for adduction of the digits, which is the action that would be used to hold a piece of paper between the fingers. The median nerve supplies cutaneous innervation to the lateral three and a half fingers and the thenar eminence and lateral two lumbricals. These muscles function to oppose the thumb and flex the MP joints, respectively. The musculocutaneous nerve is responsible for innervation of the anterior compartment of the arm, and muscular nerve fibers of this nerve would not be damaged by a wound in the distal forearm. The radial nerve supplies the dorsum of the hand, with sensation and extension function of the forearm muscles, and

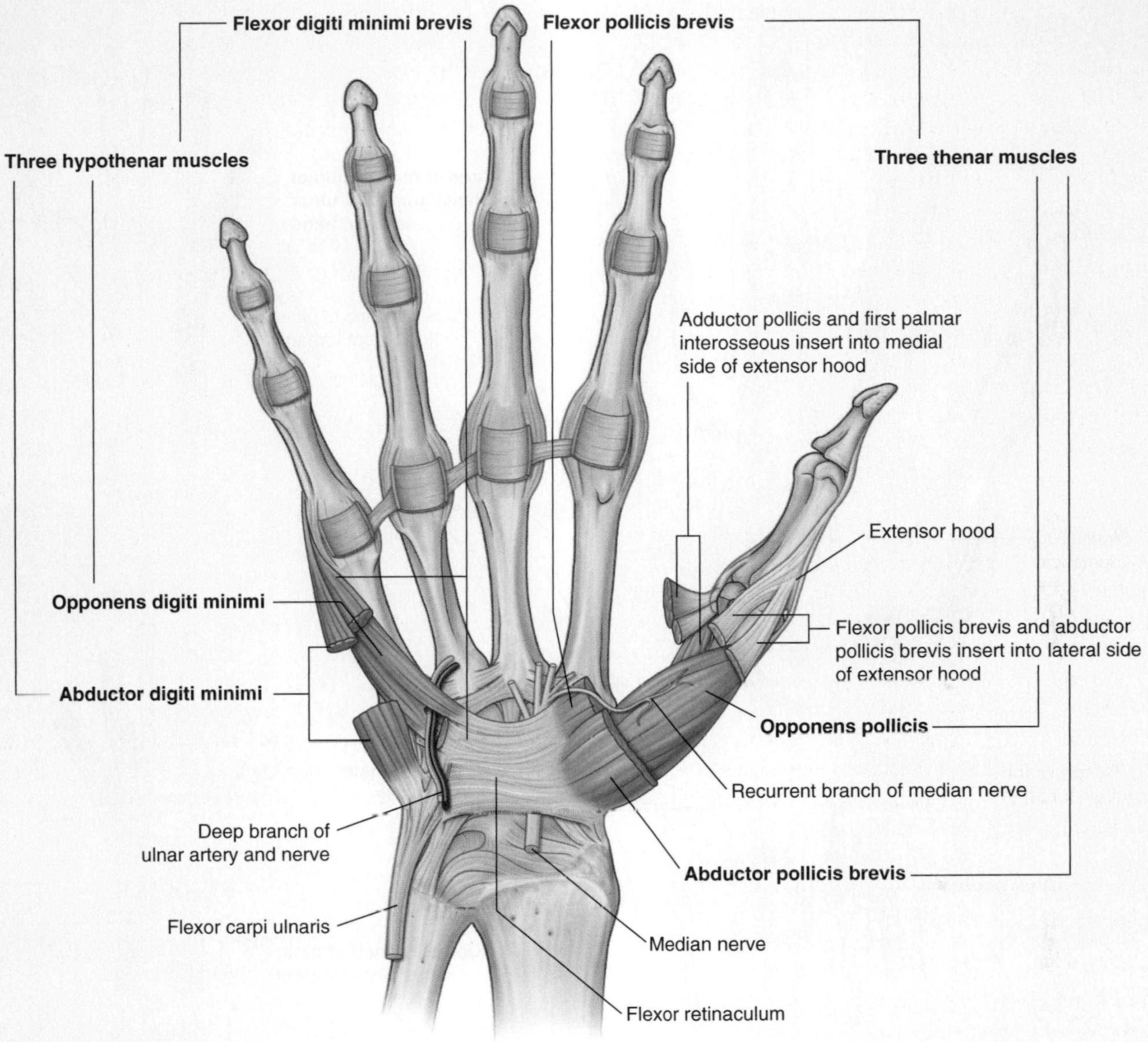

GAS Fig. 7-103

damage will not lead to this array of symptoms (*GAS* Fig. 7-109).
GAS 814, 815; N 464; McM 159

151 B. The muscle that attaches into the intertubercular sulcus of the humerus is the latissimus dorsi. Nerve supply is via the thoracodorsal nerve, which is a branch of the posterior cord and is made up of roots C6-8. Nerves C2, C3 and C4 are not part of the brachial plexus but of the cervical plexus and will supply the "strap" muscles. Nerves C4 and C5 are the main contributions to the phrenic nerve, and C5 does not contribute to the formation of the thoracodorsal nerve.
GAS 728; N 416; McM 115

152 C. Anterior dislocation of the humerus may damage the nerves located in the axilla or cause tears in the rotator cuff muscles. Internal rotation is the primary function of subscapularis muscle; with this being the only action impaired it is the most likely damaged muscle, probably as a result of injury to the upper and/or lower subscapular nerves that innervate this muscle. The infraspinatus and trees minor muscles are external rotators, and the supraspinatus muscle is the abductor of the arm from 0 to 15 degrees. The pectoralis major is a flexor, adductor, and medial rotator and would not likely be damaged during a shoulder dislocation.
GAS 712; N 411; McM 136

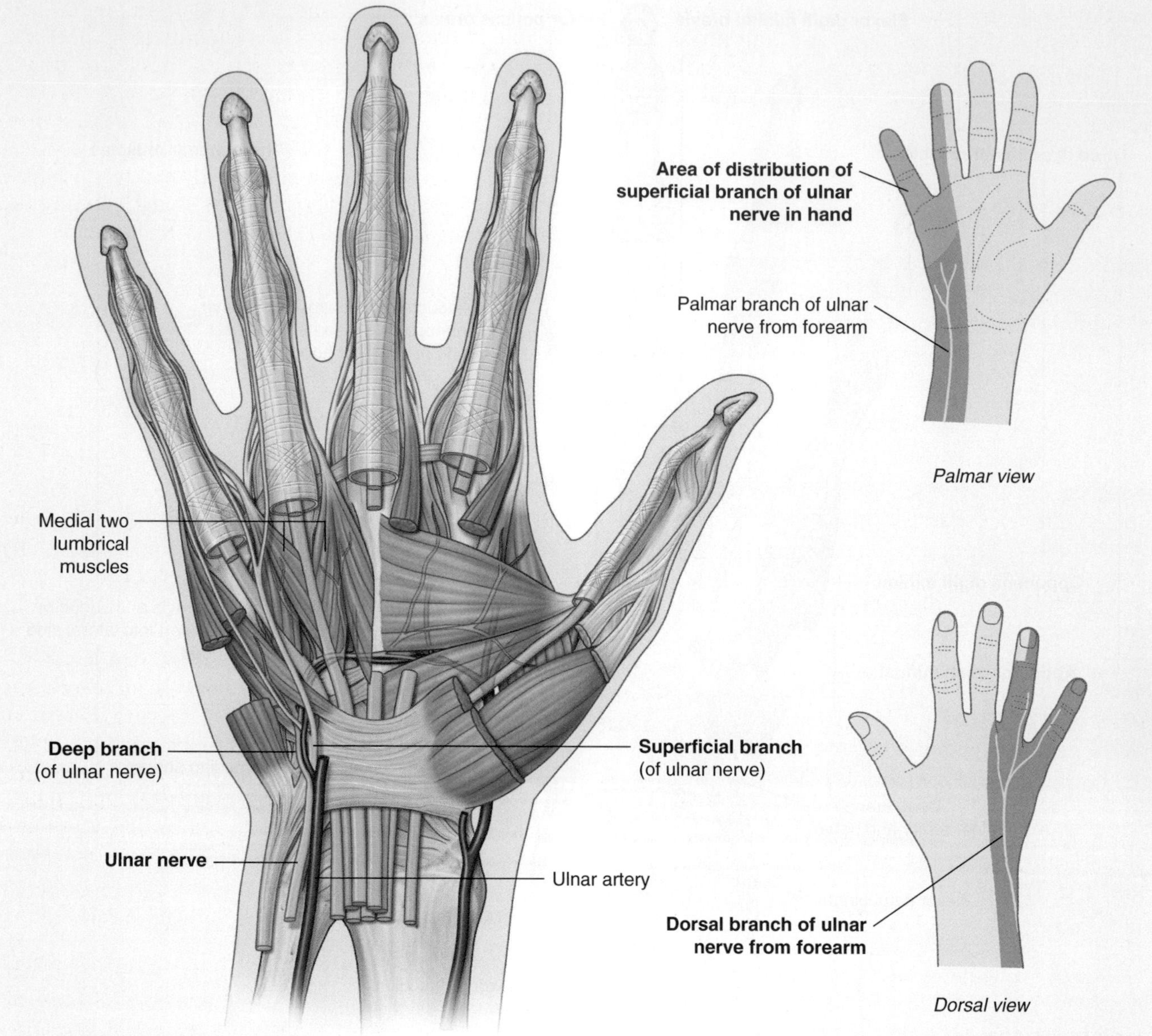

GAS **Fig. 7-109**

153 A. The nerve responsible for innervation of the interosseus muscles that are weakened in this patient is the deep branch of the ulnar nerve. Innervation of the muscles responsible for opposition of the thumb is via the recurrent branch of the median nerve. Both of these nerves are formed by the C8 and T1 ventral rami, which combine to form the inferior trunk of the brachial plexus. Damage to either the median or ulnar nerves would not produce both of these symptoms. Median nerve damage would involve all of the flexors of the wrist except the flexor carpi ulnaris and most digits except for the interphalangeal joints of the 4th and 5th fingers. It will also result in loss of function of the thumb entirely. Ulnar nerve damage will result in weakness of the medial half of flexor digitorum profundus (4th and 5th interphalangeal joint flexion), as well as the intrinsic muscles of the hand except for the lateral two lumbricals.

GAS 814; N 416; McM 157

154 C. The patient likely has damage to the ulnar nerve, which affected both the interossei and medial two lumbricals. The lumbricals extend the interphalangeal joints of the ring and little fingers, while the interossei are responsible for abduction and adduction of the digits. The dorsal interossei are responsible for abduction, while the palmar interossei are responsible for adduction of the digits. The extensor digit minimi is responsible for extension of the little finger only and if damaged will not affect the ring finger. If the extensor digitorum were damaged it would lead to weakness of all four digits, not only the ring and little fingers.

GAS 814; N 488; McM 159

155 **A.** Flexion of the elbow is achieved by contraction of the biceps brachii, brachialis, and brachioradialis muscles. The brachialis muscle is the major flexor of the elbow joint and together with the brachioradialis will continue to achieve flexion if the biceps brachii is damaged. The flexor carpi ulnaris and radialis produce flexion of the wrist, and the flexor digitorum superficialis and profundus produce flexion of the digits at the metacarpophalangeal and interphalangeal joints, respectively. The pronator teres and supinator are responsible for pronation and supination, respectively. The coracobrachialis does not cross the elbow joint and acts only on the shoulder, while the triceps brachii is the elbow extensor.

GAS 755; N 417; McM 150

156 **E.** Opposition, a complex movement, begins with the thumb in the extended position and initially involves abduction and medial rotation of the first metacarpal. This is produced by the action of the opponens pollicis muscle at the carpometacarpal joint by the flexor pollicis brevis muscle and then by flexion at the metacarpophalangeal joint. The opponens pollicis and flexor pollicis brevis muscles are supplied by the recurrent branch of the median nerve (C8, T1). The median nerve is the principal nerve of the anterior compartment of the forearm and the thenar muscles of the hand. It passes through the carpal tunnel with the tendons of the flexor digitorum profundus, flexor digitorum superficialis, and flexor pollicis longus to supply the thenar muscles of the hand. Abduction and adduction of the fingers is done by the palmar and dorsal interossei muscles, which are supplied by the median nerve. The extensor indicis extends the index finger. The ring and little fingers are flexed by the medial two tendons of the flexor digitorum superficialis (supplied by the median nerve) and the medial two tendons of the flexor digitorum profundus (supplied by the ulnar nerve).

GAS 817; N 452; McM 159

157 **D.** The scaphoid is the most frequently fractured carpal bone. Fracture often results from a fall on the palm when the hand is abducted, the fracture occurring across the narrow part ("waist") of the scaphoid. Pain occurs primarily on the lateral side of the wrist, especially during dorsiflexion and abduction of the hand. If the only blood supply to the scaphoid enters the bone distally, avascular necrosis (pathological death of bone resulting from inadequate blood supply) of the proximal fragment of the scaphoid may occur and produce degenerative joint disease of the wrist. Thumb metacarpal fractures are usually caused by an axial blow directed against the partially flexed metacarpal. Tenosynovitis is an infection of the digital synovial sheaths. Symptoms of tenosynovitis include pain, swelling, and difficulty moving the particular joint where the inflammation occurs. Carpometacarpal joint arthritis is a degenerative joint disease affecting the first carpometacarpal joint.

GAS 79; N 488; McM 159

158 **C.** The long thoracic nerve arises from the upper three ventral rami to the brachial plexus (C5 to C7) and supplies the serratus anterior, which protracts the scapula. The diaphragm is innervated by the phrenic nerve, which also arises from ventral rami (C3-C5).

GAS 727, 741; N 413; McM 140

159 **D.** The lateral epicondyle is the common extensor origin. Most of the extensor muscles of the forearm originate from this area. Putting those muscles in action will exacerbate pain on the lateral epicondyle, a condition nicknamed "tennis elbow." Radial and lateral deviations have no effect because the movement is at the wrist joint. Flexion exacerbates pain on the medial epicondyle if the patient has "golfer's elbow."

GAS 752, 785, 768; N 427; McM 145

160 **A.** Injuries to superior parts of the brachial plexus (C5-C6) usually result from an excessive increase in the angle between the neck and shoulder during a difficult delivery. Injury to the superior trunk of the plexus is apparent by the characteristic position of the limb ("waiter's position"), in which the limb hangs by the side in medial rotation. Injuries to the lower trunk of the brachial plexus (Klumpke paralysis) are much less common. These events injure the inferior trunk of the brachial plexus (C8 and T1) and may avulse the roots of the spinal nerves from the spinal cord. The short muscles of the hand are affected, and a claw hand results (*GAS* Fig. 7-52A).

GAS 738; N 452; McM 159

161 **C.** Carpal tunnel syndrome is a relatively common condition that causes pain, numbness, and a tingling sensation in the hand and fingers. Carpal tunnel syndrome is caused by compression of the median nerve, which supplies the thenar muscles and

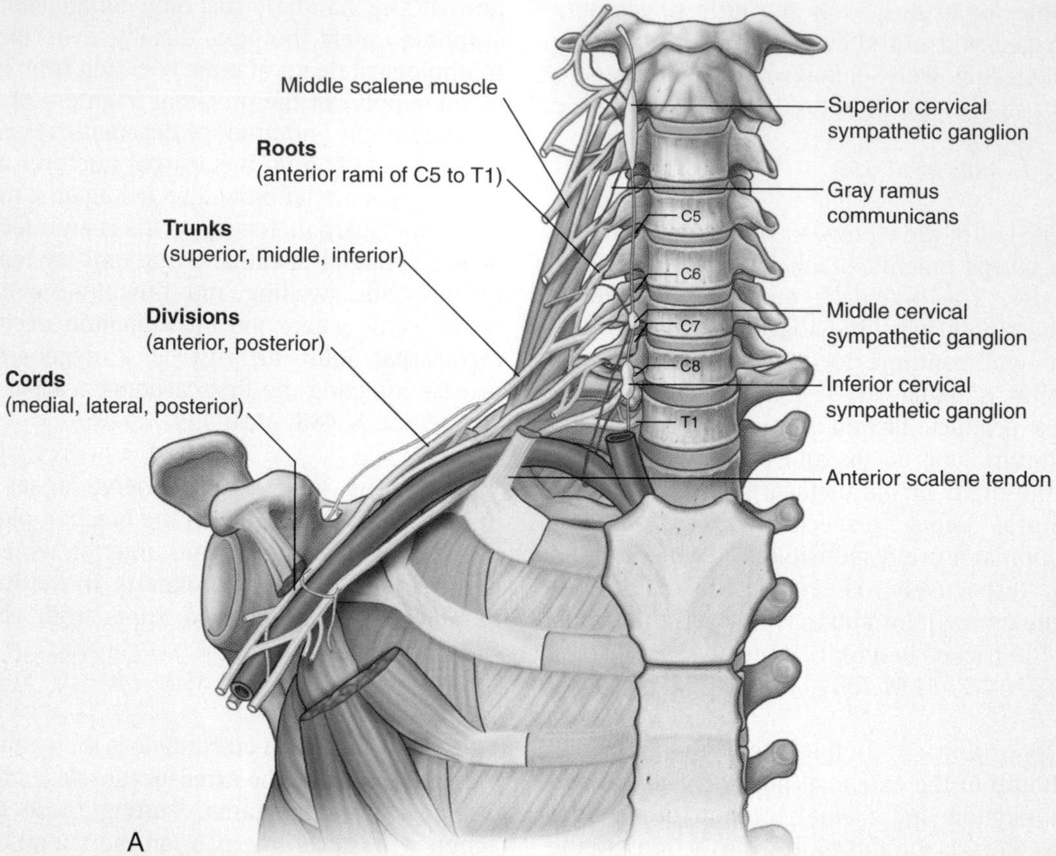

***GAS* Fig. 7-52A**

the first and second lumbricals. Dorsal and palmar interossei and the hypothenar muscles are supplied by the ulnar nerve. The flexor muscles of the forearm are supplied by the median nerve before it passes through the carpal tunnel.

GAS 798; N 449; McM 159

162 D. Recurrent branch of the median is the correct answer. This nerve, which is a branch of the median nerve, is given off after the median nerve passes through the carpal tunnel. The nerve supplies the thenar muscles. The opponens pollicis muscle, which is part of the thenar muscle group, is used while buttoning a shirt, an action that requires thumb opposition. The deep branch of the ulnar nerve supplies motor innervations to all the intrinsic muscles of the hand except the lateral two lumbricals and sensation to the medial one and a half fingers on both the palmar and dorsal sides. The patient can still grip a paper between the second and third digits, a function largely performed by the interossei muscles, which are innervated by the deep branch of the ulnar nerve. The deep branch of the radial nerve is motor to the long extensors of the wrist and fingers.

GAS 817; N 452; McM 157

163 E. Inability to adduct the thumb is the correct answer because the ulnar nerve travels superficial to the flexor retinaculum and innervates the adductor pollicis muscle, which adducts the thumb. Pronation of the forearm is carried out by muscles innervated by the median nerve, and abduction of the thumb is performed by muscles innervated by the median and radial nerves. Flexion and opposition of the thumb are performed by muscles innervated by the median nerve and would not be injured, as the median nerve travels deep to the flexor retinaculum.

GAS 814; N 452; McM 157

164 D. The supraspinatus is innervated by the suprascapular nerve (C5, C6) and the nerve continues through the spinoglenoid notch and innervates the infraspinatus. The supraspinatus initiates abduction of the arm up to the first 15 to 20 degrees. The subscapular nerve supplies the subscapularis and teres major muscles, which are medial rotators of the arm. The axillary nerve supplies the deltoid and teres minor muscles and also a patch of skin on the lateral side of the shoulder. The deltoid abducts the arm beyond 20 degrees, and the teres minor muscle, although a lateral rotator, does not abduct the arm.

The radial nerve supplies muscles in the posterior compartments of the arm and forearm, which are extensors of the elbow, wrist, and fingers in that order. The upper subscapular nerve supplies the subscapularis, a medial rotator of the arm.
GAS 717, 742; N 413; McM 138

165 C. With the involvement of the thenar muscles, lymph drains initially to the epitrochlear nodes and then to the lateral (humeral) nodes. The posterior axillary nodes receive lymph from the upper back and shoulder. The subclavian nodes receive lymph from all the axillary nodes. The anterior axillary nodes (pectoral nodes) receive lymph from most of the breast and the upper side of the anterolateral chest wall. All anterior, lateral, posterior, and medial axillary nodes drain to the central axillary nodes.
GAS 748; N 403; McM 364

166 A. "Nursemaid's elbow," a condition commonly found in children below 5 years of age, is caused by a sharp pull of the child's hand. In children, the anular ligament, which holds the head of the radius in place, is lax and allows the radial head to sublux when the hand is pulled. Also the radial head is small, so the anular ligament does not have a good "grip" on the hand. The joint capsule of the radioulnar joint is not attached to the radius; rather it passes around the neck of the radius inferiorly to attach to the coronoid process of the ulna. The interosseous membrane binds the radius and ulna together and does not maintain stability of the joint. The radial collateral ligament attaches the lateral side of the head of the radius to the lateral condyle of the humerus. The ulnar collateral ligament attaches the medial side of the ulnar head to the medial condyle of the humerus.
GAS 766; N 424; McM 146

167 A. The patient has a classic claw hand due to the damage of the deep branch of the ulnar nerve by the fractured hamate at Guyon's canal. This nerve supplies the intrinsic muscles of the hand except the lateral two lumbricals and the thenar muscles. This nerve also supplies cutaneous innervations to the medial one and a half fingers (ring and little fingers) in the palmar and dorsal sides. The lumbricals and interossei insert at the back of the fingers via the dorsal (extensor) hood. This hood extends from the metacarpophalangeal joint to the distal phalanx. Through this mechanism, the muscles flex the metacarpophalangeal joint and extend the interphalangeal joint. With damage to the deep branch of the ulnar nerve, this function is lost. The result is that there will be flexion of the interphalangeal joints and extension of the metacarpophalangeal joint, giving the appearance as shown in the photograph.
GAS 816; N 464; McM 159

168 D. In thoracic outlet syndrome—sometimes caused by a cervical rib or a cervical band—ventral rami or trunks of the brachial plexus can be compressed by these structures as they travel from the neck to the axilla. In this case the inferior trunk of the brachial plexus is being compressed by a cervical rib. The anterior division of the inferior trunk continues as the medial cord of the brachial plexus. The medial brachial cutaneous nerve (medial cutaneous nerve of the arm) and medial antebrachial cutaneous nerve (medial cutaneous nerve of the forearm) are branches of the medial cord of the plexus, with the ulnar nerve as its terminal branch. Additionally, there is medial cord contribution to the median nerve. Compression of the inferior cord of the brachial plexus therefore presents with numbness and paraesthesia on the medial part of the arm, forearm, and hand.
GAS 150; N 415; McM 140

169 A. Tenovaginitis stenosans occurs after swelling or nodular growth of the flexor tendon, which interferes with it gliding through the pulley and producing a snap or click on active extension or flexion. Mallet finger presents with permanent flexion of the distal phalanx from the lateral band of the extensor digitorum avulsion. Boutonnière deformity is due to avulsion of the central band of the extensor digitorum tendon, which presents as abnormal flexion of the middle phalanx and hyperextension of the distal phalanx. Boxer's fracture affects the metacarpals of the second and third digits commonly. Dupuytren's contracture is progressive fibrosis of the palmar aponeurosis and fascia leading to progressive shortening and thickening, eventually leading to permanent partial flexion of the metacarpophalangeal and proximal interphalangeal joints.
GAS 802; N 448; McM 157

170 B. Ganglion cysts are outpouchings of the joint capsule or tendons and may occur anywhere in the hand or feet. They contain synovial-like fluid and are pliable to touch. They commonly occur on the dorsum of the hand and may be surgically treated if necessary. The others are all solid tumors and cannot be drained.
GAS 790, 800-801; N 440; McM 158

171 A. Handlebar or ulnar neuropathy causes sensory loss of both palmar and dorsal aspects of the medial one and a half digits. Abduction of the thumb is by the abductor pollicis longus supplied by the radial nerve and the abductor pollicis brevis supplied by the median nerve. Extensors of the thumb are supplied by the radial nerve. Median nerve palsy can result in thenar muscle atrophy. A Tinel's sign might be observed near the hamate at Guyon's canal but not laterally at the scaphoid.

GAS 814-816; N 464; McM 159

172 B. Pronator syndrome is due to damage of the median nerve as it passes between the two heads of a hypertrophied pronator teres muscle. It will present with loss of opposition, atrophy of the thenar muscles, and flexion difficulty of the digits and sensory loss of the lateral three and a half digits. Hypertrophy of the supinator muscle will affect the deep branch of the radial nerve that continues distally as the posterior interosseous nerve. A medial supracondylar fracture might affect the ulnar nerve. Tennis elbow affects only the common extensor muscle origin and will not cause flexor or opposition difficulties of the digits and thumb, respectively (*GAS* Fig. 7-83).

GAS 777; N 463; McM 151

173 C. The anterior interosseous nerve runs distally and anterior to the interosseous membrane supplying the deep forearm flexors (except the ulnar part of the flexor digitorum profundus muscle, which sends tendons to the fourth and fifth fingers), it passes deep to and supplies the pronator quadratus muscle, hence the weakness in pronation and wrist flexion (*GAS* Fig. 7-87).

GAS 784; N 463; McM 151

174 E. Loss of ulnar nerve innervations eventually leads to atrophy of the interossei muscles, which presents as guttering between the metacarpals. Since the median nerve is intact there is no thenar atrophy. Similarly, if the wrist extensors, which are supplied by radial nerve, are intact, then no wrist drop is observed. Radial deviation is not seen due to action of the extensor carpi ulnaris supplied by the radial nerve.

GAS 814-816; N 464; McM 145

175 B. The lunate is the most commonly dislocated carpal bone. It helps to form the floor of the carpal arch. When it is dislocated, it is displaced into the carpal tunnel compressing the median nerve. The patient will then present with dysesthesia over the palm and palmar aspect of the thumb, index and middle fingers, and weakness in thumb opposition. The other options are not symptoms of injury solely to the median nerve.

GAS 792-795; N 439; McM 122

176 A. The deficits describe ulnar nerve damage close to its entry into the forearm. The ulnar nerve passes behind the medial epicondyle and is relatively unprotected, making this area prone to nerve injury. In the forearm, via its muscular branches, it innervates the flexor carpi ulnaris muscle and the medial half of the flexor digitorum profundus muscle. In the hand the deep branch of the ulnar nerve innervates the hypothenar muscles, adductor pollicis, abductor digiti minimi, flexor digiti minimi brevis, third and fourth lumbricals, opponens digiti minimi, and palmaris brevis muscles. The sensory innervation is to the fifth and medial half of the fourth digit and corresponding part of the hand, which can explain the deficits experienced by the patient.

GAS 784; N 463; McM 151

177 D. The lunate is compressing the median nerve. The pisiform compressing the ulnar nerve is incorrect as the ulnar nerve innervates the skin on the medial one and a half digits. Hook of hamate compressing the ulnar artery is also incorrect. The hook of the hamate forms part of Guyon's canal; compression of the ulnar artery will not produce the deficits described because of the collateral circulation and anastomoses that exist with the radial artery. The scaphoid compressing the radial artery is also incorrect because there is collateral circulation from the palmar arches to compensate for radial artery occlusion. The trapezoid is not compressing the superficial radial nerve because the superficial branch of the radial nerve supplies the radial side and ball of the thumb and radial side of the index finger via its lateral and medial branches.

GAS 792, 817; N 452; McM 168

178 D. In the midshaft region of the humerus the radial nerve runs in the radial groove; fracture of the humerus at this point will likely impinge directly on the radial nerve, producing a sensory deficit along the posterior aspect of the forearm. The lateral aspect of the forearm is innervated by the lateral antebrachial cutaneous nerve of the forearm, which comes from the musculocutaneous nerve. These nerves may not be affected by a midshaft fracture of the humerus because they are well separated from the bone by muscle. The medial aspect of the arm and forearm is supplied by the intercostobrachial nerve and the medial antebrachial cutaneous nerve that takes its origin from the medial cord of the brachial plexus where it runs superficially, making it extremely difficult to injure both nerves during a midshaft fracture of the humerus. The lateral and posterior aspect of the forearm is an unlikely choice because the

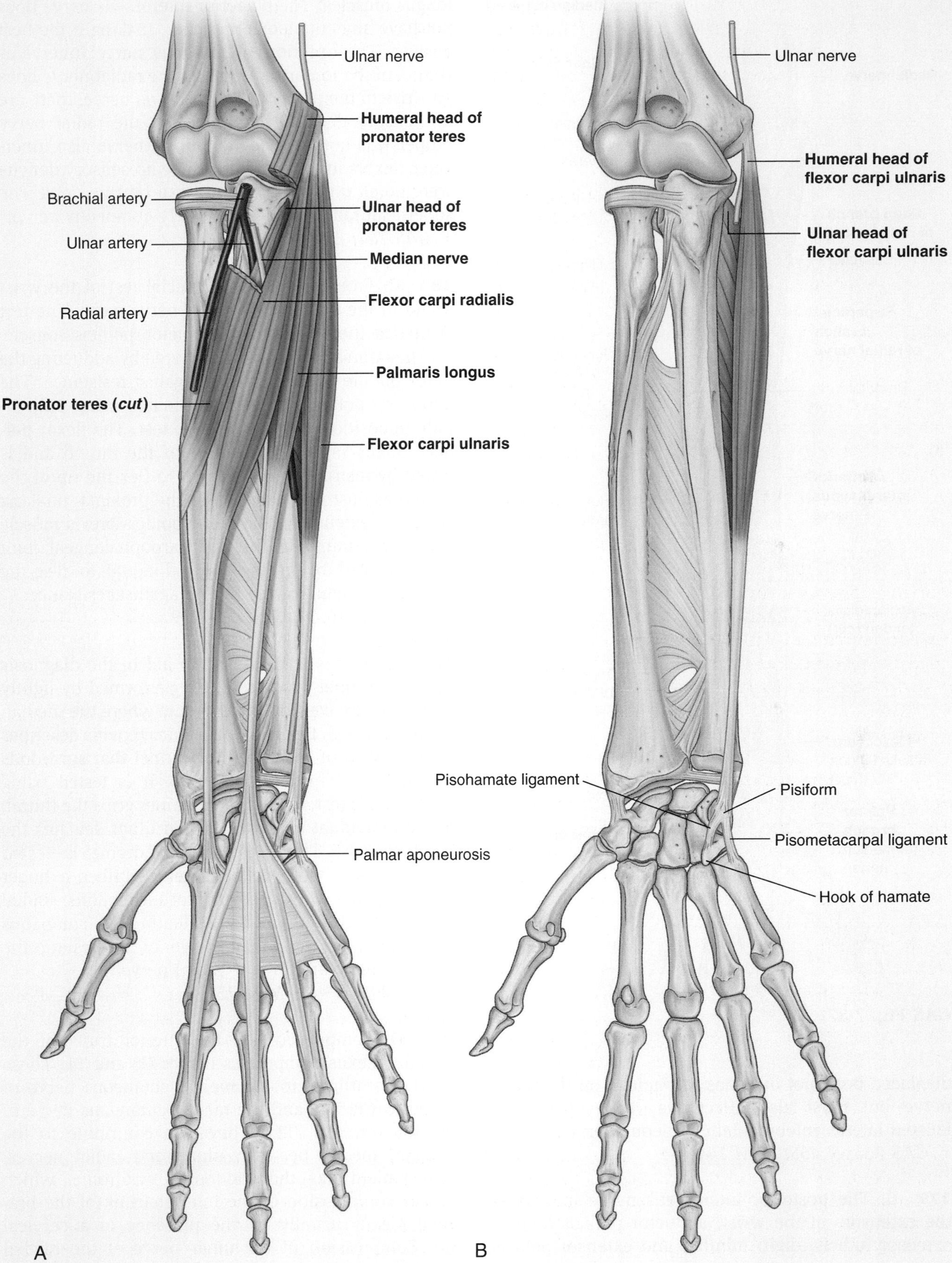

Ulnar nerve
Humeral head of pronator teres
Brachial artery
Ulnar head of pronator teres
Ulnar artery
Median nerve
Flexor carpi radialis
Radial artery
Palmaris longus
Pronator teres (cut)
Flexor carpi ulnaris
Palmar aponeurosis
A
Ulnar nerve
Humeral head of flexor carpi ulnaris
Ulnar head of flexor carpi ulnaris
Pisohamate ligament
Pisiform
Pisometacarpal ligament
Hook of hamate
B

GAS Fig. 7-83

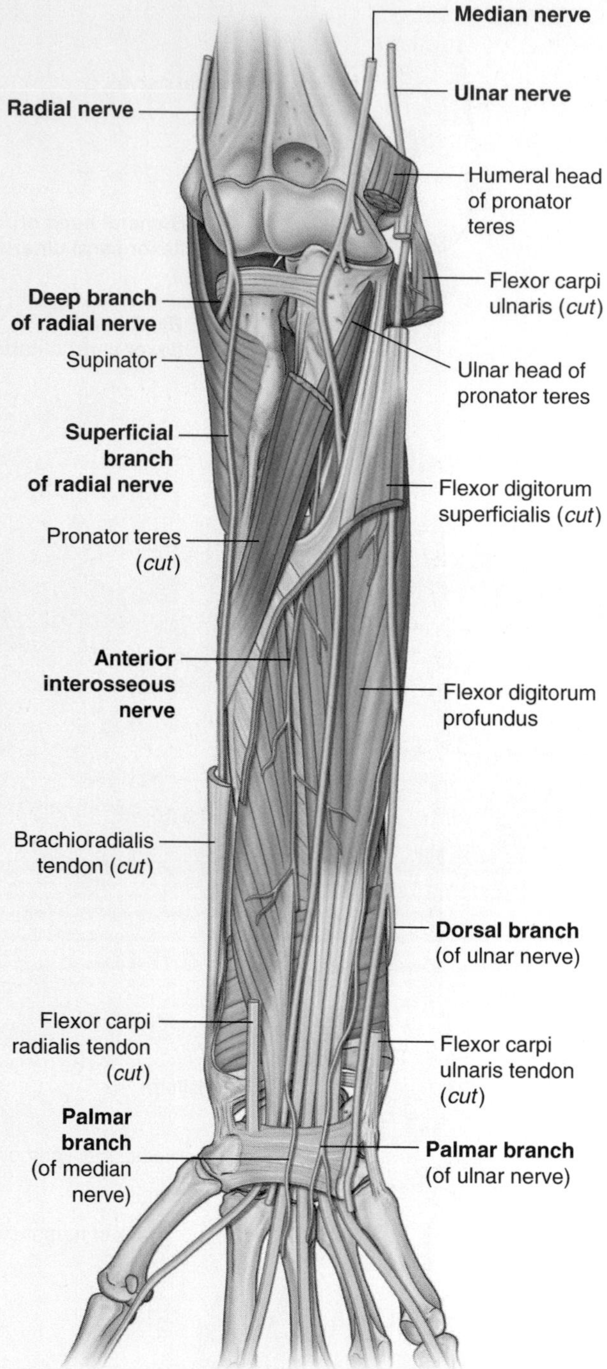

GAS Fig. 7-87

displaced bone not only has to impinge on the radial nerve but must also affect the very superficially located lateral antebrachial cutaneous nerve as well.
GAS 763; N 465; McM 144

179 B. The posterior interosseus nerve innervates the extensors of the wrist, abductor pollicis longus, extensor indicis, digiti minimi, and extensor pollicis longus muscles. The posterior interosseus nerve does not have any cutaneous branches, making it the best answer. The anterior interosseous nerve innervates flexors of the forearm. Although the radial nerve does give rise to the posterior interosseous nerve, there are no sensory deficits mentioned, so the radial nerve proper was not affected. The ulnar nerve also innervates flexors in the hand but since no sensory deficits were noted ulnar nerve injury can be ruled out. The superficial radial nerve is a purely cutaneous nerve.
GAS 784, 787; N 466; McM 152

180 C. Froment's test is a special test of the wrist to aid in the diagnosis of ulnar nerve palsy. The test evaluates the function of adductor pollicis muscle. The first dorsal interosseous is tested by adducting the index middle and ring fingers against resistance. The opponens pollicis muscle is evaluated using pulp-to-pulp opposition and the squeeze test. The flexor pollicis longus muscle is a flexor of the thumb and is tested by instructing the patient to flex the tip of the thumb against resistance while the proximal phalanx is held in extension. The flexor pollicis brevis muscle flexes the thumb at the metacarpophalangeal joint and is tested by asking the individual to flex the proximal phalanx of the thumb against resistance.
GAS 814-816; N 452; McM 159

181 A. Tinel's sign is used to aid in the diagnosis of carpal tunnel syndrome. It is performed by lightly percussing above the carpal tunnel where the median nerve is located. De Quervain's tenosynovitis describes tenosynovitis of the sheath or tunnel that surrounds tendons that control the thumb. It is tested using Finkelstein's test, where the examiner grips the thumb of the individual being tested and ulnar deviates the hand sharply. Thoracic outlet syndrome is tested using Adson's test. Mallet finger describes a finger deformity due to extensor digitorum tendons. Radial nerve damage is tested by evaluating the cutaneous distribution of the radial nerve or by testing the muscles innervated by the radial nerve.
GAS 798; N 449; McM 157

182 D. Compression on the inferior trunk of the brachial plexus compresses nerves C8 and T1. These nerves contribute to the medial cutaneous nerve of the arm (C8, T1) and the medial cutaneous nerve of the forearm (C8, T1). They also contribute to the median, medial pectoral, ulnar, and radial nerves. This patient has thoracic outlet syndrome, which causes compression of the inferior trunk of the brachial plexus usually by the presence of a cervical rib. Compression of the ulnar nerve at the medial epicondyle, radial nerve at the neck of the radius, or median nerve in the carpal tunnel would cause motor deficits not present in this patient.

GAS 738, 747; N 416; McM 129

183 **B.** The scaphoid is the most commonly fractured carpal bone as a result of the relationship with the styloid process of the radius in the distal forearm. When a person falls as described in this question, the scaphoid gets pushed against the styloid process, usually at the narrowest ("waist") part of the scaphoid and fractures as a result of the forces transmitted through the bones.

GAS 797; N 454; McM 122

184 **A.** The acromioclavicular and coracoclavicular ligaments are critical to the stability of the shoulder. In particular, the coracoclavicular ligament provides much of the weight-bearing support for the upper limb on the clavicle. The acromioclavicular joint ligament attaches the acromion (of the scapula) to the clavicle and the coracoclavicular ligament attaches the coracoid process to the clavicle. Interruption of these ligaments would cause dislocation of the acromioclavicular joint as seen in the radiograph. The sternoclavicular joint exists between the manubrium and the proximal end of the clavicle and is unrelated to either the injury or the radiograph. The coracoacromial ligament extends between the acromion and the coracoid process of the scapula. The transverse scapular ligament lies above the suprascapular notch and converts it into a foramen through which the suprascapular nerve runs (*GAS* Fig. 7-24).

GAS 706; N 408; McM 136

185 **B.** The radiograph shows a fracture of the humerus at the surgical neck. The bruising and dimpling of the upper arm would result from this injury. The axillary nerve leaves the brachial plexus as a terminal branch of the posterior cord. It passes through the quadrangular space and wraps around the head of the humerus on its way to provide innervation to the teres minor, the deltoid, and the portion of skin over the lower aspect of the deltoid that is known as the "sergeant's patch." The radial nerve travels in the radial groove along the shaft of the humerus and would be injured in a fracture of the shaft of the humerus. The ulnar nerve would be injured in a fracture of the medial epicondyle. The median nerve travels too deep to be injured here and could be compressed at the carpal tunnel or at the cubital fossa. The musculocutaneous nerve is likewise

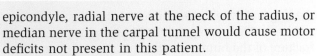

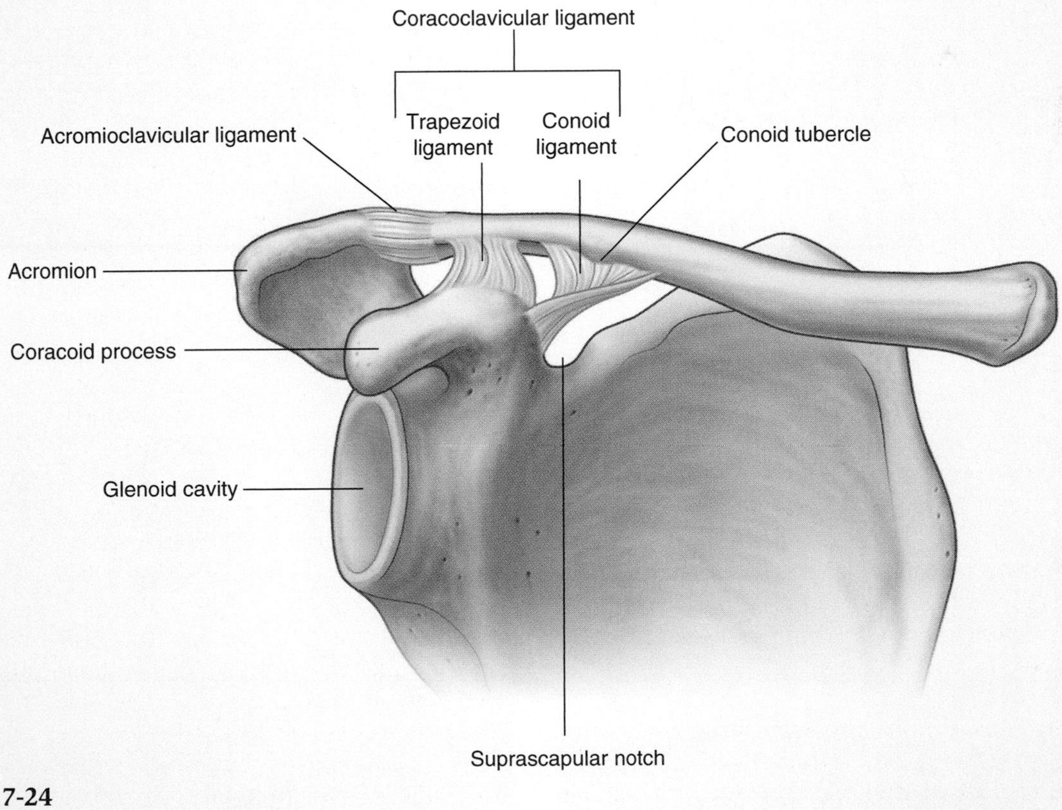

GAS **Fig. 7-24**

within the tissue and will not be affected by this injury.

GAS 704-705; N 418; McM 136

186 C. The median nerve and brachial artery were injured. Injury to the median nerve is indicated by the weakness of pronation, wrist flexion, and grip strength. The median nerve innervates the muscles that govern or carry out these movements. The brachial artery is near the median nerve and can also be injured. Flexion at the distal interphalangeal joints of the ring and little fingers indicates that the ulnar nerve is intact. The radiograph indicates a supracondylar fracture of the humerus, which is the region in which the median nerve passes. A fracture at the surgical neck would injure the axillary nerve and posterior circumflex humeral artery. A fracture of the shaft of the humerus would injure the radial nerve and deep brachial artery. The superficial radial nerve and artery would be damaged by injury over or in the anatomical snuffbox.

GAS 756, 761, 768; N 434; McM 149

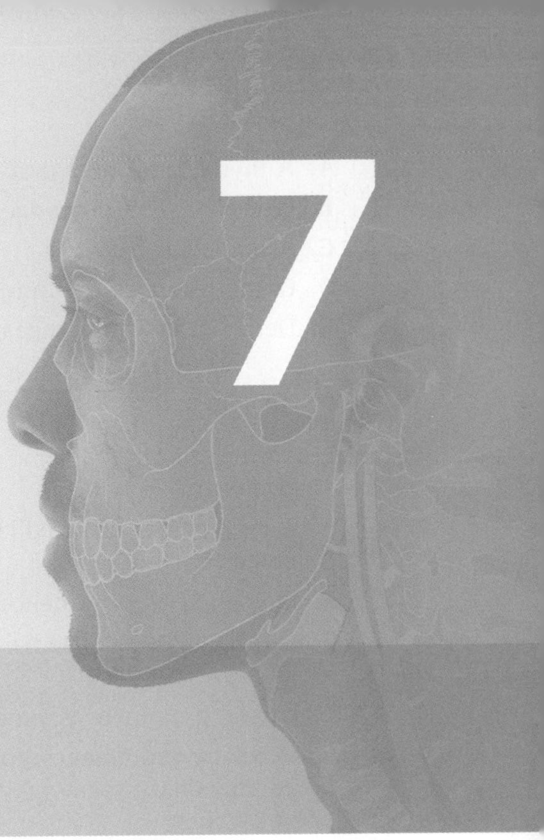

7

HEAD AND NECK

QUESTIONS

1 A 2-month-old male infant presents with a small pit at the anterior border of his left sternocleidomastoid muscle, with mucus dripping intermittently from the opening. The pit extended to the tonsillar fossa as a branchial fistula. Which of the following embryologic structure(s) is (are) involved in this anomaly?

- ▢ **A.** Second pharyngeal arch
- ▢ **B.** Second pharyngeal pouch and groove
- ▢ **C.** Third pharyngeal pouch
- ▢ **D.** Thyroglossal duct
- ▢ **E.** Second pharyngeal pouch and cervical sinus

2 A 2-day-old female infant was born with a cleft palate. The major portion of the palate develops from which of the following embryonic structures?

- ▢ **A.** Lateral palatine process
- ▢ **B.** Median palatine process
- ▢ **C.** Intermaxillary segment
- ▢ **D.** Median nasal prominences
- ▢ **E.** Frontonasal eminence

3 A 3-day-old male infant has a small area of the right iris missing, and a diagnosis of coloboma of the iris is made. Which of the following is the most likely embryologic cause of the coloboma?

- ▢ **A.** Failure of the retinal/choroid fissure to close
- ▢ **B.** Abnormal neural crest formation
- ▢ **C.** Abnormal interactions between the optic vesicle and ectoderm
- ▢ **D.** Posterior chamber cavitation
- ▢ **E.** Weak adhesion between the inner and outer layers of the optic vesicle

4 Early closure of the fontanelles of the infant skull can result in compression of the brain, restricting brain growth. Which of the following fontanelles is located at the junction of the sagittal and coronal sutures and at what age does this fontanelle typically close?

- ▢ **A.** Posterior fontanelle, which closes at about 2 years
- ▢ **B.** Mastoid fontanelle, which closes at about 16 months
- ▢ **C.** Lambdoid fontanelle, which closes at 8 months to 1 year
- ▢ **D.** Sphenoidal fontanelle, which closes at 3 years
- ▢ **E.** Anterior fontanelle, which closes at 18 months

5 A 3-year-old boy is admitted to the hospital because of a soft anterior midline cervical mass. When he is asked to protrude his tongue, the mass in the neck is observed to move upward. Which of the following is the most likely diagnosis?

- ▢ **A.** A thyroglossal duct cyst
- ▢ **B.** Defect in sixth pharyngeal arch
- ▢ **C.** A branchial cyst
- ▢ **D.** Cystic fistula of the third pharyngeal arch
- ▢ **E.** Defect in first pharyngeal arch

6 A 2-day-old male infant has a noticeable gap in his upper lip. The diagnosis is a cleft lip. Failure of fusion of which of the following structures is the most likely cause of this anomaly?

- ▢ **A.** Lateral nasal and maxillary prominences/processes
- ▢ **B.** Medial nasal prominences/processes
- ▢ **C.** Lateral nasal and medial nasal prominences/processes
- ▢ **D.** Lateral prominences/processes
- ▢ **E.** Maxillary prominences/processes and the intermaxillary segment

7 A 3-day-old male infant has a noticeably small mandible. A computed tomography (CT) scan and physical examinations reveal hypoplasia of the mandible, cleft palate, and defects of the eye and ear. Abnormal development of which of the following pharyngeal arches will most likely produce such symptoms?

- ▢ **A.** First arch
- ▢ **B.** Second arch
- ▢ **C.** Third arch
- ▢ **D.** Fourth arch
- ▢ **E.** Sixth arch

8 A 5-day-old male infant has an abnormally large head. A CT scan examination reveals enlarged lateral and third ventricles but a fourth ventricle of normal size. Stenosis of the cerebral aqueduct (of Sylvius) is suspected. Which of the following conditions will be characteristic of these symptoms?

- ▢ **A.** Nonobstructive hydrocephalus
- ▢ **B.** Anencephaly
- ▢ **C.** Obstructive hydrocephalus
- ▢ **D.** Meroanencephaly
- ▢ **E.** Holoprosencephaly

9 A 3-month-old male infant has a lump in his neck. A biopsy of the lump shows it to be thymic tissue. Based on embryonic origin, which of the following additional structures is most likely to have an ectopic location?

- ▢ **A.** Jugulodigastric lymph node
- ▢ **B.** Lingual tonsil
- ▢ **C.** Parathyroid gland
- ▢ **D.** Submandibular gland
- ▢ **E.** Thyroid gland

10 A 3-month-old male infant is under observation in the pediatric clinic. The patient has congenital hypoparathyroidism, thyroid hypoplasia, and no thymus. Abnormal development of which of the following pharyngeal pouches or arches will most likely produce these defects?

- ▢ **A.** First and second
- ▢ **B.** Second and third
- ▢ **C.** Third and fourth
- ▢ **D.** Fourth
- ▢ **E.** Fourth and sixth

11 Cleft lip, with or without cleft palate, occurs about once in 1000 births. Which of the following is considered to be the most important causative factor in the production of this anomaly?

- ▢ **A.** Riboflavin deficiency
- ▢ **B.** Infectious disease
- ▢ **C.** Mutant genes
- ▢ **D.** Cortisone administration during pregnancy
- ▢ **E.** Irradiation

12 A 5-week-old male infant is born without a thymus or inferior parathyroid glands. Which of the following pharyngeal arches is most likely involved?

- ▢ **A.** First
- ▢ **B.** Second
- ▢ **C.** Third
- ▢ **D.** Fourth
- ▢ **E.** Fifth

13 A 5-day-old female infant was born with a laryngeal defect. The greater cornuae and the inferior part of the hyoid bone were absent at birth. Failure of development of which of the following embryonic structures most likely led to these defects?

- ▢ **A.** Maxillary prominence
- ▢ **B.** Mandibular prominence
- ▢ **C.** Second pharyngeal arch
- ▢ **D.** Third pharyngeal arch
- ▢ **E.** Fourth pharyngeal arch

14 A 22-year-old woman visits the outpatient clinic with a painless swelling on the right side of her neck. A CT scan examination reveals a well-defined cystic mass at the angle of the mandible, just anterior to the

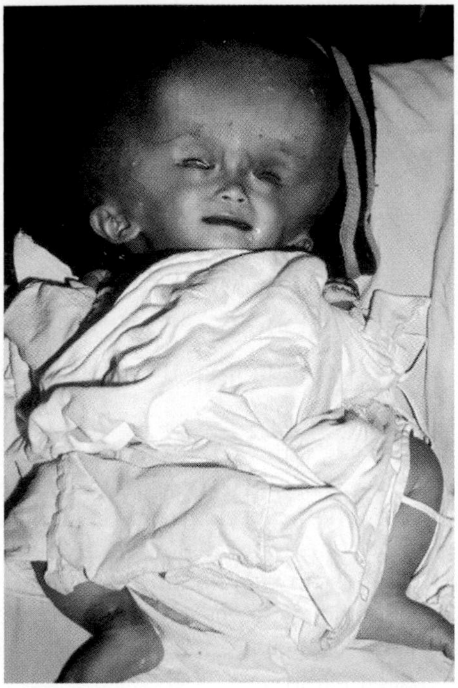

Fig. 7-1

sternocleidomastoid muscle. What is the most likely diagnosis?

- ☐ **A.** Dermoid cyst
- ☐ **B.** Inflamed lymph node
- ☐ **C.** Accessory thyroid tissue
- ☐ **D.** Thyroglossal duct cyst
- ☐ **E.** Lateral cervical cyst

15 A 5-day-old infant is diagnosed with a noncommunicating hydrocephalus (Fig. 7-1). Which of the following is most likely to lead to such a condition?

- ☐ **A.** Obstruction in the circulation of the cerebrospinal fluid (CSF)
- ☐ **B.** Excess production of CSF
- ☐ **C.** Increased size of the head
- ☐ **D.** Disturbances in the resorption of CSF
- ☐ **E.** Failure of the neural tube to close

16 A 5-day-old infant was born with a normal Apgar score. One month later the external acoustic meatus was atretic. Which of the following conditions was the most likely cause of this defect?

- ☐ **A.** Otic pit did not form
- ☐ **B.** Development of the first pharyngeal pouch was affected
- ☐ **C.** Meatal plug did not canalize
- ☐ **D.** Auricular hillocks did not develop
- ☐ **E.** The tubotympanic recess degenerated

17 A 50-year-old woman complained of pain over her chin and lower lip. A few days later, small vesicles appeared over the same area and soon began erupting. She was diagnosed with a dermatomal herpes zoster inflammation (shingles). Which of the following nerves was most likely to contain the virus in this case?

- ☐ **A.** Auriculotemporal
- ☐ **B.** Buccal
- ☐ **C.** Lesser petrosal
- ☐ **D.** Mental
- ☐ **E.** Infraorbital

18 A 68-year-old woman is suffering from excruciating, sudden bouts of pain over the area of her midface. Physical examination indicates that she has tic douloureux (trigeminal neuralgia). Which ganglion is the location of the neural cell bodies of the nerve mediating the pain?

- ☐ **A.** Geniculate
- ☐ **B.** Trigeminal (semilunar or Gasserian)
- ☐ **C.** Inferior glossopharyngeal
- ☐ **D.** Otic
- ☐ **E.** Pterygopalatine

19 A 17-year-old girl is admitted to the hospital with signs of cavernous sinus thrombosis, as revealed by radiographic and physical examinations. Thrombophlebitis in the "danger area" of the face can spread to the cavernous sinus and involve the ophthalmic branch of the trigeminal nerve. Which of the following symptoms will most likely be present during physical examination?

- ☐ **A.** Pain in the hard palate
- ☐ **B.** Anesthesia of the upper lip
- ☐ **C.** Pain from the eyeball
- ☐ **D.** Pain over the lower eyelid
- ☐ **E.** Tingling sensation over the buccal region of the face

20 A 34-year-old man is admitted to the hospital with severe headaches, dizziness, and vomiting. Imaging studies reveal a tumor at the hypoglossal canal. Which of the following muscles will most likely be affected?

- ☐ **A.** Geniohyoid
- ☐ **B.** Mylohyoid
- ☐ **C.** Palatoglossus
- ☐ **D.** Genioglossus
- ☐ **E.** Thyrohyoid

21 A 45-year-old woman is admitted to the hospital with severe headaches, dizziness, and vomiting. Radiologic examination reveals an intracranial tumor. Upon physical examination the patient has dryness of the nasal and paranasal sinuses, loss of lacrimation, and loss of taste from the anterior two thirds of the tongue. Which of the following structures is most likely involved with the tumor?

- ▢ **A.** Auriculotemporal nerve
- ▢ **B.** Lesser petrosal nerve
- ▢ **C.** Facial nerve
- ▢ **D.** Inferior salivatory nucleus
- ▢ **E.** Pterygopalatine ganglion

22 A 17-year-old girl has suffered from a painful discoloration of her hand for the past year. A magnetic resonance imaging (MRI) scan revealed "thoracic outlet" syndrome. Which symptom would most likely result from this syndrome?

- ▢ **A.** Problems with respiration because of pressure on the phrenic nerve
- ▢ **B.** Reduced blood flow to the thoracic wall
- ▢ **C.** Reduced venous return from the head and neck
- ▢ **D.** Numbness in the upper limb
- ▢ **E.** Distention of the internal jugular vein

23 A 31-year-old woman is admitted to the hospital after an automobile collision. An MRI examination reveals a large hematoma inferior to the right jugular foramen. Physical examination reveals right pupillary constriction (miosis), ptosis of the eyelid, and anhydrosis (loss of sweating) of the face. Which of the following ganglia is most likely affected by the hematoma?

- ▢ **A.** Submandibular
- ▢ **B.** Trigeminal (semilunar or Gasserian)
- ▢ **C.** Superior cervical
- ▢ **D.** Geniculate
- ▢ **E.** Ciliary

24 A 35-year-old man is admitted to the hospital with severe headaches. A CT scan evaluation reveals a tumor in the infratemporal fossa. Physical examination reveals loss of general sensation from the anterior two thirds of his tongue, but taste and salivation are intact. Which of the following nerves is most likely affected by the tumor?

- ▢ **A.** Lingual proximal to its junction with the chorda tympani
- ▢ **B.** Chorda tympani
- ▢ **C.** Inferior alveolar
- ▢ **D.** Lesser petrosal
- ▢ **E.** Glossopharyngeal

25 A 70-year-old man is admitted to the hospital with chronic headache and enlarged lymph nodes. A CT scan shows a tumor at the jugular foramen. Which of the following would be the most likely neurologic deficit?

- ▢ **A.** Loss of tongue movements
- ▢ **B.** Loss of facial expression
- ▢ **C.** Loss of sensation from the face and the scalp
- ▢ **D.** Loss of hearing
- ▢ **E.** Loss of gag reflex

26 A 40-year-old unconscious man is admitted to the emergency department after being hit in the head with a baseball. A CT scan examination reveals a fractured pterion and an epidural hematoma. Branches of which of the following arteries are most likely to be injured?

- ▢ **A.** External carotid
- ▢ **B.** Superficial temporal
- ▢ **C.** Maxillary
- ▢ **D.** Deep temporal
- ▢ **E.** Middle meningeal

27 An unconscious 48-year-old woman is admitted to the hospital. CT scan reveals a tumor in her brain. When she regains consciousness, her right eye is directed laterally and downward, with complete ptosis of her upper eyelid, and her pupil is dilated. Which of the following structures was most likely affected by the tumor to result in these symptoms?

- ▢ **A.** Oculomotor nerve
- ▢ **B.** Optic nerve
- ▢ **C.** Facial nerve
- ▢ **D.** Ciliary ganglion
- ▢ **E.** Superior cervical ganglion

28 A 55-year-old man is admitted to the hospital after an injury sustained at work in a factory. He presents with severe scalp lacerations, which were sutured. After 3 days the wound is inflamed, swollen, and painful. Between which tissue layers is the infection most likely located?

- ▢ **A.** The periosteum and bone
- ▢ **B.** The aponeurosis and the periosteum
- ▢ **C.** The dense connective tissue and the aponeurosis
- ▢ **D.** The dense connective tissue and the skin
- ▢ **E.** The dermis and the epidermis

29 A 36-year-old woman is admitted to the hospital with severe head injuries after a car crash. During neurologic examination her uvula is found to be deviated to the right. Which nerve is most likely affected to result in this deviation?

- ☐ **A.** Left vagus
- ☐ **B.** Right vagus
- ☐ **C.** Right hypoglossal
- ☐ **D.** Left glossopharyngeal
- ☐ **E.** Right glossopharyngeal

30 A 22-year-old man is admitted to the emergency department and intubated. An endotracheal tube is passed through an opening between the vocal folds. What is the name of this opening?

- ☐ **A.** Piriform recess
- ☐ **B.** Vestibule
- ☐ **C.** Ventricle
- ☐ **D.** Vallecula
- ☐ **E.** Rima glottidis

31 A 55-year-old man has a complaint of left-sided tooth pain in his upper jaw. A dental examination reveals no abnormalities of his teeth. During physical examination tapping on his left maxilla elicits sharp pain on the left side of his face, including his maxillary teeth on that side. The patient reports that he has no allergies. Which of the following conditions will be the most likely diagnosis?

- ☐ **A.** Sphenoid sinusitis
- ☐ **B.** Anterior ethmoidal sinusitis
- ☐ **C.** Posterior ethmoidal sinusitis
- ☐ **D.** Maxillary sinusitis
- ☐ **E.** Frontal sinusitis

32 A 70-year-old man is admitted to the hospital with severe headaches. During the physical examination he has difficulty coughing and swallowing. An MRI scan shows a tumor affecting a cranial nerve. Which nerve is most likely affected?

- ☐ **A.** Mandibular
- ☐ **B.** Maxillary
- ☐ **C.** Glossopharyngeal
- ☐ **D.** Vagus
- ☐ **E.** Hypoglossal

33 A 7-year-old boy with a high fever is brought to the pediatrician. During physical examination the patient complains of pain in his ear. His throat appears red and inflamed, confirming the diagnosis of pharyngitis. Which of the following structures provided a pathway for the infection to spread to the tympanic cavity (middle ear)?

- ☐ **A.** Choanae
- ☐ **B.** Internal acoustic meatus
- ☐ **C.** External acoustic meatus
- ☐ **D.** Pharyngotympanic tube
- ☐ **E.** Pharyngeal recess

34 A 33-year-old woman is unconscious when she is admitted to the hospital after she fell, hitting her head. The physician in the emergency department performs a pupillary light reflex test. The integrity of which of the following nerves is being checked?

- ☐ **A.** Optic and facial
- ☐ **B.** Optic and oculomotor
- ☐ **C.** Maxillary and facial
- ☐ **D.** Ophthalmic and oculomotor
- ☐ **E.** Ophthalmic and facial

35 A 48-year-old man complains of diplopia (double vision). On neurologic examination he is unable to adduct his left eye and lacks a corneal reflex on the left side. Where is the most likely location of the lesion resulting in the symptoms?

- ☐ **A.** Inferior orbital fissure
- ☐ **B.** Optic canal
- ☐ **C.** Superior orbital fissure
- ☐ **D.** Foramen rotundum
- ☐ **E.** Foramen ovale

36 A 34-year-old man complains of hyperacusis (sensitivity to loud sounds). Injury to which of the following cranial nerves is most likely responsible?

- ☐ **A.** Hypoglossal
- ☐ **B.** Facial
- ☐ **C.** Accessory
- ☐ **D.** Vagus
- ☐ **E.** Glossopharyngeal

37 A 34-year-old man who swims regularly presents to your office with an external ear canal infection (otitis externa). The patient coughs during inspection of the external auditory meatus with a speculum. The cough results from the irritation of which nerve that innervates an area of the external auditory meatus?

- ☐ **A.** Vestibulocochlear
- ☐ **B.** Vagus
- ☐ **C.** Trigeminal
- ☐ **D.** Facial
- ☐ **E.** Accessory

38 A 29-year-old woman underwent a thyroidectomy. Postoperatively, the patient presented with hoarseness. Which of the following nerves was most likely injured during the operation?

- ▢ **A.** Internal laryngeal
- ▢ **B.** External laryngeal
- ▢ **C.** Recurrent laryngeal
- ▢ **D.** Superior laryngeal
- ▢ **E.** Glossopharyngeal

39 A 48-year-old man presents with a constricted right pupil that does not react to light. His left pupil and vision in both eyes are normal. These findings are most likely due to a lesion involving which of the following right-sided structures?

- ▢ **A.** Oculomotor nerve
- ▢ **B.** Superior cervical ganglion
- ▢ **C.** Nervus intermedius
- ▢ **D.** Edinger-Westphal nucleus
- ▢ **E.** Trigeminal (semilunar, Gasserian) ganglion

40 A 55-year-old woman is diagnosed with a tumor at the base of the skull, resulting in a decrease in tear production. Which of the following nerves is most likely injured?

- ▢ **A.** Chorda tympani
- ▢ **B.** Deep petrosal
- ▢ **C.** Greater petrosal
- ▢ **D.** Lesser petrosal
- ▢ **E.** Nasociliary

41 A 24-year-old man is admitted to the hospital after a street fight. Radiographic examination reveals an inferior (blow-out) fracture of the orbit. Orbital structures would most likely be found inferiorly in which of the following spaces?

- ▢ **A.** Ethmoidal sinus
- ▢ **B.** Frontal sinus
- ▢ **C.** Maxillary sinus
- ▢ **D.** Nasal cavity
- ▢ **E.** Sphenoidal sinus

42 A 35-year-old woman is hospitalized due to cavernous sinus thrombosis resulting from an infection on her face. Which of the following is the most direct route for spread of infection from the face to the cavernous sinus?

- ▢ **A.** Pterygoid venous plexus
- ▢ **B.** Superior ophthalmic vein
- ▢ **C.** Frontal venous plexus
- ▢ **D.** Basilar venous plexus
- ▢ **E.** Parietal emissary vein

43 A 7-year-old boy was suffering from a severe infection of the middle ear (otitis media), which spread to the mastoid air cells (mastoiditis). Surgery was required but resulted in the following: right corner of the mouth drooping, unable to close his right eye, food collection in his right oral vestibule. Which nerve was injured?

- ▢ **A.** Glossopharyngeal
- ▢ **B.** Vagus
- ▢ **C.** Facial
- ▢ **D.** Maxillary division of the trigeminal nerve
- ▢ **E.** Mandibular division of the trigeminal nerve

44 The arterial circle (of Willis) contributes greatly to cerebral arterial circulation when one primary artery becomes occluded by atherosclerotic disease. Which of the following vessels does not contribute to the circle?

- ▢ **A.** Anterior communicating artery
- ▢ **B.** Posterior communicating artery
- ▢ **C.** Middle cerebral artery
- ▢ **D.** Internal carotid artery
- ▢ **E.** Posterior cerebral artery

45 A 45-year-old woman is admitted to the hospital for severe ear pain. Physical examination reveals chronic infection of the mastoid air cells (mastoiditis). The infection can erode the thin layer of the bone between the mastoid air cells and the posterior cranial fossa and spread most commonly into which of the following venous structures?

- ▢ **A.** Superior sagittal sinus
- ▢ **B.** Inferior sagittal sinus
- ▢ **C.** Straight sinus
- ▢ **D.** Cavernous sinus
- ▢ **E.** Sigmoid sinus

46 A 63-year-old man with hearing loss in his left ear complains of a loss of taste and drooling from the left side of his mouth. A CT scan shows a tumor compressing the nerve exiting the skull through which of the following openings?

- ▢ **A.** Foramen ovale
- ▢ **B.** Foramen rotundum
- ▢ **C.** Internal acoustic meatus
- ▢ **D.** Jugular foramen
- ▢ **E.** Superior orbital fissure

47 A 70-year-old man has a biopsy of a growth on his lower lip. The biopsy reveals a squamous cell carcinoma. Which lymph nodes will most likely be first involved in the spread of the cancer cells?

- ☐ **A.** Occipital
- ☐ **B.** Parotid
- ☐ **C.** Retropharyngeal
- ☐ **D.** Jugulodigastric
- ☐ **E.** Submental

48 A 54-year-old man is admitted to the hospital due to severe headaches. A CT examination reveals an internal carotid artery aneurysm inside the cavernous sinus. Which of the following nerves would be typically affected first?

- ☐ **A.** Abducens nerve
- ☐ **B.** Oculomotor nerve
- ☐ **C.** Ophthalmic nerve
- ☐ **D.** Maxillary nerve
- ☐ **E.** Trochlear nerve

49 A 24-year-old man had a third molar (wisdom tooth) extracted from his lower jaw. This resulted in the loss of general sense and taste sensation from the anterior two thirds of the tongue. This loss was most likely due to injury of which of the following nerves?

- ☐ **A.** Auriculotemporal
- ☐ **B.** Chorda tympani
- ☐ **C.** Lingual
- ☐ **D.** Mental
- ☐ **E.** Inferior alveolar

50 A 56-year-old woman is admitted to the hospital with rheumatoid arthritis of her temporomandibular joint (TMJ) and severe ear pain. An image from her radiographic examination is shown in Fig. 7-2. Which of the following nerves is most likely responsible for conducting the pain sensation?

- ☐ **A.** Facial
- ☐ **B.** Auriculotemporal
- ☐ **C.** Lesser petrosal
- ☐ **D.** Vestibulocochlear
- ☐ **E.** Chorda tympani

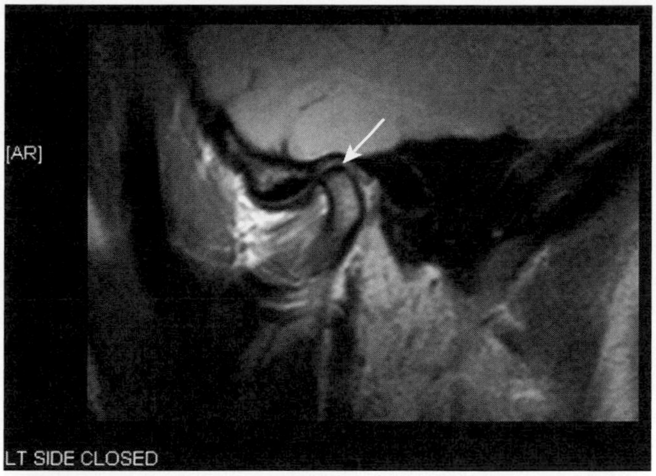

Fig. 7-2

51 Where is the location of the postganglionic parasympathetic neural cell bodies that directly innervate the parotid gland?

- ☐ **A.** Trigeminal (semilunar, Gasserian) ganglion
- ☐ **B.** Inferior salivatory nucleus
- ☐ **C.** Superior cervical ganglion
- ☐ **D.** Otic ganglion
- ☐ **E.** Submandibular ganglion

52 The arachnoid villi allow cerebrospinal fluid to pass between which two of the following spaces?

- ☐ **A.** Choroid plexus and subdural space
- ☐ **B.** Subarachnoid space and superior sagittal sinus
- ☐ **C.** Subdural space and cavernous sinus
- ☐ **D.** Superior sagittal sinus and jugular vein
- ☐ **E.** Epidural and subdural space

53 A 22-year-old woman is admitted to the hospital with an injury to her eye. The corneal reflex is tested and found to be present. Which of the following nerves is responsible for the afferent limb of this reflex?

- ☐ **A.** Frontal
- ☐ **B.** Lacrimal
- ☐ **C.** Nasociliary
- ☐ **D.** Oculomotor
- ☐ **E.** Optic

54 A 21-year-old man was brought to the emergency department because of severe epistaxis (nosebleed) from the nasal septum. This area, known as Kiesselbach's (or Little's) area, involves mostly anastomoses between which of the following arteries?

- ☐ **A.** Ascending palatine and ascending pharyngeal
- ☐ **B.** Posterior superior alveolar and accessory meningeal
- ☐ **C.** Lateral branches of posterior ethmoidal and middle meningeal
- ☐ **D.** Septal branches of the sphenopalatine and superior labial

☐ **E.** Descending palatine and tonsillar branches of the pharyngeal

55 An 11-year-old boy is examined by an otorhinolaryngologist for his swollen palatine tonsils. The palatine tonsils are located between the anterior and posterior tonsillar pillars. Which of the following muscles form these pillars?

☐ **A.** Levator veli palatini and tensor veli palatini

☐ **B.** Palatoglossus and palatopharyngeus

☐ **C.** Styloglossus and stylopharyngeus

☐ **D.** Palatopharyngeus and salpingopharyngeus

☐ **E.** Superior and middle pharyngeal constrictors

56 A 35-year-old woman is under general anesthesia. Before laryngeal intubation the rima glottidis is opened by which pair of muscles?

☐ **A.** Posterior cricoarytenoids

☐ **B.** Lateral cricoarytenoids

☐ **C.** Thyroarytenoids

☐ **D.** Transverse arytenoids

☐ **E.** Cricothyroids

57 A 32-year-old woman asks you what is the soft, thin ridge of tissue that she can feel running forward across the masseter muscle toward her upper lip. You reassure her that is perfectly normal. Which of the following is the most likely structure she is feeling?

☐ **A.** Facial artery

☐ **B.** Maxillary artery

☐ **C.** Parotid duct

☐ **D.** Marginal mandibular branch of the facial nerve

☐ **E.** Facial vein

58 A 43-year-old man is diagnosed with laryngeal carcinoma. A surgical procedure is performed and the tumor is successfully removed from the larynx. The right ansa cervicalis is anastomosed with the right recurrent laryngeal nerve to reinnervate the muscles of the larynx and restore phonation. Which of the following muscles will most likely be paralyzed after this operation?

☐ **A.** Sternocleidomastoid

☐ **B.** Platysma

☐ **C.** Sternohyoid

☐ **D.** Trapezius

☐ **E.** Cricothyroid

59 A 67-year-old woman is admitted to the emergency department with a severe swelling on the right side of her neck. An MRI examination reveals an abscess. The abscess is surgically removed from the middle of the posterior cervical triangle on the right side. During recovery the patient notices that her shoulder droops and she can no longer raise her right hand above her head to brush her hair. Which of the following nerves has most likely been iatrogenically injured?

☐ **A.** Accessory

☐ **B.** Ansa cervicalis

☐ **C.** Facial

☐ **D.** Hypoglossal

☐ **E.** Suprascapular

60 A 20-year-old man is admitted to the emergency department with a stab wound in the superior region of his neck. A radiographic examination reveals that the wound has not affected any major structures. Physical examination reveals that the patient has lost sensation from the skin over the angle of the jaw. Which of the following nerves is most likely injured?

☐ **A.** Supraclavicular

☐ **B.** Transverse cervical

☐ **C.** Great auricular

☐ **D.** Greater occipital

☐ **E.** Lesser occipital

61 A 6-year-old boy, whose medical history includes a complicated delivery, has a continuously tilted head posture, with the right ear near the right shoulder and the face turned upward and to the left. Which of the following muscles was most likely damaged during birth?

☐ **A.** Anterior scalene

☐ **B.** Omohyoid

☐ **C.** Sternocleidomastoid

☐ **D.** Trapezius

☐ **E.** Platysma

62 A 35-year-old woman is admitted to the emergency department after a violent automobile crash. The patient's upper airway is obstructed with blood and mucus, and a midline tracheostomy inferior to the thyroid isthmus is performed. Which of the following vessels are most likely to be present at the site of incision and will need to be cauterized?

☐ **A.** Middle thyroid vein and inferior thyroid artery

☐ **B.** Inferior thyroid artery and inferior thyroid vein

☐ **C.** Inferior thyroid vein and thyroidea ima artery

☐ **D.** Cricothyroid artery and inferior thyroid vein

- E. Left brachiocephalic vein and inferior thyroid artery

63 A 34-year-old woman is admitted to the hospital with a large mass at her thyroid gland. Ultrasound examination suggests a benign tumor, which is confirmed with a biopsy. Twenty-four hours following a partial thyroidectomy, in which the inferior thyroid artery was also ligated, the patient speaks with a hoarse voice and has difficulty in breathing on exertion. Which of the following nerves was most likely injured during the surgical procedure?

- A. Internal branch of superior laryngeal
- B. Ansa cervicalis
- C. Ansa subclavia
- D. Recurrent laryngeal
- E. External branch of superior laryngeal

64 A 55-year-old woman is admitted to the hospital with difficulty swallowing. Physical examination reveals that the patient has episodes of severe headaches and frequently aspirates fluids when drinking them. A radiographic examination reveals a skull base tumor occupying the space behind the jugular foramen. Involvement of which of the following structures is most likely responsible for the findings in the patient?

- A. Ansa cervicalis
- B. Cervical sympathetic trunk
- C. External laryngeal nerve
- D. Hypoglossal nerve
- E. Vagus nerve

65 A 55-year-old woman is admitted to the hospital with severe hypertension. Examination reveals hypertension (190/110 mm Hg) and hypercholesterolemia (250 mg/dL). During physical examination she complains of headaches and dizziness. An arteriogram reveals 90% occlusion of both common carotid arteries. A carotid endarterectomy is performed and large atherosclerotic plaques are removed. During a postoperative physical examination on the right side, it was noted that her tongue deviated toward the right when she was asked to protrude it. Which of the following nerves was most likely injured during the procedure?

- A. Right glossopharyngeal
- B. Right hypoglossal
- C. Left hypoglossal
- D. Left lingual
- E. Left vagus

66 A 34-year-old woman is admitted to the hospital with a large mass in her lower anterior neck. Ultrasound examination reveals a benign tumor of her thyroid gland. Twenty-four hours following a partial thyroidectomy, it was noted that the patient frequently aspirates fluid into her lungs. Upon examination it was determined that the area of the piriform recess above the vocal fold of the larynx was anesthetized. Which of the following nerves was most likely iatrogenically injured?

- A. External branch of the superior pharyngeal
- B. Hypoglossal
- C. Internal branch of the superior laryngeal
- D. Lingual
- E. Recurrent laryngeal

67 A 38-year-old man is admitted to the hospital with a large mass in his lower anterior neck. Ultrasound examination reveals a benign tumor of his thyroid gland. Twenty-four hours following a partial thyroidectomy, it was noted that the patient could not abduct the true vocal cords due to a nerve injury during the operation. Which of the following muscles was most likely denervated?

- A. Posterior cricoarytenoid
- B. Lateral cricoarytenoid
- C. Thyroarytenoid
- D. Arytenoid
- E. Cricothyroid

68 A 46-year-old woman is admitted to the hospital with a large mass in her lower anterior neck. Ultrasound examination suggests a benign tumor of her thyroid gland, which is confirmed with a biopsy. During the procedure to remove the tumor the superior thyroid artery is identified and used as a landmark in order not to damage its small companion nerve. Which of the following nerves is most likely to accompany the superior thyroid artery?

- A. Cervical sympathetic trunk
- B. External branch of the superior laryngeal
- C. Inferior root of the ansa cervicalis
- D. Internal branch of the superior laryngeal
- E. Recurrent laryngeal

69 A 3-year-old girl ruptured her tympanic membrane (eardrum) when she inserted a pencil into her external ear canal. Physical examination revealed pain in her ear and a few drops of blood in the external auditory meatus. There was the concern that there might possibly have been an injury to the nerve that principally innervates the external surface of the tympanic membrane. Which of the following tests is most likely to be performed during physical examination to check for injury to this nerve?

- ☐ **A.** Check the taste in the anterior two thirds of the tongue
- ☐ **B.** Check the sensation to the pharynx and palate
- ☐ **C.** Check if there is paraesthesia at the TMJ
- ☐ **D.** Check for sensation in the larynx
- ☐ **E.** Check for sensation in the nasal cavity

70 A 27-year-old woman is admitted to the emergency department after she was thrown from a motor scooter. Radiographic evaluation reveals a type I LeFort fracture and comminuted fracture of the mandible and TMJ. Despite reconstructive surgery, the patient develops hyperacusis (sensitivity to loud sounds) due to facial nerve paralysis. Which of the following muscles is most likely paralyzed?

- ☐ **A.** Posterior belly of digastric
- ☐ **B.** Stapedius
- ☐ **C.** Tensor tympani
- ☐ **D.** Stylohyoid
- ☐ **E.** Cricothyroid

71 A 43-year-old man is admitted to the emergency department with a fracture of the base of his skull. A thorough physical examination reveals that a number of structures have been injured, suggesting that the right greater petrosal nerve has been injured. Which of the following symptoms needs to be identified during physical examination to confirm the diagnosis of greater petrosal nerve injury?

- ☐ **A.** Partial dryness of the mouth due to lack of salivary secretions from the submandibular and sublingual glands
- ☐ **B.** Partial dryness of the mouth due to lack of salivary secretions from the parotid gland
- ☐ **C.** Dryness of the right cornea due to lack of lacrimal gland secretion
- ☐ **D.** Loss of taste sensation from the right anterior two thirds of the tongue
- ☐ **E.** Loss of general sensation from the right anterior two thirds of the tongue

72 A 12-year-old girl is admitted to the emergency department with a middle ear infection. Physical examination reveals a long history of chronic middle ear infections that have produced a lesion in the tympanic plexus in the middle ear cavity. Since the preganglionic parasympathetic fibers that pass through the plexus have been lost, which of the following conditions will be detectable during physical examination?

- ☐ **A.** Diminished mucus in the nasal cavity
- ☐ **B.** Diminished mucus on the soft palate
- ☐ **C.** Diminished saliva production by the parotid gland
- ☐ **D.** Diminished saliva production by the submandibular and sublingual glands
- ☐ **E.** Diminished tear production by the lacrimal gland

73 A 38-year-old woman is admitted to the dental clinic with acute dental pain. The attending dentist found penetrating dental caries (tooth decay) affecting one of the mandibular molar teeth. Which of the following nerves would the dentist need to anesthetize to treat the caries in that tooth?

- ☐ **A.** Lingual
- ☐ **B.** Inferior alveolar
- ☐ **C.** Buccal
- ☐ **D.** Mental
- ☐ **E.** Mylohyoid

74 A 59-year-old man is admitted to the emergency department with acute pain on his mandible. An MRI examination reveals an acute inflammation of the temporomandibular joint due to arthritis. Which of the following muscles will most likely be affected by the inflammatory process of this joint?

- ☐ **A.** Temporalis
- ☐ **B.** Medial pterygoid
- ☐ **C.** Masseter
- ☐ **D.** Lateral pterygoid
- ☐ **E.** Buccinator

75 A 56-year-old woman complains of diplopia (double vision) when walking down stairs. A lesion of which of the following nerves is most likely responsible for this patient's complaint?

- ☐ **A.** Optic
- ☐ **B.** Oculomotor
- ☐ **C.** Abducens
- ☐ **D.** Trochlear
- ☐ **E.** Frontal

76 A 43-year-old man is admitted to the hospital complaining of diplopia (double vision) when walking down stairs. During physical examination of the extraocular muscles the patient experiences diplopia, and when he is asked to turn his right eye inward toward his nose and look down, he is able to look inward but not down. Which nerve is most likely involved?

- ☐ **A.** Abducens
- ☐ **B.** Nasociliary
- ☐ **C.** Oculomotor, inferior division

- ▢ **D.** Oculomotor, superior division
- ▢ **E.** Trochlear

77 A 44-year-old woman is being treated for Raynaud's disease. A sympathetic blocking drug is administered in high doses. Which of the following conditions will most likely be expected to occur as an adverse effect of the drug?

- ▢ **A.** Exophthalmos and dilated pupil
- ▢ **B.** Enophthalmos and dry eye
- ▢ **C.** Dry eye and inability to accommodate for reading
- ▢ **D.** Wide open eyelids and loss of depth perception
- ▢ **E.** Ptosis and miosis

78 A 47-year-old woman is admitted to the hospital with signs of cavernous sinus thrombosis. Radiographic examination reveals a pituitary tumor involving the cavernous sinus, confirming the initial diagnosis (Fig. 7-3). During physical examination it is suspected that the right abducens nerve of the patient has been damaged by the tumor. In which direction will the physician most likely ask the patient to turn her right eye to confirm the abducens nerve damage, assuming she is unable to perform this task?

- ▢ **A.** Inward
- ▢ **B.** Outward
- ▢ **C.** Downward
- ▢ **D.** Down and out
- ▢ **E.** Down and in

79 An 8-year-old boy is admitted to the hospital with a drooping right eyelid (ptosis) (Fig. 7-4). The initial diagnosis is Horner's syndrome. Which of the following additional signs on the right side would confirm the diagnosis?

- ▢ **A.** Constricted pupil
- ▢ **B.** Dry eye
- ▢ **C.** Exophthalmos
- ▢ **D.** Pale, blanched face
- ▢ **E.** Sweaty face

80 A 32-year-old woman is admitted to the hospital with headaches and dizziness. During physical examination it is noted that the patient has partial ptosis (drooping eyelid). Which of the following muscles is most likely paralyzed?

- ▢ **A.** Orbicularis oculi, lacrimal part
- ▢ **B.** Orbicularis oculi, palpebral part
- ▢ **C.** Levator palpebrae superioris
- ▢ **D.** Superior oblique
- ▢ **E.** Superior tarsal (of Müller)

81 A 16 year-old boy is admitted to the hospital with fever, a confused mental state, and drowsiness. During physical examination it is noted that the boy suffers from severe acne. Radiologic examination reveals cavernous sinus thrombosis. Which of the following routes of entry to the cavernous sinus would most likely be responsible for the infection and thrombosis?

- ▢ **A.** Carotid artery
- ▢ **B.** Mastoid emissary vein

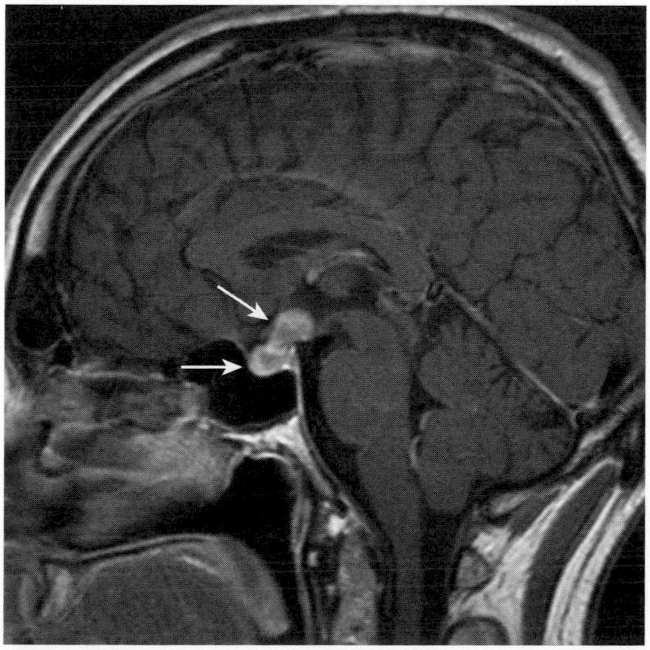

Fig. 7-3

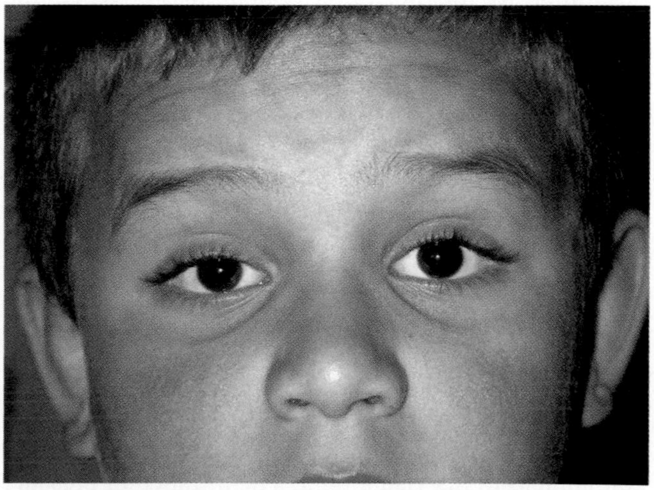

Fig. 7-4

- ▢ **C.** Middle meningeal artery
- ▢ **D.** Ophthalmic vein
- ▢ **E.** Parietal emissary vein

82 A 68-year-old man is admitted to the emergency department after an acute cerebral vascular accident (stroke). Radiologic studies reveal that the primary damage was to the anterior inferior cerebellar artery, resulting in a small hemorrhage of the artery at its origin from the main trunk. Which of the following nerves will most likely be immediately affected by the hemorrhage?

- ▢ **A.** Optic nerve
- ▢ **B.** Oculomotor nerve
- ▢ **C.** Trochlear nerve
- ▢ **D.** Trigeminal nerve
- ▢ **E.** Abducens nerve

83 A 5-year-old boy is admitted to the hospital with otitis media. Otoscopic examination reveals a bulging and inflamed eardrum. It is decided to incise the tympanic membrane to relieve the painful pressure and allow drainage of the infectious fluid associated with otitis media. Which of the following is the best location to make an opening (myringotomy) for drainage?

- ▢ **A.** The anterior superior quadrant of the eardrum
- ▢ **B.** The posterior superior quadrant of the eardrum
- ▢ **C.** Directly through the site of the umbo
- ▢ **D.** The anterior inferior quadrant of the eardrum
- ▢ **E.** A vertical incision should be made in the eardrum, from the 12 o'clock position of the rim of the eardrum to the 6 o'clock position of the rim

84 A 56-year-old man is diagnosed with an extradural tumor in the posterior cranial fossa. When the patient protruded his tongue during physical examination, the tongue deviated to the right. Which of the following muscles and nerves are most likely injured?

- ▢ **A.** Right hypoglossal nerve and right genioglossus
- ▢ **B.** Left hypoglossal nerve and left genioglossus
- ▢ **C.** Right hyoglossus and left styloglossus
- ▢ **D.** Right geniohyoid and first cervical nerve
- ▢ **E.** Contralateral vagus and hypoglossal nerves

85 A 62-year-old man is admitted to the hospital with blurred vision. Taking of his history and performance of a physical examination reveals a long history of gradual loss of his visual field. The intraocular pressure is high, and a diagnosis of glaucoma is made. Which of the following spaces first receives the aqueous humor secreted by the epithelium of the ciliary body?

- ▢ **A.** Anterior chamber
- ▢ **B.** Posterior chamber
- ▢ **C.** Pupil
- ▢ **D.** Vitreous
- ▢ **E.** Lacrimal sac

86 A 17-year-old girl is admitted to the hospital with tonsillitis. A tonsillectomy is performed and the patient complains postoperatively of ear pain. Which of the following nerves was most likely injured during the surgical procedure?

- ▢ **A.** Auriculotemporal
- ▢ **B.** Lesser petrosal
- ▢ **C.** Vagus
- ▢ **D.** Glossopharyngeal
- ▢ **E.** Chorda tympani

87 A 49-year-old woman is admitted to the hospital with headaches and dizziness. Radiologic examination reveals a tumor in the jugular canal. Upon physical examination, when the right side of the pharyngeal wall is touched with a tongue depressor, the uvula deviates to the left and the left pharyngeal wall contracts upward. When the left pharyngeal wall is touched, the response is similar. Which of the following nerves is most likely to have been injured by the tumor?

- ▢ **A.** Right glossopharyngeal
- ▢ **B.** Left glossopharyngeal
- ▢ **C.** Right mandibular
- ▢ **D.** Left hypoglossal
- ▢ **E.** Right vagus

88 A 45-year-old man is admitted to the emergency department with severe dyspnea. During physical examination there is swelling in the floor of his mouth and pharynx and his airway is nearly totally occluded. In addition, there is a swelling in his lower jaw and upper neck. His physical history indicates that one of his lower molars was extracted a week ago and he had been feeling worse every day since. Which of the following conditions will be the most likely diagnosis?

- ▢ **A.** Quinsy
- ▢ **B.** Torus palatinus
- ▢ **C.** Ankyloglossia
- ▢ **D.** Ranula
- ▢ **E.** Ludwig's angina

89 A 5-year-old girl is admitted to the hospital with an upper respiratory tract infection. During physical examination her sense of hearing appears to be poor. Her right ear is painful, and upon otoscopic examination a golden brown fluid can be observed through the tympanic membrane. Which is the most likely direct route for the spread of an infection from the upper respiratory tract to the middle ear cavity?

- ▢ **A.** Pharyngotympanic tube
- ▢ **B.** Choanae
- ▢ **C.** Nostrils
- ▢ **D.** Facial canal
- ▢ **E.** Internal acoustic meatus

90 A 54-year-old man is admitted to the hospital with severe pain in his nasal cavity. Radiographic examination reveals a carcinoma in his nasal cavity. In which of the following locations would the carcinoma block the hiatus of the maxillary sinus?

- ▢ **A.** Inferior meatus
- ▢ **B.** Middle meatus
- ▢ **C.** Superior meatus
- ▢ **D.** Nasopharynx
- ▢ **E.** Sphenoethmoidal recess

91 A 54-year-old man is diagnosed with an aneurysm of the basilar artery close to the cavernous sinus. An anterior approach to the sella turcica through the nasal cavity is performed. Through which of the following routes is the surgeon most likely to gain access to the cranial cavity?

- ▢ **A.** Cribriform plate
- ▢ **B.** Cavernous sinus
- ▢ **C.** Frontal sinus
- ▢ **D.** Maxillary sinus
- ▢ **E.** Sphenoidal sinus

92 A 10-year-old girl is admitted to the hospital with tonsillitis. A tonsillectomy is performed and the tonsils are removed. On physical examination 1 week later the patient has absence of the gag reflex on the left when the posterior part of the tongue is depressed. The sensory portion of which of the following nerves was most likely injured?

- ▢ **A.** Facial
- ▢ **B.** Glossopharyngeal
- ▢ **C.** Mandibular
- ▢ **D.** Maxillary
- ▢ **E.** Hypoglossal

93 A 56-year-old woman has just undergone a complete thyroidectomy. After she recovers from the anesthesia a hoarseness of her voice is noted that persists for 3 weeks. Subsequent examination shows a permanently adducted vocal fold on the right side. Surgical trauma to the innervation of which of the following muscles is most likely to be responsible for the position of the right vocal fold?

- ▢ **A.** Aryepiglottic
- ▢ **B.** Posterior cricoarytenoid
- ▢ **C.** Thyroarytenoid
- ▢ **D.** Transverse arytenoids
- ▢ **E.** Vocalis

94 A 45-year-old man with a complaint of ear pain, difficulty hearing in one ear, nose bleeds, and difficulty breathing through the nose is diagnosed with postnasal carcinoma. Otoscopic examination reveals fluid in the middle ear cavity. Hypertrophy of which of the following structures would be most likely to compromise the drainage of the auditory tube

- ▢ **A.** Lingual tonsil
- ▢ **B.** Palatine tonsil
- ▢ **C.** Pharyngeal tonsil
- ▢ **D.** Superior constrictor muscle
- ▢ **E.** Uvula

95 While at summer camp, a 10-year-old boy develops severe pharyngitis and swollen tonsils. Infection may spread from the nasopharynx to the middle ear cavity along the derivative of which embryonic pharyngeal pouch?

- ▢ **A.** First
- ▢ **B.** Second
- ▢ **C.** Third
- ▢ **D.** Fourth
- ▢ **E.** Sixth

96 A 25-year-old medical student discovers that his alarm has not worked and he is running late. Desperate to get to his biochemistry lecture in time, yet unbearably hungry, he quickly throws some bread in the toaster as he gets ready. Despite the toast burning a little, he eats it quickly and rushes out the door. The burnt parts of the toast scratch the roof of his mouth, leaving him with a stinging sensation there. What nerve is collecting this sensation from the hard palate?

- ▢ **A.** Posterior superior alveolar nerve
- ▢ **B.** Inferior alveolar nerve
- ▢ **C.** Lingual nerve
- ▢ **D.** Greater palatine nerve
- ▢ **E.** Lesser palatine nerve

97 A 32-year-old woman underwent a thyroidectomy. Two months postoperatively, it was observed that the patient had lost the ability to notice the presence of foreign objects in the laryngeal vestibule. Which of the following nerves was most likely injured?

- ▢ **A.** Internal laryngeal nerve
- ▢ **B.** External laryngeal nerve
- ▢ **C.** Glossopharyngeal nerve
- ▢ **D.** Hypoglossal nerve
- ▢ **E.** Recurrent laryngeal nerve

98 A 4-year-old boy suffering from ankyloglossia is brought to the speech therapist. The examining physician recommends that the child be admitted for operation by a pediatric surgeon. Which of the following surgical procedures would be most appropriate for this condition?

- ▢ **A.** Removal of pterygomandibular raphe
- ▢ **B.** Resection of the pterygoid hamulus bilaterally
- ▢ **C.** Cutting the lingual frenulum
- ▢ **D.** Repair of the palate
- ▢ **E.** Removal of the central segment of the hyoid bone

99 An 8-year-old boy was suffering from a severe infection of the right middle ear. Within the course of a week, the infection had spread to the mastoid antrum and the mastoid air cells. The organisms did not respond to antibiotics, so the surgeon decided to perform a radical mastoid operation. Following the operation, it was noticed that the boy's face was distorted. The mouth was drawn upward to the left, and he was unable to close his right eye. Saliva tended to accumulate in his right cheek and dribble from the corner of his mouth. What structure was most likely damaged during the operation?

- ▢ **A.** Mandibular nerve
- ▢ **B.** Parotid duct
- ▢ **C.** Vagus nerve
- ▢ **D.** Facial nerve
- ▢ **E.** Glossopharyngeal nerve

100 An 8-year-old boy had a mastoidectomy due to an infection that did not respond to antibiotics. Postoperatively he had Bell's palsy (facial paralysis), and one of the features was the accumulation of saliva in the vestibule of his oral cavity and dribble from the corner of his mouth. Which of the following muscles was most likely paralyzed?

- ▢ **A.** Zygomaticus major
- ▢ **B.** Orbicularis oculi
- ▢ **C.** Buccinator
- ▢ **D.** Levator palpebrae superioris
- ▢ **E.** Orbicularis oris

101 A 32-year-old man is admitted to the emergency department with visual problems. Radiographic examination reveals a tumor of the adenohypophysis (anterior pituitary gland). Physical examination reveals a loss of the lateral halves of the fields of vision of both eyes (bitemporal hemianopia or "tunnel vision"). Which of the following structures was most likely compressed by the tumor?

- ▢ **A.** Optic nerve
- ▢ **B.** Optic chiasm
- ▢ **C.** Optic tract
- ▢ **D.** Oculomotor
- ▢ **E.** Abducens nerve

102 A 45-year-old woman is admitted to the emergency department with vision problems when she walks down stairs. During physical examination the patient exhibits weakness of her downward medial gaze. Cerebral arteriography and an MRI indicate that a nerve is being compressed by an arterial aneurysm just inferior to the tentorium cerebelli. Which of the following arteries and nerves is most likely being compressed?

- ▢ **A.** Internal carotid artery/abducens nerve
- ▢ **B.** Middle cerebral artery/oculomotor nerve
- ▢ **C.** Posterior cerebral artery/ophthalmic nerve
- ▢ **D.** Basilar artery/ophthalmic nerve
- ▢ **E.** Superior cerebellar artery/trochlear nerve

103 A 72-year-old woman is admitted to the emergency department with tenderness in the upper right thorax, painful to compression. During physical examination the patient presents with slight ptosis of her right eyelid. The right pupil is constricted more distinctly than the contralateral pupil. Which of the following is the most likely diagnosis?

- ▢ **A.** Raynaud's disease
- ▢ **B.** Frey's syndrome
- ▢ **C.** Bell's palsy
- ▢ **D.** Quinsy
- ▢ **E.** Pancoast tumor

104 A 32-year-old man is admitted to the hospital with severe headache and visual problems. The dilator pupillae muscle, the smooth muscle cell fibers of the superior tarsal muscle (of Müller, part of the levator palpebrae superioris), and the smooth muscle cells of the blood vessels of the ciliary body are supplied by efferent nerve fibers. Which of the following structures contains the neural cell bodies of these fibers?

- ▢ **A.** Pterygopalatine ganglion
- ▢ **B.** Intermediolateral nucleus (lateral horn) C1 to C4
- ▢ **C.** Geniculate ganglion
- ▢ **D.** Nucleus solitarius
- ▢ **E.** Superior cervical ganglion

105 A 22-year-old man is admitted to the hospital after he was hit in the right eye with a frozen fish, thrown playfully by a friend while they were passing through the seafood section of the market. During physical examination considerable swelling and discoloration of the eyelids was observed. In addition, the patient could not turn his pupil laterally from forward gaze, indicating probable muscle entrapment. Which of the following bones was most likely fractured?

- ▢ **A.** Orbital plate of the frontal bone
- ▢ **B.** Lamina papyracea of the ethmoid bone
- ▢ **C.** Orbital plate of the maxilla
- ▢ **D.** Cribriform plate of the ethmoid bone
- ▢ **E.** Greater wing of the sphenoid bone

106 A 57-year-old man is admitted to the emergency department with dizziness and severe headaches. A CT scan evaluation reveals a tumor in the superior orbital fissure. Upon physical examination the patient's eyeball is fixed in an abducted position, slightly depressed, and the pupil is dilated. In addition, the upper lid is droopy. When the patient is asked to move the pupil toward the nose, the pupil rotates medially. Consensual corneal reflexes are normal. Which of the following nerves is most likely affected?

- ▢ **A.** Trochlear nerve
- ▢ **B.** Oculomotor nerve
- ▢ **C.** Abducens nerve and sympathetic nerve plexus accompanying the ophthalmic artery
- ▢ **D.** Ophthalmic nerve and short ciliary nerve
- ▢ **E.** Superior division of oculomotor nerve and the nasociliary nerve

107 A 57-year-old man is transported to the emergency department after falling from a tree. A CT scan reveals a fracture of the cribriform plate (Fig. 7-5). Which of the following conditions will most likely be present during the physical examination?

- ▢ **A.** Entrapment of the eyeball
- ▢ **B.** Anosmia
- ▢ **C.** Hyperacusis

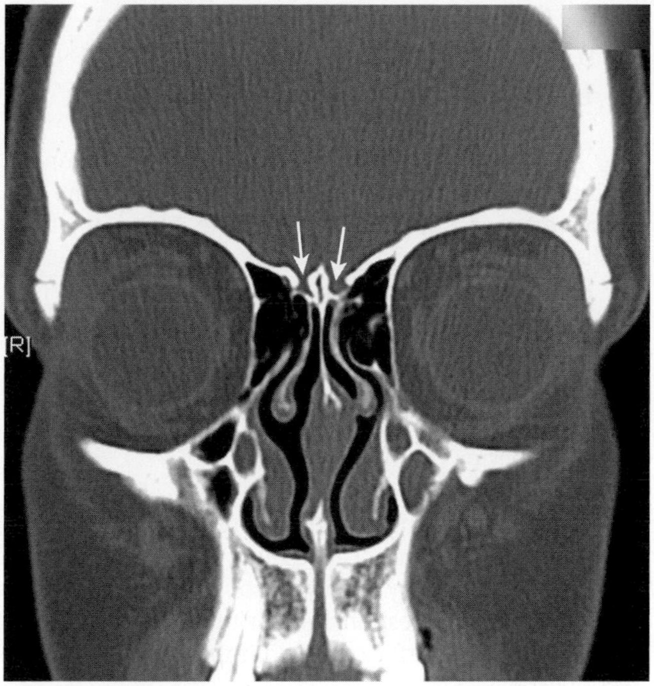

Fig. 7-5

- ▢ **D.** Tinnitus
- ▢ **E.** Deafness

108 A 45-year-old woman is admitted to the hospital with swelling on the side of her face of 2 months duration. Radiographic examination reveals a parotid gland tumor. An operative procedure is performed in which the tumor is removed. Three months postoperatively the patient complains that her face sweats profusely when she tastes or smells food, and a diagnosis is made of Frey's syndrome (gustatory sweating). Which of the following nerves was most likely injured during the procedure?

- ▢ **A.** Buccal
- ▢ **B.** Inferior alveolar
- ▢ **C.** Auriculotemporal
- ▢ **D.** Facial
- ▢ **E.** Lingual

109 A 54-year-old man is to undergo bilateral thyroidectomy. During this procedure there is the possibility of bilateral paralysis of muscles that can open the airway. If a particular nerve is injured bilaterally, there is significant risk of asphyxiation postoperatively unless the patient is intubated or the airway is opened surgically. Which of the following muscle pairs opens the airway?

- ▢ **A.** Cricothyroids
- ▢ **B.** Posterior cricoarytenoids

- ▢ **C.** Arytenoids
- ▢ **D.** Thyroarytenoids
- ▢ **E.** Lateral cricoarytenoids

110 An 11-year-old boy with swollen palatine tonsils is examined by an otolaryngologist. Which of the following arteries supplies most of the blood to these tonsils?

- ▢ **A.** Ascending pharyngeal
- ▢ **B.** Facial
- ▢ **C.** Lingual
- ▢ **D.** Descending palatine
- ▢ **E.** Superior thyroid

111 A 55-year-old man with severe ear pain visits an otorhinolaryngologist because his tympanic membrane has been ruptured by a foreign object. Which of the following nerves is responsible for the sensory innervation of the inner surface of the tympanic membrane?

- ▢ **A.** Glossopharyngeal
- ▢ **B.** Auricular branch of facial
- ▢ **C.** Auricular branch of vagus
- ▢ **D.** Great auricular
- ▢ **E.** Lingual

112 A 45-year-old man was suffering from trigeminal neuralgia (tic douloureux). The pain was so severe that the patient had considered suicide as a way to escape the pain. Even light, gentle stimuli to the skin between the lower eyelid and the upper lip resulted in severe, agonizing pain. It was decided to lesion the nerve branch involved by injecting alcohol into the nerve. To reach the nerve, the needle will most likely need to be inserted through which of the following openings?

- ▢ **A.** Foramen ovale
- ▢ **B.** Foramen spinosum
- ▢ **C.** Infraorbital foramen
- ▢ **D.** Mandibular foramen
- ▢ **E.** Foramen magnum

113 A 32-year-old woman is undergoing a thyroidectomy. Postoperatively the patient suffers from loss of sensation within the larynx from the vocal folds upward to the entrance into the larynx, allowing for aspiration of liquids into the airway. Which of the following nerves is most likely injured?

- ▢ **A.** Internal laryngeal nerve
- ▢ **B.** External laryngeal nerve
- ▢ **C.** Glossopharyngeal nerve
- ▢ **D.** Hypoglossal nerve
- ▢ **E.** Recurrent laryngeal nerve

114 A 55-year-old man is admitted to the emergency department after slipping on wet pavement and falling. Physical examination reveals that the patient has a hematoma that formed in the danger zone of the scalp, spreading to the area of the eyelids. Which of the following layers is regarded as the "danger zone"?

- ▢ **A.** Loose, areolar layer
- ▢ **B.** Skin
- ▢ **C.** Galea aponeurotica
- ▢ **D.** Pericranium
- ▢ **E.** Subcutaneous layer

115 A 45-year-old woman is admitted to the hospital with a severe headache. The patient is diagnosed with hypertension and arrhythmias. To reduce the patient's blood pressure, massage is initiated at a pressure point located deep to the anterior border of the sternocleidomastoid muscle at the level of the superior border of the thyroid cartilage. Which of the following structures is targeted by the massage?

- ▢ **A.** Carotid sinus
- ▢ **B.** Carotid body
- ▢ **C.** Thyroid gland
- ▢ **D.** Parathyroid gland
- ▢ **E.** Inferior cervical ganglion

116 A 59-year-old painter fell from the scaffolding and was admitted to the emergency department unconscious. An emergency tracheostomy is performed, and brisk arterial bleeding suddenly occurs from the midline incision over the trachea. Which of the following vessels was most likely cut accidentally?

- ▢ **A.** Inferior thyroid branch of thyrocervical trunk
- ▢ **B.** Cricothyroid branch of the superior thyroid artery
- ▢ **C.** Thyroidea ima artery
- ▢ **D.** Middle thyroid vein
- ▢ **E.** Jugular arch connecting the anterior jugular veins

117 A 21-year-old male baseball player is brought to the emergency department after having severe dizziness. During physical examination the patient demonstrates lack of equilibrium and memory impairment. A 3-cm wound is noted in his scalp from an injury suffered in a game several weeks earlier. A lumbar puncture does not reveal blood in the CSF. Which of the following is the most likely diagnosis?

- ☐ **A.** The middle meningeal artery was torn, resulting in epidural hematoma
- ☐ **B.** There is a fracture in the pterion with injury to the adjacent vasculature
- ☐ **C.** The injury resulted in the bursting of a preexisting aneurysm of the anterior communicating artery of the cerebral circle
- ☐ **D.** A cerebral vein is torn
- ☐ **E.** The cavernous sinus has a thrombus

118 A 63-year-old man had his prostate gland tumor removed 2 years before his present admission to the hospital, complaining of various neurologic problems including headaches. Radiographic examination reveals that the cancer has spread from the pelvis to the posterior cranial fossa by way of the internal vertebral venous plexus (of Batson). During physical examination the patient's right shoulder droops noticeably lower than the left, he exhibits considerable weakness in turning his head to the left, and his tongue points to the right when he attempts to protrude it directly from his mouth. There are no other significant findings. Which of the following nerves are most likely affected?

- ☐ **A.** Right vagus, right accessory, and right hypoglossal nerves
- ☐ **B.** Left accessory, right glossopharyngeal, right vagus, and left hypoglossal nerves
- ☐ **C.** Left hypoglossal, right trigeminal, and left glossopharyngeal nerves
- ☐ **D.** Right accessory and right hypoglossal nerves
- ☐ **E.** Left facial, left accessory, right accessory, and vagus nerves

119 A 3-month-old male infant is admitted to the hospital because he cries continuously. During physical examination it is observed that the infant has a dry right eye. Upon the basis of imaging studies, the neuro-ophthalmologist diagnoses a lesion at the neural cell bodies of the preganglionic axons of the fibers that terminate in the pterygopalatine ganglion. Which of the following structures contains the neural cell bodies of the preganglionic axons?

- ☐ **A.** Superior cervical ganglion
- ☐ **B.** Edinger-Westphal nucleus
- ☐ **C.** Superior salivatory nucleus
- ☐ **D.** Inferior salivatory nucleus
- ☐ **E.** Nucleus ambiguus

120 A 14-year-old girl has been suffering from peritonsillar abscess (quinsy) on the right side of her oropharynx. During surgical removal of the pathologic tissue, or during incision and drainage of the area, which of the following arteries will be at greatest risk?

- ☐ **A.** Lingual
- ☐ **B.** A branch of facial
- ☐ **C.** Superior laryngeal artery
- ☐ **D.** Ascending pharyngeal artery
- ☐ **E.** Descending palatine artery

121 A 17-year-old girl visits a dermatologist because of severe facial acne. During physical examination a rather obvious and painful lesion on the side of her nose was found. The patient was given antibiotics and warned not to press or pick at the large, inflamed swelling. If she were to squeeze, prick, or incise such a lesion in the area between the eye and the upper lip, or between the eye and the side of the nose, the infection could spread to the cavernous sinus. Which of the following pathways of spread of infection would be most typical?

- ☐ **A.** Nasal venous tributary to angular vein, to superior ophthalmic vein, then to cavernous sinus
- ☐ **B.** Retromandibular vein to supraorbital vein, then to inferior ophthalmic vein, then to cavernous sinus
- ☐ **C.** Dorsal nasal vein to superior petrosal vein, then inferior ophthalmic vein to cavernous sinus
- ☐ **D.** Facial vein to maxillary vein, then middle meningeal vein to cavernous sinus
- ☐ **E.** Transverse facial vein to superficial temporal vein to emissary vein to cavernous sinus

122 A 73-year-old man visits the outpatient clinic with a complaint of progressive, painless loss of vision. Radiographic examination reveals thrombophlebitis of the cavernous sinus. Through which of the following structures must a thrombus pass to cause the symptoms of this patient?

- ☐ **A.** Subarachnoid space
- ☐ **B.** Central artery of the retina
- ☐ **C.** Central vein of the retina
- ☐ **D.** Optic chiasm
- ☐ **E.** Ciliary ganglion

123 A 67-year-old man visits the outpatient clinic with complaints of deteriorating vision. A form of glaucoma is diagnosed in which the aqueous humor does not drain properly into the scleral venous sinus at the iridoscleral angle of the eyeball. The aqueous fluid is secreted by the epithelium of the ciliary body directly into which of the following spaces?

- ☐ **A.** Iridoscleral angle
- ☐ **B.** Posterior chamber

- ☐ **C.** Pupil
- ☐ **D.** Vitreous body
- ☐ **E.** Lacrimal sac

124 A 2-month-old female infant is hospitalized with hydrocephalus. MRI reveals a ventricular system that is entirely dilated. Which of the following conditions will most likely lead to this type of clinical picture?

- ☐ **A.** Lack of absorption through arachnoid granulations into venous system
- ☐ **B.** Occlusion of cerebral aqueduct (of Sylvius)
- ☐ **C.** Blockage of the left foramina of Luschka
- ☐ **D.** Congenital absence of the cisterna magna
- ☐ **E.** Closure of the interventricular foramina of Monro

125 A 54-year-old man was admitted to the emergency department after he was struck by an automobile. Radiographic examination revealed a fracture through the crista galli of the anterior cranial fossa, resulting in slow, local bleeding. Which of the following is the most likely source of bleeding?

- ☐ **A.** Middle meningeal artery
- ☐ **B.** The great cerebral vein of Galen
- ☐ **C.** Superior sagittal sinus
- ☐ **D.** Straight sinus
- ☐ **E.** Superior ophthalmic vein

126 During a routine ophthalmologic exam, the globe, the retina, and the cornea of each eye are tested. Which of the following nerves must be functioning properly if the patient is to be able to turn the eye laterally (abduction) without difficulty and without upward or downward deviation?

- ☐ **A.** Superior division of oculomotor, ophthalmic nerve, abducens nerve
- ☐ **B.** Trochlear nerve, abducens nerve, nasociliary nerve
- ☐ **C.** Inferior division of oculomotor, trochlear, abducens
- ☐ **D.** Oculomotor and ophthalmic nerves
- ☐ **E.** Superior division of oculomotor, trochlear, and abducens nerves

127 A 34-year-old woman is admitted to the hospital because of hoarseness for the past 3 months. Radiologic examination reveals a cancerous growth in her larynx with no evidence of metastasis. In addition, the area in which the tumor is growing is characterized by very limited lymphatic drainage. Which of the following locations is most likely to contain a tumor with these characteristics?

- ☐ **A.** Anterior commissure of the vocal ligaments
- ☐ **B.** Interarytenoid fold
- ☐ **C.** Laryngeal ventricle
- ☐ **D.** Cricothyroid ligament
- ☐ **E.** Middle segment of the vocal cord

128 A 55-year-old man is admitted to the hospital with a complaint of severe headaches. A lumbar puncture reveals traces of blood in the CSF. Which of the following conditions has most likely occurred in this patient?

- ☐ **A.** Fracture of the pterion with vascular injury
- ☐ **B.** A ruptured "berry" aneurysm
- ☐ **C.** Leakage of branches of the middle meningeal vein within the temporal bone
- ☐ **D.** A tear of the cerebral vein at the entrance to the superior sagittal sinus
- ☐ **E.** Occlusion of the internal carotid artery by a clot generated in the left atrium

129 A 55-year-old man is admitted to the neurosurgical clinic for a scheduled removal of a tumor in the left jugular canal. Postoperatively, the patient has no gag reflex when the ipsilateral pharyngeal wall is stimulated, although the pharynx moved upward and a gag reflex resulted when the right pharyngeal wall was stimulated. The uvula was deviated to the right and the left vocal cord had drifted toward the midline. Which of the following structures will contain the neural cell bodies for the motor supply of the paralyzed muscles?

- ☐ **A.** Nucleus solitarius
- ☐ **B.** Trigeminal motor nucleus
- ☐ **C.** Dorsal motor nucleus
- ☐ **D.** Nucleus ambiguus
- ☐ **E.** Superior or inferior ganglia of vagus

130 A 65-year-old man is admitted to the emergency department after his head hit the dashboard in an automobile collision. Radiographic and physical examinations reveal that the inferior alveolar nerve is injured at its origin. Which of the following muscles would most likely be paralyzed as a result?

- ☐ **A.** Geniohyoid
- ☐ **B.** Hyoglossus
- ☐ **C.** Mylohyoid
- ☐ **D.** Stylohyoid
- ☐ **E.** Palatoglossus

131 An unconscious 64-year-old man is admitted to the hospital. A CT scan examination reveals that the patient has suffered a cerebral vascular accident (stroke), with a small hematoma produced by the superior cerebellar artery. Which of the following nerves will most likely be affected by the hematoma?

- ▢ **A.** Trochlear nerve
- ▢ **B.** Abducens nerve
- ▢ **C.** Facial nerve
- ▢ **D.** Vestibulocochlear nerve
- ▢ **E.** Glossopharyngeal nerve

132 A 65-year-old man is admitted to the hospital 3 weeks after a "small bump of his head," according to his narrative. He suffered the accidental bump from a low-hanging branch while driving his tractor through the apple orchard during harvesting season. During physical examination the patient displays mental confusion and poor physical coordination. Radiologic examination reveals an intracranial thrombus probably due to leakage from a cerebral vein over the right cerebral hemisphere. From what type of bleeding is the patient most likely suffering?

- ▢ **A.** Subarachnoid bleeding
- ▢ **B.** Epidural bleeding
- ▢ **C.** Intracerebral bleeding into the brain parenchyma
- ▢ **D.** Subdural bleeding
- ▢ **E.** Bleeding into the cerebral ventricular system

133 A 27-year-old man is admitted to the hospital after a middleweight boxing match. During physical examination the strength and symmetry of strength in opening the jaws are tested. Which of the following muscles is the most important in jaw protrusion and depressing the mandible?

- ▢ **A.** Anterior portion of temporalis
- ▢ **B.** Lateral pterygoid
- ▢ **C.** Medial pterygoid
- ▢ **D.** Masseter
- ▢ **E.** Platysma

134 A 31-year-old mother visits the pediatric outpatient clinic with her 6-month-old baby girl complaining that her baby is not developing quickly and has no teeth. Which of the following teeth are expected to appear first?

- ▢ **A.** Superior medial incisors at 8 to 10 months of age
- ▢ **B.** Inferior medial incisors at 6 to 8 months of age
- ▢ **C.** Superior lateral incisors at 8 to 10 months of age
- ▢ **D.** Inferior lateral incisors at 12 to 14 months of age
- ▢ **E.** First molar at 6 to 8 months of age

135 A 56-year-old man visits the outpatient clinic with a complaint of severe headaches and ear pain. Radiologic examination reveals a tumor in the middle ear cavity, invading through the bony floor. Which of the following structures will most likely be affected?

- ▢ **A.** The cochlea and lateral semicircular canal
- ▢ **B.** The internal carotid artery
- ▢ **C.** The sigmoid venous sinus
- ▢ **D.** The internal jugular bulb
- ▢ **E.** The aditus ad antrum of the mastoid region and the facial nerve

136 A 52-year-old man is admitted to the emergency department with a bullet wound in the infratemporal fossa. During physical examination it is observed that the patient has lost unilateral sensation of hot, cold, pain, and pressure from the front part of the tongue, but taste and salivary function are preserved. Which of the following is the most likely diagnosis?

- ▢ **A.** The facial nerve was transected distal to the origin of the chorda tympani
- ▢ **B.** Receptors for hot, cold, pain, and pressure are absent in the patient's tongue
- ▢ **C.** The glossopharyngeal nerve has been injured in the pharynx
- ▢ **D.** The superior laryngeal nerve was obviously severed by the bullet
- ▢ **E.** The lingual nerve was injured at its origin near the foramen ovale

137 A 12-year-old boy is admitted to the emergency department with signs of meningitis. To determine the specific type of meningitis (i.e., viral or bacterial), it is necessary to aspirate CSF with a lumbar puncture for laboratory examination. However, before performing a lumbar puncture, it must be established that the CSF pressure is not elevated. What condition in the eye would indicate that CSF pressure is too elevated for a lumbar puncture to be performed?

- ▢ **A.** Papilledema
- ▢ **B.** Separation of the pars optica retinae anterior to the ora serrata
- ▢ **C.** The foveal centralis exhibits hemorrhage from medial retinal branches
- ▢ **D.** Obvious opacity of the lens
- ▢ **E.** Pitting or compression of the optic disc

138 A 65-year-old woman is admitted to the hospital with signs of cavernous sinus thrombosis. Radiographic examination reveals an aneurysm of the internal carotid artery within the cavernous sinus. During physical examination what sign would one expect to see first if nerve compression has occurred within the cavernous sinus?

- ☐ **A.** Inability to gaze downward and medially on the affected side
- ☐ **B.** Complete ptosis of the superior palpebra (upper eyelid)
- ☐ **C.** Bilateral loss of accommodation and loss of direct pupillary reflex
- ☐ **D.** Ipsilateral loss of the consensual corneal reflex
- ☐ **E.** Ipsilateral paralysis of abduction of the pupil

139 A 54-year-old man is admitted to the emergency department with a fracture at the frontozygomatic suture suffered in an automobile collision. During physical examination the upper eyelid of the patient exhibits multiple lacerations and the sclera contains small fragments from his broken glasses. What site would be preferable for needle insertion to anesthetize the orbital contents and then the area of the eyelid injury?

- ☐ **A.** Into the sclera in the limbic region and also into the infraorbital foramen
- ☐ **B.** Into the lacrimal fossa and also beneath the lateral bulbar conjunctiva
- ☐ **C.** Into the supraorbital foramen and also into the lacrimal caruncle
- ☐ **D.** Through the upper eyelid deeply toward the orbital apex and also between the orbital septum and the palpebral musculature laterally
- ☐ **E.** Directly posteriorly through the anulus tendineus and superior orbital fissure

140 A 45-year-old male construction worker slips and falls on a nail protruding from a board. The nail penetrates the skin overlying the submental triangle lateral to the midline. Which of the following muscles would be the last to be penetrated?

- ☐ **A.** Platysma
- ☐ **B.** Mylohyoid
- ☐ **C.** Anterior belly of the digastric
- ☐ **D.** Geniohyoid
- ☐ **E.** Genioglossus

141 A 55-year-old woman has undergone facial surgery for the excision of a malignant parotid tumor. Postoperatively, marked weakness is seen in the musculature of the patient's lower lip. Which of the following nerves was most likely injured during the parotidectomy?

- ☐ **A.** Marginal mandibular branch of facial
- ☐ **B.** Zygomatic branch of facial
- ☐ **C.** Mandibular division of the trigeminal nerve
- ☐ **D.** Buccal branch of facial
- ☐ **E.** Buccal nerve

142 A 15-year-old boy is admitted to the emergency department with severe headache and hydrocephalus. Radiographic examination reveals a craniopharyngioma occupying the sella turcica, primarily involving the suprasellar space. Which of the following is the most likely cause of this tumor?

- ☐ **A.** Persistence of a small portion of Rathke's pouch
- ☐ **B.** Abnormal development of pars tuberalis
- ☐ **C.** Abnormal development of the foramina of Monro
- ☐ **D.** Abnormal development of the alar plates that form the lateral wall of diencephalon
- ☐ **E.** Abnormal development of diencephalon

143 A 1-day-old male infant presents with a telencephalic vesicle; the eyes are fused, and a single nasal chamber is present in the midline. In addition an MRI examination reveals that the olfactory bulbs and tracts and the corpus callosum are hypoplastic. Which of the following is the most likely diagnosis?

- ☐ **A.** Holoprosencephaly
- ☐ **B.** Smith-Lemli-Opitz syndrome
- ☐ **C.** Schizencephaly
- ☐ **D.** Exencephaly
- ☐ **E.** Meningoencephalocele

144 A 1-day-old infant presents with meningohydroencephalocele. Which of the following bones is most commonly affected?

- ☐ **A.** Squamous part of temporal bone
- ☐ **B.** Petrous part of temporal bone
- ☐ **C.** Squamous part of occipital bone
- ☐ **D.** Sphenoid bone
- ☐ **E.** Ethmoid bone

145 A 1-day-old infant was born with the vault of the skull undeveloped, leaving the malformed brain exposed. A diagnosis of exencephaly is made. What is the most common embryologic cause of this condition?

- ☐ **A.** Toxoplasmosis infection
- ☐ **B.** Failure of closure of the cephalic part of the neural tube

- ▢ **C.** Ossification defect in the bones of the skull
- ▢ **D.** Caudal displacement of cerebellar structures
- ▢ **E.** Maternal alcohol abuse

146 A 6-month-old infant is admitted to the emergency department with hydrocephalus. Upon physical examination a spina bifida cystica is noted. MRI reveals a caudal displacement of the cerebellar vermis through the foramen magnum. Which of the following is the most likely diagnosis?

- ▢ **A.** Chiari II malformation
- ▢ **B.** Holoprosencephaly
- ▢ **C.** Smith-Lemli-Opitz syndrome
- ▢ **D.** Schizencephaly
- ▢ **E.** Exencephaly

147 A 1-year-old boy was admitted to the hospital because of the parents' suspicion that the child was deaf. An MRI examination showed abnormal development of the membranous and bony labyrinths, leading the physician to the diagnosis of congenital deafness. Which of the following conditions can lead to congenital deafness?

- ▢ **A.** Infection with rubella virus
- ▢ **B.** Failure of the second pharyngeal arch to form
- ▢ **C.** Failure of the dorsal portion of first pharyngeal cleft
- ▢ **D.** Abnormal development of the auricular hillocks
- ▢ **E.** Failure of the dorsal portion of first pharyngeal cleft and second pharyngeal arch

148 A 3-month-old male infant is brought to the hospital by his parents because of white patches in his eyes. An ophthalmoscopic examination shows a congenital cataract. Which of the following conditions can cause a congenital cataract?

- ▢ **A.** Infection with rubella virus
- ▢ **B.** Choroid fissure fails to close
- ▢ **C.** Persistent hyaloid artery
- ▢ **D.** Toxoplasmosis infection
- ▢ **E.** Cytomegalovirus infection

149 A newborn infant exhibits absence of the ocular lens and is admitted to the pediatric intensive care unit. Laboratory examination reveals a mutation in the *PAX6* gene. Which of the following conditions is the most likely diagnosis?

- ▢ **A.** Cyclopia
- ▢ **B.** Coloboma
- ▢ **C.** Anophthalmia
- ▢ **D.** Aphakia and aniridia
- ▢ **E.** Microphthalmia

150 A 2-month-old infant presents with small and flat maxillary, temporal, and zygomatic bones. In addition, the patient has anotia and a dermoid tumor in the eyeball. Which of the following conditions is the most likely diagnosis?

- ▢ **A.** Hemifacial microsomia
- ▢ **B.** Treacher Collins syndrome
- ▢ **C.** Robin sequence
- ▢ **D.** DiGeorge syndrome
- ▢ **E.** Velocardiofacial syndrome

151 A 3-month-old infant is diagnosed with abnormal face, thymic hypoplasia, cleft palate, hypocalcemia, and a ventricular septal defect. Which of the following genes is defective?

- ▢ **A.** *22q11*
- ▢ **B.** *Sonic Hedgehog*
- ▢ **C.** *PAX 2*
- ▢ **D.** *PAX 6*
- ▢ **E.** *47XXY*

152 A 3-day-old male infant has a noticeably small mandible. A CT scan and physical examination reveal hypoplasia of the mandible, underdevelopment of the bones of the face, downward-slanting palpebral fissures, defects of the lower eyelids, and deformed external ears. Abnormal development of which of the pharyngeal arches will most likely produce such symptoms?

- ▢ **A.** First arch
- ▢ **B.** Second arch
- ▢ **C.** Third arch
- ▢ **D.** Fourth arch
- ▢ **E.** Sixth arch

153 A 1-year-old infant is admitted to the hospital with fever. His parents explain that the infant fell several times in the playground the day before. Meningitis is suspected and radiographic examination reveals a sinus infection. Which of the following sinuses is present at this age?

- ▢ **A.** Frontal sinus
- ▢ **B.** Maxillary sinus
- ▢ **C.** Sphenoid sinus
- ▢ **D.** Middle ethmoidal air cells
- ▢ **E.** Posterior ethmoidal air cells

154 A newborn infant presents with severe brain abnormalities. The calvaria is defective and the brain is protruding from the cranium. A rudimentary brainstem and some functioning neural tissue are present. A diagnosis is made of meroencephaly. Which of the following is the most likely cause of this condition?

- ☐ **A.** Failure of the rostral neuropore to close in the fourth week
- ☐ **B.** Cytomegalovirus infection
- ☐ **C.** Failure of the hypophyseal diverticulum to develop
- ☐ **D.** Failure of the neural arch to develop
- ☐ **E.** Abnormal neural crest formation

155 A 55-year-old man is admitted to the emergency department with fever of 4 days' duration. Radiographic examination reveals the presence of an infection that is spreading from the retropharyngeal space to the posterior mediastinum. Between which of the following fascial layers is the infection most likely located?

- ☐ **A.** Between alar and prevertebral
- ☐ **B.** Between alar and pretracheal
- ☐ **C.** Between pretracheal and prevertebral
- ☐ **D.** Between buccopharyngeal and alar
- ☐ **E.** Between buccopharyngeal and prevertebral

156 A 24-year-old man is admitted to the hospital after a street fight. Radiographic examination reveals an inferior blow-out fracture of the orbit. Which of the following nerves is particularly vulnerable with this type of injury?

- ☐ **A.** Infraorbital
- ☐ **B.** Supratrochlear
- ☐ **C.** Frontal
- ☐ **D.** Inferior alveolar
- ☐ **E.** Optic

157 A 67-year-old man visits the outpatient clinic with hearing problems. During physical examination a Rinne's test for hearing is performed by placing a tuning fork on his head to test for bone conduction. Upon what specific point should the tuning fork be placed to test conduction?

- ☐ **A.** Temporal bone
- ☐ **B.** Frontal bone
- ☐ **C.** Mastoid process
- ☐ **D.** External occipital protuberance
- ☐ **E.** Vertex of the head

158 A 55-year-old man is admitted to the emergency department with a complaint of pain when chewing over the previous 3 months. Physical examination reveals the patient suffers from odynophagia and hoarseness in his speech. Radiographic examination reveals a tumor at the tracheoesophageal groove. Which of the following nerves is most likely affected by the tumor?

- ☐ **A.** Recurrent laryngeal
- ☐ **B.** Internal laryngeal
- ☐ **C.** Vagus
- ☐ **D.** External laryngeal
- ☐ **E.** Phrenic

159 A 34-year-old man is admitted to the emergency department after falling off his motorbike, suffering an injury to his head because he was not wearing a helmet. The patient has multiple lacerations in the skin over the frontal bone. Which of the following veins could most likely provide a pathway of transmission of infection from the veins of the scalp to the underlying dural venous sinuses?

- ☐ **A.** Supratrochlear vein
- ☐ **B.** Diploic veins
- ☐ **C.** Anterior cerebral veins
- ☐ **D.** Superior sagittal sinus
- ☐ **E.** Supraorbital vein

160 A 65-year-old man is admitted to the emergency department after an episode of a transient ischemic attack. Radiographic examination reveals an aneurysm in the region between the posterior cerebral artery and superior cerebellar artery. Which of the following nerves will most likely be compressed from the aneurysm?

- ☐ **A.** Trochlear
- ☐ **B.** Abducens
- ☐ **C.** Oculomotor
- ☐ **D.** Vagus
- ☐ **E.** Optic

161 A 36-year-old female racquetball player is admitted to the hospital after being struck in the orbital region. Radiographic examination reveals a blow-out fracture of the medial wall of the orbit. Physical examination also reveals that the pupil of the affected eye cannot be turned laterally. Which of the following muscles is most likely injured or trapped?

- ☐ **A.** Lateral rectus
- ☐ **B.** Medial and inferior recti
- ☐ **C.** Medial rectus
- ☐ **D.** Medial rectus and superior oblique
- ☐ **E.** Inferior rectus

162 A 16-year-old female volleyball player is admitted to the hospital after being hit in the eye with a ball spiked at the net. Radiographic examination reveals a blow-out fracture of the inferior wall of the orbit. Physical examination also reveals that the pupil of her eye cannot be turned upward. Which of the following muscle(s) is (are) most likely injured?

- ▢ **A.** Inferior rectus and inferior oblique
- ▢ **B.** Medial and inferior recti
- ▢ **C.** Inferior oblique
- ▢ **D.** Medial rectus, inferior rectus, and inferior oblique
- ▢ **E.** Inferior rectus

163 A 36-year-old man is admitted to the emergency department with a painful skin rash on the dorsum of his nose. Physical examination reveals that a herpetic lesion is affecting the dorsum of the nose and the eyeball. Which of the following nerves is most likely to be responsible for transmission of the virus to the eye?

- ▢ **A.** Nasociliary
- ▢ **B.** Supratrochlear
- ▢ **C.** Infraorbital
- ▢ **D.** Posterior ethmoidal
- ▢ **E.** Anterior ethmoidal

164 A 22-year-old man is admitted to the emergency department after he was injured in a street fight (Fig. 7-6). Radiographic examination reveals that he has suffered a forehead fracture, resulting in black and swollen eyes. Because the patient is in severe pain, an anesthetic solution is injected into his orbit. Which of the following nerves is most likely to be anesthetized?

- ▢ **A.** Ophthalmic
- ▢ **B.** Infraorbital
- ▢ **C.** Anterior ethmoidal
- ▢ **D.** Frontal
- ▢ **E.** Optic

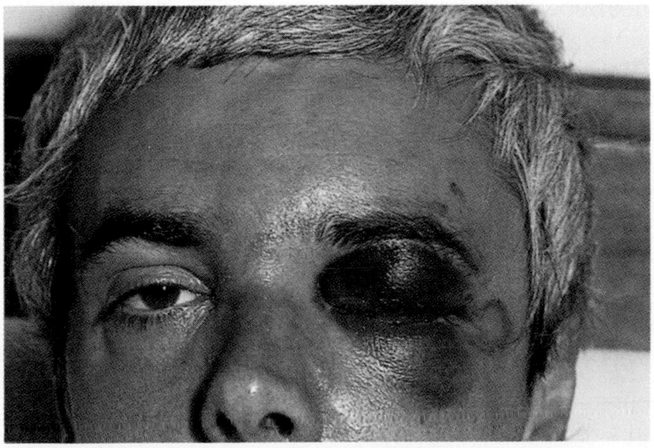

Fig. 7-6

165 A 34-year-old woman is admitted to the emergency department after her right cheekbone and bony orbit hit the dashboard in an automobile crash. Physical examination reveals that the patient has lost the ability for the affected eye to be directed downward when the pupil is in the adducted position. An MRI examination reveals a torn nerve. What is the most common location at which this nerve will be injured?

- ▢ **A.** As it pierces the dura of the tentorium cerebelli in the tentorial notch
- ▢ **B.** At the cavernous sinus
- ▢ **C.** At the sella turcica
- ▢ **D.** At the inferior orbital fissure
- ▢ **E.** At the superior orbital fissure

166 A 56-year-old woman is admitted to the hospital with eye pain. During physical examination the patient complains of excruciating pain when she performs any movement of the eye. An MRI examination reveals that the optic nerve is inflamed. What is the most likely explanation?

- ▢ **A.** The anular tendon (of Zinn) is inflamed
- ▢ **B.** The inflammation has affected the nerves innervating the eye muscles
- ▢ **C.** The muscles are contracting due to generalized inflammation
- ▢ **D.** The nasociliary nerve is affected
- ▢ **E.** The ophthalmic artery is constricted

167 A 7-day-old infant is admitted to the pediatric intensive care unit with microphthalmia. Which of the following is the most likely cause of this condition?

- ▢ **A.** Infection with rubella virus
- ▢ **B.** Choroid fissure failed to close
- ▢ **C.** Persistent hyaloid artery
- ▢ **D.** Toxoplasmosis infection
- ▢ **E.** Epstein-Barr virus infection

168 A 2-month-old male infant is admitted to the hospital after falling from his stroller. During physical examination the infant shows signs of facial nerve injury. What is the most common place for facial nerve injury in an infant?

- ▢ **A.** At the stylomastoid foramen
- ▢ **B.** Posterior to the parotid gland
- ▢ **C.** Anterior to the parotid gland
- ▢ **D.** Proximal to the stylomastoid foramen

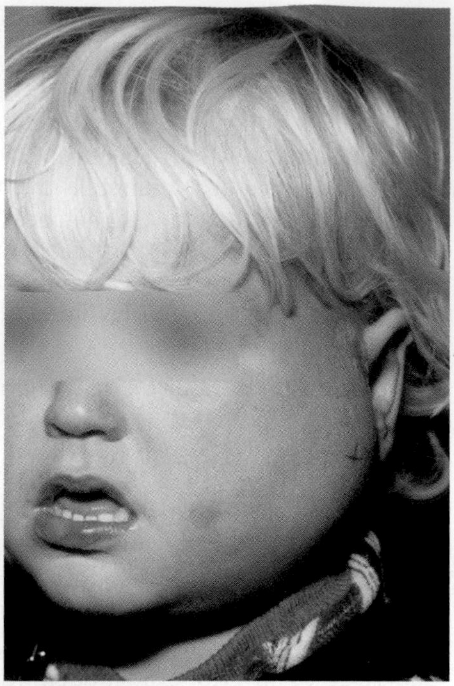

Fig. 7-7

☐ **E.** Mandibular involvement of zygomatic and buccal branches

169 A 6-year-old boy is admitted to the hospital with high fever and pain over the parotid gland (Fig. 7-7). A diagnosis of parotiditis (mumps) is established, and the boy is sent back home. Which of the following nerves is responsible for painful sensations from the region of the parotid gland?

☐ **A.** Facial
☐ **B.** Auriculotemporal
☐ **C.** Lesser petrosal
☐ **D.** Lingual
☐ **E.** Chorda tympani

170 A 55-year-old woman presents to the ENT clinic with episodes of vertigo, fluctuating hearing loss, ringing of the right ear, and feeling or fullness or pressure in her ear. The clinical diagnosis suggests Ménière's disease. Which of the following structures is most likely affected by the edema associated with Ménière's disease?

☐ **A.** Middle ear
☐ **B.** Endolymphatic sac
☐ **C.** Semicircular canals
☐ **D.** Cochlea
☐ **E.** Helicotrema

171 A 55-year-old woman visits the outpatient clinic with swelling in her neck. Ultrasound examinations reveal a thyroid gland tumor. Three days after thyroidectomy air bubbles are seen on the CT of her brain. Which of the following is the most likely cause of the air bubbles?

☐ **A.** Injury to inferior thyroid artery
☐ **B.** Injury to inferior and superior thyroid arteries
☐ **C.** Injury to superior thyroid artery and vein
☐ **D.** Injury to superior and middle thyroid veins
☐ **E.** Injury to superior, middle, and inferior thyroid veins

172 A 32-year-old man is admitted to the emergency department unconscious after a serious car crash. During an emergency cricothyroidotomy an artery is accidentally injured. Two days later the patient shows signs of aspiration pneumonia. Which of the following arteries was most likely injured?

☐ **A.** Superior thyroid
☐ **B.** Inferior thyroid
☐ **C.** Cricothyroid
☐ **D.** Superior laryngeal
☐ **E.** Suprahyoid

173 A 22-year-old woman is admitted to the emergency department unconscious after falling over the handlebars of her bicycle. An emergency tracheotomy is performed to insert a tracheotomy tube. What is the most common tracheal cartilage level at which a tracheotomy incision is performed?

☐ **A.** First to second
☐ **B.** Second to third
☐ **C.** Third to fourth
☐ **D.** Fourth to fifth
☐ **E.** Fifth to sixth

174 A 36-year-old woman is admitted to the hospital with severe head injuries after a car crash. During neurologic examination it is noted that her palate elevates asymmetrically, being pulled up toward the right. Which of the following muscles is paralyzed?

☐ **A.** Left levator veli palatini
☐ **B.** Left tensor veli palatini
☐ **C.** Right levator veli palatini
☐ **D.** Right tensor veli palatini
☐ **E.** Right tensor veli palatini and left levator veli palatini

175 A 45-year-old man presents to the outpatient clinic after stumbling and hitting his head on a table in a restaurant. Photographs were taken of the patient's eyes during neurologic examination (Fig. 7-8). Which

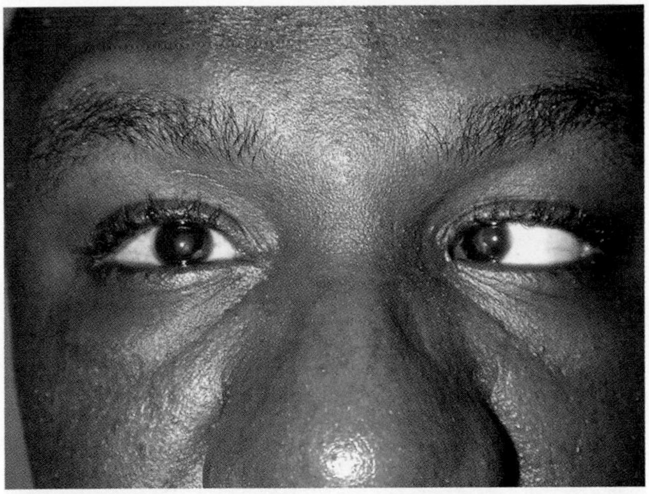

Fig. 7-8

of the following nerves to the left eye was most likely injured?

- ▢ **A.** Trochlear
- ▢ **B.** Abducens
- ▢ **C.** Oculomotor
- ▢ **D.** Optic
- ▢ **E.** Oculomotor and abducens

176 A 32-year-old woman is admitted to the hospital after losing consciousness and collapsing in the middle of the street. A neurologic examination reveals absence of the accommodation reflex of her right eye. Which of the following is most likely involved in the pathology in this patient?

- ▢ **A.** Superior salivatory nucleus
- ▢ **B.** Superior cervical ganglion
- ▢ **C.** Nervus intermedius
- ▢ **D.** Edinger-Westphal nucleus
- ▢ **E.** Trigeminal ganglion

177 A 32-year-old man is admitted to the hospital with nausea, vomiting, and severe headache. An MRI examination reveals an acoustic neuroma (Fig. 7-9). Which of the following nerves is most likely compressed by the tumor?

- ▢ **A.** Facial
- ▢ **B.** Oculomotor
- ▢ **C.** Vagus
- ▢ **D.** Hypoglossal
- ▢ **E.** Abducens

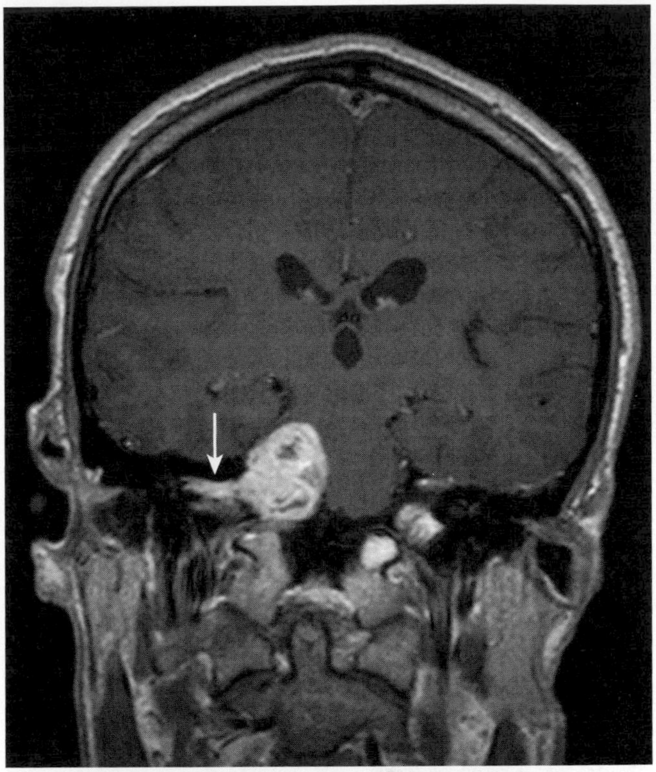

Fig. 7-9

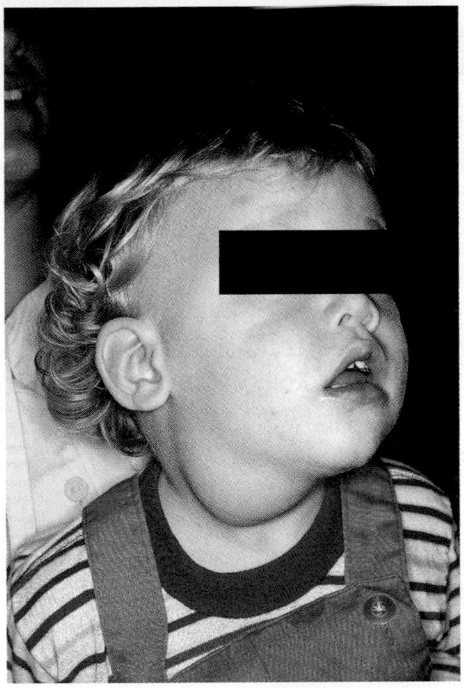

Fig. 7-10

178 A 3-year-old boy is brought to the outpatient clinic with swelling of the side of his neck. Physical examination reveals a congenital mass of tissue anterior to the superior third of the sternocleidomastoid muscle (Fig. 7-10). The swelling is asymptomatic, non-painful, and soft fluctuant. Which of the following is the most likely diagnosis?

- ▢ **A.** Branchial cleft cyst
- ▢ **B.** Ruptured sternocleidomastoid muscle

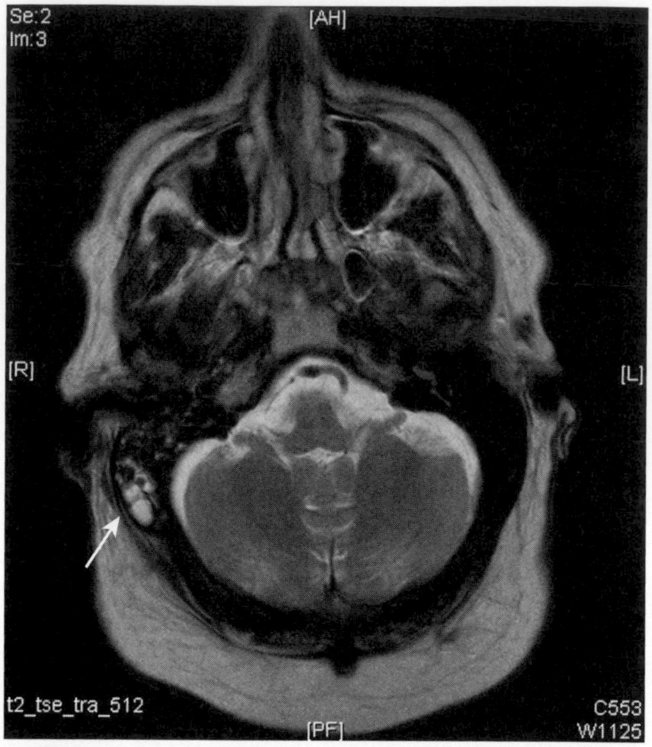

Fig. 7-12

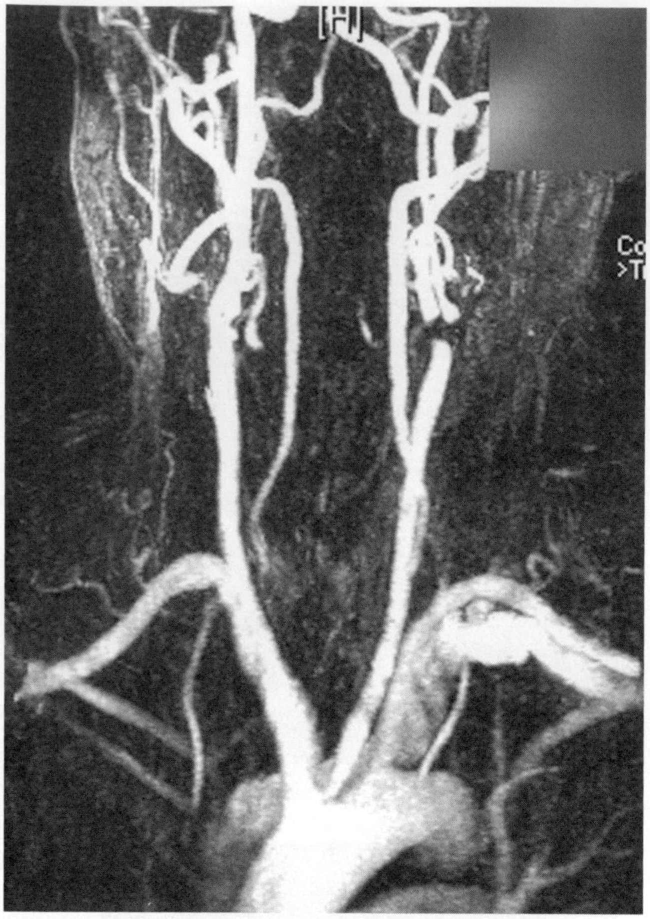

Fig. 7-11

▢ **C.** Lymph node inflammation

▢ **D.** Torticollis

▢ **E.** External carotid artery aneurysm

179 A 68-year-old woman visits the outpatient clinic with a complaint of chronic dizziness and headaches and a history of multiple transient ischemic attacks. Cranial and cervical angiography (Fig. 7-11) reveals an occluded vessel. Which of the following vessels is most likely occluded?

▢ **A.** External carotid

▢ **B.** Internal carotid

▢ **C.** Common carotid

▢ **D.** Vertebral

▢ **E.** Superior thyroid

180 A 9-year-old girl is admitted to the emergency department with painful swelling behind her ear. An MRI examination reveals mastoiditis (Fig. 7-12). Which of the following structures is most likely to be affected by the inflammation?

▢ **A.** Transverse sinus

▢ **B.** Petrous part of the temporal bone

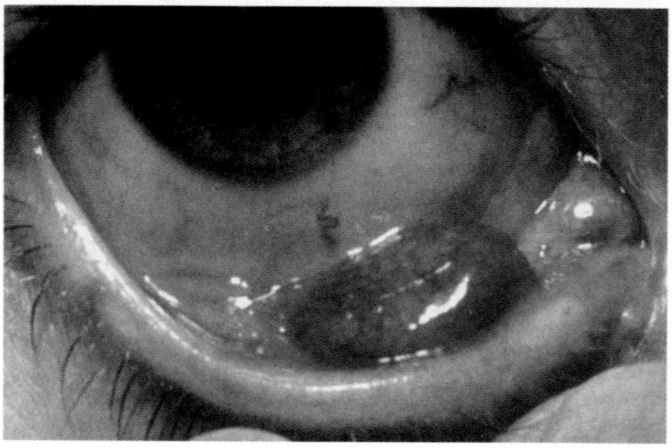

Fig. 7-13

▢ **C.** Inner ear

▢ **D.** Occipital sinus

▢ **E.** Internal carotid artery

181 A 34-year-old woman is admitted to the emergency department with a painful eye. Physical examination reveals a lump in the lower eyelid that consists of debris (Fig. 7-13). A diagnosis of a chalazion is made. Which of the following structures is most likely blocked by the chalazion?

▢ **A.** Lacrimal ducts

▢ **B.** Tarsal glands

▢ **C.** Sclera

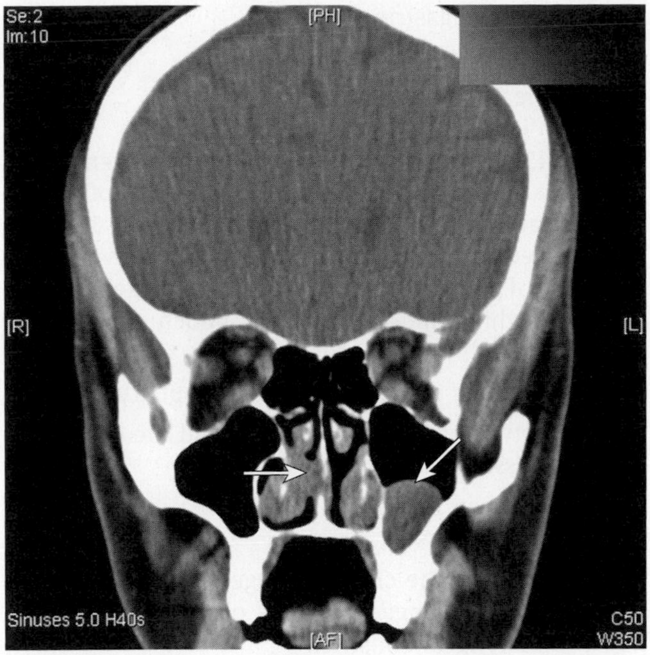

Fig. 7-14

- ☐ **D.** Pupil
- ☐ **E.** Nasolacrimal duct

182 A 45-year-old man is admitted to the hospital with breathing problems. During physical examination the patient shows signs of unilateral nasal airway obstruction. A CT scan reveals a nasal polyp obstructing the airway (Fig. 7-14). Drainage from which of the following structures is also obstructed?

- ☐ **A.** Sphenoid sinus
- ☐ **B.** Maxillary sinus and nasolacrimal duct
- ☐ **C.** Ethmoidal sinus
- ☐ **D.** Frontal sinus
- ☐ **E.** Nasolacrimal duct

183 A 58-year-old man is admitted to the ENT clinic with progressive unilateral hearing loss and ringing in the affected ear (tinnitus) of 4 months duration. MRI reveals a tumor at the cerebellopontine angle. Which of the following nerves is most likely affected?

- ☐ **A.** Vagus
- ☐ **B.** Hypoglossal
- ☐ **C.** Vestibulocochlear
- ☐ **D.** Glossopharyngeal
- ☐ **E.** Trigeminal

184 A newborn infant is delivered with forceps after a difficult delivery. Upon physical examination of the newborn a cephalohematoma is noted from rupture of small periosteal arteries. Between which of the following layers of tissue does the blood accumulate?

- ☐ **A.** Between skin and dense connective tissue layer
- ☐ **B.** Between loose connective tissue layer and galea aponeurotica
- ☐ **C.** Between galea aponeurotica and pericranium
- ☐ **D.** Between pericranium and calvaria
- ☐ **E.** In the subcutaneous layer

185 An unconscious 54-year-old woman is admitted to the hospital. A CT scan reveals a tumor in her brain, producing a transtentorial herniation. When she regains consciousness, her right eye is directed laterally and downward, with complete ptosis of her upper eyelid and pupillary dilation. Which of the following lobes of the brain is affected by the tumor?

- ☐ **A.** Parietal
- ☐ **B.** Temporal
- ☐ **C.** Occipital
- ☐ **D.** Frontal
- ☐ **E.** Parietal and temporal

186 A 54-year-old man is admitted to the hospital with severe headaches. A CT scan reveals a tumor in his brain occupying a portion of the anterior cranial fossa. Which of the following is responsible for the sensation of pain from headache in this case?

- ☐ **A.** Meningeal branches of the maxillary nerve
- ☐ **B.** Meningeal branches of the mandibular nerve
- ☐ **C.** Meningeal branches of the ethmoidal nerve
- ☐ **D.** Tentorial nerve
- ☐ **E.** C2 and C3 fibers

187 A 55-year-old woman is admitted to the emergency department with chest pain (angina). An electrocardiogram (ECG) examination reveals an acute myocardial infarction (heart attack). A series of medications is administered to the patient, including sublingual nitroglycerin for reducing her blood pressure. Which of the following structures is most likely to be the route of absorption of this drug?

- ☐ **A.** Deep lingual vein
- ☐ **B.** Submandibular duct
- ☐ **C.** Sublingual duct
- ☐ **D.** Lingual vein
- ☐ **E.** Sublingual vein

188 A 35-year-old man is admitted to the hospital with severe pain in the area of his right submandibular gland. Radiographic examination reveals a tumor of the gland. The submandibular gland and its duct are removed. Which of the following nerves is most prone to injury in this type of procedure?

- ☐ **A.** Buccal
- ☐ **B.** Lingual
- ☐ **C.** Inferior alveolar
- ☐ **D.** Nerve to mylohyoid
- ☐ **E.** Glossopharyngeal

189 A 22-year-old man is admitted to the emergency department with a sinus infection. Radiographic examination reveals posterior ethmoidal cell infection. During history taking the patient complains of progressive loss of vision. Which of the following structures is most likely affected?

- ☐ **A.** Ophthalmic artery
- ☐ **B.** Nasociliary nerve
- ☐ **C.** Anterior ethmoidal nerve
- ☐ **D.** Trochlear nerve
- ☐ **E.** Abducens nerve

190 A 55-year-old male farmer is admitted to the emergency department after falling from the hayloft in his barn. Radiographic examination reveals a small, depressed fracture of the skull vertex and thrombosis of the superior sagittal sinus. A day later the patient loses consciousness. What is the most likely cause of his loss of consciousness?

- ☐ **A.** Obstruction of CSF resorption
- ☐ **B.** Obstruction of the cerebral aqueduct (of Sylvius)
- ☐ **C.** Laceration of the middle meningeal artery
- ☐ **D.** Fracture of the cribriform plate with CSF rhinorrhea
- ☐ **E.** Aneurysm of the middle cerebral artery

191 Accompanied by his parents, an 11-year-old boy visits the outpatient clinic with a history of recurrent infections of his palatine tonsils (tonsillitis). Which of the following lymph nodes is most likely to first become visibly enlarged during tonsillitis?

- ☐ **A.** Submandibular
- ☐ **B.** Parotid
- ☐ **C.** Jugulodigastric
- ☐ **D.** Submental
- ☐ **E.** Preauricular

192 A 45-year-old man is admitted to the emergency department with a red, painful eye. During physical examination it is noted that the conjunctiva of the affected eye is infected. Which of the following lymph node groups would be first involved if the infection spread?

- ☐ **A.** Submandibular
- ☐ **B.** Parotid
- ☐ **C.** Jugulodigastric
- ☐ **D.** Submental
- ☐ **E.** Preauricular

193 A 45-year-old woman visits the outpatient clinic with past history of dysphagia, nighttime fits of coughing, repeated chest infections, and a palpable swelling in her neck. Radiographic examination reveals the presence of a persistent congenital pharyngeal pouch. Between which muscles is this pouch most likely located?

- ☐ **A.** Between styloglossus and stylopharyngeus
- ☐ **B.** Between palatoglossal arch and median glossoepiglottic fold
- ☐ **C.** Between upper and middle pharyngeal constrictors
- ☐ **D.** Between the cricopharyngeal and thyropharyngeal portions of inferior pharyngeal constrictor
- ☐ **E.** Between the middle and inferior pharyngeal constrictors

194 A 5-year-old boy fell from a tree and was admitted to the emergency department unconscious. When an emergency tracheostomy was performed, profuse dark venous bleeding suddenly occurred from the midline incision over the trachea. Which of the following vessels was most likely accidentally cut?

- ☐ **A.** Superior thyroid vein
- ☐ **B.** Inferior thyroid vein
- ☐ **C.** Left brachiocephalic vein
- ☐ **D.** Middle thyroid vein
- ☐ **E.** Jugular arch connecting the anterior jugular veins

195 A 55-year-old woman visits the outpatient clinic complaining of unilateral neck pain, sore throat, and ear pain. Radiographic examination reveals Eagle's syndrome, in which the styloid process and stylohyoid ligament are elongated and calcified. Which of the following nerves is most likely affected by Eagle's syndrome in this patient?

- ☐ **A.** Vagus
- ☐ **B.** Facial
- ☐ **C.** Glossopharyngeal
- ☐ **D.** Hypoglossal
- ☐ **E.** Vestibulocochlear

196 A 62-year-old man visits the outpatient clinic complaining of spontaneous lacrimation during eating. Which of the following nerves has developed a lesion to cause this condition?

- ☐ **A.** Facial nerve proximal to the geniculate ganglion
- ☐ **B.** Greater petrosal nerve
- ☐ **C.** Lesser petrosal nerve
- ☐ **D.** Lacrimal nerve
- ☐ **E.** Chorda tympani

197 A 54-year-old woman is admitted to the emergency department after experiencing sudden problems with vision over the past 5 days. MRI reveals that an aneurysm of one of the arteries at the base of the brain is compressing the optic chiasm. Which of the following arteries will most likely be involved?

- ☐ **A.** Middle cerebral
- ☐ **B.** Anterior communicating
- ☐ **C.** Anterior cerebral
- ☐ **D.** Superior cerebellar
- ☐ **E.** Posterior superior cerebellar

198 A 22-year-old woman visits the outpatient clinic with a sinus infection of 2 weeks duration. Physical examination reveals that the patient has focal inflammation, with mucosal edema in the inferior nasal meatus. Drainage from which of the following structures is most likely to be obstructed by this inflammation and edema?

- ☐ **A.** Anterior ethmoidal air cells
- ☐ **B.** Frontonasal duct
- ☐ **C.** Maxillary sinus
- ☐ **D.** Middle ethmoidal air cells
- ☐ **E.** Nasolacrimal duct

199 A 40-year-old woman suffers severe head trauma in a car crash. After radiographic examination she is diagnosed with a fracture of the temporal bone resulting in a lesion of the facial nerve proximal to the origin of the chorda tympani in the posterior wall of the tympanic cavity. Which of the following functions would most likely remain intact in this patient?

- ☐ **A.** Control of muscles in lower half of face
- ☐ **B.** Control of secretions by submandibular gland
- ☐ **C.** Taste sensation from anterior two thirds of tongue
- ☐ **D.** Tear production by the lacrimal gland
- ☐ **E.** Voluntary closure of the eyelid

200 Cardiac pain is referred in some cases to the mandible and the region of the temporomandibular joint. Cutaneous sensation over the angle of the mandible is normally supplied by which of the following nerves?

- ☐ **A.** Cervical branch of facial
- ☐ **B.** Great auricular nerve
- ☐ **C.** Mandibular branch of trigeminal nerve
- ☐ **D.** Mandibular branch of facial nerve
- ☐ **E.** Transverse cervical nerve

201 A 72-year-old man with enlarged cervical lymph nodes has a malignant tumor of the cecum in the right lower quadrant of his abdomen. Which of the following lymph nodes of the neck is most frequently associated with malignant tumors of the gastrointestinal tract?

- ☐ **A.** Left inferior deep cervical
- ☐ **B.** Left supraclavicular
- ☐ **C.** Right inferior deep cervical
- ☐ **D.** Right supraclavicular
- ☐ **E.** Jugulodigastric

202 A 60-year-old man presents with swelling in his neck. A biopsy shows a benign tumor in the piriform recess of his larynx. The mucosa of the piriform recess must be anesthetized during removal of the tumor. Which nerve supplies general sensation to the mucous membrane of the laryngeal vestibule and piriform recesses?

- ☐ **A.** External laryngeal
- ☐ **B.** Glossopharyngeal
- ☐ **C.** Hypoglossal
- ☐ **D.** Inferior laryngeal
- ☐ **E.** Internal laryngeal

203 A young man and woman are hiking in a wilderness area and discover the body of a man apparently in his 20s. He appears to have been dead for a few days, but animal predation was minimal. A postmortem examination was performed by the county medical examiner, and no evidence of penetrating wounds (bullet, lacerations, etc.) was found. A plain radiograph showed a fractured hyoid bone, but the calvaria and other bones appeared to be intact. Which of the following is the most likely cause of death?

- ☐ **A.** Myocardial infarction (heart attack)
- ☐ **B.** A fall from a height that resulted in fatal internal bleeding
- ☐ **C.** Subdural hematoma
- ☐ **D.** Strangulation
- ☐ **E.** Ingestion of a poisonous substance

204 A 40-year-old woman presents with severe headaches and dizziness. An MRI reveals a brain tumor, and a biopsy confirms it as an advanced melanoma. She dies 2 months later. Pigmented lesions are not seen on her skin or scalp at the time of diagnosis or during postmortem examination. Which of the following is the most likely source of the malignant melanoma cells?

- ▢ **A.** Superior sagittal sinus
- ▢ **B.** Sphenoidal sinus
- ▢ **C.** Retina of the eye
- ▢ **D.** Pituitary gland
- ▢ **E.** Thymus

205 A 3-month-old girl was admitted to the pediatric clinic after her parents noticed a small pit on the anterior border of sternocleidomastoid with mucus dripping intermittently from its opening. Which embryologic structure is involved in this anomaly?

- ▢ **A.** Persistence of the second pharyngeal arch
- ▢ **B.** Persistence of the proximal part of the second pharyngeal groove
- ▢ **C.** Persistence of the third pharyngeal pouch
- ▢ **D.** Thyroglossal duct
- ▢ **E.** Persistence of the third pharyngeal groove and cervical sinus

206 A neonate was noted to have low-set ears and an abnormal face, including a small mandible. He also had minor cardiac anomalies and a cleft palate, which necessitated assistance with feeding. Now 3 years old, he has had several episodes of otitis media and a recent seizure related to hypocalcemia. Chromosome analysis reveals a deletion in the long arm of chromosome 22. Failure of neural crest cells to migrate normally into which area(s) best explains the recurrent infections and hypocalcemia?

- ▢ **A.** First pharyngeal arch
- ▢ **B.** Third and fourth pharyngeal pouches
- ▢ **C.** The developing heart
- ▢ **D.** Second pharyngeal pouch
- ▢ **E.** First, second, and third pharyngeal arches

207 A 2-month-old girl is scheduled for reconstruction of a unilateral upper cleft lip. Failure of fusion of which structures is the most likely cause of this congenital defect?

- ▢ **A.** Lateral nasal and maxillary prominences/processes
- ▢ **B.** Right and left medial nasal prominences/processes
- ▢ **C.** Lateral nasal and medial nasal prominences/processes
- ▢ **D.** Lateral nasal prominences/processes
- ▢ **E.** Maxillary prominence/process and the intermaxillary segment

208 A 6-month pregnant woman visits her obstetrician for a routine prenatal checkup. Ultrasound examination reveals polyhydramnios and spina bifida. Which of the following conditions may also be expected to be found during the ultrasound examination of the fetus?

- ▢ **A.** Anencephaly
- ▢ **B.** Bilateral renal agenesis
- ▢ **C.** Agenesis of the vagina
- ▢ **D.** Hydrocephalus
- ▢ **E.** Omphalocele

209 A 4-month-old girl has a small area of the right iris missing. An ophthalmologist recognizes a defect in the inferior sector of the iris and the pupillary margin, which gives the pupil a keyhole appearance. Examination reveals that the defect also involves the ciliary body and retina. What is the embryologic cause of this condition?

- ▢ **A.** Failure of the retinal/optic fissure to close
- ▢ **B.** Abnormal neural crest formation
- ▢ **C.** Abnormal interactions between the optic vesicle and ectoderm
- ▢ **D.** Posterior chamber cavitation
- ▢ **E.** Weak adhesion between the inner and outer layers of the optic cup

210 A 26-year-old male boxer is brought to the emergency department after being knocked out by his rival. CT examination reveals severe trauma to the articular disc and fracture of the neck of the mandible. This could result in injury to a muscle that developed from which of the following embryonic structures?

- ▢ **A.** First pharyngeal pouch
- ▢ **B.** Second pharyngeal pouch
- ▢ **C.** First pharyngeal arch
- ▢ **D.** First pharyngeal cleft
- ▢ **E.** Second pharyngeal arch

211 A 2-day-old infant boy is admitted to the pediatric surgery department for correction of a large defect in the occipital bone (cranium bifidum). Imaging reveals that the defect contains meninges and part of the brain, including the ventricular system, protruding through it. What is the most likely diagnosis?

- ▢ **A.** Cranial meningocele
- ▢ **B.** Encephalocele
- ▢ **C.** Meroencephaly

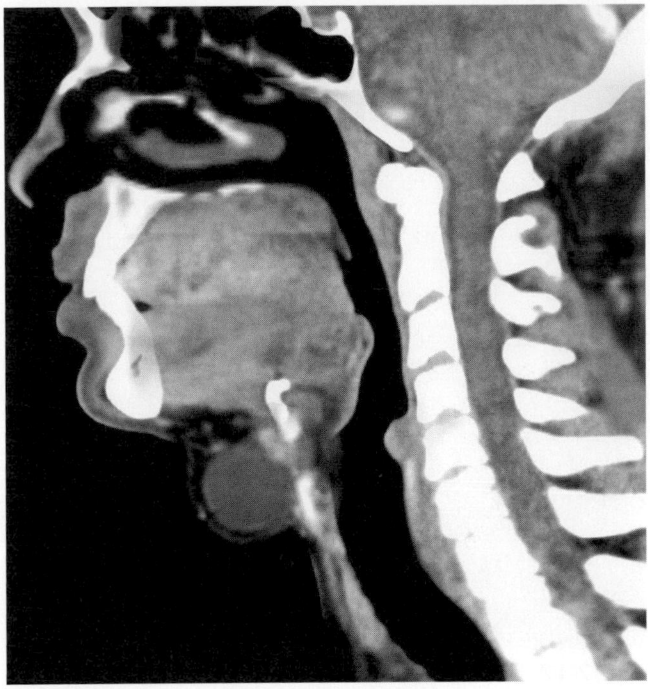

Fig. 7-15

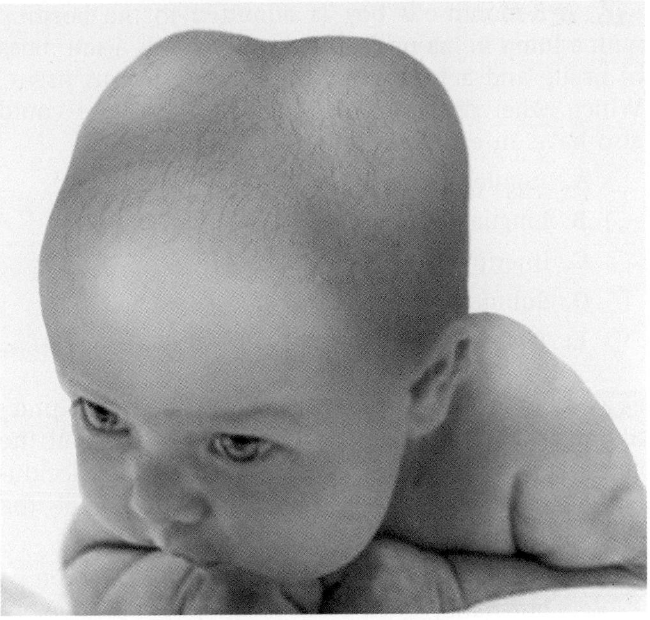

Fig. 7-16

- D. Meningohydroencephalocele
- E. Microcephaly

212 A 30-year-old man has had a mass in his neck for several years and became worried when his sister was diagnosed with lymphoma. Examination of his neck reveals a soft, midline mass about 2 cm in diameter. CT reveals a well-defined fluid-filled mass (Fig. 7-15). Persistence of which embryologic structure most likely accounts for this mass?

- A. Second pharyngeal cleft
- B. Foramen cecum
- C. Thyroglossal duct
- D. Third pharyngeal pouch
- E. Cervical sinus

213 A newborn boy is diagnosed with Treacher Collins syndrome (mandibulofacial dysostosis). Physical examination reveals down-slanting palpebral fissures, defects of the lower eyelids, and deformed external ears. Abnormal development of which pharyngeal arch will most likely produce such symptoms?

- A. First
- B. Second
- C. Third
- D. Fourth
- E. Sixth

214 A neonate is observed by the pediatric team to have bilateral swelling on both sides of the head (Fig. 7-16). On physical examination the swellings do not cross the suture lines and transillumination of the skull appears to be normal. Neurologic examination is normal. Which of the following is most likely responsible for this patient's symptoms?

- A. Intracranial bleeding
- B. Blockage of the interventricular foramen
- C. Failure of cleavage of the prosencephalon
- D. Collection of blood beneath the periosteum of the bone
- E. Collection of edema fluid above the periosteum of the bone

215 A 2-month-old female infant is admitted to the hospital with convulsions. A CT scan shows hydrocephalus and several areas of intracranial calcifications. Physical examination shows severe chorioretinitis. What is the most likely cause of these symptoms?

- A. The mother was treated with tetracyclines during pregnancy
- B. The mother was infected with rubella during the first trimester of pregnancy
- C. The mother was infected with CMV during the first trimester of pregnancy
- D. The mother was infected with *Treponema pallidum* during pregnancy exhibiting congenital syphilis
- E. The mother was infected with *Toxoplasma gondii* during the first trimester of pregnancy

216 A 3-month-old boy is admitted to the hospital with a lump in his neck. A CT scan reveals a soft mass of tissue and a biopsy reveals ectopic thymus tissue. Which other developmentally related structure could also have an ectopic location?

- ▢ **A.** Jugulodigastric lymph node
- ▢ **B.** Lingual tonsil
- ▢ **C.** Inferior parathyroid gland
- ▢ **D.** Submandibular gland
- ▢ **E.** Thyroid gland

217 A 1-year-old girl was brought to the family practitioner by her mother who was concerned about the yellowish brown discoloration of the child's deciduous teeth. What is the most likely cause of the discoloration?

- ▢ **A.** The mother continued to smoke during the pregnancy
- ▢ **B.** The mother was treated with tetracycline during the pregnancy
- ▢ **C.** Poor calcification of dentin due to calcium deficiency during the pregnancy
- ▢ **D.** The mother was infected with rubella during the pregnancy
- ▢ **E.** The mother continued to use alcohol during the pregnancy

218 A low birthweight neonatal girl is admitted to the intensive care unit with patent ductus arteriosus. During physical examination it is noted that the baby has bilateral cataracts. Which of the following will be the most likely cause?

- ▢ **A.** The mother was taking thalidomide during pregnancy
- ▢ **B.** The mother was infected with rubella during the first trimester of pregnancy
- ▢ **C.** The mother was infected with cytomegalovirus during the first trimester of pregnancy
- ▢ **D.** The mother used cocaine during pregnancy
- ▢ **E.** The mother was infected with *Toxoplasma gondii* during the first trimester of pregnancy

219 At birth, a neonatal boy was noted to have multiple craniofacial abnormalities and a cleft palate. CT studies (including the 3D reconstruction shown in Fig. 7-17) are obtained when the infant is 1 year old for surgery planning. What other abnormality would most likely be found with appropriate investigations?

- ▢ **A.** Hyperthyroidism
- ▢ **B.** Hypoplasia of the hyoid bone

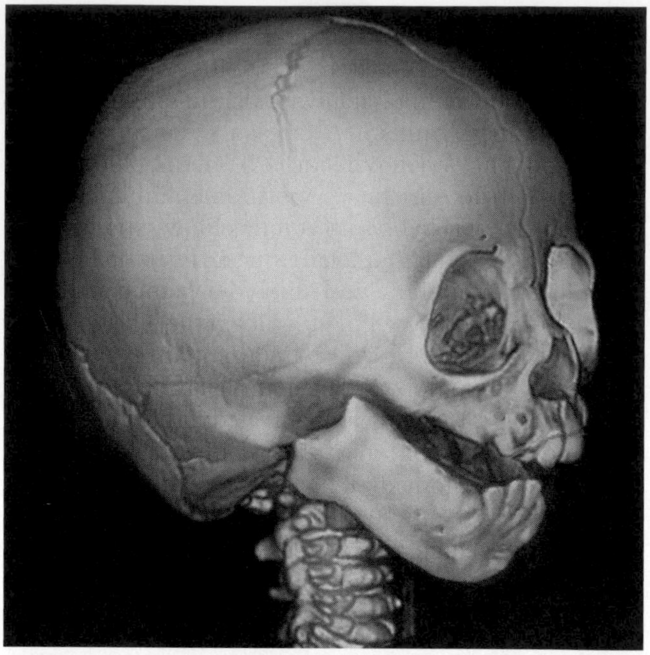

Fig. 7-17

- ▢ **C.** Malformation of laryngeal cartilages
- ▢ **D.** Hypoplasia of the thymus gland
- ▢ **E.** Hearing loss

220 A 14-year-old boy is brought to the family medicine clinic because of an enlarged mass on the left side of his neck. He had an upper respiratory infection 3 weeks ago that resolved uneventfully. Examination reveals a soft fluid-filled mass on the left side of the neck at the level of the laryngeal prominence. Axial CT with contrast shows a well-defined, 4-cm diameter, fluid-filled mass with a thin rim (Fig. 7-18). A diagnosis of a branchial cyst is made. Which embryologic structure is most likely contributing to this mass?

- ▢ **A.** First pharyngeal pouch
- ▢ **B.** Second pharyngeal arch
- ▢ **C.** Third pharyngeal pouch
- ▢ **D.** Cervical sinus
- ▢ **E.** Thyroglossal duct

221 A neonatal boy has hypoplasia of the mandible and zygomatic bones, slanted palpebral fissures, and malformed external ears. What is the name of his condition?

- ▢ **A.** Pierre Robin syndrome
- ▢ **B.** DiGeorge syndrome
- ▢ **C.** Fetal alcohol syndrome (FAS)
- ▢ **D.** Chiari I malformation
- ▢ **E.** Treacher Collins syndrome

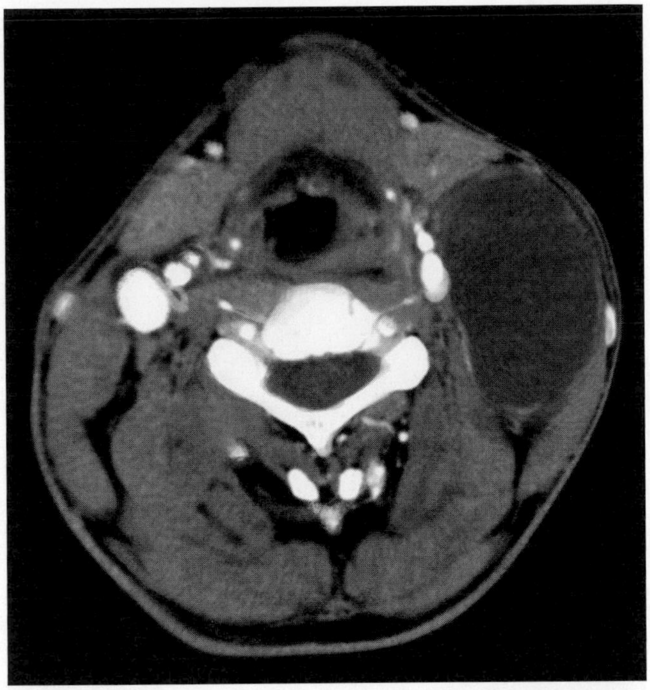

Fig. 7-18

222 A severe mandibular fracture in a 22-year-old woman requires surgical reconstruction. Postoperatively, she complains of numbness of the lower lip and chin. Which nerve was most likely injured?

- ☐ **A.** Auriculotemporal
- ☐ **B.** Buccal
- ☐ **C.** Lesser petrosal
- ☐ **D.** Mental
- ☐ **E.** Infraorbital

223 A 22-year-old man presents with severe facial trauma after a car crash. A CT scan of the head reveals multiple fractures of the facial bones. Following surgery to correct his facial fractures, he asserts that he cannot taste anything on the tip of his tongue. Which ganglion contains the neuron cell bodies of taste fibers from this part of the tongue?

- ☐ **A.** Trigeminal
- ☐ **B.** Geniculate
- ☐ **C.** Inferior glossopharyngeal
- ☐ **D.** Submandibular ganglion
- ☐ **E.** Pterygopalatine

224 A 21-year-old man has suspected intracranial inflammation from an infection. A CT scan showed an abscess compressing the ophthalmic branch of the trigeminal nerve. Which of the following would be a plausible complaint of this individual?

- ☐ **A.** Pain in the hard palate
- ☐ **B.** Anesthesia of the upper lip
- ☐ **C.** Painful eyeball
- ☐ **D.** Pain over the lower eyelid
- ☐ **E.** Tingling sensation over the buccal region of the face

225 A 72-year-old man presents at the clinic with difficulty when eating. An MRI showed a tumor of the brainstem affecting the contents of the hypoglossal canal. Which of the following muscles would be affected by such a tumor?

- ☐ **A.** Geniohyoid
- ☐ **B.** Mylohyoid
- ☐ **C.** Palatoglossus
- ☐ **D.** Genioglossus
- ☐ **E.** Stylohyoid

226 An MRI performed on a 71-year-old man who presents at the clinic confirms the presence of a brain tumor. Additionally, he complains that the right side of his nasal cavity is dry and irritated, and he frequently uses drops in his right eye, as it is always dry. The tumor probably involves which cranial nerve nucleus?

- ☐ **A.** Inferior salivatory nucleus
- ☐ **B.** Dorsal vagal nucleus
- ☐ **C.** Superior salivatory nucleus
- ☐ **D.** Edinger-Westphal nucleus
- ☐ **E.** Nucleus ambiguus

227 A 23-year-old right-handed pitcher for a Major League Baseball team presents to the clinic for evaluation concerning a constellation of symptoms. A CT scan demonstrates hypertrophied scalene muscles on the right side. The diagnosis is thoracic outlet syndrome. Which symptom is consistent with this diagnosis?

- ☐ **A.** Problems with respiration because of pressure on the phrenic nerve
- ☐ **B.** Reduced blood flow to the thoracic wall
- ☐ **C.** Reduced venous return from the head and neck
- ☐ **D.** Numbness in the upper extremity
- ☐ **E.** Distension of the internal jugular vein

228 After undergoing a thyroidectomy for a cancerous nodule, a 29-year-old woman develops a postoperative hematoma in her neck. Physical examination reveals partial ptosis of her eyelid and pupillary constriction on the side of the hematoma. The hematoma is most likely compressing which ganglion to result in the symptoms?

- ▢ **A.** Submandibular
- ▢ **B.** Trigeminal
- ▢ **C.** Superior cervical
- ▢ **D.** Geniculate
- ▢ **E.** Ciliary

229 A 26-year-old man suffers a traumatic injury to the midface region. Physical examination reveals intact taste and salivation but no general sensation from his anterior tongue. Which nerve was probably injured?

- ▢ **A.** Lingual proximal to its junction with the chorda tympani
- ▢ **B.** Chorda tympani
- ▢ **C.** Inferior alveolar
- ▢ **D.** Lingual distal to its junction with the chorda tympani
- ▢ **E.** Glossopharyngeal

230 An 82-year-old man is being evaluated preoperatively for a tumor in the posterior cranial fossa. MRI demonstrated perineural spread of the tumor along nervous tissue at the jugular foramen. Which deficit would you expect?

- ▢ **A.** Loss of tongue movements
- ▢ **B.** Loss of facial expression
- ▢ **C.** Loss of sensation from the face and the scalp
- ▢ **D.** Loss of hearing
- ▢ **E.** Loss of gag reflex

231 The goalkeeper of a soccer team accidentally hit his head against the goal post while trying to reach for the ball. He was confused for several minutes and later resumed playing. Four hours later, he was found unconscious and was immediately rushed to the emergency department. A CT scan of his head shows a hemorrhage (Fig. 7-19, arrows). The vessel that was ruptured to produce this hemorrhage enters the skull through which of the following openings?

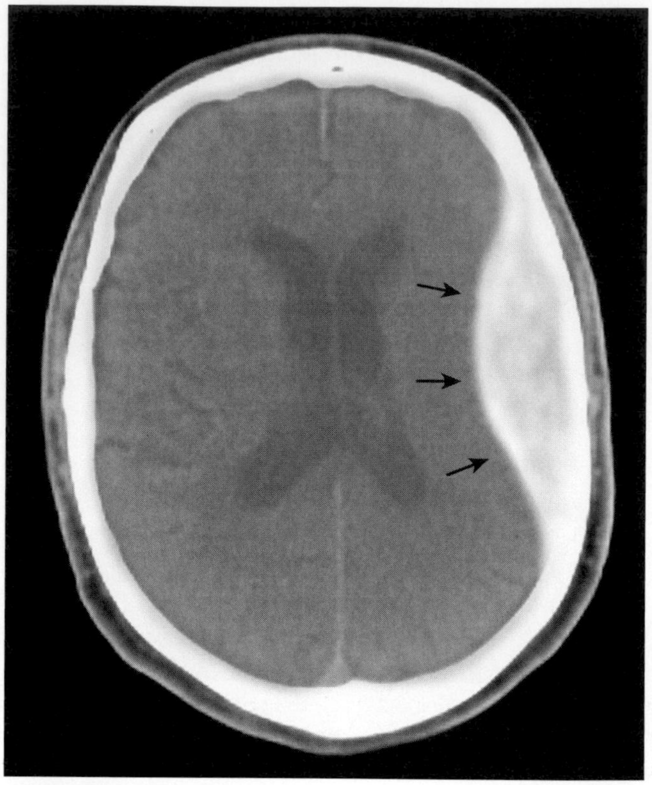

Fig. 7-19

- ▢ **A.** Foramen spinosum
- ▢ **B.** Foramen ovale
- ▢ **C.** Jugular foramen
- ▢ **D.** Hypoglossal canal
- ▢ **E.** Foramen lacerum

232 Found unconscious by her husband, a 55-year-old woman is brought to the hospital with a constellation of symptoms that suggests a ruptured aneurysm. Physical examination of the right eye reveals ptosis, dilated pupil, and the eye deviated inferolaterally. Angiography most likely reveals a hematoma compressing which structure?

- ▢ **A.** Oculomotor nerve
- ▢ **B.** Optic nerve
- ▢ **C.** Facial nerve
- ▢ **D.** Ciliary ganglion
- ▢ **E.** Superior cervical ganglion

233 A 20-year-old construction worker presented to the emergency department with an occipital scalp laceration. The wound was closed. Three days later he presents at the clinic with a tender erythematous infected wound that has spread anteriorly on the scalp. Between which layers of the scalp has the infection spread?

- ▢ **A.** The periosteum and bone
- ▢ **B.** The aponeurosis and the periosteum
- ▢ **C.** The dense connective tissue and the aponeurosis
- ▢ **D.** The dense connective tissue and the skin
- ▢ **E.** The dermis and the epidermis

234 A 73-year-old patient presents at the clinic with neck pain, hoarseness, and weight loss of 6 months duration. During laryngoscopy a large tumor is identified on one of the true vocal folds. The ENT specialist is unable to pass the scope through the opening between the folds. What is the name of this opening?

- ▢ **A.** Piriform recess
- ▢ **B.** Vestibule
- ▢ **C.** Ventricle
- ▢ **D.** Vallecula
- ▢ **E.** Rima glottidis

235 An 82-year-old man presents to the ENT clinic for evaluation of a neck mass. Visual examination with a flexible laryngoscope reveals a tumor in the piriform recess. In taking a biopsy, the physician must be careful not to injure which nerve?

- ▢ **A.** Mandibular
- ▢ **B.** Maxillary
- ▢ **C.** Glossopharyngeal
- ▢ **D.** Internal laryngeal
- ▢ **E.** Hypoglossal

236 A pediatrician is consulted to evaluate a 3-year-old girl who was admitted for a severe throat infection. Examination reveals a bulging and red tympanic membrane. What is the embryologic origin of the structure that allowed the infection to spread from the pharynx to the middle ear cavity?

- ▢ **A.** Second pouch
- ▢ **B.** First groove
- ▢ **C.** Second groove
- ▢ **D.** First pouch
- ▢ **E.** Third pouch

237 Upon neurologic evaluation of a comatose head trauma patient, the physician performs an examination to evaluate the cranial nerves. A light is directed into the right eye and the pupil constricts. This confirms which two nerves are intact?

- ▢ **A.** Optic and facial
- ▢ **B.** Optic and oculomotor
- ▢ **C.** Maxillary and facial
- ▢ **D.** Ophthalmic and oculomotor
- ▢ **E.** Ophthalmic and facial

238 A 27-year-old unconscious woman is admitted to the emergency department. Examination reveals the right pupil is dilated and unresponsive to light. A CT scan reveals a large aneurysm of the superior cerebellar artery just after it branches off from the basilar, compressing the nerve responsible for the symptoms. Which nerve is being compressed?

- ▢ **A.** Oculomotor
- ▢ **B.** Trigeminal
- ▢ **C.** Facial
- ▢ **D.** Vagus
- ▢ **E.** Abducens

239 Physical examination of an 88-year-old man reveals inability to abduct his right eye and an absent corneal reflex on the same side. These symptoms might indicate a growth in which part of the skull?

- ▢ **A.** Inferior orbital fissure
- ▢ **B.** Optic canal
- ▢ **C.** Superior orbital fissure
- ▢ **D.** Foramen rotundum
- ▢ **E.** Foramen ovale

240 A 72-year-old woman presents at the clinic with a herpes zoster oticus. Upon questioning, she complains that she must hold the phone away from her ear because it sounds too loud. Which cranial nerve is affected by this infection to result in the hyperacusis?

- ▢ **A.** Hypoglossal
- ▢ **B.** Facial
- ▢ **C.** Spinal accessory
- ▢ **D.** Vagus
- ▢ **E.** Glossopharyngeal

241 A 70-year-old man presents to his otologist for evaluation of sudden hearing loss. Upon examination the physician visualizes a large amount of cerumen (earwax) in the external auditory meatus and removes it to fully evaluate the tympanic membrane. During this process the patient begins to cough. The cough results from stimulation of an area of the meatus that is innervated by which nerve?

- ▢ **A.** Vestibulocochlear
- ▢ **B.** Vagus
- ▢ **C.** Trigeminal
- ▢ **D.** Facial
- ▢ **E.** Accessory

242 A 30-year-old woman underwent a total thyroidectomy for a cancerous thyroid nodule. Three weeks after the procedure she complains of unresolved hoarseness. Which nerve was most likely traumatized during the operation?

- ▢ **A.** Internal laryngeal
- ▢ **B.** External laryngeal
- ▢ **C.** Recurrent laryngeal
- ▢ **D.** Superior laryngeal
- ▢ **E.** Glossopharyngeal

243 An 82-year-old man receives a home visit from his family practitioner, who notices that the man's pupils are unequally dilated. Which test would the physician use to determine which eye had the problem and whether it was a sympathetic or oculomotor nerve lesion?

- ▢ **A.** Startle reflex
- ▢ **B.** Blink reflex
- ▢ **C.** Pupillary light reflex
- ▢ **D.** H-test
- ▢ **E.** Vision test (reading chart)

244 A 22-year-old baseball player is hit in the eye by a baseball. On examination he was able to move his eye normally and see distant objects but was unable to focus on close objects. Injury to which of the following nerve structures would most likely be the cause of his condition?

- ▢ **A.** Trochlear nerve and abducens nerve
- ▢ **B.** Oculomotor nerve and abducens nerve
- ▢ **C.** Superior cervical ganglion and long ciliary nerves
- ▢ **D.** Short ciliary nerves and ciliary ganglion
- ▢ **E.** Infratrochlear nerve and ciliary ganglion

245 Herpetic lesions of the forehead require expeditious treatment because the infection can spread to the cavernous sinus, leading to intracranial complications. Which venous structure is the most likely route of transmission of this infectious process to the cavernous sinus?

- ▢ **A.** Pterygoid venous plexus
- ▢ **B.** Ophthalmic vein
- ▢ **C.** Superior petrosal sinus
- ▢ **D.** Basilar venous plexus
- ▢ **E.** Parietal emissary vein

246 An 87-year-old woman underwent surgery to remove a vestibular schwannoma (tumor at the internal acoustic meatus). Resection was successful but resulted in the following findings postoperatively: drooping of the right corner of the mouth, inability to close the right eye, and food collection in the right oral vestibule. Which cranial nerve was injured during the surgery?

- ▢ **A.** IX
- ▢ **B.** X
- ▢ **C.** VII
- ▢ **D.** V2
- ▢ **E.** V3

247 A 51-year-old man complains of hearing loss in his left ear, poor balance, a loss of taste, and drooling from the left side of his mouth. A CT scan shows a tumor on the left side of the posterior cranial fossa. Where would the tumor be located to result in the symptoms?

- ▢ **A.** Foramen ovale
- ▢ **B.** Foramen rotundum
- ▢ **C.** Internal acoustic meatus
- ▢ **D.** Jugular foramen
- ▢ **E.** Superior orbital fissure

248 A 50-year-old woman with a history of cigarette smoking and alcohol abuse presents to the clinic with a lower lip lesion. Biopsy of her lower lip reveals a squamous cell carcinoma. Which lymph nodes will most likely be first affected by the spread of the tumor cells?

- ▢ **A.** Occipital
- ▢ **B.** Parotid
- ▢ **C.** Retropharyngeal
- ▢ **D.** Jugulodigastric
- ▢ **E.** Submental

249 An 84-year-old man presents to the emergency department complaining of double vision. Physical examination reveals inability to abduct his right eye. In which of the locations indicated in the arteriogram (Fig. 7-20) will an aneurysm most likely be located to cause the nerve compression resulting in these symptoms/signs?

- ▢ **A.** A
- ▢ **B.** B

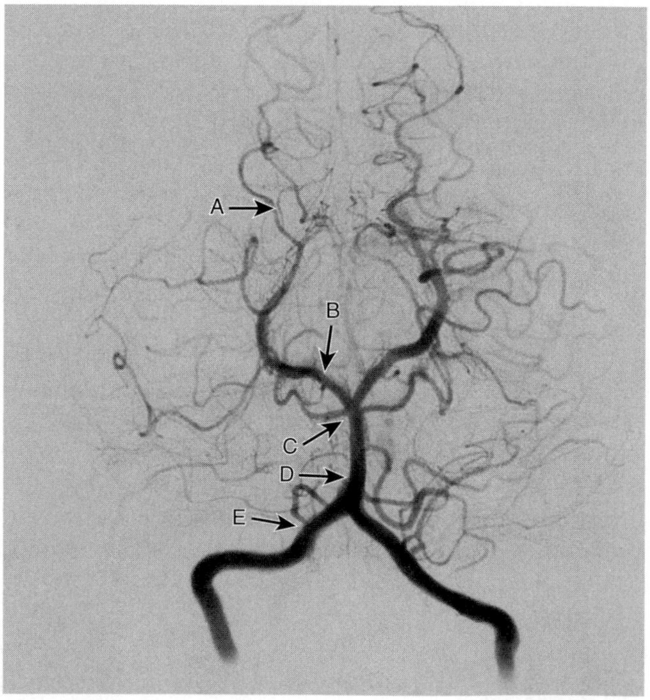

Fig. 7-20

- ☐ **C.** C
- ☐ **D.** D
- ☐ **E.** E

250 A 3-year-old boy is being evaluated for painful swelling on the right side of his face. Imaging (Fig. 7-21) reveals an obstructed and enlarged structure (arrows) and inflammation of the associated salivary gland. Which of the following nerves is most likely responsible for the pain?

- ☐ **A.** Facial
- ☐ **B.** Auriculotemporal
- ☐ **C.** Lingual
- ☐ **D.** Vagus
- ☐ **E.** Chorda tympani

251 Following thyroidectomy, a 44-year-old female soprano has persistent problems with phonation. Fiberoptic laryngoscopy reveals that the vocal folds look normal and meet in the midline. A diagnosis of surgical injury of the left superior laryngeal nerve is established. Which of the following additional abnormal findings would be expected in this nerve injury?

- ☐ **A.** Decreased/absent sensation above the vocal folds
- ☐ **B.** Decreased/absent sensation below the vocal folds
- ☐ **C.** Poorly coordinated swallowing reflex
- ☐ **D.** Bilateral weakness/paralysis of the posterior cricoarytenoid muscles
- ☐ **E.** Weakness/paralysis of the left posterior cricoarytenoid muscle

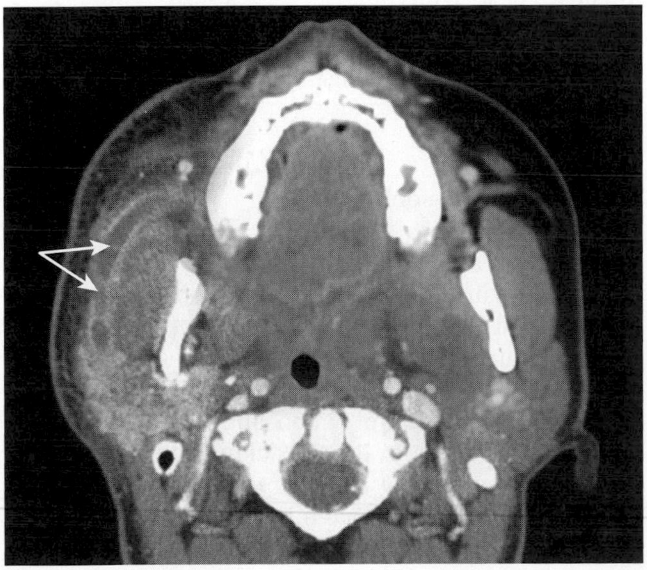

Fig. 7-21

252 A 59-year-old man is recovering after resection of a brainstem tumor. Postoperative imaging reveals a nonobstructive (communicating) hydrocephalus. Between which structures is malabsorption most likely to occur?

- ☐ **A.** Choroid plexus and subdural space
- ☐ **B.** Subarachnoid space and superior sagittal sinus
- ☐ **C.** Subdural space and cavernous sinus
- ☐ **D.** Superior sagittal sinus and jugular vein
- ☐ **E.** Epidural and subdural space

253 A 52-year-old man with a growing lump on the side of his face and neck for the past several months visits his doctor because of the recent development of pain along with other new neurologic symptoms. Based on the mass in the CT image (Fig. 7-22), which of the following neurologic abnormalities will most likely be present on examination as a direct result of the growing mass?

- ☐ **A.** Contralateral deviation of the uvula during elevation of the soft palate
- ☐ **B.** Ipsilateral deviation on protraction of the tongue
- ☐ **C.** Ipsilateral pupillary constriction and partial ptosis
- ☐ **D.** Ipsilateral weakness in elevation of the mandible
- ☐ **E.** Ipsilateral weakness in tight closure of the eyelids

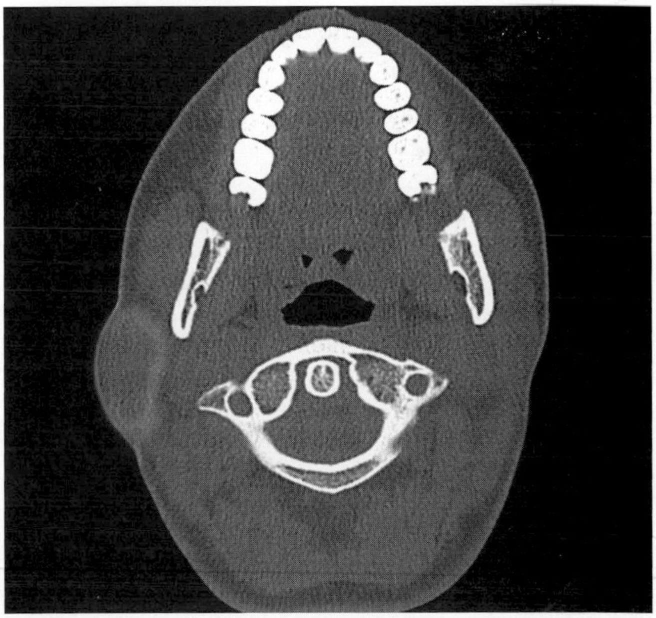

Fig. 7-22

254 A 55-year-old man with a history of cocaine abuse is brought to the emergency department because of severe uncontrolled epistaxis. Flexible nasal endoscopy reveals the source of bleeding to be in Kiesselbach's area. Anastomotic connections between which arteries are involved in this condition?

- ▢ **A.** Descending palatine and ascending pharyngeal
- ▢ **B.** Posterior superior alveolar and accessory meningeal
- ▢ **C.** Lateral branches of posterior ethmoidal and middle meningeal
- ▢ **D.** Branches of sphenopalatine, superior labial, and anterior ethmoidal
- ▢ **E.** Descending palatine and tonsillar branches of the ascending pharyngeal

255 A 49-year-old woman is admitted to the ENT department. Physical examination reveals swollen palatine tonsils and a tonsillectomy is performed. Which nerve coursing along the tonsillar bed needs to be spared during the surgery?

- ▢ **A.** Vagus
- ▢ **B.** Hypoglossal
- ▢ **C.** Glossopharyngeal
- ▢ **D.** Internal laryngeal
- ▢ **E.** External laryngeal

256 A 39-year-old man presents to an ENT specialist with hoarseness. Laryngoscopy shows nodules on the vocal cords with normal movement. Which muscle functions to open the rima glottidis?

- ▢ **A.** Posterior cricoarytenoids
- ▢ **B.** Lateral cricoarytenoids
- ▢ **C.** Thyroarytenoids
- ▢ **D.** Transverse arytenoids
- ▢ **E.** Cricothyroids

257 A 61-year-old man was admitted to the hospital after being found unconscious by his daughter. Shortly afterwards, he regained consciousness and physical examination showed that he was unable to shrug his shoulder on the right side and turn his head to the left. A CT scan demonstrated a large aneurysm of an artery compressing the nerve responsible for his symptoms. In which artery is the aneurysm?

- ▢ **A.** Superior cerebellar
- ▢ **B.** Posterior cerebral
- ▢ **C.** Anterior inferior cerebellar
- ▢ **D.** Posterior inferior cerebellar
- ▢ **E.** Basilar

258 Following a small brainstem stroke of limited size, a 64-year-old diabetic woman has uncoordinated swallowing and difficulty with phonation. The cranial nerve responsible for the dysfunction will most likely also produce which of the following symptoms?

- ▢ **A.** Weakness/paralysis of muscles of mastication on one side
- ▢ **B.** Weakness/paralysis of muscles of facial expression on one side
- ▢ **C.** Hearing loss and balance problems
- ▢ **D.** Decreased/absent sensation in the oropharynx
- ▢ **E.** Decreased/absent cough reflex

259 Following thyroidectomy for multiple benign thyroid nodules in a 44-year-old woman, a diagnosis of surgical injury to the left external laryngeal nerve is established. This may result in which of the following symptoms and signs?

- ▢ **A.** Inability to abduct the vocal fold
- ▢ **B.** Monotone, easily fatigued voice with poor pitch control
- ▢ **C.** Decreased/absent sensation above the vocal folds
- ▢ **D.** Decreased/absent sensation below the vocal folds
- ▢ **E.** Decreased/absent cough reflex

260 A physician is performing a cranial nerve examination on a 49-year-old patient. Oral examination revealed that the patient's uvula is deviated to the right. When the left side of the pharyngeal mucosa is touched, the gag reflex is weaker than when the mucosa on the right side is touched. Which nerve is most likely injured to cause these symptoms?

- ▢ **A.** Left vagus
- ▢ **B.** Left glossopharyngeal
- ▢ **C.** Right vagus
- ▢ **D.** Left V3
- ▢ **E.** Right glossopharyngeal

261 A 40-year-old woman comes to the physician because of pain in the region of her left jaw, left-sided earache, and headache for 3 days. The patient has not had any trauma to her face or jaw but says she often grinds her teeth. She is concerned because she is a singer, and it is painful when she opens her mouth wide to sing. There is also a clicking sound when she opens her mouth. Physical examination shows the left side of the jaw deviating slightly to the left on elevation. The area around the left mandibular condyle is painful on palpation. Mandibular depression is difficult to perform because of pain. This movement also elicits an audible clicking sound. There is tightness indicative of a muscle spasm along the left mandibular ramus. Palpation shows no other area of tightness. Spasms of which of the following muscle are most likely associated with this condition?

- ▢ **A.** Buccinator
- ▢ **B.** Masseter
- ▢ **C.** Mylohyoid
- ▢ **D.** Posterior belly of the digastric
- ▢ **E.** Lateral pterygoid

262 During a test of the cough reflex a 62-year-old woman inhales air containing different amounts of particles that will adhere to mucus primarily in the trachea. Blockade of afferent neurons in which cranial nerve will most likely suppress this woman's cough reflex?

- ▢ **A.** Glossopharyngeal
- ▢ **B.** Hypoglossal
- ▢ **C.** External laryngeal
- ▢ **D.** Trigeminal
- ▢ **E.** Vagus

263 A neurologist strokes a wisp of cotton across a patient's left cornea without a response. The neurologist then strokes the cotton across the patient's right cornea and both eyes blink. The most likely explanation of these findings is damage to which of the following cranial nerve on the left?

- ▢ **A.** Optic
- ▢ **B.** Oculomotor
- ▢ **C.** Trigeminal
- ▢ **D.** Abducens
- ▢ **E.** Facial

264 A 12-year-old girl is brought to the physician by her parents because of a sore neck for 4 days. Her temperature is 37.7° C (99.9° F). Physical examination shows a tender swelling anterior to, and just above, the thyroid notch of the neck. The physician explains that there is a cyst in the tract along which the thyroid gland descended. All of the tract tissue must be removed between which of the following two structures to treat this patient's condition?

- ▢ **A.** Left lobe of thyroid gland and tonsillar fossa
- ▢ **B.** Right lobe of thyroid gland and epiglottis
- ▢ **C.** Right lobe of thyroid gland and hyoid bone
- ▢ **D.** Thyroid isthmus and foramen cecum
- ▢ **E.** Thyroid isthmus and piriform recess

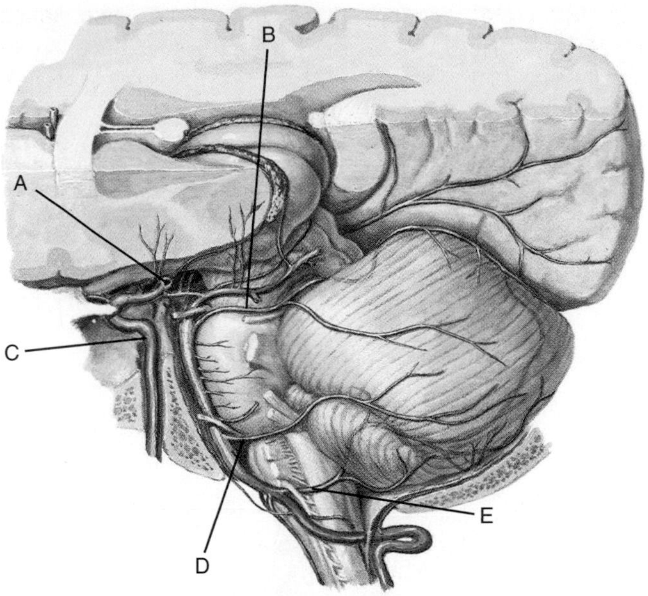

Fig. 7-23

265 A 34-year-old man complains of diplopia that becomes worse when reading a newspaper or walking down the stairs. Physical examination in the neurosurgery outpatient clinic reveals weakness of downward movement of the left eye. A CT scan reveals a large aneurysm in one of the arteries of the posterior cerebral circulation compressing the nerve resulting in the symptoms. In which artery in the diagram (Fig. 7-23) is the aneurysm?

- ▢ **A.** A
- ▢ **B.** B
- ▢ **C.** C
- ▢ **D.** D
- ▢ **E.** E

266 A 63-year-old woman presents with ptosis of the left eye. On examination the left eye is abducted and depressed and the light reflex is absent. Angiography reveals an aneurysm (arrow, Fig. 7-24) of an artery compressing the nerve responsible for the symptoms. Which of the following describes the location of the aneurysm?

- ▢ **A.** ICA in the cavernous sinus
- ▢ **B.** Division of the ICA into middle and anterior cerebral arteries
- ▢ **C.** Left vertebral artery at the junction with the basilar artery
- ▢ **D.** Union of left and right vertebral arteries forming basilar artery
- ▢ **E.** Basilar artery between the left superior cerebellar and posterior cerebral arteries

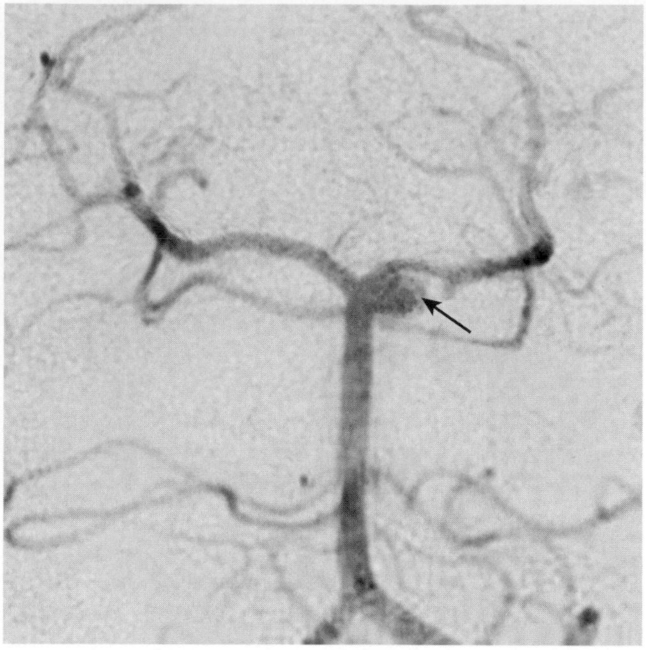

Fig. 7-24

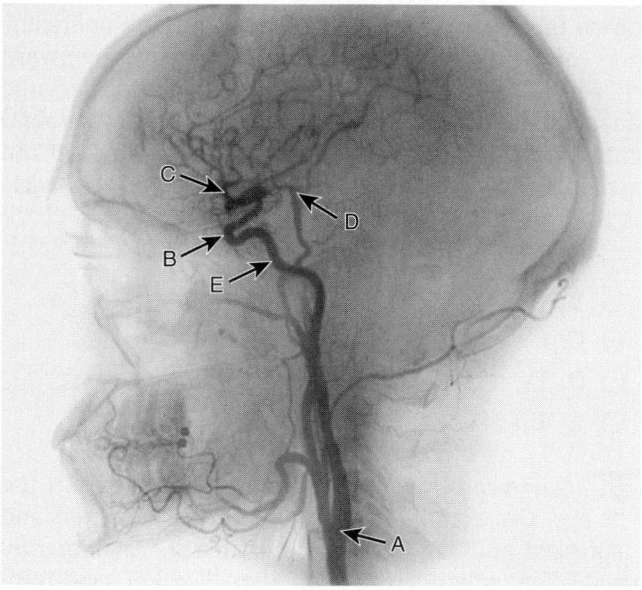

Fig. 7-25

267 A 75-year-old woman presents to the emergency department complaining of double vision. Physical examination reveals inability to abduct her right eye. In which of the locations indicated in the arteriogram (Fig. 7-25) would an aneurysm most likely be located to cause the nerve compression resulting in these symptoms/signs?

- ▢ **A.** PCA
- ▢ **B.** ICA
- ▢ **C.** External carotid artery

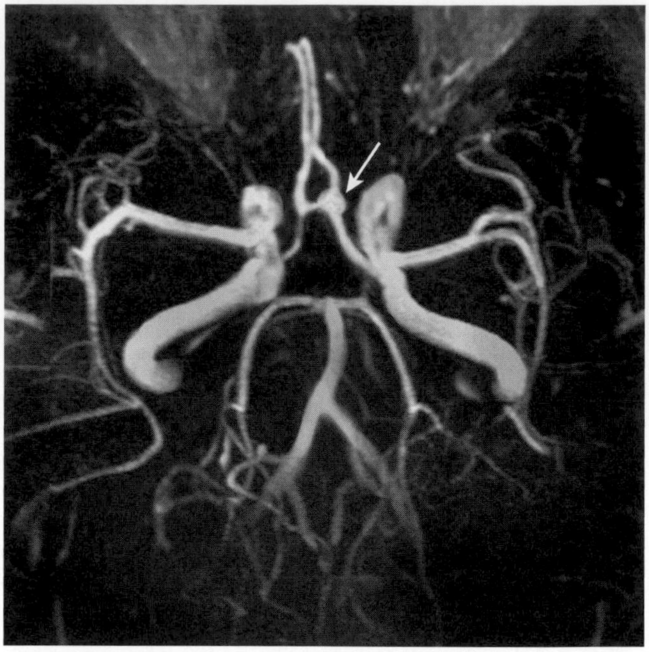

Fig. 7-26

- ▢ **D.** Anterior cerebral artery
- ▢ **E.** Posterior communicating artery

268 A 49-year-old man is seen in the emergency department because of headaches and dizziness for the past couple of months. Imaging studies reveal a saccular (berry) aneurysm (Fig. 7-26, arrow). An aneurysm at this location would most likely cause nerve compression resulting in which of the following additional findings on neurologic examination?

- ▢ **A.** Inability to abduct the eye
- ▢ **B.** Inability to depress the adducted eye
- ▢ **C.** Loss of corneal sensation
- ▢ **D.** Ptosis
- ▢ **E.** Visual field deficits

269 A 16-year-old boy presents to the emergency department with pain and blurred vision following a blow to his left eye with a baseball bat. On examination, when asked to gaze upwards his eyes move as seen in the photograph (Fig. 7-27B). Imaging studies reveal a fracture, as indicated by the arrow in the image (Fig. 7-27A). Which of the following muscles is most likely affected?

- ▢ **A.** Levator palpebrae superioris
- ▢ **B.** Inferior oblique
- ▢ **C.** Inferior rectus
- ▢ **D.** Medial rectus
- ▢ **E.** Superior rectus

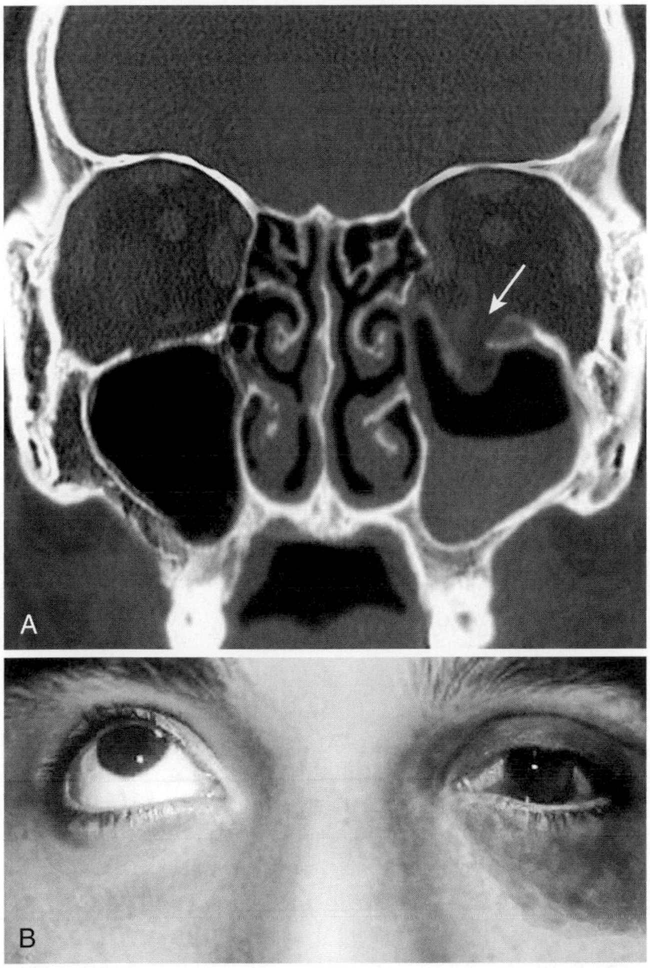

Fig. 7-27AB

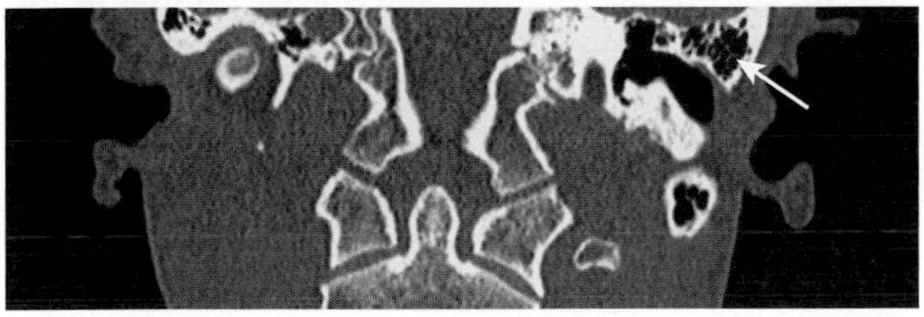

Fig. 7-28

270 A 10-year-old child appearing acutely ill is seen in the emergency department because of severe ear pain, headache, and fever for the past five days. Physical examination reveals a red and bulging tympanic membrane with a purulent effusion, and tenderness over the area indicated by the arrow in the coronal CT (Fig. 7-28). Assuming that this area is now infected, which of the following venous channels is most at risk for thrombosis as a direct result of proximity to the infected/inflamed bone?

- ▢ **A.** Cavernous sinus
- ▢ **B.** Pterygoid venous plexus
- ▢ **C.** Sigmoid sinus
- ▢ **D.** Straight sinus
- ▢ **E.** Superior petrosal sinus

271 A 12-year-old boy complains of symptoms suggestive of sinusitis. During the physical examination the physician taps the area slightly superior to the midportion of the patient's eyebrows and this maneuver elicits pain. Which anatomic area is the physician most likely examining?

- ▢ **A.** Maxillary sinus
- ▢ **B.** Temporal bone
- ▢ **C.** Frontal sinus
- ▢ **D.** Sphenoid sinus
- ▢ **E.** Ethmoid sinus

272 A physician palpates the mastoid process of an adolescent complaining of pain behind the ear. Which bone is the physician palpating?

- ▢ **A.** Occipital
- ▢ **B.** Zygomatic
- ▢ **C.** Temporal
- ▢ **D.** Parietal
- ▢ **E.** Sphenoid

273 A physician performs an ophthalmoscopic examination on a 45-year-old man and can clearly observe the macula lutea and optic disc. He also sees several branching arteries emanating from the optic disc. These arteries are most likely derived from which of the following?

- ▢ **A.** Central retinal artery
- ▢ **B.** Long posterior ciliary artery
- ▢ **C.** Short posterior ciliary artery
- ▢ **D.** Ophthalmic artery
- ▢ **E.** Anterior ciliary artery

274 While at a party, an intoxicated teenage girl asks her friend to pierce the tragus of her left ear. While attempting to pass a needle through the tragus, the friend slips and the needle deeply punctures the skin directly anterior to the tragus. The next morning the teenager awakens to find that she has no feeling on the left temporal side of her scalp up to the vertex of her head. Which of the following nerves is most likely damaged?

- ▢ **A.** Lesser occipital
- ▢ **B.** Greater occipital
- ▢ **C.** Auriculotemporal
- ▢ **D.** Zygomaticotemporal
- ▢ **E.** Great auricular

275 A 27-year-old woman is found to have unilateral facial paralysis. An MRI of her head reveals a small tumor located at the internal acoustic meatus. Which of the following cranial nerves is most likely being compressed by the tumor?

- ▢ **A.** V
- ▢ **B.** VI
- ▢ **C.** VII
- ▢ **D.** IX
- ▢ **E.** X

276 A patient with a brain tumor near the crista galli and cribriform plate of the ethmoid bone most likely experiences which of the following symptoms?

- ▢ **A.** Paralysis of facial muscles
- ▢ **B.** Loss of vision
- ▢ **C.** Difficulty swallowing
- ▢ **D.** Loss of smell
- ▢ **E.** Loss of hearing

277 A 20-year-old man fell off a motorcycle and sustained a head injury. A CT scan of his head revealed a fracture of the sella turcica. Which of the following bones was most likely damaged in this patient?

- ▢ **A.** Sphenoid
- ▢ **B.** Temporal
- ▢ **C.** Occipital
- ▢ **D.** Ethmoid
- ▢ **E.** Frontal

278 A 21-year-old man shaved his head with a razor blade and sustained a deep cut to the scalp. An infection occurred at the site of the cut. The man did not seek medical attention and the infection eventually subsided. Three weeks later he woke up with a severe headache and nausea. He was brought to the emergency department and found to have an infection of the superior sagittal sinus. Which of the following veins was most likely responsible for this patient's current infection?

- ▢ **A.** Intercavernous
- ▢ **B.** Inferior sagittal
- ▢ **C.** Diploic
- ▢ **D.** Basilar
- ▢ **E.** Emissary

279 A 20-year-old man was in a bar fight and sustained a deep laceration to his face after being slashed with a broken glass bottle. Physical examination revealed a deep, 10-cm laceration running obliquely across his right cheek. He is now unable to close his right eye and cannot smile on the right side. Which additional structure was most likely damaged in this patient?

- ▢ **A.** Vertebral artery
- ▢ **B.** Common carotid artery
- ▢ **C.** Parotid gland
- ▢ **D.** Lateral pterygoid muscle
- ▢ **E.** Temporalis muscle

280 A 25-year-old man sustains a blow to the back of the head during a fight and is brought to the emergency department unconscious. A CT scan of the head reveals a fracture in the occipital bone extending superiorly from the foramen magnum. Which of the following is transmitted through the foramen magnum?

- ▢ **A.** Cranial nerve I
- ▢ **B.** Cranial nerve IX
- ▢ **C.** Cranial nerve X
- ▢ **D.** Cranial nerve XI
- ▢ **E.** Cranial nerve XII

281 An otherwise healthy 11-year-old girl with recurrent upper respiratory tract infections undergoes bilateral tonsillectomy. While performing the procedure, the surgeon accidentally damages the nerve that lies in the tonsillar fossa, deep to the palatine tonsil. Which of the following is most likely to result from this injury?

- ▢ **A.** Loss of sensation on the posterior one third of the tongue
- ▢ **B.** Loss of taste on the anterior two thirds of the tongue
- ▢ **C.** Paralysis of the constrictor muscles of the pharynx
- ▢ **D.** Paralysis of the muscles of the soft palate
- ▢ **E.** Paralysis of the muscles of the tongue

282 A 70-year-old patient with sudden-onset hoarseness is found to have a small carcinoma of the mucosa overlying the right vocalis muscle. Which of the following is most likely located immediately lateral to this muscle?

- ▢ **A.** Lateral cricoarytenoid muscle
- ▢ **B.** Aryepiglottic muscle
- ▢ **C.** Posterior cricoarytenoid muscle
- ▢ **D.** Oblique arytenoids muscle
- ▢ **E.** Thyroarytenoid muscle

283 A 34-year-old woman bursts through the doors of the emergency department. She is straining to take a breath but can only mouth, "I can't breathe" before collapsing. She is placed on a stretcher. Her tongue is swollen and protruding from her mouth. The patient has only minimal air movement with bag-mask ventilation. Oxygen saturation is approximately 80%. Attempts at oral intubation are unsuccessful due to massive soft tissue edema of her pharynx. A decision is made to perform a cricothyrotomy. After palpation of the neck to identify the appropriate landmarks, an incision should most likely be made at which of the following locations?

- ▢ **A.** The cricothyroid membrane, which is located at the junction of the clavicle and the sternum
- ▢ **B.** The cricothyroid membrane, which is located between the thyroid cartilage and the cricoid cartilage below
- ▢ **C.** The thyrohyoid membrane, which is located between the thyroid cartilage (Adam's apple) and the hyoid bone above
- ▢ **D.** The sternal notch, which is located at the junction of the clavicle and the sternum
- ▢ **E.** The trachea, which is located below the cricoid cartilage

284 A patient is rushed to the emergency department and requires insertion of an endotracheal tube. Because the physician needs to insert the tube immediately, the patient is not given anesthesia. As the physician inserts the tube, he strikes the epiglottis, which causes the patient to grimace. Which of the following cranial nerves most likely allows the patient to sense pain from the larynx?

- ▢ **A.** Vagus
- ▢ **B.** Glossopharyngeal
- ▢ **C.** Vestibulocochlear
- ▢ **D.** Hypoglossal
- ▢ **E.** Facial

285 A 55-year-old man complains of progressive hearing loss and a continuous strange noise in his right ear that he noticed several months ago. On physical examination he has right-sided hearing loss, asymmetric smile, and decreased corneal reflex in his right eye. A CT scan reveals a large intracranial tumor. Which of the following will most likely be the location of the tumor?

- ▢ **A.** Between the medulla and the cerebellar hemisphere
- ▢ **B.** Above the diaphragma sellae
- ▢ **C.** Over the lateral hemispheric fissure
- ▢ **D.** Between the cerebellum and the lateral pons
- ▢ **E.** Between the cerebellar peduncles

286 A 28-year-old woman visits the ENT physician because of a painful infection of her outer ear. During physical examination the ENT physician inserts a speculum into the external auditory meatus in close contact with its posterior wall. The patient starts coughing and complains of feeling dizzy. Irritation of which of the following nerves was most likely stimulated by the speculum?

- ▢ **A.** Vestibulocochlear
- ▢ **B.** Vagus
- ▢ **C.** Trigeminal
- ▢ **D.** Facial
- ▢ **E.** Accessory

287 A 60-year-old man is undergoing a thyroidectomy procedure. The superior thyroid artery is ligated and special attention needs to be paid to the adjacent nerve. Which of the following muscles is innervated by this nerve?

- ▢ **A.** Thyroarytenoid
- ▢ **B.** Lateral cricoarytenoid
- ▢ **C.** Posterior cricoarytenoid
- ▢ **D.** Cricothyroid
- ▢ **E.** Aryepiglotticus

288 A 55-year-old woman presented to the emergency department with complaints of severe headaches for 2 weeks. There was no history of fever, neck stiffness, or photophobia. On examination, she was in pain and distress. Vital signs revealed blood pressure (BP) 160/89 mm Hg, pulse 110 bpm, respiration rate 16/min, temperature 36° C. Range of movement of the neck was normal, and funduscopy showed no abnormalities on the retina. A CT scan of the brain with contrast was performed and revealed a dilated branch of the basilar artery at the junction of the pons and medulla on the right side. She was referred to the neurosurgeon for assessment and further management. Which of the following statements describes clinical features with which this patient might present?

- ▢ **A.** Weak abduction and depression of the right eye
- ▢ **B.** Weak adduction of the left eye
- ▢ **C.** Weak adduction and elevation of the right eye
- ▢ **D.** Weak abduction of the right eye
- ▢ **E.** Weak abduction of the left eye

289 A 65-year-old woman presented to the emergency department with complaints of severe headaches for 2 weeks. There was no history of fever, neck stiffness, or photophobia. On examination, she was in painful distress. Vital signs revealed BP 160/89 mm Hg, pulse 110 bpm, respiration rate 16/min, temperature 36° C. Range of movement of the neck was normal and funduscopy showed no abnormalities of the retina. A CT scan of the brain with contrast revealed a dilated branch of the basilar artery at the junction of the pons and midbrain on the right side. She was referred to the neurosurgeon for assessment and further management. Which of the following statements describes clinical features with which this patient might present?

- ▢ **A.** Weak abduction of the right eye
- ▢ **B.** Blurred vision from the right eye and full ptosis of the right upper eyelid
- ▢ **C.** Loss of vision from lateral fields right eye and medial fields of left eye
- ▢ **D.** Inability to detect odors through the right nostril
- ▢ **E.** Loss of sensation of the skin over the right forehead, cheek, and mandible

290 A 60-year-old man presented to his family practitioner with complaints of numbness to the right side of the lower jaw and the inside of the cheek. Examination revealed loss of sensation over the scalp in the posterior temporal region and skin over the anterior auricle. There was weak lateral deviation of the mandible to the right. He was referred for a CT scan of the brain, which showed a mass in the medial temporal fossa. What other functions are most likely affected in this patient?

- ▢ **A.** Weak elevation of the corner of the right side of the mouth
- ▢ **B.** Loss of sensation over the upper lip and to the upper teeth
- ▢ **C.** Inability to sense a foreign body in the right eye
- ▢ **D.** Decreased secretion from the parotid gland
- ▢ **E.** Inability to abduct the right eye

291 A 40-year-old woman presented to the emergency department with complaints of swelling and pain over the left side of her face. On examination, there was tender, warm swelling over the left mandible anterior to the ear. Ultrasound revealed a hyperechoic mass within the lumen of the parotid duct, which was distended proximally. What other clinical features are most likely present in this patient?

- ▢ **A.** Weak deviation of the mandible to the right
- ▢ **B.** Complete ptosis of the left eyelid
- ▢ **C.** Numbness of the skin over the left lower mandible
- ▢ **D.** Excessive tearing
- ▢ **E.** Pain over the anterior auricle, tragus, and anterior helix

292 A 40-year-old man was brought to the emergency department after falling through a glass window to the ground 5 feet below. He complained of pain from multiple lacerations across his body, particularly from a laceration to the left cheek. On examination, he was comfortable with stable vital signs. There were multiple superficial lacerations on his upper and lower limbs but no deformities of bones or joints were evident. There was a 5-cm longitudinal laceration over the left jaw. Gentle exploration of the wound revealed that it was deep and a foreign body was present. A CT scan of the head confirmed that a 3 × 2 cm foreign body, possibly glass, was lodged between the two heads of the lateral pterygoid muscle. Which of the following clinical findings are most likely to be found in this patient?

- ▢ **A.** Weak elevation of the jaw
- ▢ **B.** Weak deviation of the jaw to the right side
- ▢ **C.** Numbness over the skin of the tragus and helix of the left ear
- ▢ **D.** Numbness over the skin and mucosa of the anterior cheek
- ▢ **E.** Decreased volume of saliva

293 A 30-year-old man was brought to the emergency department after being involved in a head-on collision with another car. He did not wear a seat belt and was found unconscious in the driver's seat, from which he had to be extricated. Examination revealed that he was poorly responsive with a low blood pressure, tachycardia, and several lacerations about his face and body. There was an obvious deformity of the face but "step-off" defects were palpated over the root of the nose and the glabella. There was also clear fluid draining from the nasal cavity. Once the patient was stabilized, a CT of the skull was performed and revealed a fracture in the middle region of the anterior cranial fossa. Which of the following complaints will the patient most likely complain of once he regains consciousness?

- ▢ **A.** Blurred vision
- ▢ **B.** Diplopia
- ▢ **C.** Anosmia
- ▢ **D.** Blindness
- ▢ **E.** Dry left eye

294 A 30-year-old man was brought to the emergency department after being involved in a head-on collision with another car. He did not wear a seat belt and was found unconscious in the driver's seat, from which he had to be extricated. Examination revealed a poorly responsive patient with low BP, tachycardia, and several lacerations about his face and body. Once the patient was stabilized, a CT of the skull was done, revealing a fracture near the apex of the orbit with narrowing of the opening to the orbit in the area. Which of the following functions will most likely be maintained or spared in this patient?

- ▢ **A.** Secretions from the right lacrimal gland
- ▢ **B.** Ability to detect a foreign body on the cornea
- ▢ **C.** Sensation over the anterior scalp
- ▢ **D.** Sensation to the upper eyelid
- ▢ **E.** Ability to abduct the eye

295 A 30-year-old man was brought to the emergency department after being involved in a head-on collision with another car. He did not wear a seat belt and was found unconscious in the driver's seat, from which he had to be extricated. Examination revealed a poorly responsive patient with a low BP, tachycardia, and several lacerations about his face and body. Examination revealed a bony deformity of the right mandible where abnormal mobility of the bone was palpated approximately along the ramus. Once the patient was stabilized, a CT of the skull was performed, revealing a displaced, transverse fracture of the ramus, just proximal to the angle of the mandible. Which of the following will most likely be affected?

- ▢ **A.** Elevation of the jaw
- ▢ **B.** Lateral deviation of the jaw to the left side
- ▢ **C.** Salivation; sensation and taste from the anterior tongue
- ▢ **D.** Sensation from skin over anterior cheek and tongue
- ▢ **E.** Salivation; sensation from posterior temporal skin and tragus of the ear

296 A 20-year-old man was brought to the emergency department after the motorcycle he was driving was struck by a car. He was unable to recall all events of the incident and complained of pain to right side of the head and face, lower back, right elbow, and right knee. On examination, he was alert and oriented. There were multiple abrasions to his upper and lower limbs but no neurologic deficits were evident. There was a tender 6 × 6 cm swelling over the right temporal bone and a laceration to the superior aspect of the helix of the right ear. A CT scan of the head and brain was done, revealing a minimally displaced fracture of the floor of the middle cranial fossa involving the pterygoid canal. Which of the following describes all fiber types that are most likely affected in this injury?

- ▢ **A.** Presynaptic parasympathetic
- ▢ **B.** Postsynaptic sympathetic; presynaptic parasympathetic
- ▢ **C.** Postsynaptic sympathetic; postsynaptic parasympathetic
- ▢ **D.** Special sensory; postsynaptic parasympathetic
- ▢ **E.** General sensory; postsynaptic parasympathetic

297 A 20-year-old man presented to the emergency department with complaints of fever, swelling over the right side of the temple of his head, and headache for 5 days. He had a history of trauma 1 week before presentation, when he was struck from his motorcycle by a car and suffered a minimally displaced open fracture of right temporal bone. The wound was irrigated and debrided and after 24 hours of neurologic observation in hospital, he was discharged. On examination, he was in painful distress. There was a tender swelling over the right temporal bone where sutured skin appeared flushed (erythematous). Neurologic examination produced findings consistent with neuritis (irritation) of the nerve passing through the distal part of the facial canal. Which of the following functions is likely to be spared by this lesion?

- ▢ **A.** Taste from the anterior two thirds of the tongue
- ▢ **B.** Movements of the right side of the face
- ▢ **C.** Secretions from the submandibular gland
- ▢ **D.** Secretions from the sublingual gland
- ▢ **E.** Secretions from the lacrimal gland

298 A 20-year-old woman presented to the emergency department after being thrown from her horse during an equestrian competition. She denied loss of consciousness but complained of pain on the left side of her face, hand, and elbow, as well as double vision. On examination, there was a tender swelling over the superolateral aspect of the left eye, and a defect in the bone was palpable. There was significant periorbital edema and bruising of the inferior skin of the eye. Pupillary light reflexes were normal, and funduscopy showed no abnormalities of the retina. A CT scan of the head and face revealed a comminuted, depressed fracture of the frontal process of the left zygomatic bone involving the orbit. Which of the following describes the most likely consequence of her injury?

- ▢ **A.** Weak abduction of the eye
- ▢ **B.** Diplopia
- ▢ **C.** Blurred vision
- ▢ **D.** Decreased secretions from the left lacrimal gland
- ▢ **E.** Partial ptosis

299 A 30-year-old man was brought to the emergency department with complaints of severe pain to the right eye and double vision. While playing a game of cricket, he was struck in the face just below the eye. On examination, there was periorbital edema and bruising of the skin around the eye and tenderness over the inferior orbital margin. A defect of the bone along this margin was palpated. A CT scan of the brain and face revealed a displaced fracture of the inferior margin and floor of the orbit along the suture line between the zygomatic and maxillary bones. Which of the following best explains this patient's symptoms?

- ▢ **A.** Partial ptosis of the upper eyelid
- ▢ **B.** Complete ptosis of the upper eyelid
- ▢ **C.** Inability to elevate the abducted eyeball
- ▢ **D.** Inability to depress the abducted eyeball
- ▢ **E.** Inability to produce tears

300 A 40-year-old woman presented to her family practitioner with complaints of vertigo and nausea and reduced hearing through her left ear for 3 months. She also complained of a dry mouth and dryness of the left eye. CT scan of the head showed thickening of the bones of the skull. Which of the following areas was most likely affected to produce this patient's symptoms?

- ▢ **A.** Petrous temporal bone
- ▢ **B.** Infratemporal fossa
- ▢ **C.** Facial canal
- ▢ **D.** Middle ear
- ▢ **E.** Inner ear

301 A 15-year-old boy was brought to the emergency department with complaints of right ear pain. While attempting to clean his itchy ear with a swab, his little brother bumped into his elbow, causing the stick to penetrate deeply into the ear. On examination with the otoscope, the tympanic membrane was pearly white and there was no cone of light visible. There was clotted blood in the external auditory meatus. Rinne's test was positive (bone conduction was better than air conduction). Which of the following best describes the nerves responsible for the perception of pain from the injured area?

- ▢ **A.** Auriculotemporal and great auricular nerves
- ▢ **B.** Facial, glossopharyngeal, and vagus nerves
- ▢ **C.** Lesser occipital and great auricular nerve
- ▢ **D.** Chorda tympani and glossopharyngeal nerve
- ▢ **E.** Tympanic plexus and lesser petrosal nerve

302 A 20-year-old woman delivered an infant girl at term after an uneventful pregnancy. Upon examination of the infant, the intern noticed that the iris of the left eye had a defect inferolaterally, so the pupil appeared to have an extended opening. The mother of the infant was reassured that this would not likely cause any significant visual impairment, as the defect was very small. Which of the following explains the defect noticed in the infant's eye?

- ▢ **A.** Failed induction of surface ectoderm by the neuroectoderm
- ▢ **B.** Failed obliteration of the intraretinal space
- ▢ **C.** Failed closure of the choroid fissure
- ▢ **D.** Optic cup does not overlap the developing lens
- ▢ **E.** Lens vesicle remains connected to surface ectoderm

303 A 30-year-old woman presented to her physician with complaints of nasal congestion and headache for 2 days. Her symptoms were associated with clear fluid from her nostrils (rhinorrhea). Examination revealed that she was febrile (38° C) and the nasal mucosa was erythematous with swelling of the conchae. There was tenderness over the forehead above the root of the nose and the areas on either side of the glabella. She was diagnosed with an upper respiratory tract infection. Which of the following structures is the most likely passage for the spread of infection in this patient?

- ▢ **A.** Pharyngotympanic tube
- ▢ **B.** Ethmoidal infundibulum
- ▢ **C.** Nasolacrimal duct
- ▢ **D.** Spheno-ethmoidal recess
- ▢ **E.** Superior nasal meatus

304 A 20-year-old woman delivered an infant girl at term after an uneventful pregnancy. She admitted to the use of alcohol and tobacco throughout the pregnancy. Upon examination of the infant, the intern discovered that there was a deformity of the face in which a groove connected the medial canthus of the right eye to the right corner of the upper lip. There was a clear, watery discharge from the groove. A defect in which of the following developmental processes most likely resulted in the deformity seen in this infant?

- ▢ **A.** Fusion of maxillary processes to each other
- ▢ **B.** Fusion of medial nasal prominences to each other
- ▢ **C.** Migration of ectoderm between maxillary and lateral nasal prominences
- ▢ **D.** Fusion of the maxillary and lateral nasal processes
- ▢ **E.** Fusion of the intermaxillary segment with the maxillary processes

305 A 20-year-old woman delivered an infant boy at term after an uneventful pregnancy. On examination of the infant, the intern noted that the corners of the eyes were downward slanting and the pinnae and the mandible were underdeveloped. The mother of the infant stated that he had difficulty with breastfeeding and feeding by bottle because he was unable to create the suction needed to feed, and the milk often refluxed through his nose. She also stated that the father of the child had similar facial abnormalities. Which of the following is the most likely cause of the deformities seen in this infant?

- ☐ **A.** Failed fusion of lateral nasal prominences and maxillary processes
- ☐ **B.** Lack of fusion of medial nasal prominences
- ☐ **C.** Failed migration of neural crest cells to the first pharyngeal arch
- ☐ **D.** Failed migration of neural crest cells to the third and fourth pharyngeal pouches
- ☐ **E.** Failed migration of ectoderm between maxillary and lateral nasal prominences

306 A 40-year-old woman presented to the neighborhood clinic with complaints of a constant, worsening headache for 4 months that was unresponsive to pain medication. The pain was worse on the right side. She denied having fever, neck stiffness, or aversion to light. On examination, there was no motor weakness of the upper or lower limbs. A CT scan of the brain with contrast revealed a berry aneurysm of the right superior cerebellar artery. Which of the following will most likely be identified during physical examination of this patient?

- ☐ **A.** Lack of accommodation, adduction of the right eye
- ☐ **B.** Blurred vision, complete ptosis, abduction of the right eye
- ☐ **C.** Partial ptosis, adduction and downward rotation of the right eye
- ☐ **D.** Complete ptosis, abduction and upward rotation of the right eye
- ☐ **E.** Complete ptosis, abduction and downward rotation of the right eye

307 A 20-year-old woman delivered an infant boy at term by cesarean section (C-section). During the third trimester an abdominal ultrasound revealed enlarged ventricles of the fetal brain. On examination, the circumference of the infant's head was 40 cm (normal range, 34 to 36 cm). He showed decreased movement of the limbs and seemed drowsy. A CT scan of the brain with contrast medium showed dilatation of all the ventricles. Which of the following is likely to be the cause of the infant's condition

- ☐ **A.** Narrowing of the median aperture
- ☐ **B.** Narrowing of the lateral aperture
- ☐ **C.** Abnormality of arachnoid granulations
- ☐ **D.** Lack of choroid plexus in the lateral ventricles
- ☐ **E.** Increased blood flow in the cerebral arteries

308 A 64-year-old man has a parotidectomy because of a malignant tumor in his parotid gland. About a year after the surgery he notices that when he sees appetizing food he sweats on the side of his face where the tumor was removed. Where are the nerve cell bodies for the nerve fibers that are now innervating his sweat glands?

- ☐ **A.** Ciliary ganglion
- ☐ **B.** Pterygopalatine ganglion
- ☐ **C.** Otic ganglion
- ☐ **D.** Submandibular ganglion
- ☐ **E.** Superior salivatory nucleus

ANSWERS

1 E. The child in this case suffers from a fistula that indicates an open malformation. This implies that the defect must be due to failure of closure for both an internal and an external structure. This excludes the second pharyngeal arch and third pharyngeal pouch from being the answers alone. A branchial fistula results from failure of closure of both the second pharyngeal pouch and the cervical sinus, the cervical sinus being the consolidation of the second through fourth pharyngeal clefts, all being external structures. The thyroglossal duct extends from the thyroid to the tongue and failure of its closure would not result in an external defect. The second pharyngeal groove merges with the third and fourth pharyngeal grooves to form the cervical sinus. Failure of closure of the second groove alone would not present with an open fistula.

GAS 1016; N 64; McM 28-35

2 A. The largest part of the palate is formed by the secondary palate, which is embryologically derived from the lateral palatine processes. The median palatine process gives rise to the smaller primary palate, located anteriorly. The intermaxillary segment gives rise to the middle upper lip, premaxillary part of the maxilla, and the primary palate. The median nasal prominences merge with each other and the maxillary prominences to give rise to the intermaxillary segment. The frontonasal eminence gives rise to parts of the forehead, nose, and eyes.

GAS 1089, 1077; N 62, 64; McM 1, 9

3 A. A coloboma of the iris is caused by failure of the retinal fissure to close during the sixth week. Abnormal neural crest formation would lead to abnormal development of choroid, sclera, and cornea because these are derived from neural crest cells. Abnormal interaction between the optic vesicle and ectoderm would lead to abnormal development of the entire eye because a lens placode may fail to develop or develop abnormally. The iris would not be affected by abnormal development of the posterior chamber. Weak adhesion between the layers of the optic vesicle leads to congenital retinal detachment.

GAS 947; N 83; McM 54

4 E. The anterior fontanelle is located at the junction of the sagittal and coronal sutures and closes at around 18 months of age. The posterior fontanelle is located at the junction of the sagittal suture and lambdoid suture, and it closes at around 2 to 3 months. The mastoid fontanelle is located at the junction of the squamous suture and the lambdoid suture, and it closes at the end of the first year. The sphenoidal fontanelle is located at the junction of the squamous suture and the coronal suture and closes at around 2 to 3 months. There is a lambdoid suture but not a lambdoid fontanelle.

GAS 860, 864; N 9; McM 14

5 A. Thyroglossal duct cysts occur due to retention of a remnant of the thyroglossal duct along the path followed by the descending thyroid gland during development. The path begins at the foramen cecum of the tongue and descends in the midline to the final position of the thyroid. The sixth pharyngeal arch provides origin to muscles and cartilage of the neck and would produce a midline mass connected to the tongue. A branchial cyst or fistula would not be present in the midline. The first pharyngeal arch gives rise to muscles of mastication and the malleus and incus. The third pharyngeal arch provides origin to the stylopharyngeus muscle and hyoid bone.

GAS 1020; N 64; McM 33

6 E. The most common cause of cleft lip is failure of fusion of the maxillary process and the intermaxillary segment. Defects located between the lateral nasal prominences and the maxillary processes would affect the development of the nasolacrimal duct. Failure of fusion of the medial nasal prominences would produce a median cleft lip, a rare congenital anomaly. The lateral and median nasal processes both arise from the nasal placodes and do not undergo subsequent fusion. The lateral nasal prominences do not fuse with each other.

GAS 1077; N 46; McM 80

7 A. The listed symptoms are typical of first pharyngeal (brachial) arch syndrome because the first arch normally gives rise to muscles of mastication, mylohyoid, anterior belly of the digastric, tensor tympani, tensor veli palatini, malleus, and the incus. Abnormal development of the second arch would affect the muscles of facial expression, the stapes, and parts of the hyoid bone. Abnormal development of the third pharyngeal arch would affect only the stylopharyngeus muscle and parts of the hyoid bone. Abnormal development of the fourth and sixth arch would affect various muscles and cartilages of the larynx and pharynx and would not produce the hypoplastic mandible characteristic of first arch syndrome.

GAS 977, 961, 1009; N 48-49, 74, 94; McM 35, 39, 61

8 C. Obstructive hydrocephalus, in this case resulting from obstruction of the cerebral aqueduct (of Sylvius), refers to a condition in which flow of cerebrospinal fluid (CSF) is obstructed within the ventricular system. This leads to pressure increasing in the CSF upstream from the obstruction, expanding the lateral and third ventricles. Nonobstructive hydrocephalus is due to either excessive CSF production or ineffective CSF reabsorption. This would lead to enlargement of all ventricular chambers. Anencephaly, also known as meroanencephaly, is a partial absence of the brain and is due to defective closure of the anterior neuropore. Holoprosencephaly is a failure of cleavage of the forebrain and would result in a single fused ventricle.

GAS 877-878; N 147; McM 72, 81

9 C. Both the inferior parathyroid glands and the thymus are derived from the third pharyngeal (brachial) pouch. Therefore, an ectopic thymus is likely to be associated with ectopic parathyroid tissue, indicating abnormal development of the third pharyngeal pouch. The lingual tonsil develops from an aggregation of lymph nodules on the tongue and is not associated with development of the thymus. The submandibular gland develops from endodermal buds in the floor of the stomodeum and is not associated with development of the thymus. The thyroid gland arises from an outpocketing of the floor of the primitive oral cavity, descending along the route of the thyroglossal duct, and it is not associated with development of the thymus. Development of the lymph nodes is also not associated with development of the thymus.

GAS 1022; N 78; McM 30

10 C. The defect is likely in the development of third and fourth pharyngeal pouches because the superior parathyroid glands are derived from the fourth pouch, whereas the inferior parathyroid glands are derived from the third pouch. In addition, the third pouch gives rise to the thymus, and the parafollicular cells of the thyroid gland are derived from the fourth pharyngeal pouch. The first pouch gives rise to the tympanic membrane and cavity. The second pouch gives rise to the palatine tonsils and tonsillar sinus.

GAS 1022; N 78; McM 30

11 C. Whereas all forms of clefts are considered to have a multifactorial etiology, cleft lip in particular seems to have a strong genetic factor. This has been determined using studies of twins. The other listed factors may or may not play a role in the development of a cleft lip, but genetics remains the most important determining factor.

GAS 1077; N 46; McM 80

12 C. Absence of the thymus and inferior parathyroid glands would be due to defective development of the third pharyngeal pouch, their normal site of origin. The first pouch gives rise to the tympanic membrane and cavity. The second pouch gives rise to the palatine tonsils and tonsillar sinus. The fourth pharyngeal pouch gives rise to the superior parathyroid glands and the parafollicular cells of the thyroid gland. The fifth pharyngeal pouch contributes to the formation of the parafollicular cells of the thyroid gland.

GAS 1022; N 78; McM 30

13 D. The third pharyngeal arch gives rise to the greater cornuae and lower part of the hyoid bone, in addition to the stylopharyngeus muscle. The maxillary prominence is important in the development of the cheeks and upper lip. The mandibular prominence is important in development of the mandible. The second pharyngeal arch gives rise to the lesser cornu and upper part of the hyoid bone. The fourth pharyngeal arches, while extensively involved in development of the cartilage and muscles of the larynx, play no part in the development of the hyoid bone.

GAS 1091; N 15; McM 48

14 E. A lateral cervical cyst is caused by remnants of the cervical sinus and would present anterior to the sternocleidomastoid. A dermoid cyst is a cystic teratoma that often occurs near the lateral aspect of the eyebrow. A swollen lymph node is likely to present with pain. Accessory thyroid tissue is normally situated along the route of descent of the thyroglossal duct, either in the posterior tongue or along the midline of the neck. A cyst of the thyroglossal duct would be found in locations similar to where accessory thyroid tissue is found.

GAS 1016; N 64; McM 28-35

15 A. Noncommunicating hydrocephalus, also known as obstructive hydrocephalus, is due to an obstruction to flow of CSF within the ventricular system. Excess production of CSF or disturbed resorption of CSF gives rise to communicating or nonobstructive hydrocephalus. An increased size of the head can occur as a result of hydrocephalus but would not be a causative factor for hydrocephalus. Failure of the neural tube to close may lead to anencephaly or spina bifida, depending on the portion of the tube affected, but would not result in hydrocephalus.

GAS 877-878; N 147; McM 72, 81

16 C. A normal APGAR score indicates that the child appeared normal and healthy at birth, based on skin color, heart rate, reflexes, muscle tone, and breathing (Appearance, Pulse, Grimace, Activity, and Respiration). An atretic external acoustic canal occurs due to failure of the meatal plug to canalize, an event that normally occurs in late fetal life. Failure of the otic pit to form results in an absent otic vesicle and absence of the membranous labyrinth. The first pharyngeal pouch gives rise to the tympanic membrane and cavity, and abnormal development would not affect the external acoustic meatus. Failure of the auricular hillocks to develop results in failure of the external ear to develop. A degenerated tubotympanic recess would not lead to an atretic external acoustic meatus.

GAS 956; N 95; McM 60

17 D. The chin and lower lip area are supplied by the mental nerve, a branch of the inferior alveolar nerve, which in turn is a branch of the mandibular division of the trigeminal nerve (CN V3). The auriculotemporal nerve supplies the TMJ, the temporal region, the parotid gland, and the ear. The buccal nerve is sensory to the internal surface of the cheek. The lesser petrosal nerve is a parasympathetic nerve and would not be affected by herpes zoster, a disease of the dorsal root ganglia. The infraorbital nerve provides sensory innervation to the upper lip.

GAS 986; N 50; McM 38

18 B. The trigeminal ganglion, also known as the semilunar or Gasserian ganglion, is the location of the sensory neuron cell bodies of the trigeminal nerve (CN V). Tic douloureux (trigeminal neuralgia) is a condition in which pain occurs over the area of distribution of trigeminal nerve branches. The geniculate ganglion is found on the facial nerve (CN VII) and receives sensory fibers for taste and transmits preganglionic parasympathetic fibers. The inferior glossopharyngeal ganglion is part of the glossopharyngeal nerve (CN IX), not the trigeminal nerve, and is not the site of the cell bodies mediating the pain. The otic ganglion, located on the mandibular division of the trigeminal nerve, contains postganglionic parasympathetic cell bodies for parotid secretion. The pterygopalatine ganglion, located in the pterygopalatine fossa, also contains postganglionic parasympathetic cell bodies for lacrimation and mucosal secretion.

GAS 921; N 123; McM 75

19 C. The ophthalmic branch of the trigeminal nerve (CN V1) supplies sensory innervation to the eyeball, leading to pain when damaged. Pain in the hard palate and lower eyelid and anesthesia of the upper lip would be carried by the maxillary branch of the trigeminal nerve (CN V2). Paraesthesia over the buccal portion of the face would be mediated by the maxillary division of the trigeminal nerve.

GAS 914; N 52; McM 75

20 D. A tumor at the hypoglossal canal would compress the hypoglossal nerve (CN XII) and affect the genioglossus, a muscle it supplies. The palatoglossus is innervated by the vagus nerve (CN X), and the thyrohyoid is innervated by the ansa cervicalis (C1 to C3). The geniohyoid is supplied by C1, which runs with the hypoglossal nerve after it passes through the hypoglossal canal, and would therefore be unaffected. The mylohyoid is supplied by the nerve to mylohyoid, a branch of the mandibular division of the trigeminal nerve (CN V3).

GAS 1097-1098; N 59; McM 48

21 C. The superior salivatory nucleus is the autonomic nucleus for the facial nerve (CN VII). Parasympathetic fibers carried by the greater petrosal branch of the facial nerve are responsible for supply of the lacrimal gland and sinuses, via the pterygopalatine ganglion. The geniculate ganglion contains the cell bodies for taste from the anterior two thirds of the tongue carried by the chorda tympani branch of the facial nerve. This branch also carries the parasympathetic supply for the submandibular and sublingual salivary glands. The auriculotemporal nerve provides sensory innervation to the temporal regions of the head, the TMJ, and general sensation from the ear. The inferior salivatory nucleus provides preganglionic parasympathetic fibers carried by the glossopharyngeal nerve (CN IX) that synapse in the otic ganglion, providing parotid stimulation. The pterygopalatine ganglion includes fibers that innervate only lacrimation and the nasal sinuses, but not taste on the anterior two thirds of the tongue (*GAS* Fig. 8-84).

GAS 911; N 124; McM 39

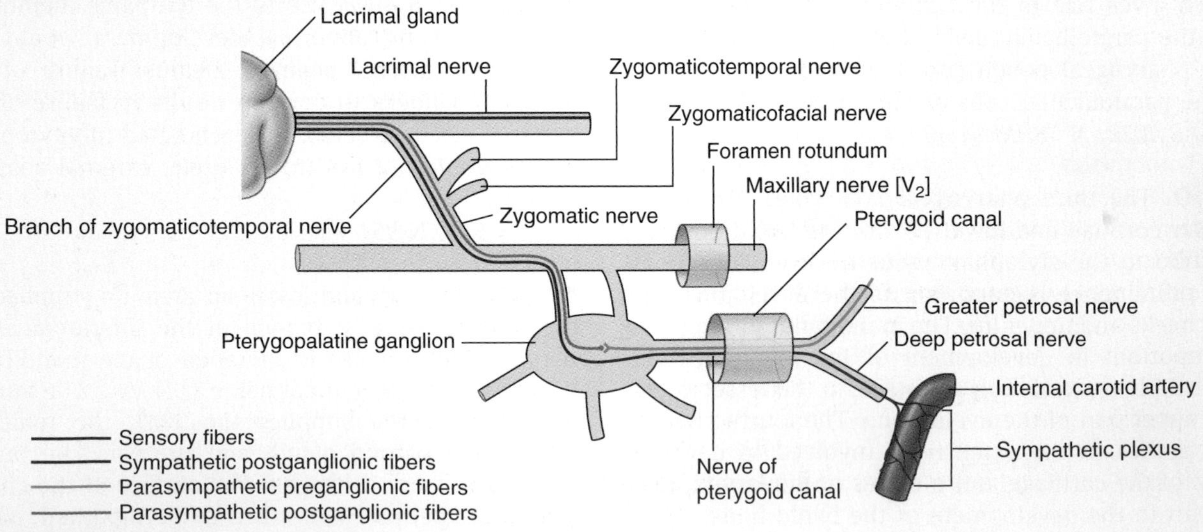

***GAS* Fig. 8-84**

22 D. Thoracic outlet syndrome is characterized by the presence of a cervical rib, accessory muscles, or connective tissue bands that constrict the limited dimensions of the thoracic outlet. The cervical rib is usually located on the C7 vertebra and can impinge on the brachial plexus, resulting in loss of some feeling to the upper limb. There would be no impingement on the phrenic nerve because it leaves C3 to C5 directly parallel with the vertebral column. The syndrome does not include reduction of blood flow to the thoracic wall because of extensive anastomoses between the vessels that supply blood to the anterior thoracic wall. Venous return from the head and neck is mainly through the internal jugular vein and would not be affected because of this vein's location near the midline of the body; thus, it would not be occluded or distended.

GAS 150; N 182, 186; McM 216

23 C. The superior cervical ganglion (SCG), which is the uppermost part of the sympathetic chain, supplies sympathetic innervation to the head and neck. The usual symptoms for SCG injury, commonly known as Horner's syndrome, are miosis, ptosis, and anhydrosis in the head and neck region. Postganglionic sympathetic nerves usually run alongside the arteries leading into the head and neck region. The submandibular ganglion does not carry sympathetic nerves to areas of the head and neck. The trigeminal ganglion includes only cell bodies from afferent sensory nerves from the head. The geniculate ganglion includes cell bodies for taste sensation from the anterior two thirds of the tongue, carried by the facial nerve; it also transmits parasympathetic innervation to many sections of the head and face. The ciliary ganglion provides parasympathetic innervation to the eye and also has some sympathetic fibers coursing through but not synapsing; thus, it would not account for the symptoms of the face.

GAS 1036; N 132; McM 47

24 A. The chorda tympani joins the lingual nerve in the infratemporal fossa, and a lesion to the lingual nerve before it joins the chorda tympani would account for the loss of general sensation, with no loss to the special sense of taste and saliva production. If the chorda tympani were injured, the patient would present with a loss of taste (from the anterior two thirds of tongue) and a decrease in saliva production because the submandibular and sublingual salivary glands would be denervated. The inferior alveolar nerve provides sensory innervation to the mandibular teeth, but no such loss is present. The lesser petrosal nerve innervates postganglionic neurons supplying the parotid gland, but no loss of salivation is present. The glossopharyngeal nerve provides taste innervation to the posterior third of the tongue and sensation related to the gag reflex, but there is no deficit present in this patient.

GAS 1101; N 46; McM 76

25 E. The jugular foramen is the route of exit for three nerves (glossopharyngeal [CN IX], vagus [CN X], and spinal accessory [CN XI] nerves) and one vein (internal jugular vein) from the cranial cavity. The glossopharyngeal nerve provides the sensory input for the gag reflex, whereas the vagus nerve provides the motor output. Nerve compression within this foramen would lead to a loss of both systems and thus no gag reflex. Tongue movements are almost entirely supplied by the hypoglossal nerve (CN XII), which exits the skull through the hypoglossal canal. The facial nerve (CN VII) innervates the muscles of the face and would not be affected by this injury. Loss of sensation from the face and scalp would be present only if there was involvement of the trigeminal nerve. Loss of hearing would be present with any compression of the vestibulocochlear nerve (CN VIII). The vestibulocochlear nerve was formally called the *auditory nerve* but *vestibulocochlear* clearly refers to its dual function and hearing.

GAS 870; N 13; McM 11

26 E. The middle meningeal artery is a branch of the maxillary artery and courses between the dura mater and skull close to the area of the pterion. Any fracture or impact trauma to this location typically results in a laceration of the middle meningeal artery resulting in an epidural hematoma. The external carotid artery ends behind the mandible by dividing into the maxillary and the superficial temporal arteries, and neither of these arteries directly affects the meninges of the brain. The deep temporal arteries do not penetrate the bony skull and thus would not contribute to an epidural hematoma (*GAS* Fig. 8-33).

GAS 990; N 102; McM 42

27 A. An injury to the oculomotor nerve (CN III) would cause the eye to point downward and laterally due to the unopposed contractions of the muscles innervated by the trochlear (CN IV) and abducens (CN VI) nerves (superior oblique and lateral rectus muscles, respectively). The oculomotor nerve also provides innervation to the levator palpebrae superioris; thus, any injury will cause complete ptosis or inability to raise the eyelid. The constriction of the pupil is provided by parasympathetic nerves via the oculomotor nerve. The optic nerve is responsible only

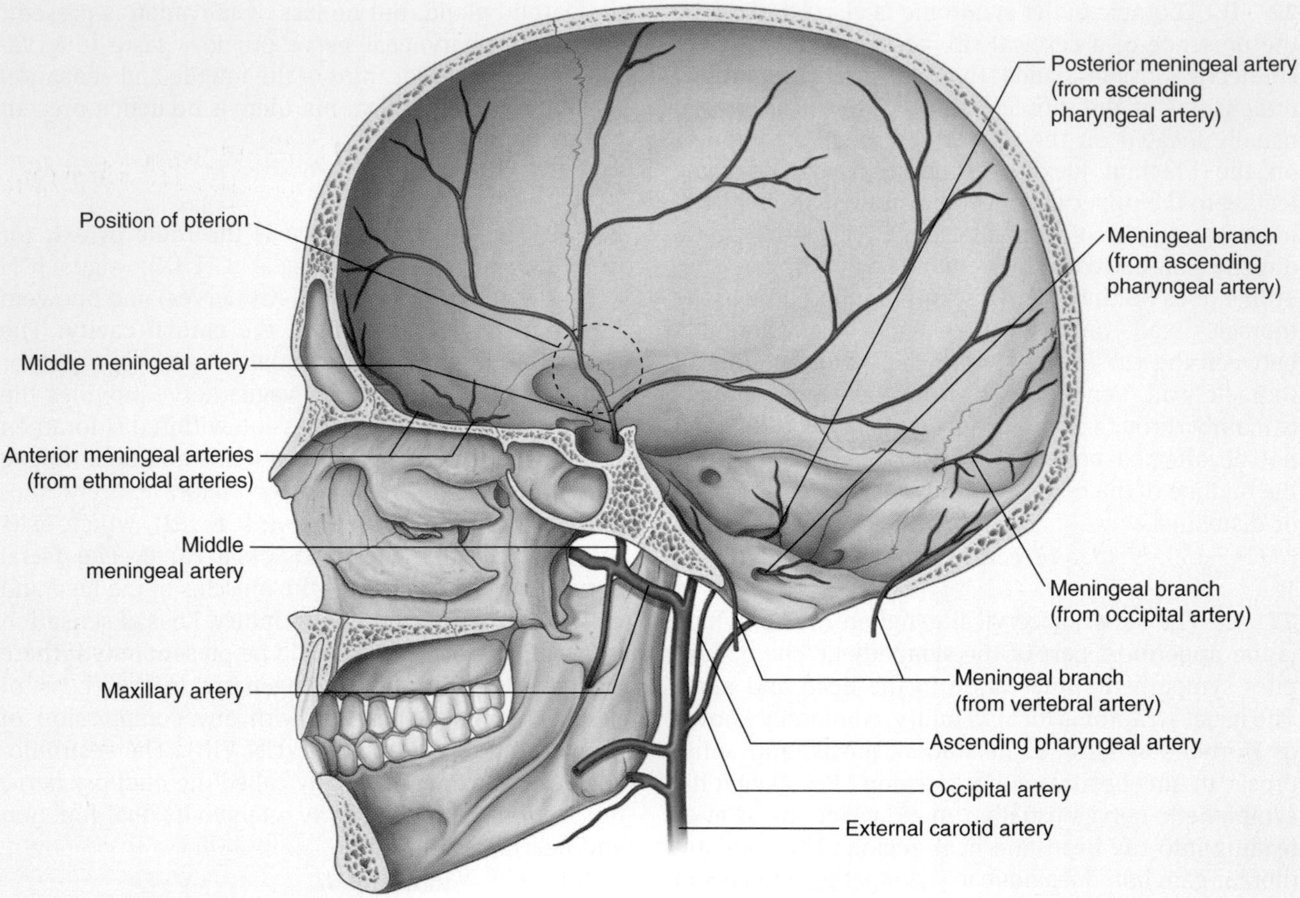

GAS **Fig. 8-33**

for the sensory aspect of light via the retina in the eye. The facial nerve innervates the facial muscles, including the orbicularis oculi, which closes the eylid for the blink reflex. The ciliary ganglion could be damaged in this patient, but the loss of parasympathetic supply will not adequately explain the ptosis of the eyelid. The superior cervical ganglion provides sympathetic innervation to the head and neck including the smooth muscle in the upper lid (superior tarsal muscle of Müller), but no loss of sympathetics is evident in this patient.

GAS 901-902; N 55; McM 55, 57, 81

28 B. The scalp is divided into five layers: skin, dense connective tissue, aponeurosis, loose connective tissue, and periosteum. A handy mnemonic is SCALP (skin, connective tissue, aponeurosis, loose connective tissue, and periosteum). Typically, infections will be located in the loose connective tissue because of the ease with which infectious agents spread via the many veins located in this region. This area is usually referred to as the "danger zone" of the scalp mainly because scalp infections here can be transmitted into the skull via emissary veins, then via diploic veins of the bone to the cranial cavity. The periosteum and bone are tightly bound together; thus, it is not likely to find infections between these layers. The areas between the dense connective tissue and aponeurosis and between the connective tissue and the skin layers do not include connecting veins but mainly superficial veins of the head. The skin provides a very strong barrier against infections; the epidermis and dermis layers are rarely seen separated, and thus the likelihood of an infection between these areas would be rare.

GAS 922; N 3, 25; McM 5, 81, 82

29 A. An injury to the left vagus nerve (CN X) would cause the uvula to become deviated to the right. This is because the vagus nerve innervates the musculus uvulae muscle that makes up the core of the uvula. If only one side is effectively innervated, contraction of the active muscle will deviate the uvula to the contralateral side of the injury (ipsilateral side

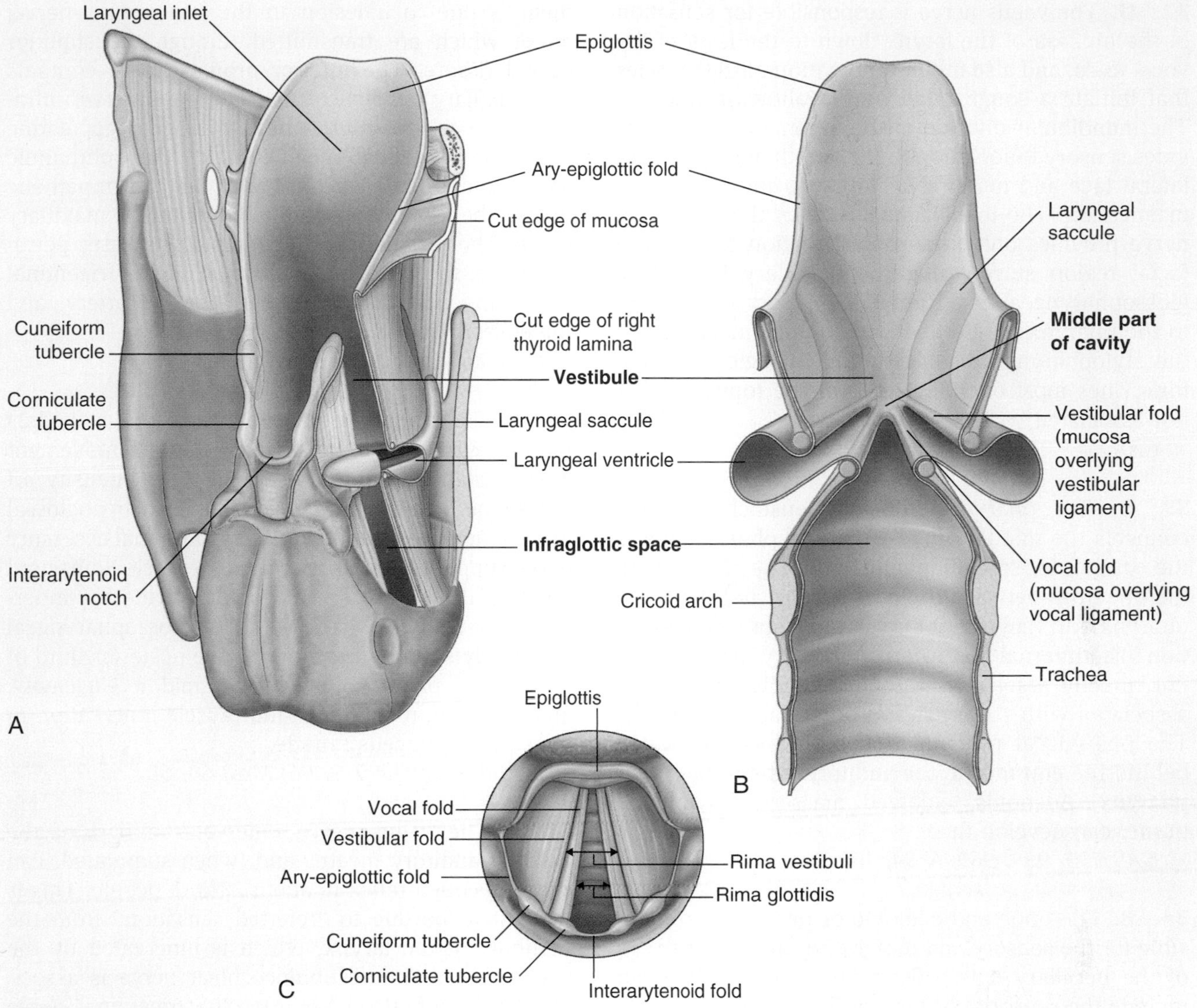

GAS **Fig. 8-217ABC**

of the uninjured vagus nerve). In addition, the intact levator veli palatini will pull the uvula to the intact side. The right and left hypoglossal nerves innervate the tongue muscles and would not affect the uvula. The glossopharyngeal nerve supplies sensory innervation to the oropharynx and nasopharynx, but not motor innervation to these areas.

GAS 901; N 71, 127; McM 47

30 E. The rima glottidis is the opening between the vocal folds and the arytenoid cartilages on the right and left sides. The piriform recess is the recess lateral to the laryngeal opening of the laryngopharynx. The vestibule is the region between the epiglottis and rima glottidis. The ventricle is the area between the true and false vocal cords. The vallecula is a bilateral recess anterior to the epiglottis just posterior to the tongue in the laryngopharynx (*GAS* Fig. 8-217).

GAS 1060; N 80; McM 49

31 D. Maxillary sinusitis is an infection of the maxillary sinus, which is located in the body of the maxillary bone. Sharp pain can be a major symptom of maxillary sinusitis. The difference between the remaining answer choices is the location of the sinus. The sphenoid sinus is located in the posterior nasopharynx. The ethmoidal sinuses are located laterosuperiorly to the nasal septum. The frontal sinus is located in the frontal bone in the anterior part of the face.

GAS 1074-1076; N 42-44; McM 43, 76

32 D. The vagus nerve is responsible for sensation in the mucosa of the larynx down to the level of the vocal folds, and also motor innervation of the muscles that initiate a cough reflex and swallowing (motor). The mandibular division of the trigeminal nerve provides sensory innervation to the mouth and lower and lateral face and motor innervation to the muscles of mastication. The maxillary division of the trigeminal nerve provides only sensory innervation to the midfacial region surrounding the maxillary bone. The glossopharyngeal nerve provides sensory innervation to the pharynx (gag reflex) and motor innervation to the stylopharyngeus muscle. The hypoglossal nerve innervates most of the muscles of the tongue and is not associated with the cough reflex.

GAS 900, 1052-1053; N 71; McM 45

33 D. The pharyngotympanic (eustachian) tube connects the middle ear and the nasopharynx and is the conduit for spreading infections. The choanae are the openings between the nasal cavity and the nasopharynx, but they are not involved in spreading infection. The internal and external auditory meatuses are not directly associated with the middle ear but are associated with the inner and outer ear, respectively. The pharyngeal recess is a slitlike opening located behind the entrance to the auditory tube in the nasopharynx. Adenoids, enlarged masses of lymphoid tissue, can develop there.

GAS 956, 958, 960; N 94, 100; McM 60, 61

34 B. The optic and oculomotor nerves are responsible for the sensory and motor portions, respectively, of the pupillary light reflex. The optic nerve would include the sensory portion, but the facial nerve only closes the eyelid and does not affect the pupil. The maxillary division of the trigeminal nerve only provides sensory innervation to the skin surrounding the maxillary bone. The ophthalmic division of the trigeminal nerve provides sensory innervation to the cornea for the corneal reflex, but not the light reflex.

GAS 901; N 88; McM 54

35 C. The superior orbital fissure is the opening that allows the passage of the oculomotor nerve and the trochlear nerve; the lacrimal, frontal, and nasociliary branches of ophthalmic division of the trigeminal nerve; the abducens nerve; the superior and inferior divisions of the ophthalmic vein; and the sympathetic fibers from the cavernous plexus. The sensory and motor components of the corneal reflex are the ophthalmic division of the trigeminal nerve and the oculomotor nerve, whereas the eye impairment is due to a lesion to the oculomotor nerve, all of which are transmitted through the superior orbital fissure. The inferior orbital fissure contains the maxillary division of the trigeminal nerve, infraorbital vessels, and branches of the pterygopalatine ganglion. The optic canal contains the ophthalmic artery and optic nerve, in addition to sympathetic fibers. The foramen rotundum contains the maxillary nerve. The foramen ovale contains the lesser petrosal nerve, the mandibular division of the trigeminal nerve, the accessory middle meningeal artery, and the emissary veins.

GAS 901, 934; N 85; McM 23, 25

36 B. The facial nerve innervates the stapedius muscle, which is responsible for limiting movement of the stapes, thereby reducing the intensity of the sound entering the inner ear. The hypoglossal nerve innervates tongue muscles; the spinal accessory nerve supplies the trapezius and sternocleidomastoid muscles; the vagus nerve does not provide any innervation for sound in the ear; and the glossopharyngeal nerve only supplies sensation to the posterior third of the tongue, pharynx (gag reflex), middle ear cavity, and tympanic membrane, and muscle innervation to the stylopharyngeus muscle.

GAS 895, 898-899; N 96; McM 60, 61

37 B. The vagus nerve innervates a part of the external auditory meatus and, when stimulated, can trigger a cough reflex in about 20% of people. This is thought to be due to "referred sensation" from the vestibule of the larynx, which is innervated by the vagus nerve. The vestibulocochlear nerve is associated only with the inner ear. The trigeminal nerve does provide some innervation to the external auditory meatus but does not affect the cough reflex as does the vagus nerve. The auricular branch of the facial nerve only provides a small amount of general sensory supply to the external ear; it is not associated with the cough reflex.

GAS 956; N 95; McM 60, 61

38 C. The recurrent laryngeal nerve supplies most of the motor innervation to the larynx and sensation below the true vocal folds. The thyroid gland and the recurrent laryngeal nerve are in close proximity and thus the nerve is the most likely to be injured with a thyroidectomy. Injury to the recurrent laryngeal nerve can result in speech defects, including hoarseness. The superior laryngeal nerve has two branches: the internal laryngeal nerve innervates the mucous membranes of the larynx above the vocal folds, and the external laryngeal nerve innervates the cricothyroid muscle, which tenses the vocal folds. The glossopharyngeal nerve is located superiorly to the true vocal folds and would not be affected by this procedure.

GAS 1021; N 78; McM 49

39 B. The superior cervical ganglion provides sympathetic innervation to the face and neck regions. Sympathetics travel along the branches of the internal carotid artery, and one result of stimulation of these nerves is to dilate the pupil during a sympathetic response ("flight or fight"). The oculomotor nerve would not affect the dilation of the pupil; rather, its stimulation results in the constriction (parasympathetic nerves). The nervus intermedius is the parasympathetic component to the facial nerve and affects only lacrimation of the eye. The Edinger-Westphal nucleus is the location of the cell bodies of the preganglionic parasympathetic neurons that are carried by the oculomotor nerve (not sympathetics). The trigeminal ganglion only provides sensory innervation to the face and eye but has no motor effect on the pupil.

GAS 931, 1036; N 132; McM 44

40 C. The greater petrosal nerve, a parasympathetic branch of the facial nerve, provides innervation to the lacrimal gland in the orbit. The chorda tympani provides innervation to the submandibular and sublingual glands and also taste to the anterior two thirds of the tongue. The deep petrosal nerve carries sympathetic innervation to the blood vessels and mucous glands of the head and neck. The lesser petrosal nerve provides parasympathetic innervation to the parotid gland. The nasociliary nerve provides sensory innervation to the ethmoidal sinuses and the cornea as well as innervation to the skin of the eyelids and superior nose regions.

GAS 932-933; N 124; McM 55-57

41 C. The maxillary sinus is located directly inferior to the orbit. Any trauma to the inferior bony wall of the orbit will likely displace the orbital structures in the compartment to the space below the orbit (maxillary sinus). In most people the sclera of the eyeball is stronger than in the orbital floor, so a blow-out fracture is more likely than rupture of the eyeball. The ethmoidal sinus is located superiorly and medially to the orbit, whereas the frontal sinus is located superiorly to the orbit. The nasal cavity is toward the midline and is not inferior to the orbit. The sphenoidal sinus is deeper into the facial region but is not inferior to the orbit.

GAS 1074, 1076; N 43; McM 18

42 B. The superior ophthalmic vein drains directly into the cavernous sinus. The danger area of the face is located in the triangular region from the lateral angle of the eye to the middle of the upper lip, near the nose, and is drained by the facial vein. The facial vein communicates directly with the cavernous sinus through the superior ophthalmic vein. The pterygoid venous plexus communicates with the cavernous sinus through the inferior ophthalmic vein, but it is not directly connected to the cavernous sinus. The basilar venous plexus connects the inferior petrosal sinuses and communicates with the internal vertebral venous plexus. The parietal emissary veins and frontal venous plexus do not communicate directly with the cavernous sinus.

GAS 888; N 73; McM 51

43 C. A lesion of the facial nerve is likely to lead to the symptoms described (drooping mouth, unable to close right eye, and food collection in the oral vestibule) because the muscles of facial expression are paralyzed. There is a bony prominence over the facial nerve located on the medial wall of the middle ear. Because of its close proximity, the facial nerve can be very rarely damaged due to otitis media. The other nerves listed are not located in close proximity to the middle ear and, if injured, would not present with the symptoms described.

GAS 960; N 94; McM 60, 61

44 C. The arterial circle (of Willis) receives its blood supply from the internal carotid and vertebral arteries. The actual circle is formed by the bifurcation of the basilar, posterior cerebral, posterior communicating, internal carotid, anterior cerebral, and anterior communicating arteries. The middle cerebral artery is the lateral continuation of the internal carotid artery and therefore not part of the arterial circle. Although it receives its blood supply from the arterial circle (of Willis), it does not actually form any part of the circle (*GAS* Fig. 8-38A).

GAS 883; N 141; McM 68

45 E. The sigmoid venous sinus empties into the internal jugular vein and drains the cranial vault. It runs along the posterior cranial fossa near the suture between the temporal and occipital bones just lateral to the mastoid air cells. The superior sagittal sinus lies within the superior aspect of the longitudinal fissure, between the two cerebral hemispheres. The inferior sagittal sinus runs inferior to the superior sagittal sinus within the falx cerebri and joins the great cerebral vein (of Galen) to form the straight sinus. The straight sinus drains the great cerebral vein

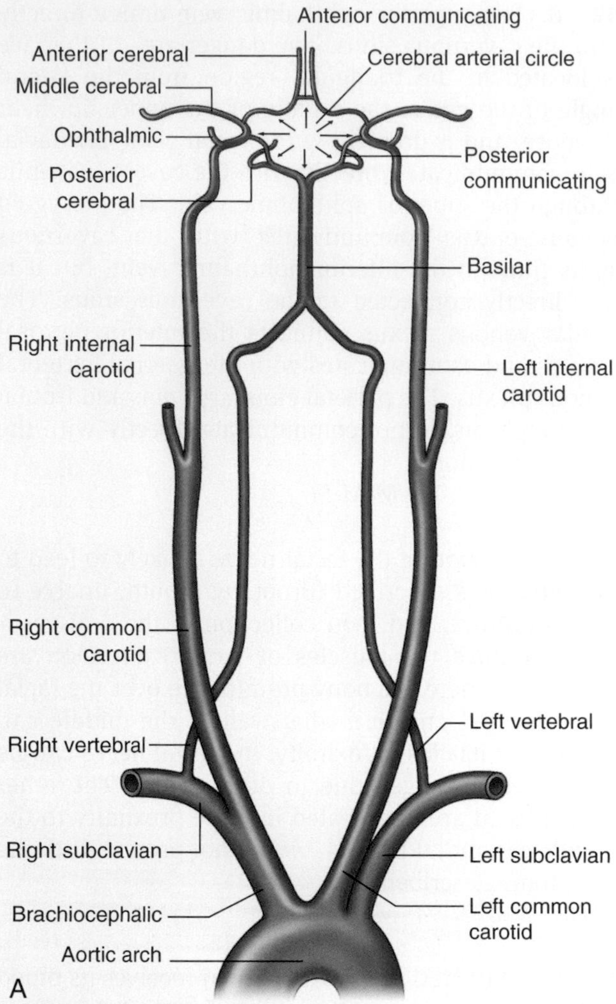

GAS **Fig. 8-38A**

(of Galen) into the confluence of sinuses. The cavernous sinus is located within the middle cranial fossa and receives the ophthalmic veins, the greater petrosal sinus, and other venous vessels (*GAS* Fig. 8-44).

GAS 887; N 99; McM 53

46 **C.** The tumor is compressing the facial nerve, which runs through the internal acoustic meatus along with the vestibulocochlear nerve. The facial nerve provides the sensation of taste to the anterior two thirds of the tongue via the chorda tympani and also mediates all of the facial muscles, except the muscles of mastication. The mandibular branch of the trigeminal nerve courses through the foramen ovale and mediates motor to the muscles of mastication and sensory to the lower third of the face. The maxillary branch of the trigeminal branch passes through the foramen rotundum and is sensory to the middle third of the face. The jugular foramen has the glossopharyngeal, vagus, and accessory nerves coursing through it. Finally, the superior orbital fissure has the ophthalmic branch of the trigeminal nerve coursing through it, along with the oculomotor, trochlear, and abducens nerves.

GAS 898-899; N 94; McM 61

47 **E.** The submental lymph nodes drain approximately the anterior two thirds of the mouth and tongue, including the lower lips. The occipital nodes serve the inferoposterior aspect of the head. The parotid nodes lie anterior to the ear and serve the region of the lateral aspect of the eye, the parotid gland, and anterior ear. The retropharyngeal nodes lie posterior to the pharynx and drain the posterior aspect of the throat and pharynx. The jugulodigastric node is a large node posterior to the parotid gland and just below the angle of the mandible, and it receives lymph from much of the face and scalp and is commonly enlarged in tonsillitis.

GAS 920; N 75; McM 13

48 **A.** The abducens nerve would be affected first due to aneurysmal dilation of the internal carotid artery (ICA) because the nerve runs in closest proximity to the artery within the cavernous sinus. The other nerves running in the wall of the cavernous sinus are the oculomotor nerve, trochlear nerve, and both the maxillary and ophthalmic branches of the trigeminal nerve. Each of these nerves, however, courses along, or within, the lateral walls of the cavernous sinus and may not be immediately affected by an aneurysm of the ICA (*GAS* Fig. 8-45).

GAS 888; N 105; McM 51

49 **C.** The lingual nerve is the most likely nerve damaged because there is loss both of taste and general sensory supply to the anterior two thirds of the tongue, which is innervated by the lingual nerve, which at this point has been joined by the chorda tympani. The chorda tympani would be a likely choice; however, it carries only taste and does not mediate other general sensation to the tongue. The auriculotemporal nerve is a posterior branch of the mandibular division of the trigeminal nerve and innervates skin near the ear and temporal region. The mental nerve is the terminal branch of the inferior alveolar nerve and innervates the skin of the chin.

GAS 1101; N 50; McM 35

50 **B.** The auriculotemporal nerve is a posterior branch of the mandibular division of the trigeminal nerve. It encircles the middle meningeal artery and courses medially to the TMJ and then ascends up near the auricle. Because this nerve supplies the TMJ and

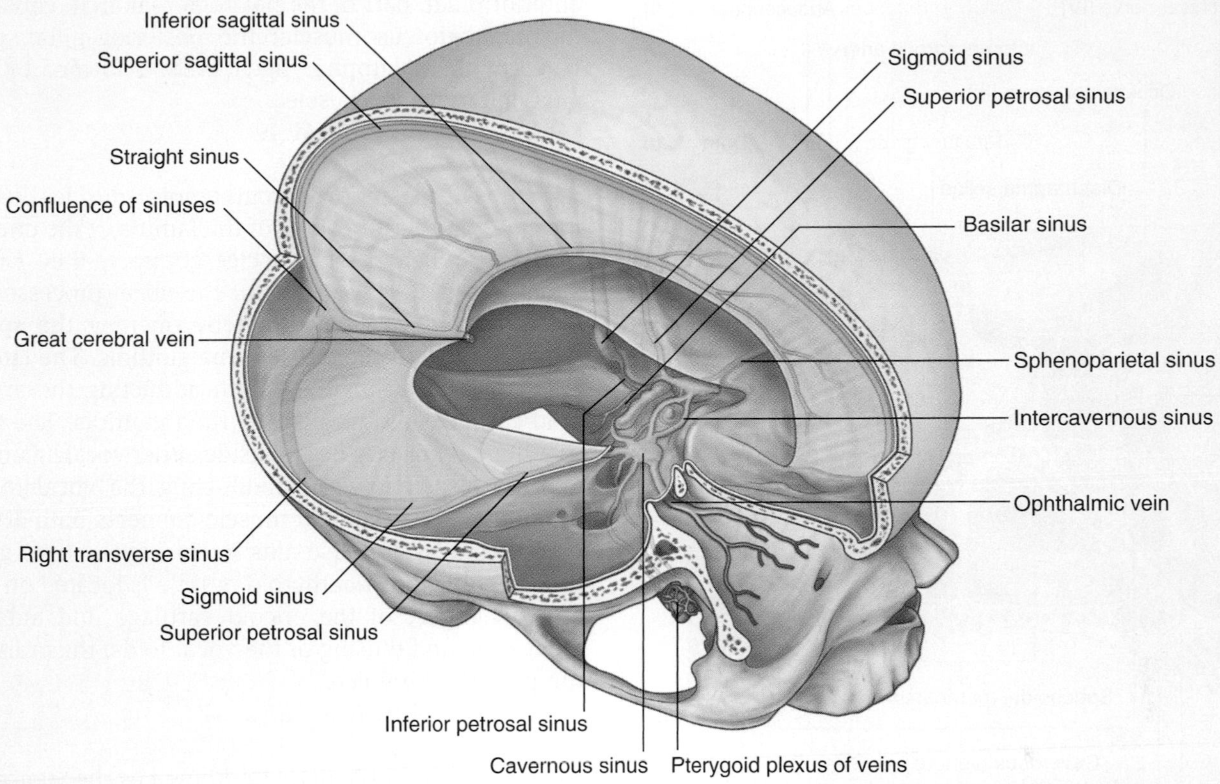

GAS **Fig. 8-44**

skin of the external auditory canal, pain from the joint can be referred to the ear as in this case. The facial nerve courses over the ascending ramus of the mandible, passing superficial to the masseter muscle and below the TMJ through the parotid gland, and would not be involved in this problem. The lesser petrosal nerve courses through the middle cranial fossa and exits through the foramen ovale, where it joins the otic ganglion. The vestibulocochlear nerve exits the cranial cavity through the internal acoustic meatus and innervates structures in the inner ear. Finally, the chorda tympani is a branch of the facial nerve and joins the mandibular division of the trigeminal nerve anterior to the TMJ.

GAS 985-986; N 50; McM 29

51 D. The otic ganglion is the location of the postganglionic parasympathetic neural cell bodies innervating the parotid gland. The ganglion lies on the mandibular division of the trigeminal nerve near the foramen ovale. The trigeminal ganglion contains cell bodies for neurons innervating sensory aspects of the face. The inferior salivatory nucleus lies within the brainstem and contains preganglionic parasympathetic neurons whose axons pass within the lesser petrosal nerve to the otic ganglion for synapse in the supply of the parotid. The superior cervical ganglion has the cell bodies of postganglionic sympathetic fibers innervating sympathetic structures to the head. The submandibular ganglia contain the cell bodies of postganglionic parasympathetic fibers innervating the sublingual and submandibular salivary glands.

GAS 889-900; N 135; McM 33

52 B. The arachnoid villi are extensions of the arachnoid mater into the superior sagittal sinus. The villi allow for proper drainage of the CSF into the venous bloodstream from the subarachnoid space in which the CSF circulates. These villi are a crucial element in maintaining proper intracranial pressure and circulation of the CSF.

GAS 876; N 103; McM 2

53 C. The afferent/sensory limb of the corneal (blink) reflex is carried by the nasociliary nerve. It is a branch of the ophthalmic division of the trigeminal nerve. The frontal and lacrimal nerves provide cutaneous supply to parts of the orbit and face, but they do not innervate the cornea. The facial nerve is the efferent limb of the corneal reflex and mediates the closing of both eyes in response to irritation of the cornea. The oculomotor nerve mediates the reopening of the

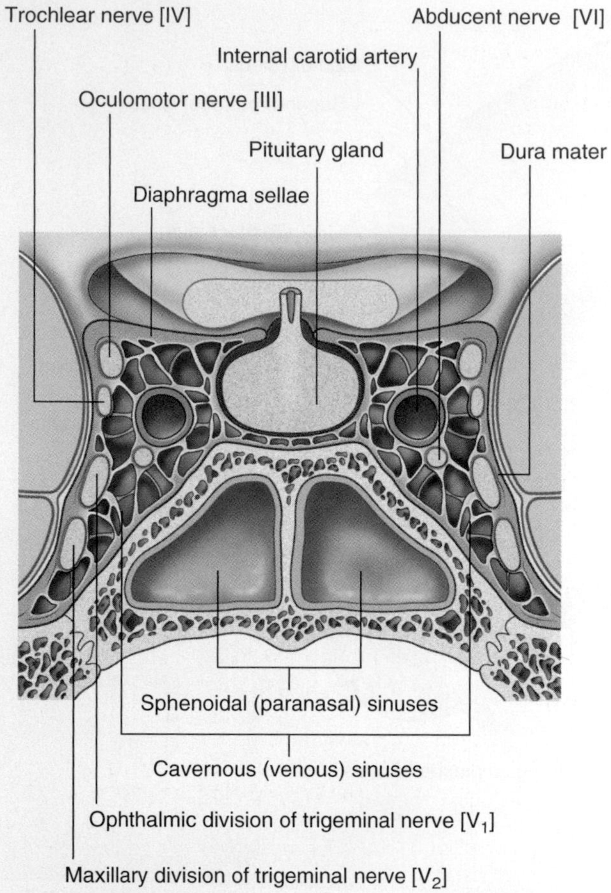

***GAS* Fig. 8-45**

eyes by contraction of the levator palpebrae superioris. The optic nerve also innervates the eye for the sense of vision and is the afferent limb of the pupillary light reflex.

GAS 901; N 88; McM 44, 54, 55

54 D. Kiesselbach's plexus (also called Little's area) is an anastomosis of four arteries on the anterior nasal septum. The four arteries are the anterior ethmoidal artery, sphenopalatine artery, superior labial artery, and greater palatine artery. The two largest contributors, however, are the septal branches of the sphenopalatine (from the maxillary artery) and superior labial arteries (branches of the facial artery, which in turn is a branch of the external carotid artery) (*GAS* Fig. 8-239AB).

GAS 998, 999; N 40; McM 42

55 B. The palatine tonsils lie in tonsillar beds with muscular (covered with mucosa) anterior and posterior pillars forming the boundaries of the bed. These pillars are formed by the palatoglossal arch, anteriorly, and the palatopharyngeal arch, posteriorly. The anterior pillar, part of the palatoglossal arch, contains the palatoglossus muscle; the posterior pillar, provided by the palatopharyngeal arch, is formed by the palatopharyngeus muscle.

GAS 1044; N 57; McM 49

56 A. The posterior cricoarytenoid muscles lie on the superoposterior aspect of the lamina of the cricoid cartilage. When these muscles contract, they cause lateral rotation (abduction) of the vocal processes of the arytenoid cartilages, thereby opening the space between the vocal folds, the rima glottidis. The lateral cricoarytenoid is involved with adducting the arytenoid cartilage and closing the rima glottidis. The thyroarytenoid muscles lie alongside either vocal ligament and are also involved in adducting the vocal folds. The transverse arytenoid muscle connects both arytenoid cartilages and also aids in closing the rima glottidis. Finally, the cricothyroid muscle is located on the anterior aspect of the cricoid cartilage and aids in elongation and tensing of the vocal folds, thus raising the pitch of the voice.

GAS 1059-1061; N 56; McM 47

57 C. The parotid duct, also known as the Stensen's duct, crosses the masseter muscle transversely and extends to the oral cavity where it opens by the upper second molar. The facial artery can be palpated in the groove anterior to the mandibular angle. The facial vein lies anterior to the artery, passing toward the angle of the lips, but does not ascend in close proximity to the masseter. All of the other vessels are located more deeply and cannot be palpated.

GAS 911; N 56; McM 40

58 C. Because of the surgical division of the ansa cervicalis, the sternohyoid muscle will most likely be paralyzed following this tumor resection. The ansa cervicalis innervates the strap muscles, including the sternohyoid, sternothyroid, and omohyoid muscles. The sternocleidomastoid is innervated by the spinal accessory nerve and will not be involved with this surgery. The platysma is located most superficially on the neck and is innervated by the cervical branch of the facial nerve. The trapezius muscle is also innervated by the spinal accessory nerve and plays no role in ansa cervicalis functions. Finally, the cricothyroid muscle is innervated by the external laryngeal branch of the vagus and would not be affected by the surgery.

GAS 1016; N 31; McM 31, 33

59 A. The spinal accessory nerve passes across the posterior triangle of the neck and innervates both the trapezius muscle and the sternocleidomastoid muscle

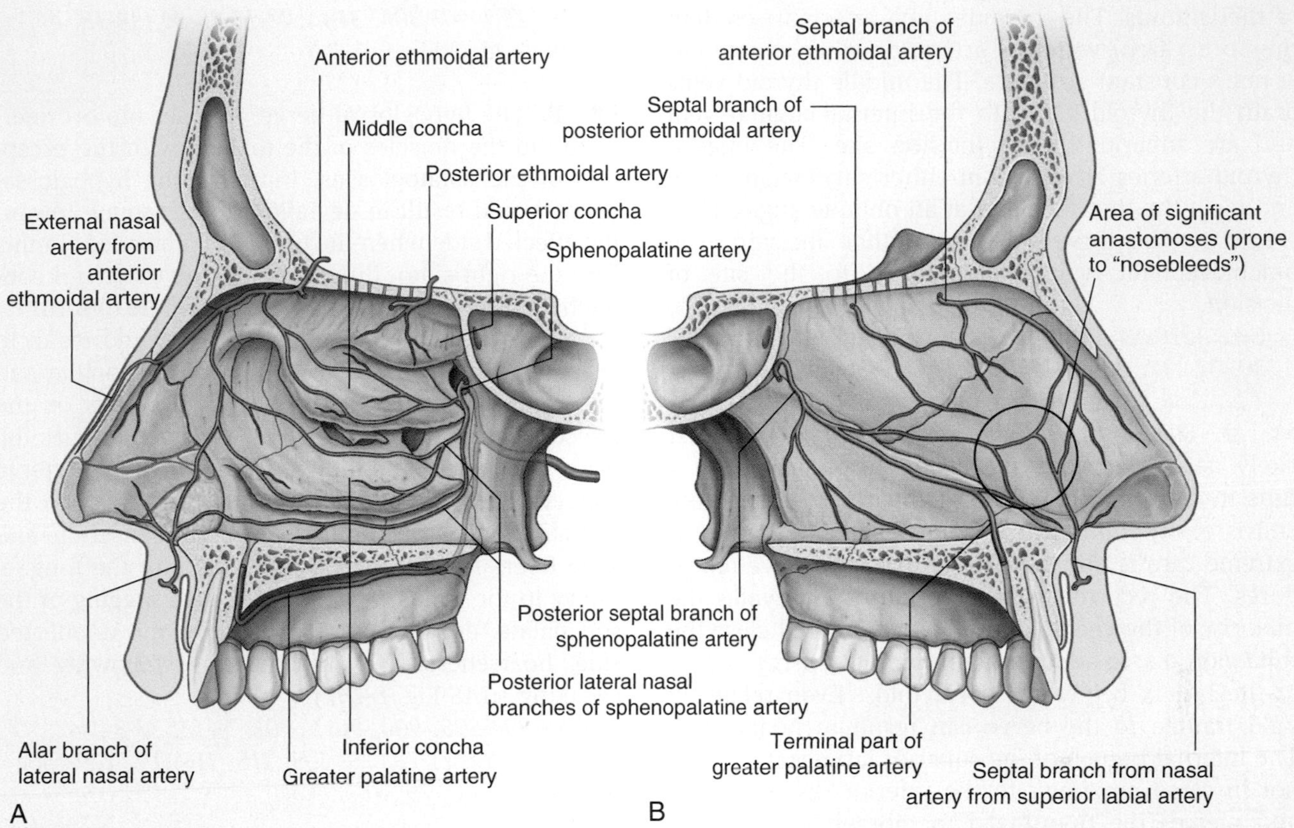

GAS **Fig. 8-239AB**

for the respective side of the body. Upon surgical division of the nerve, the patient will lose the ability to raise the ipsilateral shoulder and will demonstrate weakness in turning the head to the opposite side. The trapezius will also lose tone and the shoulder will droop. The ansa cervicalis innervates strap muscles of the neck and, if cut, would not produce drooping of the shoulder. The facial nerve does not pass through any of the triangles of the neck; however, if it were divided, paralysis would result in the muscles of facial expression. The hypoglossal nerve innervates the intrinsic muscles of the tongue, plus the genioglossus, hyoglossus, and styloglossus and, if injured, would not result in any of the patient's symptoms.

GAS 87; N 32; McM 29, 30, 32

60 C. Four nerves participate in providing cutaneous supply to the neck. The nerves are the supraclavicular, great auricular, transverse cervical, and the lesser occipital. The area over the angle of the jaw is innervated by the great auricular nerve. It ascends from spinal segments from C2 and C3 and innervates the skin over the angle of the jaw and posteroinferior to the auricle of the ear. The transverse cervical also originates from the C2-3 spinal segments but passes anteriorly to innervate the anterior and lateral aspects of the neck. The lesser occipital nerve innervates skin in the area of the back of the neck and posterior occiput. The supraclavicular nerves originate from C3-4 and innervate the more inferior aspects of the neck, the upper deltoid region, and skin inferior to the clavicles.

GAS 985-986; N 2; McM 29, 30, 31, 33

61 C. Because of its size and vulnerable position during birth, the sternocleidomastoid muscle is injured more often than other muscles of the head and neck during birth especially if the delivery is difficult. When acting alone, the action of this muscle is to turn the head to the opposite side and bend it toward the ipsilateral shoulder. When using both muscles, the head will flex toward the chest. Therefore, the most likely muscle to have been injured here is the left sternocleidomastoid muscle.

GAS 1024; N 29; McM 31, 32

62 C. The most likely structures one would encounter while performing a midline incision below the isthmus of the thyroid gland would be the inferior thyroid vein and the thyroidea ima artery. The inferior thyroid vein drains typically to the left brachiocephalic vein, which crosses superficially, just inferior to the isthmus. The thyroidea ima artery arises from the aortic arch, vertebral artery, or other source but is not a constant structure. The middle thyroid veins drain the thyroid gland to the internal jugular vein and are superior to the incision site. The inferior thyroid arteries branch from either subclavian artery and meet the thyroid gland at an oblique angle. They would not be ligated with a midline incision. The brachiocephalic veins are inferior to the site of incision.

GAS 1019; N 31, 73, 76-78, 195, 208, 234; McM 30, 32, 37, 206

63 D. The recurrent laryngeal nerve is the most likely nerve damaged during the surgery because it runs in close proximity to the inferior thyroid artery and is easily injured or transected with the artery if extreme care is not exercised during operative procedures. The recurrent laryngeal nerve innervates the majority of the vocal muscles that open and close the rima glottidis, in addition to providing sensory supply to the larynx below the vocal folds. Even relatively mild trauma to the nerve can result in hoarseness. The internal branch of the superior laryngeal nerve is not in close proximity to the inferior thyroid artery and pierces the thyrohyoid membrane to enter the pharynx. The ansa cervicalis lies lateral to the site of surgery and does not innervate any structures that, if paralyzed, would cause hoarseness.

GAS 1020, 1021, 1034, 1069; N 26, 33, 69, 71, 76-78, 82, 127, 131, 206-209, 223, 228-229, 236, 238-239; McM 35-36, 47, 49-50, 78

64 E. The vagus nerve exits the skull at the jugular foramen and is responsible for motor innervation to the smooth muscles of the trachea, bronchi, and digestive tract, in addition to the muscles of the palate, pharynx, larynx, and superior two thirds of the esophagus. The ansa cervicalis innervates the strap muscles of the neck, with the exception of the thyrohyoid muscle. The cervical sympathetic trunk does not enter into the jugular foramen; it runs behind the carotid sheath, parallel with the internal carotid artery; its carotid branch accompanies the artery into the carotid canal and carries sympathetic fibers to deep areas of the head. Damage to the external laryngeal nerve would result in paralysis of the cricothyroid muscle, presenting as an easily fatigued voice with hoarseness. Injury to the hypoglossal nerve would result in protrusion of the tongue toward the affected side and moderate dysarthria.

GAS 894-895, 900, 902, 1034; N 12, 26, 32-34, 42, 55, 61, 71-72, 76-78, 105, 115, 117-118, 126-128, 131-132, 136, 164, 203, 206-208, 224, 229, 236, 303-304, 318, ; McM 29-30, 34-35, 47, 67-69, 78, 207

65 B. The hypoglossal nerve provides motor innervation to the muscles of the tongue, with the exception of the palatoglossus. Injury to the hypoglossal nerve would result in deviation of the tongue toward the affected side when the tongue is protruded (in this case the right side), due mainly to the unilateral contraction of left genioglossus, and moderate dysarthria. Injury to the glossopharyngeal nerve would result in loss of taste in the posterior third of the tongue and a loss of soft palate sensation and gag reflex on the affected side. The inferior alveolar nerve supplies the tissues of the chin and lower teeth. The lingual nerve conveys parasympathetic preganglionic fibers to the submandibular ganglion and general sensation and taste fibers for the anterior two thirds of the tongue. Injury to the vagus nerve would cause sagging of the soft palate, deviation of the uvula to the unaffected side, hoarseness, and difficulty in swallowing and speaking (*GAS* Fig. 8-257).

GAS 894-895, 900, 901b, 902; N 12, 33-34, 42, 47, 50, 55, 59, 71-73, 75, 105, 115, 118-119, 129-130; McM 44, 67, 79, 81

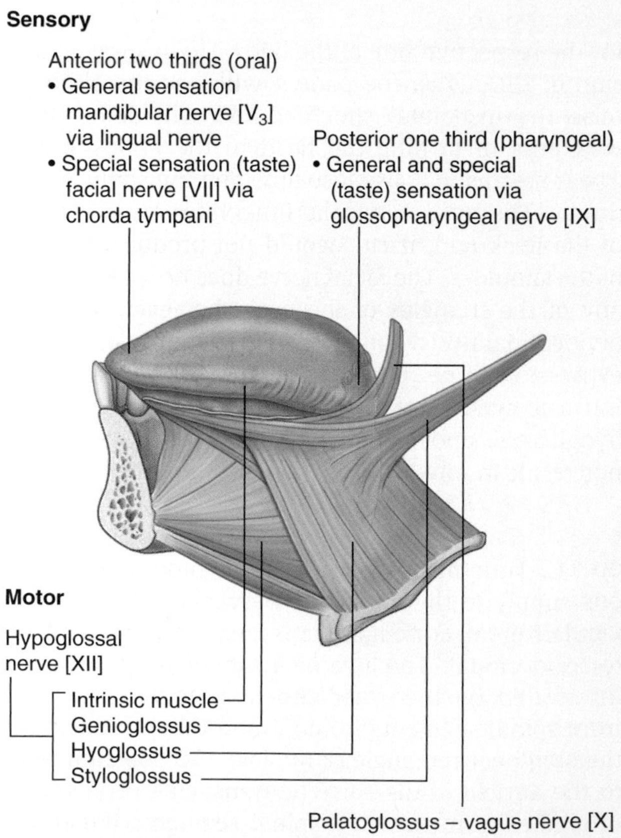

***GAS* Fig. 8-257**

66 **C.** During removal of the tumor, the internal branch of the superior laryngeal nerve was injured. Injury to this nerve results in loss of sensation above the vocal cords, at the entrance to the larynx, and loss of taste on the epiglottis. Loss of sensation in the laryngeal vestibule can precipitate aspiration of fluid into the larynx, trachea, and lungs. The pharyngeal nerve from the vagus nerve supplies motor innervation to the muscles of the pharynx, except the stylopharyngeus (glossopharyngeal nerve). Injury to the hypoglossal nerve would result in protrusion of the tongue toward the affected side and moderate dysarthria. The lingual nerve conveys parasympathetic preganglionic fibers to the submandibular ganglion and general sensation and taste fibers for the anterior two thirds of the tongue. The recurrent laryngeal provides sensory fibers to the larynx below the vocal cords and motor fibers to all of the muscles of the larynx except for the cricothyroid.

GAS 1068; N 61, 65, 67, 69, 71, 76-78, 80, 82, 127; McM 47, 78

67 **A.** The posterior cricoarytenoids are the only muscles of the larynx that abducts the vocal cords. The remaining answer choices are muscles that act in adduction of the vocal cords.

GAS 1061, 1062; N 67, 69, 80, 81, 82, 151; McM 47-49

68 **B.** The external branch of the superior laryngeal nerve courses together with the superior thyroid artery for much of its route. The cervical sympathetic trunk is located more laterally and quite posteriorly to this location. The inferior root of the ansa cervicalis is located more superficially in the anterior neck. The internal branch of the superior laryngeal nerve takes a route superior to that of the external branch and the superior thyroid artery and would be unlikely to be injured in this case. The recurrent laryngeal nerve terminates inferiorly, passing into the larynx in relation to the inferior thyroid artery or its branches.

GAS 1068; N 71, 76-78, 82, 127; McM 47, 78

69 **C.** The external surface of the tympanic membrane is innervated primarily by the auriculotemporal nerve, a branch of the mandibular division of the trigeminal nerve. Damage to this nerve would additionally result in painful movements of the TMJ because this joint receives innervation from the same nerve. Taste in the anterior two thirds of the tongue is supplied by the facial nerve and would be unaffected in this injury. (The chorda tympani could be injured, but its superior location on the medial side would make this unlikely.) The sensory innervation of the nasal cavity is supplied by the ophthalmic and maxillary divisions of the trigeminal nerve and would be unaffected by injury to the tympanic membrane. Sensory innervation to the larynx is provided by the vagus nerve, whereas the pharynx receives sensory fibers from the glossopharyngeal and vagus nerves. The palate is supplied by the maxillary divisions of the trigeminal nerve and would be unaffected by this injury.

GAS 912, 915, 985-986, 1104; N 2, 18, 46, 49-51, 71-72, 123, 126, 135; McM 29, 39-40, 59, 75-76

70 **B.** Both the stapedius and tensor tympani normally function to dampen movements of the middle ear ossicles, thereby muting sound and preventing hyperacusis. A stapedius would be the source of hyperacusis in this problem because it receives its innervation from the facial nerve. The tensor tympani receives motor innervation from the mandibular division of the trigeminal nerve. The posterior belly of the digastric and the stylohyoid receive innervation from the facial nerve, but their paralysis would not cause hyperacusis. Damaged innervation of the cricothyroid, which is supplied by the external branch of the superior laryngeal nerve, would not result in hyperacusis.

GAS 963, 969-971; N 55, 96, 119, 124, 151; McM 60-61

71 **C.** The greater petrosal nerve carries parasympathetic fibers that are involved in the innervation of the lacrimal gland, as well as the mucosal glands of the nose, palate, and pharynx. As a result, an injury to the right greater petrosal nerve would be expected to result in decreased lacrimal secretions for the right eye. The sublingual and submandibular glands receive their parasympathetic fibers from the facial nerve via the chorda tympani and the lingual nerve. They would be unaffected by this lesion. The parotid gland receives its parasympathetic secretory innervation from the glossopharyngeal nerve via the lesser petrosal and auriculotemporal nerves and would be unaffected. Taste to the anterior tongue is provided by the facial nerve via the chorda tympani, and general sensation to the anterior tongue is provided by the mandibular division of the trigeminal nerve via the lingual nerve.

GAS 969, 988, 997, 1104, 1105; N 13, 39, 53, 55, 61, 88, 96, 124-126, 132, 134, 136; McM 44, 61, 79

72 **C.** Parasympathetic innervation of the parotid gland is provided by axons carried by the glossopharyngeal nerve that emerge from the tympanic plexus of the middle ear as the lesser petrosal nerve. These preganglionic parasympathetic fibers terminate at synapses in the otic ganglion, which supplies the secretory parasympathetic innervation to the parotid gland. Glandular secretions of the nasal cavity, soft palate, and lacrimal gland all receive parasympathetic innervation from the fibers of the greater petrosal nerve and would remain intact following a tympanic plexus lesion. Axons for secretory innervation to the sublingual and submandibular glands are carried by the facial nerve, then course through the chorda tympani, before synapsing in the submandibular ganglion, with postganglionic fibers eventually reaching the glands via the lingual nerve (*GAS* Figs. 8-116 and 8-121).

GAS 964, 989; N 12-13, 50, 88, 95-96, 123-124, 126, 135; McM 44, 78-79

73 **B.** The inferior alveolar branch of the mandibular division of the trigeminal nerve provides sensory innervation to the mandibular teeth and would require anesthesia to abolish painful sensation. The lingual nerve provides taste and sensation to the anterior two thirds of the tongue and carries general sensory fibers, taste fibers, and parasympathetic fibers. It does not provide sensory innervation to the teeth. The buccal nerve provides sensory innervation to the inner surface of the cheek. The mental nerve is the distal continuation of the inferior alveolar nerve as it exits the mental foramen of the mandible and does not affect the teeth. The nerve to the mylohyoid is a motor branch of the inferior alveolar nerve that supplies the mylohyoid and the anterior belly of the digastric.

GAS 894, 896, 897-898, 901-902, 989; N 18, 47, 49-51, 58, 61, 71, 123, 132, 135; McM 42, 59, 75-76, 81

74 **D.** Part of the lateral pterygoid muscle has its insertion on the articular disc within the TMJ and would be most affected by the inflammation of this joint. The temporalis muscle inserts upon the coronoid process and retracts the jaw. The medial pterygoid muscle extends from the medial surface of the

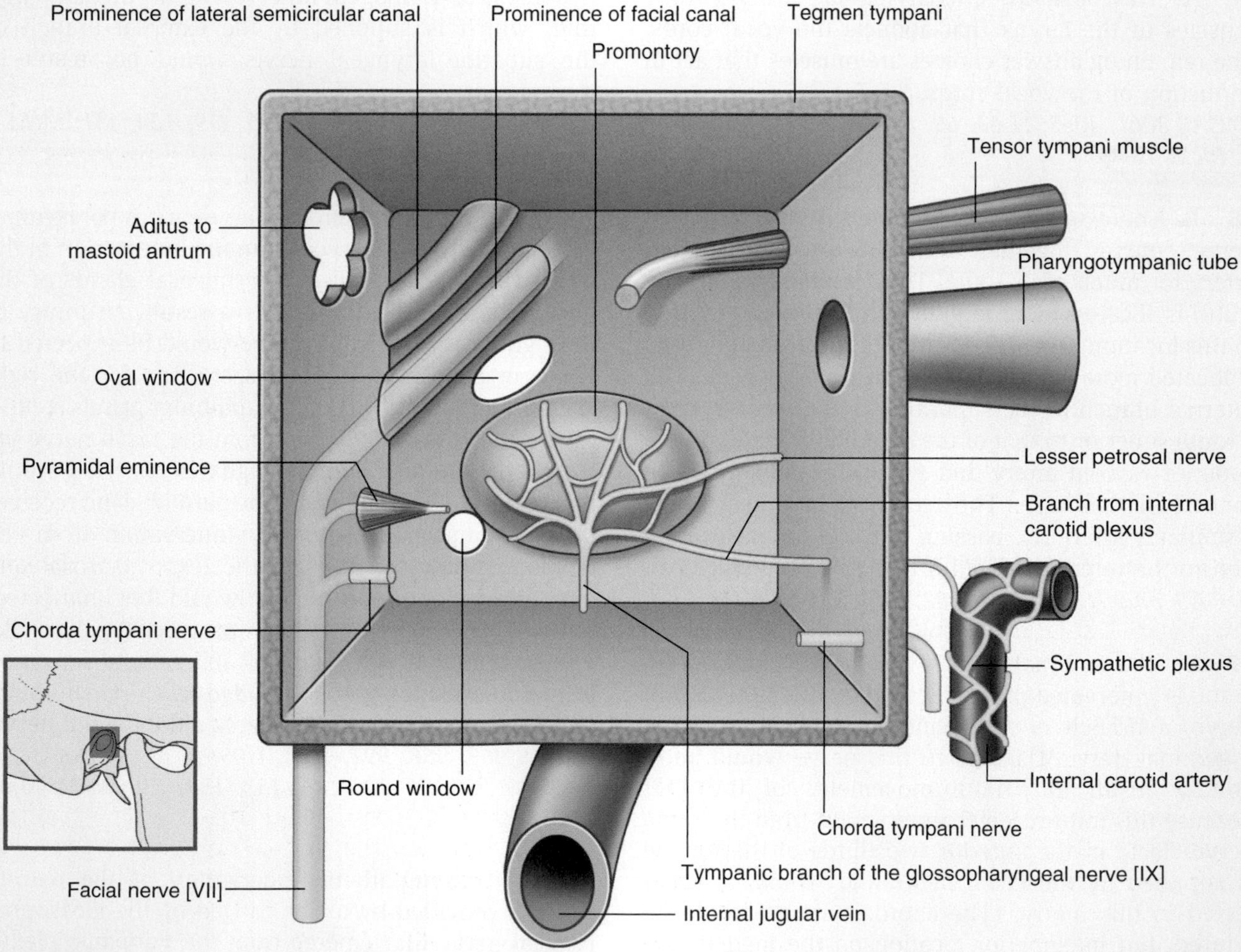

GAS **Fig. 8-116**

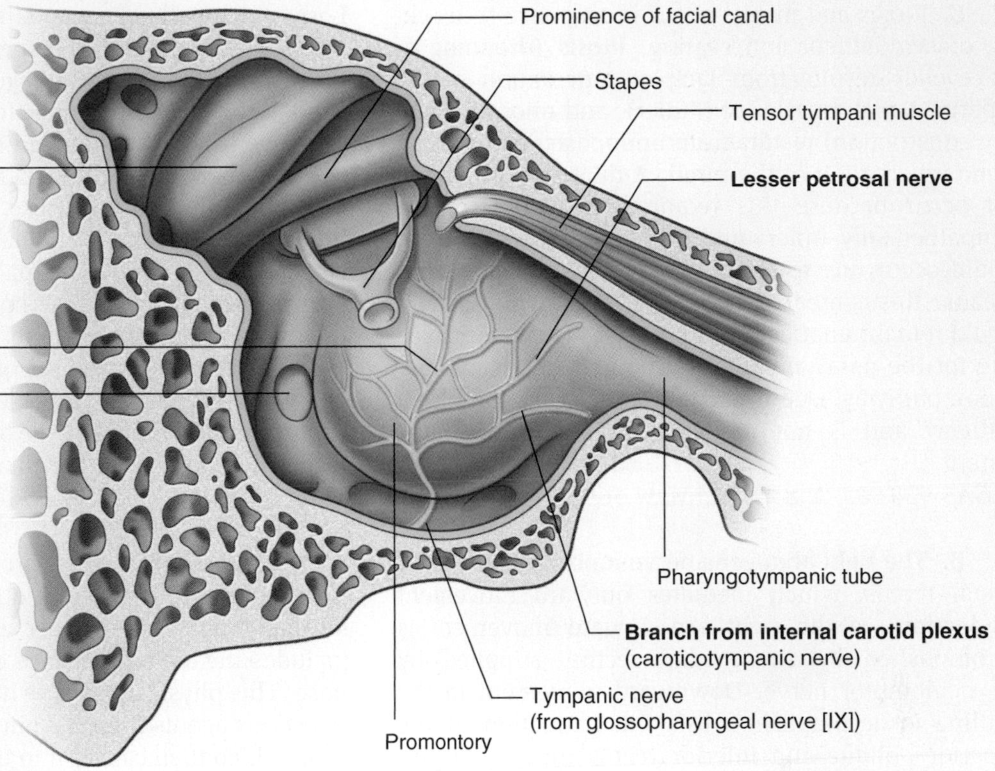

GAS **Fig. 8-121**

lateral pterygoid plate to the mandible and functions in elevation of the jaw. The masseter extends from the zygomatic arch to the lateral ramus of the mandible and elevates the jaw. The buccinator pulls back the angle of the mouth and flattens the cheek.

GAS 977, 983, 985; N 6, 42, 49-51, 151; McM 10, 19, 42-44

75 D. The trochlear nerve innervates the superior oblique muscle, which acts to move the pupil downward and laterally. It is the only muscle that can depress the pupil when the eye is adducted. When an individual walks down stairs, this eye motion is initiated, and diplopia results if it is not functioning properly. The optic nerve provides vision, and a lesion of this nerve would not result in diplopia when an affected individual walks down the stairs, but rather diminished vision or blindness. The oculomotor nerve supplies the superior, inferior, and medial rectus as well as the inferior oblique. Overall, innervation from the oculomotor nerve results in upward and inward movements of the eye, and a lesion of this nerve would not induce diplopia in an individual walking down stairs. The abducens nerve innervates the lateral rectus muscle, which abducts the eye, and damage would not induce the diplopia presented in this problem. The frontal nerve is a branch of the ophthalmic division of the trigeminal nerve and provides sensory innervation to the forehead.

GAS 894-895, 897, 901b, 902, 943-944; N 55, 85-86, 88, 105, 115-119, 122, 145; McM 53, 59, 74, 82

76 E. The superior oblique muscle turns the pupil downward from the adducted position. Inability to perform this motion, in conjunction with diplopia when walking down stairs, indicates damage to the trochlear nerve. The abducens innervates the lateral rectus, resulting in abduction of the eye. The oculomotor nerve supplies the superior, inferior, and medial rectus as well as the inferior oblique muscles. Overall, innervation from the oculomotor nerve results in upward and downward movements of the eye. Damage to this nerve would not induce diplopia when an affected individual walks down stairs. In addition, inability to gaze downward in the adducted position does not indicate oculomotor nerve damage. In this position the oculomotor nerve would be responsible for upward movement. The nasociliary nerve is a sensory nerve originating from the ophthalmic branch of the trigeminal nerve.

GAS 894-895, 897, 901b, 902, 943-945; N 55, 85-86, 88, 105, 115-119, 122, 146; McM 53, 59, 74, 82

77 **E.** Ptosis and miosis occur in response to blocking of sympathetic innervation. Ptosis (drooping of the eyelid) results from lack of innervation of the superior tarsal muscle (of Müller), and miosis (pupillary constriction) results from unopposed parasympathetic innervation of the pupil. A dilated pupil would not occur because this requires the action of the sympathetically innervated dilator pupillae. Dry eye would occur due to lacrimal gland insufficiency, but because this is mediated by parasympathetic fibers, it would remain unaffected in this case. The same holds true for the parasympathetically mediated accommodation pathway. Depth perception involves the visual pathway and is not mediated by the sympathetic system.

GAS 928-931; N 83, 132; McM 56, 81

78 **B.** The right abducens nerve innervates the right lateral rectus, which mediates outward movement (abduction) of the right eye. Inward movement is accomplished by the medial rectus, supplied by the oculomotor nerve. Downward movement in the midline is accomplished by joint activation of the superior oblique and inferior rectus muscle. Downward movement of the pupil from the adducted position is a function of the superior oblique alone, which is supplied by the trochlear nerve. Down and out motion is mediated by the combined actions of the lateral rectus and inferior rectus muscles, which are innervated by the abducens and oculomotor nerves. Downward movement of the pupil from a forward gaze is a result of combined actions of inferior rectus and superior oblique muscles, supplied by oculomotor and trochlear nerves, respectively.

GAS 894-895, 898, 901b, 902, 944; N 13, 55, 85-86, 88, 105, 115, 118, 122; McM 67, 74, 77, 80

79 **A.** Horner's syndrome involves interruption of sympathetic supply to the face. This results in ptosis (drooping eyelid), miosis (constricted pupil), and anhydrosis (lack of sweating) of the face. The eye is lubricated by the lacrimal gland, which secretes in response to parasympathetic stimulation, and would be unaffected. Exophthalmos (protrusion of the globe) is frequently caused by hyperthyroidism and is not present in Horner's syndrome. Loss of sympathetic innervation leads to unopposed vasodilatation of the vessels to the face, leading to flushing rather than paleness.

GAS 928-931; N 83, 132; McM 81

80 **E.** The superior tarsal muscle (of Müller), innervated by sympathetics, is smooth muscle that assists in elevating the eyelids and maintaining this position. Loss of sympathetic innervation will result in partial ptosis of the eyelid. The superior oblique, innervated by the trochlear nerve, moves the pupil downward from the adducted position (for example, as when the right eye gazes down toward the left foot). To test the trochlear nerve, ask the patient to look with each eye toward the tip of the nose. The orbicularis oculi, innervated by the facial nerve, is responsible for closure of the eye. The palpebral part closes the eyelids ordinarily; the lacrimal part contracts when the eye is closed more forcibly, resulting in increased tear movement across the globe (perhaps to flow down the cheeks). Damage to the levator palpebrae superioris, innervated by the oculomotor nerve, would result in complete, rather than partial, ptosis.

GAS 928-931; N 83; McM 81

81 **D.** Cavernous sinus thrombosis can often result from squeezing pimples or other infectious processes located around the danger area of the face, which includes the area of the face directly surrounding the nose. This physical pressure has the potential to move infectious agents from the pimple into the ophthalmic vein, which then carries it to the cavernous sinus. The pterygoid venous plexus and ophthalmic vein both communicate with the cavernous sinus and therefore offer a route of travel for the spread of infection, but the path provided by the superior ophthalmic vein is a more direct route. Additionally, the superior ophthalmic vein receives blood supply from the supraorbital, supratrochlear, and angular veins that supply the area around the nose and lower forehead. (Venous blood in the head can flow in either direction because these veins do not possess valves.) The emissary veins communicate between the venous sinuses and the veins of the scalp and would therefore not be involved in the spread of infection between the nose and cavernous sinus. The middle meningeal artery courses between the dura and periosteum, whereas the carotid artery, specifically the ICA, traverses through the cavernous sinus and provides origin to the ophthalmic artery. As with the middle meningeal artery, the carotid artery would not offer a route of communication between the area of infection and the cavernous sinus (*GAS* Fig. 8-65).

GAS 887-888, 920, 934; N 13, 73, 85, 87, 93, 105; McM 47, 51

82 **E.** The anterior inferior cerebellar artery (AICA) is a major supplier of the anterior inferior portion of the cerebellum. Nerves located in close proximity would likely be affected by hemorrhage of this artery. The optic, oculomotor, and trochlear nerves are all associated with the midbrain region and would likely

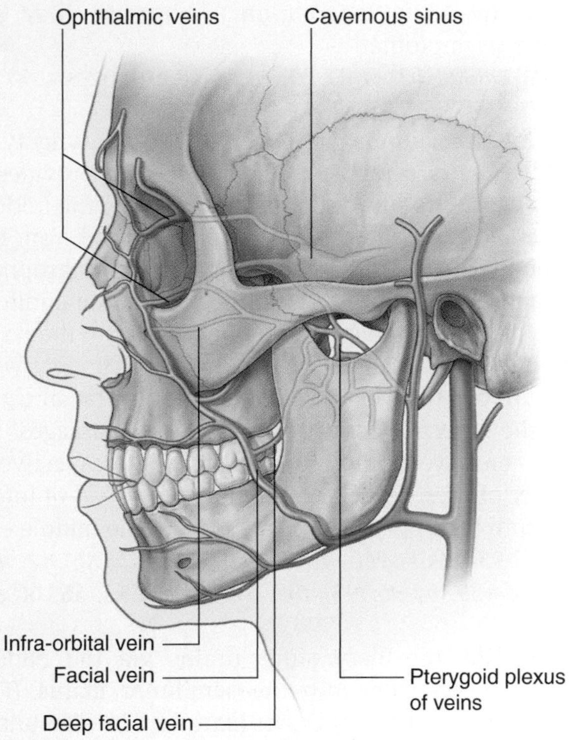

GAS **Fig. 8-65**

not suffer any damage with a possible hemorrhage. The trigeminal nerve is situated in the pons and is thus located too far rostrally to be affected. The abducens nerve is situated at the pontomedullary junction and is therefore most likely to be damaged following hemorrhage of the AICA.

GAS 882; N 137, 139-142, 144, 167; McM 68

83 D. The anterior inferior quadrant of the eardrum is the only portion of the tympanic membrane that would allow for an incision with minimal or no damage to adjacent important structures. Incision in the anterior and posterior superior quadrants of the eardrum would likely damage the malleus, which is situated immediately superior and medially to the tympanic membrane. The umbo is situated in close proximity to the handle of the malleus and might be damaged during incision. A vertical incision through the eardrum would almost certainly damage the malleus of the middle ear. Damage to the malleus from surgical incision would interfere with the auditory conduction through the middle ear cavity, and this should be avoided to prevent conductive hearing loss.

GAS 956-958, 971; N 94-96, 98; McM 44, 60-61

84 A. The hypoglossal nerve innervates the muscles of the tongue and is therefore directly involved in alteration of shape and movement of the tongue. A lesion in this nerve would cause deviation of the tongue toward the injured side, which could be observed upon protrusion of the tongue. The genioglossus is the major muscle involved in protrusion of the tongue. The genioglossus muscles arise from the inside of the mandible and pass posteriorly to insert into the deep aspect of the tongue. When the genioglossus muscles contract, they pull the tongue forward, and out of the mouth, in protrusion. If one genioglossus is paralyzed, it acts like a brake on one side of the tongue when the tongue is pulled forward, causing the tip of the tongue to point to the nonmoving side. The styloglossus muscle is responsible for retraction and elevation of the tongue.

GAS 894-895, 900, 901, 902; N 12, 33-34, 42, 47, 50, 55, 59, 71-73, 75, 105, 115, 118-119, 129-130; McM 44, 67, 79, 81

85 B. The posterior chamber receives ciliary body secretions first. The ciliary body produces aqueous humor and is located in the posterior chamber. Increased production of fluid from this site would cause an increase in intraocular pressure if drainage is inadequate. The iridoscleral angle of the anterior chamber is the location of drainage of the aqueous humor; therefore, a blockage of drainage in this location can cause increased intraocular pressure. The pupil is the connection between the anterior and posterior chamber; a collection of fluid does not occur here, for this is simply an aperture to allow light onto the retina. The vitreous body is not directly connected to the production of aqueous humor. The lacrimal sac is the upper dilated end of the nasolacrimal duct and opens up into the inferior meatus of the nasal cavity. The nasolacrimal duct has nothing to do with increased intraocular pressure.

GAS 947-948, 950; N 89-90; McM 54

86 D. The glossopharyngeal nerve mediates general somatic sensation from the pharynx, the auditory tube, and from the middle ear. Painful sensations from the pharynx, including the auditory tube, can be referred to the ear by this nerve, as in this case of tonsillectomy. The auriculotemporal nerve supplies skin of the auricle and tympanic membrane and scalp. This nerve would not be involved directly or indirectly in the operation. The lesser petrosal nerve contains preganglionic parasympathetic fibers that run in the glossopharyngeal and tympanic nerves before synapsing in the otic ganglion. The vagus nerve mediates general somatic afferent supply to the auricle and external acoustic meatus; stimulation of the meatus can trigger a gag reflex or coughing reflex. The chorda tympani mediates taste for the anterior two thirds of the tongue.

GAS 894-895, 899-900, 901, 902; N 34, 42, 55, 61, 71-72, 105, 115, 117-118, 124, 126-127, 131-132, 134-136, 207; McM 44, 67, 78

87 E. A tumor of the jugular canal would likely affect the glossopharyngeal, vagus, and accessory nerves as they exit the cranium through the jugular foramen. The uvula deviates toward the unaffected side of the pharyngeal muscles because of the pull of the unopposed levator veli palatini. In this case, the uvula deviates to the left, indicating that the left palatal muscles are unaffected whereas the right muscles are not working properly. The pharyngeal wall on the left side is also drawn upward by the nonparalyzed stylopharyngeus, supplied by the left glossopharyngeal nerve. The pharyngeal constrictor muscles, as well as muscles of the palate, are all innervated by the vagus nerve, except for the tensor veli palatini, which is supplied by the mandibular division of the trigeminal nerve. The right mandibular nerve (of the mandibular division of trigeminal nerve) provides sensory innervation to the face and motor supply to the masticatory muscles and does not innervate the muscles of the pharynx. The left hypoglossal nerve innervates the intrinsic and extrinsic muscles of the left side of the tongue. Compression or injury of this nerve would not lead to uvula deviation.

GAS 894-895, 900, 902, 1034; N 12, 26, 32-34, 42, 55, 61, 71-72, 76-78, 105, 115, 117-118, 126-128, 131-132, 136, 164, 203, 206-208, 224, 229, 236, 303-304, 318; McM 47, 53, 67-69, 78, 207

88 E. An infection of the submandibular space is usually the result of a dental infection in the mandibular molar area in the floor of the mouth (Ludwig's angina). If the patient is not treated with antibiotics promptly, the pharyngeal and submandibular swelling can lead to asphyxiation. Quinsy, also known as peritonsillar abscess, is a pus-filled inflammation of the tonsils that can occur due to tonsillitis. Ankyloglossia, which is also known as tongue-tie, is a congenital defect that results in a shortened lingual frenulum that restricts movement of the tongue. The affected person will usually have a speech impediment. Torus palatinus is a benign bony growth on the hard palate; a torus mandibularis is a similar growth on the inside of the mandible. Such growths are usually benign and would not typically cause pain. A ranula is a mucocele found on the floor of the mouth, often resulting from dehydration in older individuals, with coagulation (inspissation) of salivary secretions. It can be caused by acute local trauma; however, they are usually asymptomatic.

GAS 988, 1103; N 27-29; McM 18, 30, 32-33, 40

89 A. The auditory (eustachian or pharyngotympanic) tube is a mucosal-lined tube that provides a direct connection from the nasopharynx to the middle ear cavity. A respiratory infection can travel from the upper respiratory tract to the oropharynx or nasopharynx and then on into the middle ear via the auditory tube. The choanae are paired openings from the nasal cavity into the nasopharynx and do not connect with the auditory tube or the middle ear. The facial canal and the internal acoustic meatus are passages for facial and vestibulocochlear nerves, respectively. Neither of these is a likely site for the spread of infection from the upper respiratory tract to the middle ear.

GAS 954, 961, 966, 1046-1048, 1090; N 36, 42, 49, 57, 64-69, 94-96, 98, 100, 126; McM 52, 58, 60-61

90 B. The maxillary sinus drains via the middle meatus, specifically into the semilunar hiatus. The middle meatus and semilunar hiatus are located under the middle nasal concha. The inferior meatus drains the lacrimal secretions carried by the nasolacrimal duct, whereas the superior meatus drains the posterior ethmoidal and sphenoid sinuses. The nasopharynx and sphenoethmoidal recess are not situated in close proximity to the maxillary sinus and are therefore not involved in its drainage (*GAS* Fig. 8-235).

GAS 1069-1071; N 36-37, 43-44; McM 3, 12, 16, 44, 58

91 E. The sphenoidal sinus provides the most direct access to the pituitary gland, which is situated directly above this sinus. Neither the frontal sinus nor maxillary sinus has any direct communication with the interior of the cranial vault and would therefore not allow the surgeon a potential access point to the pituitary gland. The cribriform plate could offer a point of entry into the cranium; entry at that site would lead to damage of the olfactory cells and nerve, but it would also lead to entry into the subarachnoid space, with leakage of CSF and potential meningitis. The cribriform plates are also located too far anteriorly from the pituitary gland. The cavernous sinus is situated within the cranial vault and surrounds the pituitary gland; it is not a site for surgical entrance to the cranial cavity.

GAS 1075, 1076; N 38, 39; McM 12, 17, 25, 43, 47, 58, 73

92 B. The gag reflex is composed of both an afferent and an efferent limb. These reflexes are mediated by the glossopharyngeal and vagus nerves, respectively. Together, the glossopharyngeal and vagus nerves are responsible for the contraction of the muscles of the pharynx involved in the gag reflex. In this case the glossopharyngeal nerve was injured when the tonsils were excised, resulting in the loss of the sensory side of the reflex. The mandibular and maxillary nerves are part of the trigeminal nerve and are thus largely associated with the sensory supply of the face, sinuses, and oral cavity. The hypoglossal nerve innervates most of the muscles of the tongue. The facial nerve is involved with taste of the anterior two thirds of the tongue; however, it does not mediate the gag reflex.

GAS 1100; N 61; McM 29, 35, 36, 44, 67, 78

93 B. The recurrent laryngeal nerve is often at risk of being damaged during a thyroidectomy. Patients who have a transected or damaged recurrent laryngeal will often present with a characteristic hoarseness following surgery. The posterior cricoarytenoid is supplied by the recurrent laryngeal nerve and would thus be impaired following damage to the nerve. The posterior cricoarytenoid is the only muscle responsible for abduction of the vocal cords, and paralysis of this muscle would result in a permanently adducted position of the involved vocal cord. The other muscles listed are all adductors of the vocal cords, and paralysis of these would not lead to closure of the airway.

GAS 1062; N 80, 81, 82; McM 47-49

94 C. The pharyngeal tonsil is situated in a slitlike space, the pharyngeal recess, in the nasopharynx behind the opening of the auditory (eustachian) tube, and a pharyngeal tonsil in this location can lead to blockage of the drainage of the auditory tube. The lingual tonsil is located in the posterior aspect of the tongue, whereas the palatine tonsil is contained within the tonsillar fossa between the palatoglossal and palatopharyngeal arches. An enlargement of the lingual tonsil or the palatine tonsil will not occlude the auditory tube due to their location in the oropharynx. The superior pharyngeal constrictor would not be involved in occlusion of the auditory tube because it is located more posteriorly. The uvula is drawn upward during deglutition and prevents food from entering the nasopharynx; it does not block the auditory tube.

GAS 1047; N 36; McM 52, 360

95 A. Infection can spread from the nasopharynx to the middle ear by way of the auditory tube, which opens to both spaces. The first pharyngeal pouch is responsible for formation both of the auditory tube and middle ear (tympanic) cavity. The second pharyngeal pouch persists as the tonsillar sinus and tonsillar crypts. The third pharyngeal pouch develops into the inferior parathyroid gland and thymus, whereas the fourth pharyngeal pouch forms the remainder of the parathyroid glands and the ultimobranchial body. The sixth pharyngeal pouch is not

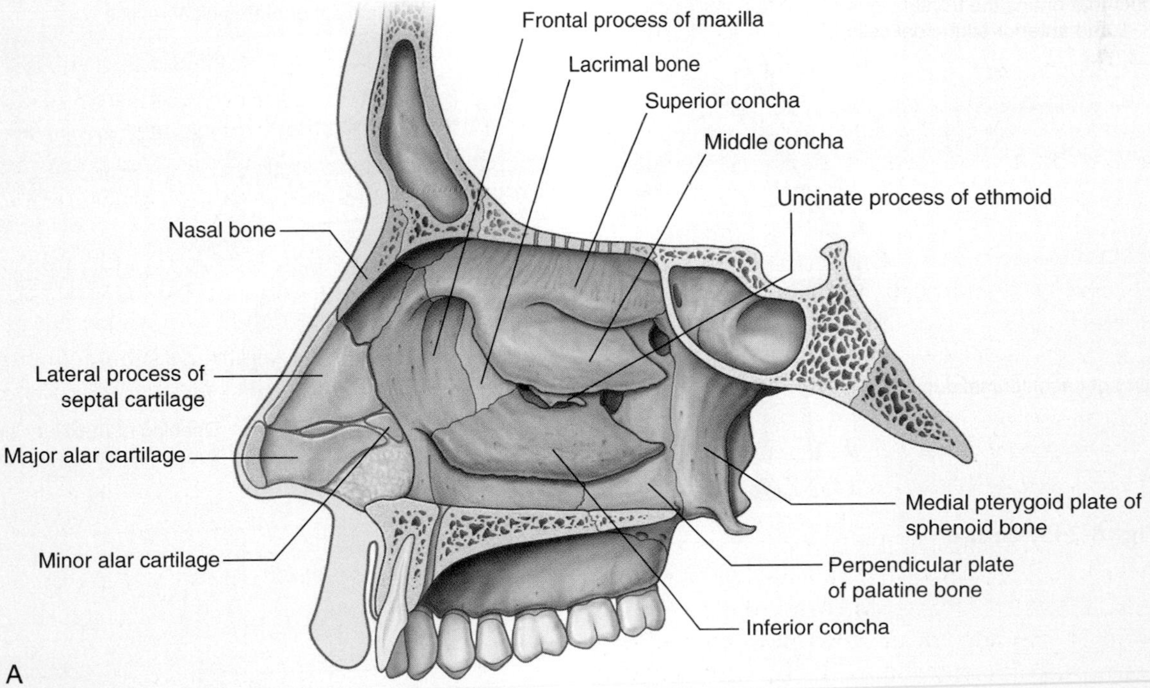

GAS Fig. 8-235

Continued

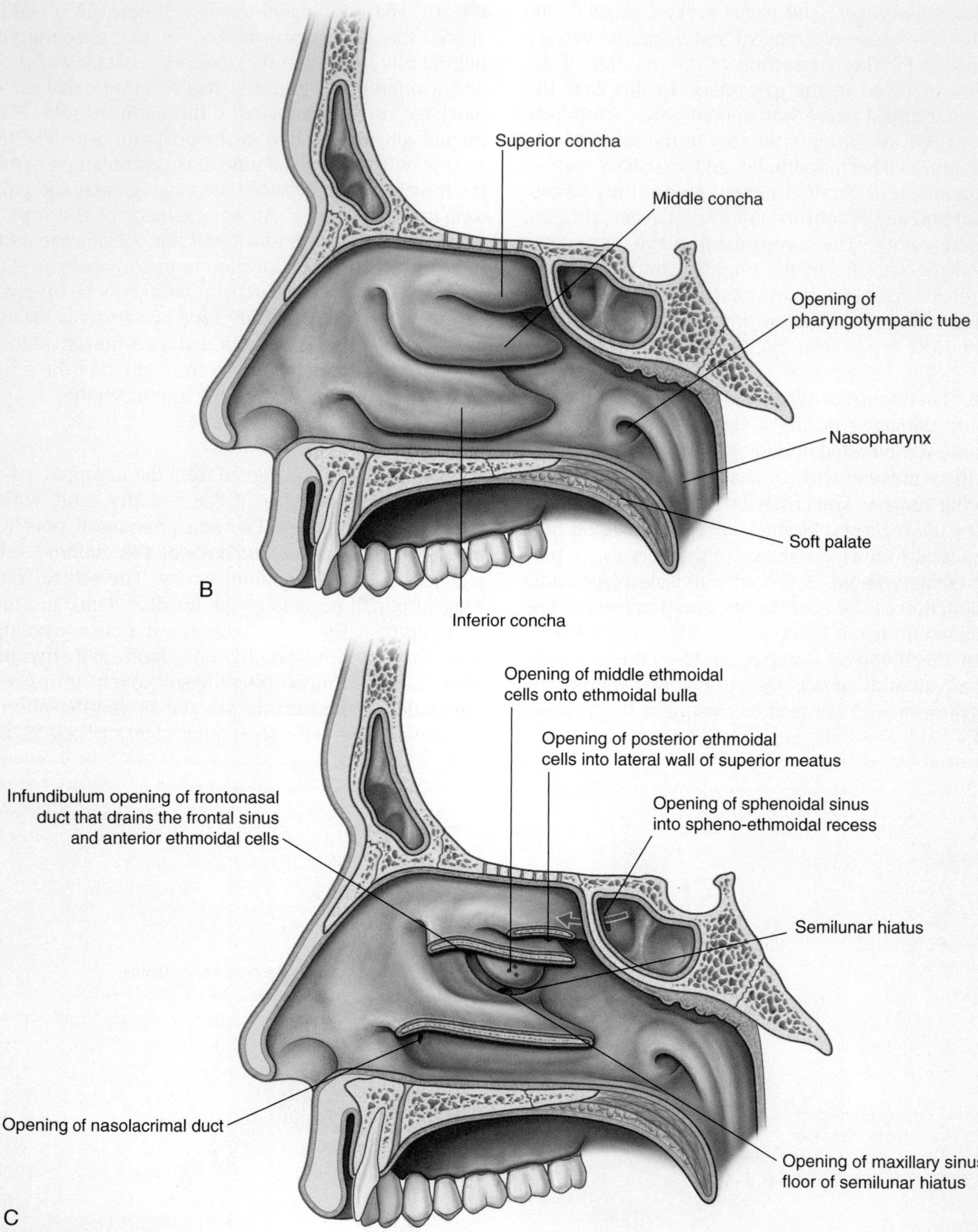
Superior concha
Middle concha
Opening of
pharyngotympanic tube
Nasopharynx
Soft palate
B
Inferior concha
Opening of middle ethmoidal
cells onto ethmoidal bulla
Opening of posterior ethmoidal
cells into lateral wall of superior meatus
Infundibulum opening of frontonasal
duct that drains the frontal sinus
and anterior ethmoidal cells
Opening of sphenoidal sinus
into spheno-ethmoidal recess
Semilunar hiatus
Opening of nasolacrimal duct
Opening of maxillary sinus in
floor of semilunar hiatus
C

GAS **Fig. 8-235, cont'd**

well defined and would therefore not contribute to the development of the auditory tube.

GAS 961; N 94; McM 45-47, 49

96 D. The greater palatine nerve is responsible for the sensory innervation of the hard palate, or the hard part of the roof of the mouth. The lesser palatine nerve supplies the soft palate and palatine tonsil but is not involved in supply to the hard palate. The posterior superior alveolar nerve supplies multiple structures, including posterior portions of the gums, cheeks, and the upper posterior teeth. However, it is not involved in nerve supply to the hard palate. The inferior alveolar nerve has several branches, including the mental nerve, incisive branch, nerve to the mylohyoid, and inferior dental branch. These nerves do not supply the roof of the mouth and thus are not involved. The lingual nerve supplies taste and general sensation to the anterior two thirds of the tongue.

GAS 995, 1112-1113; N 39, 41, 53-55, 57, 61, 71, 123, 132; McM 44, 58

97 A. Damage to the internal laryngeal nerve would result in a general loss of sensation to the larynx above the vocal cords, leaving the patient with an inability to detect food or foreign objects in the laryngeal vestibule. The external laryngeal nerve and recurrent laryngeal nerve are both at risk during thyroidectomy. Damage to the recurrent laryngeal nerve would result in paralysis of all the laryngeal muscles except the cricothyroid; it would render the patient hoarse, with a loss of sensation below the vocal cords. Loss of the external laryngeal nerve would lead to paralysis of the cricothyroid muscle and vocal weakness. Injury to the hypoglossal nerve would result in weakness or paralysis of muscle movement of the tongue.

GAS 1068; N 61, 65, 67, 69, 71, 76-78, 80, 82, 127; McM 49-50, 78

98 C. Ankyloglossia (tongue-tie) is characterized by a lingual frenulum that extends all the way to the tip of the tongue. This condition can cause problems with speech, feeding, and oral hygiene as a result of the low range of motion of the tongue. Ankyloglossia can be treated surgically by cutting the lingual frenulum. None of the other procedures described would treat this condition.

GAS 1096; N 46, 56; McM 43, 47, 49, 59

99 D. Of the answer choices listed, the left facial nerve of the patient is the most likely to be damaged during the mastoidectomy. The facial nerve exits the skull via the stylomastoid foramen, just anterior to the mastoid process. A lesion of the facial nerve is likely to cause the symptoms described as a result of paralysis of the facial muscles. Depending upon the site of injury, the patient could also lose the chorda tympani branch of the facial nerve, leading to loss of taste from the anterior two thirds of the tongue ipsilaterally as well as loss of functions of the submandibular and sublingual salivary glands. The other nerves listed are not likely to be damaged during a mastoidectomy.

GAS 970; N 96; McM 61, 39, 40, 77

100 C. Normally the tonus of the buccinator muscle prevents the accumulation of saliva and foodstuffs in the oral vestibule. Although a lesion of the facial nerve would paralyze the other muscles listed, the buccinator is the predominant muscle of the cheek.

GAS 904, 909, 911, 1092; N 24, 25, 46, 48, 50, 57, 65; McM 39-40, 43

101 B. Compression of the optic chiasm can cause bitemporal hemianopia due to compression of nerve fibers coming from the nasal (medial) hemiretinas of both eyes. The optic chiasm is located in very close proximity above the pituitary gland. Compression of an optic nerve would cause complete blindness in the affected eye. Compression of an optic tract would cause homonymous hemianopia. Compression of the oculomotor nerve would cause the eye to deviate "out and down" (paralysis of the four extraocular muscles innervated by this nerve), ptosis (paralysis of levator palpebrae), and mydriasis (paralysis of constrictor pupillae). Compression of the abducens nerve would cause paralysis of the lateral rectus muscle, leading to medial deviation (adduction) of the eye.

GAS 1135; N 105, 107, 108; McM 51, 64-65

102 E. A lesion of the trochlear nerve causes weakness of downward medial gaze. As a result, patients with trochlear nerve lesions commonly have difficulty walking down stairs. The superior cerebellar artery branches from the basilar artery just before it bifurcates into the posterior cerebral arteries. The trochlear nerve emerges from the dorsal aspect of the midbrain and can easily be compressed by an aneurysm of the superior cerebellar artery as it wraps around the midbrain. Aneurysms of the other arteries mentioned are not likely to compress the trochlear nerve, and lesions of the nerves listed are not likely to cause problems walking down stairs.

GAS 882; N 144; McM 51, 65, 67-68

103 E. A Pancoast tumor is located in the pulmonary apex, usually in the right lung. (This is because inhaled gases tend to collect preferentially in the upper right lung, in part because of the manner of branching of the tertiary bronchi.) These tumors can involve the sympathetic chain ganglia and cause Horner's syndrome (slight ptosis and miosis). The other conditions listed are not likely to cause symptoms of Horner's syndrome. Raynaud's disease, a vascular disorder that affects the extremities, is caused by excessive tone of sympathetic vasoconstriction. Frey's syndrome, a rare malady resulting from parotidectomy, is characterized by excessive facial sweating in the presence of food or when thinking about it. Bell's palsy is characterized by a lesion of the facial nerve, with weakness or paralysis of mimetic muscles. Quinsy is characterized by painful, pus-filled inflammation of the tonsils.

McM 216

104 E. The dilator pupillae, levator palpebrae superioris, and smooth muscle cells of blood vessels in the ciliary body all receive sympathetic innervation. The postsynaptic cell bodies of the sympathetic neurons that innervate these structures are located in the superior cervical ganglion. The intermediolateral cell column contains presynaptic sympathetic neurons, but it is located only at spinal cord levels T1 to L2. The other structures listed do not contain sympathetic cell bodies.

GAS 1035, 1036; N 133; McM 36

105 B. A fracture of the lamina papyracea of the ethmoid bone is likely to entrap the medial rectus muscle, causing an inability to gaze laterally. A fracture of the orbital plate of the frontal bone could perhaps entrap the superior oblique or superior rectus muscle, but this would be very unusual. A fracture of the orbital plate of the maxilla can entrap the inferior rectus or inferior oblique muscles, limiting upward gaze. A fracture of the cribriform plate could damage olfactory nerves and result in leakage of CSF through the nose (CSF rhinorrhea), with associated meningeal infection. A fracture of the greater wing of the sphenoid is not likely to entrap any extraocular muscles.

GAS 1072, 1073; N 4, 6, 8; McM 12, 17, 26

106 B. A lesion of the oculomotor nerve will cause the eye to remain in a "down and out" position. This is due to the actions of the unopposed lateral rectus (supplied by the abducens nerve) and the superior oblique (supplied by the trochlear nerve). The tertiary function of the superior oblique is to cause intorsion (internal rotation) of the eyeball, a function that is not usually seen unless the oculomotor nerve is paralyzed. The patient is also likely to present with a full or partial ptosis due to paralysis of the levator palpebrae muscle. The pupil will remain dilated because of loss of stimulation by parasympathetic fibers that innervate the constrictor pupillae muscle. Damage to the other nerves listed will not lead to the conditions described.

GAS 902; N 86, 88; McM 44, 51, 53, 55, 59, 74

107 B. The axons of olfactory nerves run directly through the cribriform plate to synapse in the olfactory bulb. Damage to this plate can damage the nerve axons, causing anosmia (loss of the sense of smell). A fracture of the cribriform plate is not likely to entrap the eyeball. Hyperacusis can occur following paralysis of the stapedius muscle. A lesion of the vestibulocochlear nerve can cause tinnitus and/or deafness.

GAS 1072, 1073; N 8; McM 11-12, 26, 51

108 C. Frey's syndrome occurs when parasympathetic axons in the auriculotemporal nerve are cut during a parotidectomy. When these postganglionic cholinergic axons grow peripherally after parotid surgery, they establish synapses upon the cholinergic sweat glands, which are innervated normally only by sympathetic fibers. As the peripheral nerves make new connections, aberrant connections can be formed between the auriculotemporal nerve and other glands (not usually innervated by the auriculotemporal nerve). This results in flushing and sweating in response to the thought, smell, or taste of food, instead of the previous, normal salivary secretion by the parotid gland.

GAS 850, 985; N 2; McM 39-40, 42, 59, 75-76

109 B. The posterior cricoarytenoid muscle is the only abductor of the larynx that opens the rima glottidis and rotates the arytenoid cartilages laterally. All of the other listed muscles have adduction as part of their function and thus are not required to maintain the airway.

GAS 1062; N 80, 81, 82; McM 47-49

110 B. The palatine tonsils are highly vascular and are primarily supplied by the tonsillar branch of the facial artery; therefore, care is taken to identify and ligate or cauterize this artery while performing a tonsillectomy. The palatine tonsil also receives arterial supply from the ascending pharyngeal, the dorsal lingual, and the lesser palatine, but the supply from the facial artery is by far the most significant.

GAS 1012, 1013, 917, 918; N 68; McM 28-32, 39-40

111 A. The inner surface of the tympanic membrane is supplied by the glossopharyngeal nerve. The auricular branches of the facial and vagus nerves and the auriculotemporal branch of the trigeminal nerve innervate the external surface of the tympanic membrane. The great auricular nerve arises from C2 and C3 and supplies the posterior auricle and skin over the parotid gland. The lingual nerve does not have anything to do with sensory supply of the tympanic membrane.

GAS 957, 959; N 96, 119; McM 23, 60

112 C. The infraorbital branch of the maxillary division of the trigeminal nerve exits the front of the skull below the orbit through the infraorbital foramen. A needle inserted into the infraorbital foramen and directed posteriorly will pass through the foramen rotundum to reach the trigeminal ganglion and the beginning of the maxillary division of the trigeminal nerve. The mandibular division of the trigeminal nerve exits the skull through the foramen ovale. The middle meningeal artery exits the infratemporal fossa through the foramen spinosum to enter the cranial cavity. The inferior alveolar branch of the mandibular division passes into the mandibular foramen to then descend in the jaw to supply the mandibular teeth. The foramen magnum is where the spinal cord exits the skull and where the spinal accessory nerve ascends into the skull after arising from the cervical spinal cord and brainstem.

GAS 935; N 4, 6, 14, 35; McM 1, 12, 21, 38

113 A. If there is an injury to the internal laryngeal nerve, there is a loss of sensation above the vocal cords. In this case, for internal laryngeal injury to occur, one must conclude that the operative field extended above the position of the thyroid gland to the level of the thyrohyoid membrane. The external laryngeal nerve can be injured during a thyroidectomy, but its injury would result in paralysis of the cricothyroid muscle and weakened voice/hoarseness. Injury of the glossopharyngeal nerve would result in more widespread symptoms, including loss of sensation from the pharynx, posterior tongue, and middle ear. Injury to the hypoglossal nerve would cause deficits in motor activity of the tongue. Damage to the recurrent laryngeal nerve would result in paralysis of most laryngeal muscles, with possible respiratory obstruction, hoarseness, and loss of sensation below the vocal cords.

GAS 1068; N 61, 65, 67, 69, 71, 76-78, 80, 82, 127; McM 49-50, 78

114 A. The loose areolar connective tissue layer is known as the "danger zone" because hematoma can spread easily from this layer into the skull by means of emissary veins that pass into and through the bones of the skull. None of the other scalp layers listed is referred to as the "danger zone."

GAS 922, 923; N 3; McM 5

115 A. The carotid sinus is a baroreceptor that can be targeted for carotid massage to decrease blood pressure. The carotid sinus receptors are sensitive to changes in pressure. For this reason, sustained compression of the carotid sinuses can lead to unconsciousness or death as the heart rate is reflexively reduced. The carotid body is a chemoreceptor, responsive to the balance of oxygen and carbon dioxide. Neither the thyroid gland nor the parathyroid gland has anything to do with acute control of blood pressure due to mechanical stimuli. The inferior cervical ganglion fuses with the first thoracic ganglion to form the stellate ganglion. It gives rise to the inferior cervical cardiac nerve and provides postganglionic sympathetic supply to the upper limb.

N 126, 131-132, 137, 207; McM 35, 45

116 C. The thyroidea ima artery is present in about 10% of people; when present it supplies the thyroid gland and ascends in the front of the trachea; therefore, it would be easily injured in an emergency tracheostomy with a midline incision over the trachea. The inferior thyroid branch of the thyrocervical trunk does not run along the front of the trachea in such a position that a midline incision could damage it. The cricothyroid branch of the superior thyroid artery passes across the cricothyroid ligament, well above the site of incision. Arterial bleeding would not result from damage to either the middle thyroid vein or the jugular venous arch.

GAS 1019; N 34, 76, 72, 78; McM 29-32

117 D. A torn cerebral vein often results in a relatively slow-bleeding subdural hematoma. Such a hematoma can be involved in gradual compression of the brain, resulting in confusion, dizziness, clumsiness, and memory loss. There would be no sign of blood in the CSF because the bleeding is into the subdural space, not the subarachnoid space. This would fit the description of symptoms in this case. Middle meningeal artery rupture results in an epidural hematoma, which is much more acute and often includes a brief period of unconsciousness followed by a lucid interval and can proceed to death if the bleeding is left untreated. Fracture of the pterion also can result in an epidural hematoma because the middle meningeal artery is the adjacent vasculature mentioned. Rupture of the anterior communicating artery would result in a subarachnoid hematoma, and there would be blood in the CSF upon lumbar puncture. In a cavernous sinus thrombosis there would be cranial nerve involvement due to compression of those nerves that run through or near the cavernous sinus, including the oculomotor, trochlear, trigeminal (maxillary and mandibular divisions), and abducens nerves.

GAS 886; N 101; McM 63

118 **D.** Paralysis of the right accessory and hypoglossal nerves is present in this patient. Drooping of the right shoulder occurs as a result of paralysis of the trapezius as a result of injury to the right accessory nerve, which supplies that muscle. Loss of the right accessory nerve would also result in weakness in turning the head to the left, a function of the right sternocleidomastoid muscle, which is supplied by this nerve. The tongue deviation to the right is due to the unopposed activity of the left tongue muscles since the right hypoglossal nerve (which innervates the right tongue muscles) is affected. The other combinations of affected cranial nerves would not produce the specific symptoms described here.

GAS 894, 895, 900, 901, 902; N 128, 129; McM 29, 32-33, 44, 65, 67, 78, 79, 81

119 **C.** The neural cell bodies whose axons synapse in the pterygopalatine ganglion are located in the superior salivatory nucleus, which is in the pons; this nucleus provides the general visceral efferent (GVE) fibers of the facial nerve for lacrimal and salivary secretion. The SCG superior cervical ganglion is a sympathetic ganglion containing postganglionic neurons and is not concerned with the pterygopalatine ganglion, which is a parasympathetic ganglion. The Edinger-Westphal nucleus is located in the midbrain and contains the cell bodies of the GVE fibers of the oculomotor nerve, which are responsible for constriction of the pupil via synapse in the ciliary ganglion and supply to the sphincter pupillae muscle and accommodation via the ciliary muscle. The inferior salivatory nucleus is located in the medulla and gives origin to GVE fibers of the glossopharyngeal nerve to the otic ganglion for secretion of saliva from the parotid gland.

GAS 850, 894, 895, 898, 899, 901, 902; N 53, 117-118, 124, 134; McM 79

120 **B.** A branch of the facial artery would be of primary concern because its branches supply the oropharynx and it is the primary source of arterial supply to the palatine tonsil. The location of the lingual artery is inferior to the oropharynx and it would be less likely to be injured in the event of a surgical procedure. The superior laryngeal artery is also located lower and would not be subject to injury by surgery in the area of the oropharynx. The ascending pharyngeal artery arises in the carotid triangle from the external carotid artery and gives rise to pharyngeal, palatine, inferior tympanic, and meningeal branches. This vessel is located inferiorly to the site of surgery. Terminal branches of the descending palatine artery could be encountered at the upper pole of the palatine tonsil, but the main stem of the vessel would not be endangered in the surgical treatment here.

GAS 1045, 1047-1048; N 47, 56-57, 60, 64, 66, 68; McM 28, 39-40, 43

121 **A.** Infection in the "danger area of the face" can lead to cavernous sinus thrombosis because infection spreads from the nasal venous tributary to the angular vein, then to the superior ophthalmic vein, which passes into the cavernous sinus. None of the other routes listed would be correct for drainage from the danger area of the face.

GAS 919-920; N 87, 105, 137, 141; McM 47, 51, 80

122 **C.** The thrombus may pass through the central vein of the retina to reach the cavernous sinus. The patient would suffer blindness because the central vein is the only vein draining the retina and if it is occluded, blindness will ensue. The subarachnoid space would not be associated with the blindness experienced. Thrombus of the central artery would not cause cavernous sinus thrombophlebitis. The optic chiasm is a neural structure that does not transmit thrombi. The ciliary ganglion is a parasympathetic ganglion; a thrombus in the cavernous sinus would not pass through it.

GAS 948; N 89, 92-93; McM 73

123 **B.** Aqueous humor is secreted by the ciliary body into the posterior chamber of the eye, just behind the iris. The humor flows through the pupil into the anterior chamber and then is filtered by a trabecular meshwork, then drained by the scleral venous sinus (also called the canal of Schlemm). The pupil is the opening in the iris, which leads from the posterior chamber to the anterior chamber. Vitreous humor, not aqueous humor, is found in the vitreous body. The lacrimal sac is involved with tears, not the secretion of aqueous humor.

GAS 947; N 89; McM 54-57, 74

124 **A.** With all of the ventricles enlarged and no obvious single site of complete ventricular obstruction, the problem must be a condition of communicating hydrocephalus, with inadequate drainage through the arachnoid granulations into the superior sagittal

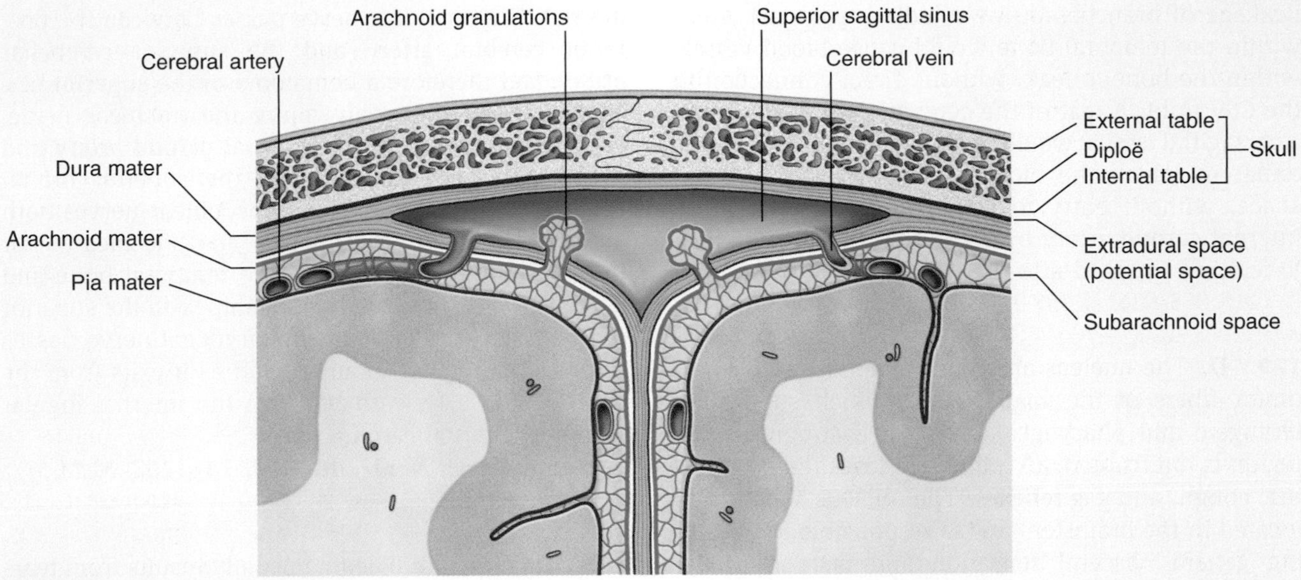

***GAS* Fig. 8-35**

sinus. There is no evidence of obstruction of CSF flow somewhere in the ventricular system. The other choices listed are all examples of noncommunicating hydrocephalus that result from obstruction, not just overproduction or filtration problems (*GAS* Fig. 8-35).

GAS 99, 877-878; N 147; McM 72

125 C. The superior sagittal sinus would most likely be the source of the bleeding because it attaches anteriorly to the crista galli and because of the slow nature of the bleed. The middle meningeal artery would not be a good answer because its location is near the pterion on the temporal aspect of the skull but its bleeding would be profuse, not slow. The great cerebral vein (of Galen) is located posteriorly in the cranial cavity and is not in the right location for an injury of this type to disrupt it. The straight dural venous sinus is also posterior, receiving the draining of the inferior sagittal sinus and the great vein (of Galen). It drains posteriorly to the confluence of sinuses (eponym: Torcular of Herophilis). The superior ophthalmic vein drains from the orbit to the cavernous sinus; further, it is located inferiorly to the crista galli and is not directly related to the superior sagittal sinus.

GAS 864, 886-887, 1083-1084; N 101-102, 104; McM 47, 52-53, 62

126 C. For proper movements of the eye to occur, all the cranial nerves that innervate the extraocular eye muscles are required (oculomotor, trochlear, and abducens nerves). The inferior division of the oculomotor innervates the inferior rectus, the medial rectus, and the inferior oblique. Lateral movement of the eye is initiated by the lateral rectus (abducens nerve), assisted thereafter by the superior oblique (trochlear nerve). The inferior rectus (inferior division of the oculomotor nerve) balances the upward deviation exerted by the superior rectus (superior division of the oculomotor nerve). The medial rectus (superior division of the oculomotor nerve) must relax to facilitate the lateral excursion. Answers A, B, and D all have branches of the trigeminal nerve, which have no role in motor movement of the eye. Finally, for answer E, the superior division innervates the superior rectus and the levator palpebrae; therefore, C is the best answer.

GAS 936-940; N 86, 92; McM 54-57

127 E. The middle of the vocal cord would be the most likely location of the tumor because there is no direct lymph drainage from this region. All other locations mentioned are drained by the lymphatics. Areas above the vocal cords are drained by the superior deep cervical nodes, and areas below the vocal cords drain to the pretracheal nodes before draining into the inferior deep cervical nodes.

GAS 1049-1050; N 74, 75; McM 359, 361

128 B. When a berry aneurysm ruptures, the blood flows into the subarachnoid space and therefore mixes with CSF; thus, blood would be present in the CSF when a lumbar puncture is performed. The pterion overlies the anterior branch of the middle meningeal vessels, and damage to these vessels would result in an epidural hematoma, with compression of the brain.

Leakage of branches of the middle meningeal artery within the temporal bone would cause blood vessels within the bone to leak, without direct connection to the CSF fluid. A tear of the cerebral vein in the superior sagittal sinus would lead to a subdural hematoma, in which the blood collects in the subdural space, without entry to CSF. The occlusion of the internal carotid artery by way of clot would not lead to leakage of blood into the CSF.

GAS 885-886; N 137-144; McM 68

129 **D.** The nucleus ambiguus gives rise to efferent motor fibers of the vagus nerve, which supply the laryngeal and pharyngeal muscles. If supply to this region is interrupted, an individual loses the swallowing, cough, and gag reflexes. The nucleus solitarius is located in the brainstem and is responsible for receiving general visceral sensation and taste from the facial, glossopharyngeal, and vagus nerves. The trigeminal motor nucleus contains motor neurons that innervate muscles of mastication, the tensor tympani, tensor veli palatini, mylohyoid, and anterior belly of the digastric. The dorsal motor nucleus contains the cell bodies of preganglionic parasympathetic fibers of the vagus nerve innervating the heart muscle and smooth musculature and glands of the respiratory and intestinal tract. The superior ganglion of the vagus contains cell bodies of general somatic afferent fibers, and the inferior ganglion of the vagus is chiefly visceral afferent in function concerning sensations (with the exclusion of painful sensation) from the heart, lungs, larynx, and alimentary tract.

GAS 850, 895-897; N 899-900; McM 78

130 **C.** Just before it passes into the mandible to supply the lower teeth and chin, the inferior alveolar nerve gives rise to the mylohyoid nerve, a motor nerve supplying the mylohyoid and anterior belly of the digastric. The geniohyoid muscle is innervated by motor fibers from spinal nerve C1 that run with the hypoglossal nerve. The hyoglossus muscle is innervated by the hypoglossal nerve. The stylohyoid muscle is innervated by the facial nerve. The palatoglossus muscle is innervated by the vagus nerve.

GAS 986-989; N 123-124, 126-127, 129, 134, 136; McM 75-79

131 **A.** The superior cerebellar artery arises near the termination of the basilar artery, passes immediately below the oculomotor nerve, and eventually winds around the cerebral peduncle, close to the trochlear nerve, as it continues on toward the upper surface of the cerebellum where it will divide into branches that anastomose with the inferior cerebellar arteries. The trochlear nerve passes between the posterior cerebral artery and the superior cerebellar artery, and therefore a hematoma of the superior cerebellar artery can easily injure the trochlear nerve, which runs alongside the internal carotid artery and then enters the orbit through the superior orbital fissure. The facial and vestibulocochlear nerves both enter the skull via the internal acoustic meatus (or internal auditory meatus) in the temporal bone and do not have an intimate relationship with the superior cerebellar artery. The glossopharyngeal nerve passes through the jugular foramen, and as it exits from the skull it passes forward between the internal jugular vein and internal carotid artery.

GAS 880-883; N 137, 139-142, 144, 167; McM 51, 65, 67-68

132 **D.** Subdural bleeding usually results from tears in veins that cross the subdural space, between the dura and the arachnoid. This bleeding may cause a gradual increase in intracranial pressure and may result in leakage of venous blood over the right cerebral hemisphere with a variable rate of progression. A subarachnoid bleed is due to rupture of an artery into the subarachnoid space surrounding the brain, between the arachnoid membrane and the pia mater. Hydrocephalus may result if the subarachnoid bleeding or subsequent fibrosis creates obstructions to CSF flow through the subarachnoid space or drainage of the CSF. Epidural bleeding results in most cases from tearing of the middle meningeal artery, and this rapidly expanding, space-occupying lesion can cause death within 12 hours. Intracerebral bleeding into the brain parenchyma is focal bleeding from a blood vessel into the brain parenchyma, most likely caused by hypertension and/or atherosclerosis. Typical symptoms include focal neurologic deficits, with abrupt onset of headache, nausea, and impairment of consciousness. Bleeding into the cerebral ventricular system may be due to trauma or hemorrhage of blood from nearby arteries, especially those related to the supply of the choroid plexus.

GAS 891-893; N 140-144; McM 65

133 **B.** The lateral pterygoid muscle is a muscle of mastication innervated by the lateral pterygoid nerve of the mandibular division of the trigeminal nerve. The lateral pterygoid acts to protrude the mandible and open the jaw. The anterior portion of temporalis is a muscle of mastication innervated by the deep temporal nerves of the mandibular division of the trigeminal nerve that elevates the mandible when contracted. The medial pterygoid muscle is a muscle of mastication innervated by the mandibular division of the trigeminal nerve. This muscle closes the jaw and works with the contralateral medial pterygoid in side-to-side (grinding) jaw movements. The masseter muscle is a muscle of mastication innervated by the mandibular division of the trigeminal nerve that specifically assists in chewing. The platysma is a thin muscle of facial expression that lies within the superficial fascia of the neck and lower face. It is innervated by the cervical branch of the facial nerve. The platysma produces a slight wrinkling of the surface of the skin of the neck in an oblique direction, depresses the lower jaw, and draws down the lower lip and angle of the mouth.

GAS 977, 983; N 6, 42, 49-51, 71, 123, 151; McM 42-44

134 B. The order of tooth eruption is a follows: inferior medial incisors (6 to 8 months), superior medial incisors (8 to 10 months), first molar (6 to 8 months), superior lateral incisors (8 to 10 months), and finally inferior lateral incisors (12 to 14 months). Teeth tend to erupt earlier in girls than in boys, and quite a range exists in the normal distribution curve.

GAS 1114-1119; N 5, 45, 62-63; McM 13

135 D. The sigmoid sinus collects venous blood from the transverse sinuses and empties it into a small cavity known as the jugular bulb, the inferior portion of which is located beneath the bony floor of the middle ear cavity. A paraganglioma is a tumor that may originate from paraganglia cells found in the middle ear and on the jugular bulb. Tumors that originate from the jugular bulb can grow to fill the entire bulb and may effectively block blood returning to the heart from that side of the brain. Blood flow from the brain is gradually diverted toward the opposite sigmoid sinus and jugular bulb, causing the opposite venous system to expand and accommodate increased blood flow. The cochlea and lateral semicircular canals are located in the inner ear and are not directly affected by such a tumor. The internal carotid artery is related to the anterior wall of the middle ear cavity and is not likely to be affected by a tumor penetrating the middle ear. The sigmoid venous sinus collects venous blood beneath the temporal bone and follows a tortuous (S-shaped) course to the jugular foramen where it becomes continuous with the internal jugular vein at the jugular bulb. The aditus ad antrum is the entrance to the mastoid antrum, which is the common cavity in the mastoid bone into which mastoid air cells open. Below the aditus ad antrum is an elevation of bone, the pyramid of the stapes, which is occupied by the stapedius muscle.

GAS 886-888; N 55, 99, 104-105; McM 69

136 E. The lingual nerve supplies sensory innervation to the mucous membrane of the anterior two thirds of the tongue, taste sensation to the anterior part of the tongue, and parasympathetic fibers to the oral salivary glands. The chorda tympani branch of the facial nerve is responsible for carrying taste fibers from the anterior two thirds of the tongue and preganglionic parasympathetic fibers for the submandibular ganglion. Injury to the lingual nerve at its origin, before it joins with the chorda tympani, will result in loss of general sensation of the tongue, but with preservation of taste and salivary function. Injury to the glossopharyngeal nerve would result in loss of general sensory and taste fibers from the posterior third of the tongue and parasympathetic supply for the parotid gland. Injury to the superior laryngeal nerve, a branch of the vagus nerve, will result in loss of sensation from the larynx above the vocal folds (*GAS* Fig. 8-146A).

GAS 1098, 1101, 1103; N 46-47, 49-51, 56, 58-59, 61, 71, 123-124, 132, 134-136; McM 29, 35, 75-76

137 A. Papilledema is optic disc swelling ("edema of the papilla") that is caused by increased intracranial pressure caused increased CSF pressure. If a lumbar puncture is performed in a patient with elevated CSF pressure and fluid is withdrawn from the lumbar cistern, the brain can become displaced caudally and the brainstem is pushed against the tentorial notch. This is a potentially fatal complication known as brain herniation. Separation of the pars optica retinae anterior to the ora serrata, or retinal detachment, may result in vision loss or blindness. A hemorrhage from medial retinal branches may result in damage to the fovea centralis and can result in macular degeneration. Opacity of the lens (cataracts) will cause gradual yellowing and may reduce the perception of blue colors. Cataracts typically progress slowly to cause vision loss and are potentially blinding if untreated. Compression of the optic disc, resulting from increased intrabulbar pressure, will lead to an excessive accumulation of serous fluid in the tissue space.

GAS 942; N 92; McM 43-44, 73

138 E. Within the cavernous sinus the abducens nerve is in intimate contact with the internal carotid artery. Therefore, an aneurysm of the internal carotid artery could quickly cause tension or compression on the abducens nerve. This would result in ipsilateral paralysis of abduction of the pupil. Inability to gaze downward and medially would be due to the trochlear nerve, which is not in the cavernous sinus. Complete ptosis would be a result of a complete lesion in

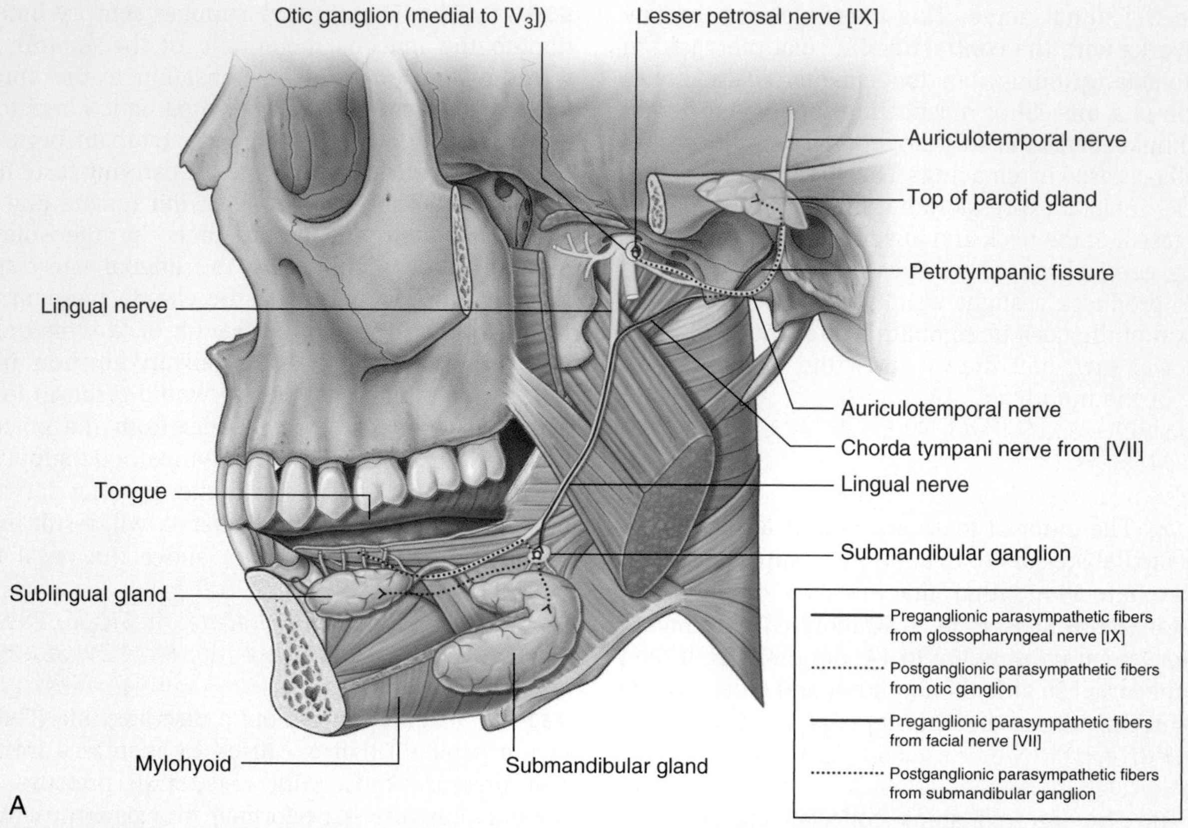

***GAS* Fig. 8-146A**

the oculomotor nerve, which is not apparent here. Bilateral loss of accommodation and loss of pupillary reflex would be the result of bilateral loss of the oculomotor nerve, which is not likely in this situation. Finally, ipsilateral loss of the consensual corneal reflex is a result of loss of both the ophthalmic division of the trigeminal nerve and the facial nerve, supplying the afferent and efferent limbs of the reflex, respectively.

GAS 888-889; N 105; McM 47, 51, 80

139 D. It is necessary to anesthetize the conjunctival covering of the sclera, which is supplied by the nasociliary branch of the ophthalmic division of the trigeminal nerve. To do that, the needle should be placed through the upper eyelid deeply toward the orbital apex to infiltrate the nasociliary nerve, and also between the orbital septum and the palpebral musculature laterally to anesthetize lateral sensory supply from the lacrimal nerve and (perhaps) twigs from the maxillary division of the trigeminal nerve. The lacrimal fossa, which is occupied by the lacrimal sac portion of the nasolacrimal duct, is too medial, whereas the supraorbital foramen is above the eye. Injections into either location would not result in anesthetizing of the sclera. Answers A and E both result in puncturing of the sclera and would most likely cause further damage to the eye.

GAS 942-946; N 13, 52, 85, 88, 122-123, 132-133; McM 44, 54, 74-75

140 E. During a puncture wound as described in this case, passing up from below the chin, the nail would first pierce the platysma, then the anterior belly of the digastric, then the mylohyoid, then the geniohyoid, and finally the genioglossus.

GAS 907, 910, 1006-1008; N 27, 29, 31; McM 28, 205

141 A. The anterior division of the facial nerve passes through the parotid gland and is therefore at risk during surgery of the parotid gland. Since this patient's symptoms involved paralysis of the muscles of the lower lip, the branch of the facial nerve that supplies these muscles, the marginal mandibular branch, is the one that has suffered the iatrogenic injury.

GAS 911, 912; N 24; McM 40

142 A. During embryologic development of the pituitary gland, an outgrowth from the roof of the pharynx (Rathke's pouch) grows cephalad and forms the anterior lobe (pars distalis) of the pituitary gland. Since this gland normally occupies the sella turcica, it is most likely a tumor derived from the Rathke's pouch that is extending up into the sella turcica and the space just above it, the suprasellar space.

GAS 866, 867; N 45; McM 47

143 A. In holoprosencephaly, loss of midline structures results in malformations of the brain and face. There is a single telencephalic vesicle, fused eyes, and a single nasal chamber. Also, there is often hypoplasia of the olfactory bulbs, olfactory tracts, and corpus callosum. Children with Smith-Lemli-Opitz syndrome have craniofacial and limb defects and 5% have holoprosencephaly. Schizencephaly is rare and is characterized by large clefts in the cerebral hemispheres, which in some cases cause a loss in brain tissue. Exencephaly is caused by failure of the cephalic part of the neural tube to close; therefore, the skull does not close, leaving the brain exposed. Meningohydroencephalocele is a deficit of the cranium involving the squamous part of the occipital bone and, in some cases, the posterior aspect of the foramen magnum. It can include the meninges if the herniation or protruding brain includes part of the ventricular system.

N 107; McM 46

144 C. Usually, deficits of the cranium involve the squamous part of the occipital bone and, in some cases, the posterior aspect of the foramen magnum. If the herniation or protruding brain includes part of the ventricular system (most likely the posterior horn of the lateral ventricles), then it is referred to as meningohydroencephalocele. The deficit in the squamous part of the occipital bone usually occurs at the posterior fontanelle of the skull.

GAS 868, 869; N 8; McM 27

145 B. The rostral neuropore closes during the fourth week of development. If this does not occur, the forebrain primordium is abnormal and the calvaria or vault fails to develop. Toxoplasmosis infection during embryologic development leads to microcephaly, in which the brain and calvaria are small in size. These patients usually have mental retardation due to an undeveloped brain. An ossification defect in the bones of the skull is often a result of hydrocephalus. Caudal displacement of the cerebellar structures would not lead to an undeveloped calvaria or vault. Maternal alcohol abuse leads to intrauterine growth restriction (IUGR), causing microcephaly and mental retardation.

N 110; McM 52

146 B. Holoprosencephaly is caused by failure of the prosencephalon to properly divide into two cerebral hemispheres. In severe cases, this is incompatible with life, but in less severe cases, such as the one presented here, babies have normal or near-normal brain development, sometimes with facial abnormalities. In this case, the child has a myelomeningocele. Almost all of these patients with this condition have a concomitant Chiari II malformation where the cerebellar vermis, fourth ventricle, and associated brainstem are herniated through the foramen magnum and into the upper cervical spinal canal.

N 106; McM 65

147 A. Congenital deafness is due to a maldevelopment of the conducting system of the middle and external ear or neurosensory structures of the inner ear. Rubella infection during a critical time of ear development can lead to a malformed spiral organ (neurosensory hearing loss) or congenital fixation of the stapes, resulting in conducting hearing loss. Failure of the second pharyngeal arch to form would lead to an ear without a stapes bone. However, in congenital deafness, there is a fixation of the stapes. Failure of the dorsal portion of the first pharyngeal cleft would lead to undeveloped malleus and incus. These are not affected in congenital deafness, however. Abnormal development of the auricular hillocks does not lead to deafness but is a marker for other potential congenital anomalies.

N 94; McM 60

148 A. With congenital cataracts, the lens appears opaque and grayish white and blindness will result. Infection by teratogenic agents such as rubella virus (German measles) can cause congenital cataracts. This infection can affect the development of the lens, which has a critical period of development between the fourth and seventh week. Choroid fissure failure would lead to coloboma, a condition that can lead to a cleft and eye abnormalities but not congenital cataracts. A persistent hyaloid artery would not lead to a cataract but rather a freely moving, wormlike structure (as interpreted by the patient) projecting on the optic disc. Toxoplasmosis infection would lead to microcephaly and eventually mental retardation due to an undeveloped brain. Similarly, cytomegalovirus would cause microcephaly and mental retardation.

N 91; McM 54

149 D. A mutation of the *PAX6* gene usually results in congenital aphakia (absence of the lens) and aniridia (absence of the iris). Cyclopia is a condition in which there is a single eye and is usually caused by a mutation of the *Sonic Hedgehog* gene *(SHH)*, leading to a loss of midline tissue and underdevelopment of the forebrain and frontonasal prominence. Coloboma occurs if the choroid fissure fails to fuse, which is usually caused by a mutation of the *PAX2* gene. Anophthalmia is a disorder in which there is a complete absence of the eye. In microphthalmia, the eye is small in development, typically less than two thirds its normal size. This condition usually results from an infection such as CMV and toxoplasmosis.
GAS 1074, 1075; N 91; McM 54

150 A. In hemifacial microsomia the craniofacial anomalies that usually occur involve small and flat maxillary, temporal, and zygomatic bones. Ear and eye anomalies also occur with this syndrome. Ear abnormalities include tumors and dermoids of the eyeball. Treacher Collins syndrome is normally characterized by malar hypoplasia (caused by undeveloped zygomatic bones), mandibular hypoplasia, down-slanted palpebral fissures, lower eyelid colobomas, and malformed ears. Robin Sequence is caused by an altered first arch structure, with the development of the mandible most affected. Infants with Robin Sequence normally have micrognathia, cleft palate, and glossoptosis. DiGeorge syndrome is a severe craniofacial defect that includes velocardiofacial syndrome and conotruncal anomalies face syndrome. It is characterized by cleft palate, cardiac defects, abnormal face, thymic hypoplasia, and hypocalcemia.
N 4, 208, 36; McM 30

151 A. Abnormal face, cardiac defects, thymic hypoplasia, cleft palate, and hypocalcemia are characteristics of DiGeorge syndrome. A deletion of the long arm of chromosome 22 (22q11) causes this developmental defect. A defect of the *Sonic Hedgehog* gene *(SHH)* can lead to cyclopia. *PAX2* and *PAX6* gene mutations lead to malformations of the eye. Specifically, *PAX2* mutations are responsible for coloboma, and *PAX6* mutations characterize congenital aphakia and aniridia. Turner syndrome (47XXY) is characterized by webbed neck and small stature.
N 4, 208, 36; McM 30

152 A. The first pharyngeal arch, which is often associated with the mandible, is responsible for development of Meckel's cartilage, malleus, incus, and mandible. Additionally, it is innervated by the trigeminal nerve, specifically the mandibular division that innervates the muscles of mastication. This patient presents with features characteristic of developmental defects in the first arch. The second pharyngeal arch gives rise to the stapes, styloid process, lesser cornu, Reichert's cartilage, and the upper half of the hyoid bone. It is innervated by the facial nerve. The third pharyngeal arch is responsible for formation of the greater cornu and the lower half of the hyoid bone and is innervated by the glossopharyngeal nerve. The fourth and sixth pharyngeal arches give rise to the laryngeal cartilages, in addition to being innervated by the vagus nerve.
N 4, 94; McM 21

153 B. The maxillary sinus arises late in fetal development and is the only sinus present at birth. The frontal and sphenoid sinuses often develop at approximately 2 years of age from the anterior ethmoid air cells and the posterior ethmoid air cells, respectively.
GAS 1002, 1003; N 76; McM 47

154 A. Meroencephaly often results from a failure of the rostral neuropore to close during the fourth week of development. The calvaria is absent, with a resultant extrusion of the brain from the cranium. Defects are often found along the vertebral column as well. Cytomegalovirus infection is a major cause of microcephaly, in which both the brain and cranium are drastically reduced in size. However, there is no extrusion of the brain from the cranium. The hypophyseal diverticulum is associated with the pituitary gland and usually regresses to leave only a remnant stalk. Failure of this diverticulum to develop would not be associated with meroencephaly. Neural crest cells give rise to a variety of cell types, and abnormal formation would likewise not be associated with meroencephaly.
N 103; McM 63

155 A. The retropharyngeal space extends from the inferior aspect of the skull to the posterior mediastinum behind the esophagus. An infection or abscess in this space could thus travel toward the posterior mediastinum. The retropharyngeal space is enclosed between the visceral fascia covering the posterior wall of the pharynx and the alar layer of the prevertebral fascia. The alar fascia is formed from bilateral anterior extensions of the prevertebral fascia. Between the alar fascia and the more posterior prevertebral fascia covering the skeletal musculature is the so-called danger space of the neck. This space is continuous superiorly to the base of the skull and continues inferiorly through the posterior mediastinum to the level of the

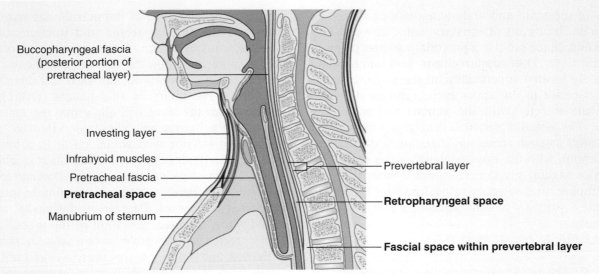

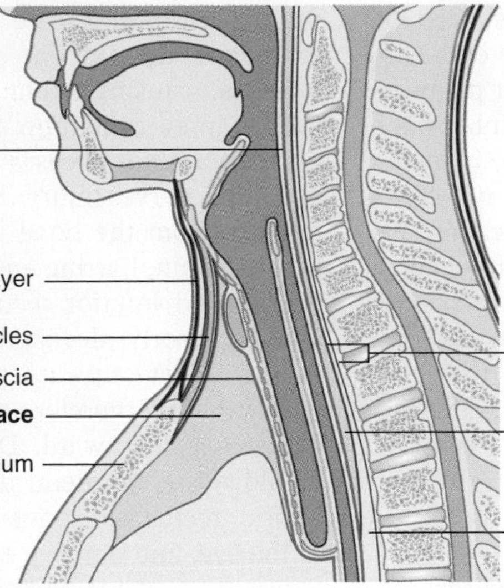

GAS **Fig. 8-159**

respiratory diaphragm. The alar fascia is continuous with the carotid sheath and provides the posterior boundary for the retropharyngeal space. Attachments of the alar fascia to the retropharyngeal fascia result in separation of the pretracheal space from the retropharyngeal space. The prevertebral fascia invests the vertebral column and the intrinsic muscles of the back. The pretracheal fascia encloses the trachea and larynx, whereas the buccopharyngeal fascia invests the superior pharyngeal constrictor and buccinator muscles (*GAS* Fig. 8-159).

GAS 1002, 1003; N 76; McM 47

156 **A.** An inferior fracture of the orbit would likely damage the infraorbital nerve. A blow-out fracture often results in a displaced orbital wall, and in this case, the inferior wall. The infraorbital nerve leaves the skull immediately inferior to the inferior aspect of the orbit, via the infraorbital foramen. Thus, this nerve is the most likely to be damaged. The frontal nerve courses superiorly over the orbital contents before dividing into the supratrochlear and supraorbital nerves. The optic nerve is located behind the eyeball and travels posteriorly away from the orbit to enter the cranium. These nerves are therefore unlikely to be damaged.

GAS 915; N 54; McM 74-76

157 **C.** Rinne's test is often employed during physical examination to determine possible conduction hearing loss. A tuning fork is struck and placed on the mastoid process. It is then placed near the external ear until the patient can no longer detect vibrations. In a normal healthy patient the air conduction will be better than the bone conduction. Rinne's test is often used in conjunction with the Weber test to rule out sensorineural hearing loss.

GAS 715, 839, 1120; N 42; McM 4, 7, 9, 16

158 **A.** The right and left recurrent laryngeal nerves loop around the right subclavian artery and the arch of the aorta, respectively. These nerves then travel superiorly in the tracheoesophageal groove to the larynx. Damage to the recurrent laryngeal nerve as a result of surgical intervention or the presence of a tumor in the tracheoesophageal groove would render the patient hoarse. This hoarseness is due to a lack of innervation by the recurrent laryngeal nerve to most of the muscles of the larynx. Damage to the internal laryngeal nerve would cause a loss of sensation above the vocal cords, in addition to a loss of taste on the epiglottis. Damage to the external laryngeal nerve, which can occur during thyroidectomy, will result in a loss of innervation to the cricothyroid muscle, with resultant vocal weakness. Patients with this lesion will often present with a fatigued voice. The vagus nerve gives rise to the recurrent laryngeal nerves; damage to this nerve, however, would result in numerous symptoms beyond just hoarseness.

GAS 1020, 1021, 1034, 1069; N 227, 228; McM 47, 49, 50, 78

159 **B.** Diploic veins are responsible for communication between the veins of the scalp and the venous sinuses of the brain. Diploic veins are situated within the layers of bone of the skull and connect the emissary veins of the scalp to the venous sinuses located between two layers of dura. The diploe are of clinical significance in that the diploic veins within this layer provide a pathway of communication between the veins of the scalp and underlying venous sinuses of the brain, by means of emissary veins. The emissary veins and diploe provide a potential vascular pathway of infection. The supratrochlear and supraorbital veins are located superficially on the scalp, immediately superior to the upper eyelid, and do not communicate directly with the venous sinuses of the brain. The anterior cerebral vein is an intracranial vein and, as such, does not maintain a direct communication with the external veins of the scalp. The superior sagittal sinus receives blood from the cerebral, diploic, and emissary veins; however, it does not provide a pathway of communication to the veins of the scalp.

GAS 886; N 26, 27; McM 11

160 **C.** The oculomotor nerve passes between the posterior cerebral artery (PCA) and the superior cerebellar artery near the junction of the midbrain and pons. The optic nerve arises near the arterial circle of Willis close to the internal carotid artery. Its location would thus prevent compression following an aneurysm at the PCA and superior cerebellar artery. Although the trochlear nerve could be compressed by the superior cerebellar artery, it would not likely be damaged by an aneurysm of the PCA. The abducens nerve is located in the pons, and the vagus is situated near the postolivary sulcus in the medulla. Neither of these nerves is likely to be compressed by the arteries mentioned here due to their more distal location.

GAS 850, 894, 895, 897, 901, 902, 943; N 2, 35, 52-55, 73; McM 74

161 **C.** A blow-out fracture of the medial wall of the orbit would likely render the medial rectus muscle nonfunctional by entrapment of the muscle between the fracture fragments of the cracked medial wall. The medial rectus is responsible for adduction of the eye, but in this case the muscle acts as a tether or anchor on the eyeball, preventing lateral excursion (abduction) of the eye. There is no nerve damage here, and the muscle is not paralyzed. The lateral rectus is responsible for abduction of the eye, and the inferior rectus rotates the eyeball downward. Damage to these muscles or their nerve supply would result in an inability to move the eye laterally and inferiorly, respectively.

GAS 939-940; N 6; McM 55, 56, 74

162 **A.** The inferior rectus and inferior oblique muscles are entrapped in the fissure between the parts of the fractured orbital floor. Normally, the superior rectus and the inferior oblique are responsible for an upward movement of the eyeball. In this case, however, the broken orbital plate of the maxilla has snared or entrapped the inferior rectus and inferior oblique muscles, causing them to act as anchors on the eyeball, preventing upward movement of the eye. The muscles are not necessarily damaged and there is no apparent nerve injury in this patient. Freeing the muscles from the bone will allow free movement of the eye again, barring any other injury. Damage to the medial and inferior recti would result in a laterally and superiorly deviated eye. The inferior oblique rotates the eye upward and laterally. Damage to this muscle would therefore cause the pupil to be directed somewhat downward. Damage to the medial rectus would result in lateral deviation of the eyeball. The inferior rectus is responsible for downward movement of the eye, and damage to this muscle would result in a superiorly deviated eyeball or an inability to gaze upward symmetrically with both eyes.

GAS 938-940; N 26, 33, 69, 71, 82, 131, 229, 236

163 **A.** A herpes rash on the dorsum of the nose is known as Hutchinson's sign. This indicates that the virus is located in cell bodies of the ophthalmic division of the trigeminal nerve. This nerve branches into nasociliary, frontal, and lacrimal branches. The nasociliary nerve has direct branches that carry sensory innervation from the eye. The nasociliary nerve also gives off the ethmoidal nerves that innervate the superior nasal mucosa, in addition to providing the origin of the dorsal nasal nerve. The supratrochlear nerve is a branch of the frontal nerve and carries sensory innervation from the skin superior to the orbit. The infraorbital nerve is a branch from the maxillary division of the trigeminal nerve and carries sensory innervation from the skin of the face between the orbit and the upper lips.

GAS 945, 946, 1075; N 101, 103; McM 44, 54, 74-75

164 **A.** Anesthetics are injected into the submuscular layer of delicate (areolar) connective tissue, the layer that contains nerves of the eyelid. This space is continuous with the "danger zone" of the scalp. A blow to the forehead can result in a hematoma known as a "black eye," with the passage of blood into the submuscular space. Infections can, likewise, pass within this space. One can insert a needle through the upper eyelid, near the orbital margin, and then direct it deeply toward the orbital apex. The anesthetic can there infiltrate the branches of the ophthalmic division of the trigeminal nerve, including its nasociliary branch, resulting in anesthesia of the area.

GAS 850, 898, 914, 915, 944-946, 1085, 1086; N 86, 88; McM 44, 59, 75

165 A. Paralysis of the trochlear nerve results in loss of ability for the affected eye to be directed downward when the pupil is in the adducted position (the primary action of the superior oblique muscle). The patient must tilt her head toward the opposite side to allow the two pupils to converge on an object on the floor. Paralysis of the trochlear nerve is not unusual when a patient's head has hit the dashboard in an automobile crash—the delicate nerve is easily torn where it pierces the dura of the tentorium cerebelli in the tentorial notch because the brain and brainstem move forward and backward with the force of impact (a "coup-contrecoup" injury).

GAS 874; N 85, 86, 122, 151; McM 44, 51-53

166 A. The dural covering of the optic nerve is connected to the anular tendon which serves as the origin of the rectus muscles; therefore, when there is an inflammation of the optic nerve, contractions of the rectus muscles can evoke severe pain.

N 85-86, 122, 151; McM 57

167 D. Toxoplasmosis infection is caused by the parasite *Toxoplasma gondii*, which is associated with undercooked meat and the feces of cats. Whereas it is a relatively common infection, once one has been exposed, one has immunity. The biggest concern is when a pregnant woman is exposed who has not been previously exposed. Congenital malformation, microphthalmia being one of the more common, can occur if the infection is passed on to the fetus.

N 13, 52, 85, 88, 122, 123, 132, 133; McM 57

168 A. At the point where the facial nerve exits the stylomastoid foramen it is most susceptible to shearing forces. In the absence of a skull fracture whereby the facial nerve can be damaged within the facial canal, the nerve is most commonly injured as it exits the stylomastoid foramen. In infants, in whom the mastoid process has not yet developed, the facial nerve lies unprotected, just beneath the skin.

GAS 870, 921, 970; N 2, 50, 52, 55, 88, 105, 122, 123, 132-136; McM 9, 14, 23, 60

169 B. The auriculotemporal nerve, a branch of the mandibular division of the trigeminal nerve (CV V3) leads into the parotid gland, and its compression in mumps can be associated with severe pain. The compressive effects are due in large part to the continuity of the facial capsule of the parotid gland with the tough layer of superficial investing fascia of the neck, a layer that is almost nondistensible. When the gland swells, sensory fibers for pain are triggered rapidly, and can be referred to the ear. None of the other nerves listed supply the parotid gland.

GAS 912, 915, 985, 986, 1104; N 88, 104, 105, 145, 146; McM 29, 38-40, 42, 59-60, 75-76

170 B. Hydrops (edema) results from accumulation of excessive fluid in the endolymphatic sac. Labyrinthine hydrops or endolymphatic hydrops is known as Ménière's disease. This disease can result in hearing loss, roaring noises in the ear, and episodic dizziness (vertigo) associated with nausea and vomiting. About 10% of patients require surgical intervention for persistent, incapacitating vertigo; others are treated with diuretics, low salt intake, and reduction of stimulants like caffeine to lower the volume of body fluids and alleviate the symptoms of Ménière's disease.

GAS 968; N 85-86, 88, 122; McM 60-61, 81

171 D. The superior thyroid vein is a tributary to the internal jugular vein; it accompanies the superior thyroid artery. The middle thyroid vein is typically a short, direct tributary to the internal jugular vein. The inferior thyroid vein usually drains vertically downward to one or both brachiocephalic veins. The superior and middle thyroid veins can be torn in thyroid surgery, perhaps admitting an air bubble (due to negative pressure in the veins) that can ascend in the internal jugular vein into the skull, with deleterious or lethal results.

GAS 1019, 1020; N 76; McM 28-30, 32-33

172 C. The cricothyroid artery is a small branch of the superior thyroid artery. It anastomoses with the cricothyroid artery of the opposite side at the upper end of the median cricothyroid ligament, a common site for establishing an emergency airway. The cricothyroid artery can be pushed into the airway during a cricothyroidotomy. The vessel(s) can bleed directly into the trachea, bleeding that can go unnoticed by medical personnel, with potentially fatal aspiration of blood by the patient.

GAS 849, 1057; N 10, 12, 24, 100, 124, 126; McM 34

173 C. An incision at the level of the third and fourth tracheal cartilages usually results in the fewest complications during a tracheostomy (or tracheotomy). The isthmus of the thyroid gland (a richly vascular structure) is usually at the level of the second tracheal cartilage and this incision is just inferior to that. However, other vascular structures such as a thyroidea ima artery or tributaries of the external jugular veins make a tracheostomy a surgical procedure to be performed with care.

GAS 1065; N 2, 18, 46, 49-51, 71-72, 123, 126, 135; McM 36, 37, 197

174 A. The uvula would move toward the intact right side. This is because the intact levator veli palatini would be unopposed by the opposite, paralyzed left levator veli palatini.

GAS 846, 982, 1044, 1106, 1108; N 98; McM 10, 47

175 B. If the left abducens nerve is injured, there will be a loss of function of the left lateral rectus muscle so the patient will be unable to abduct his left eye. The trochlear nerve supplies the superior oblique muscle, which if injured would cause the patient to lose the ability to turn the pupil downward when it is in the adducted position. As an example, the affected patient could not turn the pupil to look downward to the left if the right trochlear nerve were paralyzed. This deficiency can make it difficult for individuals to descend stairs if they have trochlear nerve palsy. If the oculomotor nerve were injured, the pupil would be directed "down and out" due to unopposed actions of the lateral rectus and superior oblique, which are innervated by the abducens and trochlear nerves, respectively. If the optic nerve were injured, the patient would have blindness in the affected eye. If the oculomotor and abducens nerves were injured, the patient would have only the actions of the superior oblique muscle, and the eye would be directed downward and outward from the position of forward gaze.

GAS 894-895, 898, 901, 902, 944; N 31, 73, 76-78, 82, 195, 208, 234; McM 51, 53, 55-57, 64, 65, 67, 68, 74, 77, 80

176 D. The accommodation reflex is performed by constriction of the pupil when trying to focus on a near object. This function is controlled by the parasympathetic nerve fibers carried in the oculomotor nerve from the Edinger-Westphal nucleus of the midbrain that synapse in the ciliary ganglion. Postganglionic axons act on the sphincter pupillae muscle to cause reduction in pupil diameter and on the ciliary muscle to cause relaxation of the suspensory ligament, allowing the lens to adopt a more spherical shape for near focusing. If there is a lack of accommodation, it means the action of the ciliary muscle is compromised. The ciliary muscle also gets parasympathetic innervation by postganglionic neurons evoked from the ciliary ganglion by GVE fibers of oculomotor nerve whose cell bodies are located in the Edinger-Westphal nucleus. The superior salivatory nucleus is

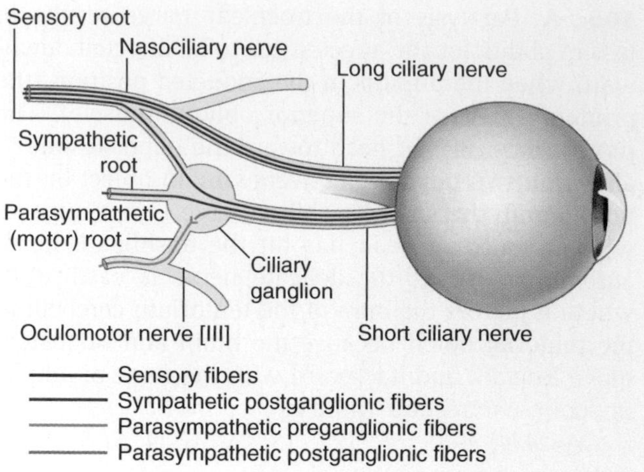

GAS **Fig. 8-103**

involved with lacrimation and salivation, not the ciliary muscle and accommodation. The superior cervical ganglion is a sympathetic ganglion; its postganglionic axons innervate the dilator pupillae muscle, which causes mydriasis, but not the miosis of accommodation. The trigeminal ganglion does not have parasympathetic fibers and does not innervate the ciliary muscle for accommodation (*GAS* Fig. 8-103).

N 72, 76; McM 79

177 A. An acoustic neuroma (vestibular schwannoma or neurolemmoma) is a benign tumor of the vestibulocochlear nerve (CN VIII), which causes compression of the facial nerve (CN VII). This nerve leads from the inner ear to the brain. Although many such tumors will not grow or grow very slowly, growth can in some cases result ultimately in brainstem compression (as in this example), hydrocephalus, brainstem herniation, and death. It is diagnosed on MRI with gadolinium contrast as shown. Extension of the neuroma into the right internal auditory meatus can be seen on the coronal MRI (see arrow in Fig. 7-9). The exact cause of the tumor is unknown; most people with acoustic neuromas are diagnosed between the ages of 30 and 60. Due to advances in microsurgery, including intraoperative monitoring of facial and cochlear function, the risks of facial paralysis and hearing loss have been greatly reduced. Many acoustic neuromas can now be treated effectively with both surgery and targeted radiation therapy (gamma knife). The outcomes for those with small acoustic neuromas are better, whereas those with neuromas larger than 2.5 cm are likely to experience significant hearing loss postsurgery.

GAS 850, 894, 895, 898, 899, 901, 902, 912, 916, 917, 921, 969-971, 1013; N 199

178 A. Pharyngeal (branchial) cleft cysts are the most common congenital cause of a neck mass. They are epithelial cysts that arise anterior to the superior third of the sternocleidomastoid muscle from a failure of obliteration of the second branchial cleft in embryonic development. The second arch grows caudally and, ultimately, covers the third and fourth arches. The buried clefts become ectoderm-lined cavities that normally involute. Occasionally this process is arrested and the entrapped remnant forms an epithelium-lined cyst, in some cases with a sinus tract to the overlying skin. Many branchial cleft cysts are asymptomatic; others may become tender, enlarged, or inflamed, or they may develop abscesses that rupture, resulting in a purulent draining sinus to the skin or pharynx. Surgery is indicated in these cases.

N 42, 49, 57, 65, 67, 68, 70, 127, 151; McM 32

179 C. The angiograph provided clearly shows that the radiopaque medium injected into the patient did not completely fill the common carotid artery. Portions of the internal and external carotid arteries are filled above the common carotid due to "back fill" provided by the collateral circulation. However, vascular supply to the brain is still compromised in this patient, leading to her symptoms.

GAS 126, 134, 135, 484, 872, 1010, 1011; N 13, 55, 85, 86, 88, 105, 115, 118, 122; McM 212

180 A. Mastoiditis is an infection of the air cells within the mastoid process of the temporal bone, often caused by untreated acute otitis media. A known complication of mastoiditis is inflammation of the transverse sinus. Necrosis of the bone due to untreated infection will often affect the transverse sinus. The petrous part of the temporal bone is unlikely to experience inflammation. Infection in the middle ear is usually the preceding event to mastoiditis rather than occurring as a result of it. The occipital sinus is located far posteriorly to the mastoid process and is unlikely to be affected. Because of its position, the internal carotid artery will not be affected by this inflammation.

GAS 958-964; N 117, 118, 122, 133; McM 60-61, 81

181 B. A chalazion is caused by an obstructed tarsal gland of the eyelid. Swellings of the lacrimal gland usually present on the upper lateral eyelid and are not indicative of a chalazion. A chalazion is not an infection within the eye, so this excludes sclera and pupil from being the correct answers. The nasolacrimal duct runs from the medially located lacrimal sacs to the inferior meatus of the nose and would be unaffected in the case of a chalazion.

GAS 932; N 13, 34, 42, 47, 50, 51, 53, 55, 71, 94, 96, 99, 105, 115, 118, 123, 124, 132, 135, 136; McM 55-57

182 B. The nasal polyp also involved the maxillary sinus, located immediately laterally to the nasal cavity. The sphenoid sinus, located posterosuperiorly to the nasopharynx, is unlikely to be affected by a nasal polyp. The ethmoidal sinuses, located medially to the orbit and lateral to the nasal cavity, are also unlikely to be affected by a nasal polyp, although this possibility cannot be ruled out. The frontal sinuses located superomedially to the eyes are unlikely to be affected by the nasal polyp. The frontonasal ducts, the communication between the frontal sinus and the nasal cavity, are also unlikely to be affected.

GAS 1074-1076; N 54; McM 3, 12, 16

183 C. A tumor at the cerebellopontine angle, such as an acoustic schwannoma, is most likely to affect first the vestibulocochlear nerve and then the facial nerve. This excludes the vagus, hypoglossal, glossopharyngeal, and trigeminal nerves from being the correct answers.

GAS 953, 970; N 3, 26, 30-31, 33-34, 55, 71-73, 76-78, 126, 129, 131-132, 134-135, 137, 139, 187, 195, 207, 229, 233; McM 11, 17, 23

184 D. Rupture of the periosteal arteries resulting in a cephalohematoma is defined as a collection of blood underneath the periosteum. On the head, it is located between the pericranium (periosteum of the skull) and the calvaria (skull). The galea aponeurotica, skin and areolar connective tissue are all located superficial to the site of bleeding and hematoma.

GAS 922-925; N 94-100; McM 5

185 B. The tentorial/uncal herniation described in this case is most likely to occur as a result of a temporal lobe tumor. The uncus is part of the temporal lobe, and when enlarged, it will be compressed against the foramen magnum. This results in the symptoms manifested by damage to the nearby oculomotor nerve. The uncus is not a part of the other named lobes.

GAS 862, 868; N 107-108; McM 9

186 C. A tumor involving the meningeal branches of the ethmoidal nerves that originate from the ophthalmic division of the trigeminal nerve is likely to cause pain from pressure and nerve injury in the anterior cranial fossa. The maxillary and mandibular divisions of the trigeminal nerve provide sensory innervation to the middle and posterior aspects of the meninges, respectively. Spinal nerve C2 and C3 fibers do not provide meningeal innervation. The tentorial nerve, a branch of the ophthalmic division of the trigeminal nerve, supplies the tentorium and the supratentorial falx cerebri.

GAS 924, 850, 894; N 2, 122-123; McM 44, 53

187 A. The deep lingual vein is located most superficially on the underside of the tongue. It is therefore the most direct route for absorption of the administered nitroglycerin. The submandibular and sublingual ducts are excretory in function and do not function to absorb a drug, such as nitroglycerin. The lingual and sublingual vein are located more deeply within the floor of the mouth and do not provide the most direct route for absorption.

GAS 1, 100; N 59; McM 29, 35

188 B. The lingual nerve initially courses directly underneath the mucosa of the floor of the mouth and superficial to the submandibular gland, specifically the submandibular duct. This nerve is therefore at risk for ligation, division, or trauma during excision of the gland and duct. The lingual nerve is part of the mandibular division of the trigeminal nerve and carries fibers from the chorda tympani, a branch of the facial nerve (CN VII). These latter fibers supply taste to the anterior two thirds of the tongue and preganglionic parasympathetic axons involved in salivary gland secretion. Fibers of the mandibular division of the trigeminal nerve (CN V3) give rise to the lingual nerve and supply general sensation to the anterior two thirds of the tongue. The lingual nerve passes deep both to the lateral pterygoid muscle and the ramus of the mandible and subsequently travels deep to the submandibular gland itself. The buccal nerve, also a branch of the mandibular division of the trigeminal nerve, supplies the mucosa of the cheek and is not in close proximity to the gland or duct. The inferior alveolar nerve, though close in proximity to the submandibular gland, travels deep to the lateral pterygoid muscle and later enters the mandibular canal to supply the lower teeth. The nerve to the mylohyoid, a branch of the inferior alveolar nerve, supplies the mylohyoid muscle and the anterior belly of the digastric. Neither of these nerves is at risk for damage during excision of the submandibular gland and duct.

GAS 1100-1101; N 59; McM 29, 35

189 A. The ophthalmic artery is a branch of the internal carotid artery and provides origin to the ocular and orbital vessels, including the central artery of the retina, which supplies the retina. The central artery of the retina is an end artery that has no anastomoses with other arterial sources; therefore, occlusion of this artery will result in loss of vision. The nasociliary nerve is a branch of the ophthalmic division of the trigeminal nerve. It is the general sensory nerve for the eye and is the afferent limb of the corneal blink reflex; it has no direct effect on vision. The anterior ethmoidal nerve is a branch of the nasociliary nerve and supplies the anterior ethmoid air cells, the nasal septum, and the lateral walls of the nasal cavity; it also supplies the skin on the bridge of the nose. The trochlear nerve is the fourth of the 12 cranial nerves and innervates the superior oblique muscle, one of the six extraocular muscles. The extraocular muscles function in the movement of the eyeball and not the perception of light. The optic nerve is the second of the 12 cranial nerves and is responsible for vision. A lesion of the optic nerve would lead to blindness; however, based on the location of the patient's infection, the optic nerve was not affected by the loss of arterial supply.

GAS 934; N 137-139; McM 56-57

190 A. CSF is mostly secreted from the choroid plexuses of the lateral, third, and fourth ventricles of the brain. The CSF enters the subarachnoid space from the fourth ventricle, via the foramina of Luschka and Magendie. The CSF then circulates in the subarachnoid space until it is finally resorbed back into the venous side of the circulation through the arachnoid granulations into the superior sagittal sinus. A thrombus of the superior sagittal sinus can to lead to an obstruction of CSF (communicating hydrocephalus) in which all of the ventricles of the brain are enlarged and the intracranial pressure is increased.

GAS 31-32; N 109-111; McM 69-71

191 C. The jugulodigastric node, also known as the tonsillar lymph node, receives drainage from the palatine tonsils, tongue, and pharynx. It is often enlarged during tonsillitis. The submandibular lymph nodes drain the back of the tongue, gums, upper lip, parts of the lower lip, and sides of the face. They drain into the deep cervical group of nodes. The parotid nodes are located superficially and deep to the parotid gland and drain aspects of the cheek, external acoustic meatus, the lateral aspects of the eyelids and posterior orbit. The submental nodes drain the tip of the tongue bilaterally, the lower lip, and floor of the mouth. Finally, the retropharyngeal lymph nodes drain the nasopharynx, nasal cavities, and auditory tubes (*GAS* Fig. 8-66).

GAS 1038-1039; N 74-75; McM 32

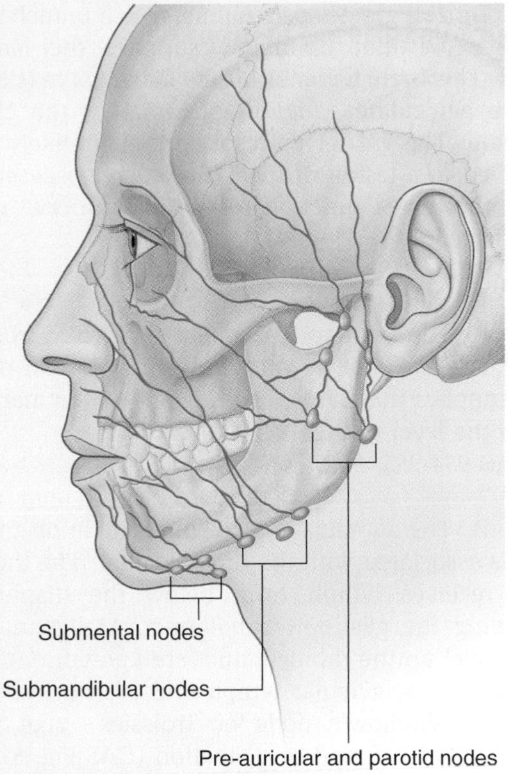

GAS Fig. 8-66

192 **B.** The preauricular lymph nodes are also known as the deep parotid nodes. They are located deep to the parotid gland and drain lymph from the posterior orbit. The submandibular nodes drain the side of the cheek and lateral aspects of the nose and lips. The superficial parotid lymph nodes lie superficially to the parotid gland and drain the lateral angles of the eyelids, aspects of the nose, and the external acoustic meatus. The jugulodigastric nodes receive drainage from all of the superior nodes of the face and also drain the tonsils. The submental lymph nodes drain the tip of the tongue and chin (*GAS* Fig. 8-72).

GAS 920, 1038-1039; N 74; McM 39-41

193 **D.** The pharyngeal (Zenker's) diverticulum is usually located between the cricopharyngeal and thyropharyngeal portions of the inferior pharyngeal constrictor. This is the most common site for development of a pharyngeal diverticulum due to the inherent weakness between the pharyngeal muscles in this location. Stasis of materials within this diverticulum can lead to inflammation, infection, and abscess. This site is also known as Killian's triangle.

GAS 1042-1045; N 77; McM 49, 52

194 **C.** The left brachiocephalic vein is the most likely vein punctured in the procedure because it

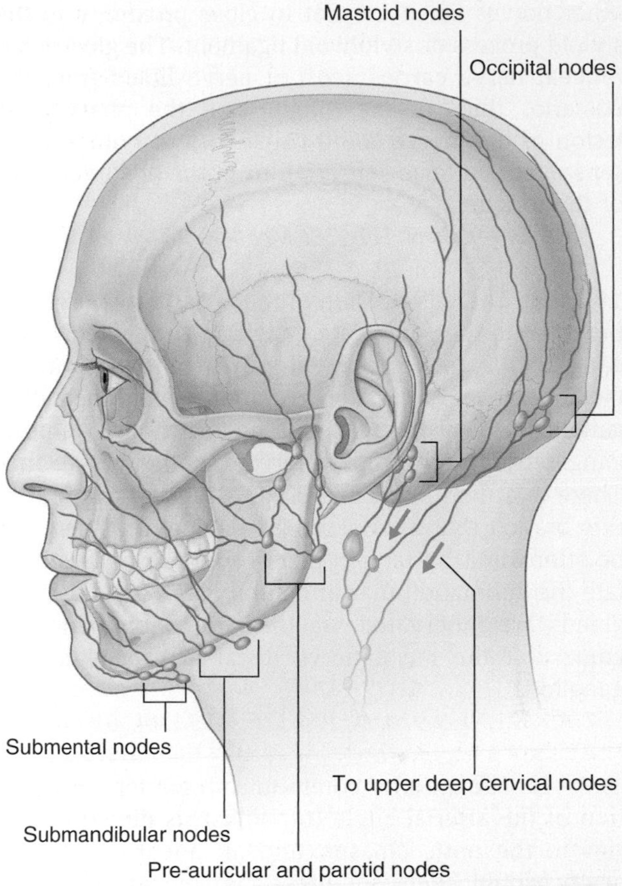

GAS Fig. 8-72

extends across the trachea from the left side of the body, joining the right brachiocephalic vein to form the superior vena cava, which is located just to the right of the midline. The superior thyroid veins drain the superior aspects of the thyroid glands and join the internal jugular veins bilaterally and superiorly to the site of incision. The middle thyroid veins drain the middle portions of the thyroid glands and also terminate in the internal jugular veins laterally, superior to the incision site. The inferior thyroid veins drain the inferior aspects of the thyroid glands and descend bilaterally to the trachea to join the right and left brachiocephalic veins, respectively. Finally, the jugular arch connecting the anterior jugular veins is quite superficial and is not typically a source of concern if encountered surgically.

GAS 133, 157, 171; N 208-209; McM 36-37

195 **C.** The glossopharyngeal nerve (CN IX) enters the posterior oropharynx by coursing between the stylohyoid ligament and the stylopharyngeus muscle. Calcification of the stylohyoid ligament can readily affect this nerve by irritation or compression. The other nerves listed are not in close proximity to the styloid process or stylohyoid ligament. The glossopharyngeal nerve carries sensory nerve fibers from the posterior third of the tongue and the pharynx. A lesion of this nerve could cause loss of both general sensation and taste sensation from the posterior third of the tongue.

GAS 899-900; N 117-118; McM 35-36

196 **A.** There is a lesion of the facial nerve (CN VII) proximal to the geniculate ganglion. At the geniculate ganglion the greater petrosal nerve branches from the facial nerve and ultimately runs to the pterygopalatine ganglion where preganglionic fibers synapse on postganglionic neurons that innervate the lacrimal gland. There is a disruption of the facial nerve proximal to this branch that allows the greater petrosal nerve to be stimulated by factors that would normally stimulate the submandibular and sublingual glands. These glands are innervated via the chorda tympani that comes off the facial nerve distal to the geniculate ganglion.

GAS 921, 969-970; N 124-126; McM 44, 61

197 **B.** The anterior communicating artery, the portion of the arterial circle (of Willis), is directly superior to the optic chiasm, and an aneurysm of this artery would likely compress the chiasm, as in this patient.

GAS 881; N 141; McM 68

198 **E.** The nasolacrimal duct is the only duct that normally drains into the inferior meatus of the nose and therefore would be affected by a focal inflammation in this region.

GAS 1078-1080; N 84; McM 54, 58

199 **D.** The greater petrosal nerve is a branch of the facial nerve that ultimately supplies the lacrimal gland. This branch comes off the facial nerve (CN VII) at the geniculate ganglion proximal to the chorda tympani. The greater petrosal nerve is unlikely to be involved in a lesion of the facial nerve as described. The other listed functions of the facial nerve would be affected by the lesion.

GAS 1104-1105; N 125; McM 44, 61, 79

200 **B.** The great auricular nerve is derived from the ventral rami of the second and third cervical nerves and supplies the skin over the angle of the mandible up to the level of the TMJ.

GAS 954-955; N 2; McM 29-32

201 **B.** The supraclavicular lymph node on the left side is associated with the thoracic duct. The thoracic duct receives lymph from below the diaphragm, including the gastrointestinal tract. Malignant cells that travel up the thoracic duct are known to involve the left supraclavicular lymph node. Historically this is called Virchow's node or Troissier's sign when enlargement is found on palpation (*GAS* Fig. 8-192).

GAS 134-135; N 74; McM 30

202 **E.** The internal branch of the superior laryngeal nerve, often called the internal laryngeal nerve, supplies the mucosa of the larynx above the vocal folds (which includes the vestibule of the larynx) and the piriform recess. The external branch of the superior laryngeal nerve (external laryngeal nerve) is motor to the cricothyroid muscle. The inferior laryngeal nerve supplies the mucosa of the larynx below the vocal folds. The glossopharyngeal nerve (CN IX) supplies sensation to the posterior third of the tongue and to

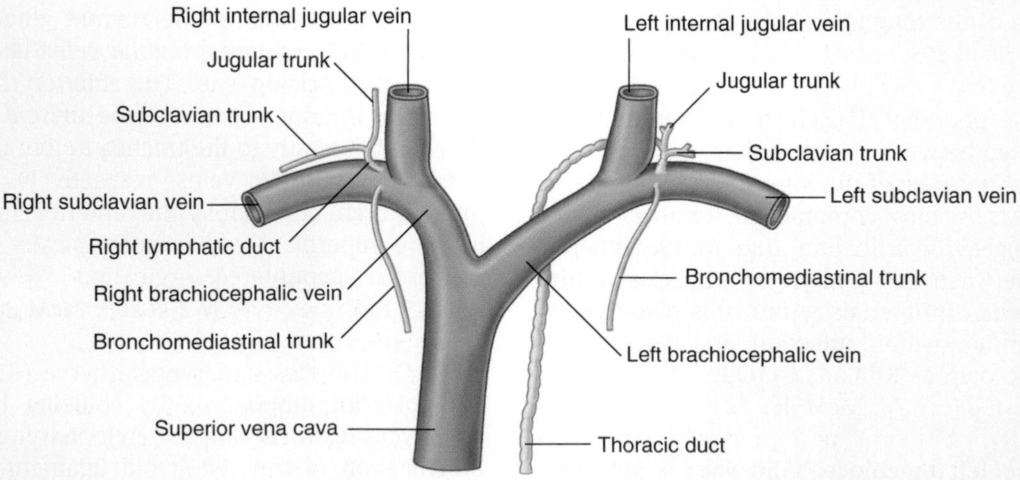

***GAS* Fig. 8-192**

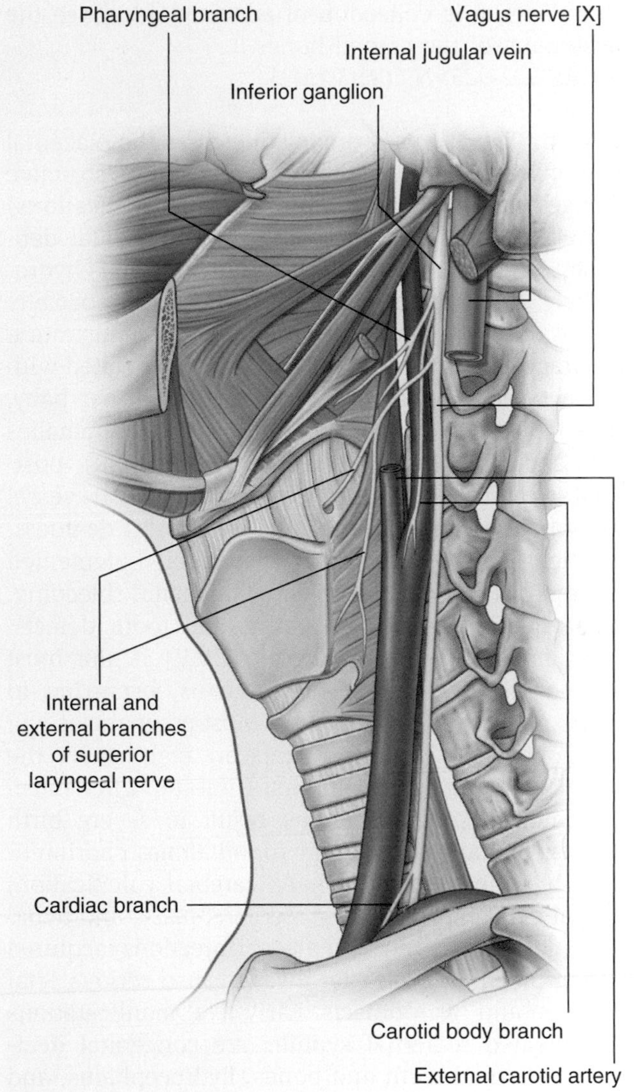

GAS **Fig. 8-169**

the pharynx. The hypoglossal nerve (CN XII) is motor (*GAS* Fig. 8-169).

GAS 1068; N 131-132; McM 48, 78

203 D. A fractured hyoid bone is evidence of strangulation. A fall from a height and subdural hematoma would likely be accompanied by fractured bones. Whereas myocardial infarction or poison remain possibilities, the medical examiner would have a high index of suspicion for strangulation because of the fractured hyoid bone.

GAS 845, 849; N 46-47; McM 31, 33

204 C. Melanocytes in the pigmented layer of the retina are a potential source of malignant melanoma cells. The tumor spreads hematogenously directly to the brain and has a very poor prognosis. None of the other listed structures contains melanocytes.

GAS 947; N 92; McM 73

205 B. Branchial sinus results from the failure of the second pharyngeal groove and the cervical sinus to obliterate. It typically opens anywhere along the inferior third of the anterior border of sternocleidomastoid. Thyroglossal duct cysts or sinuses are usually found in the median plane of the neck and found just below the hyoid or open anterior to the laryngeal cartilages.

N 26-27, 80; McM 32-33

206 B. DiGeorge syndrome occurs due to failure of differentiation of the third and fourth pouches into thymus and parathyroid glands as a result of failure of neural crest migration into the third and fourth pouches. Absence of normal T-cell development leads to poor immunity and hypocalcemia from lack of parathyroid hormone. However, the facial dimorphism is due to lack of neural crest cell involvement in first pharyngeal arch development.

N 227-228; McM 81

207 E. Cleft lip is a result of failure of the mesenchyme in the medial nasal and maxillary prominences to fuse. Unilateral cleft occurs if the maxillary prominence on the affected side fails to fuse with the intermaxillary segment, whereas bilateral cleft occurs if there is failure of fusion on both sides. Median cleft occurs from failure of formation of the intermaxillary segment from the medial nasal processes.

GAS 856; N 14, 45; McM 26, 80

208 A. Severe cases of spina bifida are often associated with anencephaly due to the fact that they all occur from different types of nonfusion defects in the neural tube. Anencephaly is usually seen in conjunction with polyhydramnios due to lack of neurologic control to initiate and complete swallowing of amniotic fluid for absorption in the gastrointestinal tract. These conditions lead to high alpha-fetoprotein levels in the amniotic fluid.

GAS 74; N 304; McM 89

209 A. Coloboma of the iris and retina is due to defective closure of the retinal fissure during the sixth week of life and may involve the ciliary body. Neural crest cells in the eye form the choroid, sclera, and corneal endothelium. Weak adhesion between the layers of the optic cup leads to congenital retinal detachment.

GAS 947; N 91-92; McM 73

210 C. The lateral pterygoid muscle attaches to the articular disc and capsule of the temporomandibular joint and as such any damage here will injure the muscle. The muscles of mastication including the lateral pterygoid muscle are derived from the first pharyngeal arch mesenchyme. The second arch forms the muscles of facial expression. The first pouch gives rise to the tubotympanic recess and the second pouch forms the tonsillar sinus. The first cleft gives rise to the external acoustic meatus.

GAS 977; N 49-51; McM 42-44

211 D. In cranium bifidum, if the protruding brain contains part of the ventricular system the condition is known as meningohydroencephalocele. It is a cranial meningocele if only meninges herniate; it is a meningoencephalocele if it also contains brain matter. Meroencephaly is the neural tube defect in which only a rudimentary brain or minor functioning neural tissue is present instead of a whole brain. Microcephaly is an abnormally small head, which is a result of an abnormally small brain.

GAS 74; N 304; McM 89

212 C. Thyroglossal duct cysts are due to the failure of obliteration of the thyroglossal duct. The thyroglossal duct is formed as the thyroid primordium descends from the posterior aspect of the tongue to its usual location. The thyroglossal duct may persist and form cysts, which are usually found in the median plane of the neck and just below the hyoid bone. The only other midline structure is the foramen cecum, which is a persistence of the proximal part of the thyroglossal duct and is above the hyoid bone.

GAS 1020; N 60, 64; McM 52

213 A. The first pharyngeal arch gives rise to the maxillary and mandibular prominences. Failure or insufficient migration of neural crest cells here leads to mandibulofacial dysostosis (Treacher Collins syndrome) in which there is malar hypoplasia, downslanting palpebral fissures, defects of the lower eyelids, and external ear deformities.

N 60, 64; McM 49

214 D. Cephalohematoma is hemorrhage between the cranium and the periosteum of the cranial bones by rupture of vessels crossing the periosteum. In contrast, subgaleal (subaponeurotic) hemorrhage is hemorrhage between the periosteum and the aponeurotic layer and more extensive with more complications. The swelling does not cross suture lines in cephalhematoma but does in subgaleal hemorrhage. Caput succedaneum is collection of edema fluid above the periosteum of the cranial bones.

GAS 922-925; N 101; McM 5

215 E. The *T. gondii* organism crosses the placental membrane and infects the fetus, causing destructive changes in the brain (intracranial calcifications) and eyes (chorioretinitis) that result in mental deficiency, microcephaly, microphthalmia, and hydrocephaly. Fetal death may follow infection, especially during the early stages of pregnancy. Administration of tetracycline to a pregnant woman is associated with stained teeth and hypoplasia of enamel in her baby. Rubella virus is associated with various anomalies such as intrauterine growth restriction (IUGR), postnatal growth retardation, cardiac and great vessel abnormalities, microcephaly, sensorineural deafness, cataract, microphthalmos, glaucoma, pigmented retinopathy, mental deficiency, neonatal bleeding, hepatosplenomegaly, osteopathy, and tooth defects. Infection with cytomegalovirus (CMV) is the most common viral infection of the fetus, occurring in approximately 1% of neonates. Most pregnancies end in spontaneous abortion (miscarriage) when the infection occurs during the first trimester. CMV infection later in pregnancy may result in severe birth defects, including IUGR, microphthalmia, chorioretinitis, blindness, microcephaly, cerebral calcification, mental deficiency, deafness, cerebral palsy, and hepatosplenomegaly. Primary maternal infections (acquired during pregnancy) nearly always cause serious fetal infection and birth defects. Early fetal manifestations of untreated maternal syphilis are congenital deafness, abnormal teeth and bones, hydrocephalus, and mental deficiency.

N 101; McM 34

216 C. In the fifth week, epithelium of the dorsal region of the third pouch differentiates into the inferior parathyroid gland while the ventral region forms the thymus. The palatine tonsil is derived from the second pharyngeal pouch. The submandibular glands appear late in the sixth week. They develop from endodermal buds in the floor of the stomodeum. The lingual tonsil develops from an aggregation of lymph nodules in the root of the tongue. Lymph nodules also develop in the mucosa of the respiratory and alimentary systems. The lymph nodes are derived from mesenchymal cells.

N 77; McM 81

217 B. Tetracycline crosses the placental membrane and is deposited in the embryo's bones and teeth at sites of active calcification. Tetracycline therapy during the fourth to ninth months of pregnancy may also cause tooth defects (e.g., enamel hypoplasia), yellow to brown discoloration of the teeth, and diminished growth of long bones. Calcification of the permanent teeth begins at birth and, except for the third molars, is complete by 7 to 8 years of age; hence, long-term tetracycline therapy during childhood can affect the permanent teeth. Rubella virus is associated with various anomalies such as intrauterine growth restriction (IGUR), postnatal growth retardation, cardiac and great vessel abnormalities, microcephaly, sensorineural deafness, cataract, microphthalmos, glaucoma, pigmented retinopathy, mental deficiency, neonate bleeding, hepatosplenomegaly, osteopathy, and tooth defects.

N 6; McM 63

218 B. Rubella virus (German measles) is associated with various anomalies such as intrauterine growth restriction (IUGR), postnatal growth retardation, cardiac and great vessel abnormalities, microcephaly, sensorineural deafness, cataract, microphthalmos, glaucoma, pigmented retinopathy, mental deficiency, neonatal bleeding, hepatosplenomegaly, osteopathy, and tooth defects. The *T. gondii* organism crosses the placental membrane and infects the fetus causing destructive changes in the brain (intracranial calcifications) and eyes (chorioretinitis) that result in mental deficiency, microcephaly, microphthalmia, and hydrocephaly. CMV infection later in pregnancy may result in severe birth defects such as IUGR, microphthalmia, chorioretinitis, blindness, microcephaly, cerebral calcification, mental deficiency, deafness, cerebral palsy, and hepatosplenomegaly. The effects of cocaine include spontaneous abortion, prematurity, IUGR, microcephaly, cerebral infarction, urogenital anomalies, neurobehavioral disturbances, and neurologic abnormalities. Thalidomide is a potent teratogen. The characteristic presenting feature is meromelia, but the defects range from amelia (absence of limbs) through intermediate stages of development (rudimentary limbs) to micromelia (abnormally small and/or short limbs).

GAS 933; N 86.5; McM 55-58

219 E. In Treacher Collins syndrome (mandibulofacial dysostosis), which is caused by an autosomal dominant gene, there is malar hypoplasia (underdevelopment of the zygomatic bones of the face) with down-slanting palpebral fissures, defects of the lower eyelids, deformed external ears, and sometimes abnormalities of the middle and internal ears. From the CT it is clear that there is no external acoustic meatus.

GAS 1074-1077; N 92.8; McM 3, 12, 17

220 D. Cervical cysts, sinuses, and fistulas may develop from parts of the second pharyngeal groove, the cervical sinus, or the second pharyngeal pouch that fail to obliterate. An ectopic thyroid gland results when the thyroid gland fails to descend completely from its site of origin in the tongue. The first pharyngeal pouch gives rise to the tympanic cavity, mastoid antrum, and pharyngotympanic tube. The second pharyngeal pouch is associated with the development of the palatine tonsil. The thymus is derived from the third pair of pharyngeal pouches, and the parathyroid glands are formed from the third and fourth pairs of pharyngeal pouches.

GAS 953, 971; N 99.1; McM 11, 17, 24

221 E. In Treacher Collins syndrome (mandibulofacial dysostosis), which is caused by an autosomal dominant gene, there is malar hypoplasia (underdevelopment of the zygomatic bones of the face) with down-slanting palpebral fissures, defects of the lower eyelids, deformed external ears, and sometimes abnormalities of the middle and internal ears. Pierre Robin sequence, an autosomal recessive disorder, is associated with hypoplasia of the mandible, cleft palate, and defects of the eye and ear. Chiari I malformation is inferior displacement of the cerebellar tonsils more than 5 mm through the foramen magnum into the cervical canal. Symptoms of fetal alcohol syndrome (FAS) are intrauterine growth restriction (IUGR), mental deficiency, microcephaly, ocular anomalies, joint abnormalities, and short palpebral fissures. Patients with DiGeorge syndrome are born without a thymus and parathyroid glands and have defects in cardiac outflow tracts. In some cases, ectopic glandular tissue has been found.

GAS 922-926; N 105.4; McM 13

222 D. The mental nerve and vessels pass through the mental foramen in the mandible. The mental nerve supplies the skin and mucous membrane of the lower lip from the mental foramen to the midline, including the skin of the chin. It is a branch of the inferior alveolar nerve, which comes off the posterior division of the mandibular division of the trigeminal nerve. The buccal nerve is a branch of the anterior division of the mandibular nerve, which supplies the skin over the buccal membrane. The auriculotemporal nerve and the great auricular nerve, a branch of the cervical plexus composed of fibers from C2 and C3 spinal nerves, innervates the parotid sheath as well as the overlying skin. The lesser petrosal nerve is the visceral motor component of the glossopharyngeal nerve (CN IX), carrying parasympathetic fibers from the tympanic plexus to the parotid gland. The infraorbital nerve innervates (sensory) the lower eyelid, upper lip, and part of the nasal vestibule and exits the infraorbital foramen of the maxilla.

GAS 307, 709, 853; N 107-109; McM 17

223 **B.** The sensory supply of the mucous membrane of the oral part (anterior two thirds), but not the region of the vallate papillae, is by the lingual nerve. General sensation is via the mandibular division of the trigeminal nerve (with cell bodies in the trigeminal ganglion) and taste via chorda tympani, from the facial nerve, which have their cell bodies in the geniculate ganglion. The submandibular and pterygopalatine ganglia contain parasympathetic fibers from chorda tympani and greater petrosal nerves, respectively.

GAS 307, 278, 969; N 2, 122-124; McM 44, 54

224 **C.** Ophthalmic nerve (ophthalmic division of the trigeminal nerve, CN V1) carries sensory branches from the eye, conjunctiva, and orbital contents, including the lacrimal gland. It also receives sensory branch from the nasal cavity, frontal sinus, ethmoidal cells, falx cerebri, dura in the anterior cranial fossa and superior part of the tentorium cerebelli, upper lid, dorsum of the nose, and anterior part of the scalp. Branches of ophthalmic nerve are lacrimal, supraorbital, supratrochlear, infratrochlear, and external nasal nerves. Maxillary nerve (CN V2) and mandibular nerve (CN V3) carry sensory information from other regions of the face.

GAS 306, 848, 085; N 59; McM 29, 35

225 **D.** The hypoglossal nerve (CN XII) passes through hypoglossal canal. All the muscles of the tongue, intrinsic and extrinsic, are supplied by the hypoglossal nerve (except palatoglossus). Extrinsic muscle supplies the genioglossus, hyoglossus, and styloglossus. Thus compression of the nerve will affect intrinsic and extrinsic muscles of the tongue.

GAS 1100-1102; N 59; McM 29, 35

226 **C.** Superior salivatory nucleus (or superior salivary nucleus) of the facial nerve is a visceromotor cranial nerve nucleus located in the pontine tegmentum. Preganglionic parasympathetic fibers arise from the nucleus and pass laterally to exit the pons with motor VII axons. Then some of the preganglionic fibers pass to the pterygopalatine ganglion via the greater petrosal (via the pterygoid canal, also known as the Vidian canal) and synapse in the pterygopalatine ganglion. Postganglionic efferent fibers travel to innervate the lacrimal gland and the mucosal glands of the nose, palate, and pharynx, whereas the other preganglionic parasympathetic fibers are also distributed partly via the chorda tympani and lingual nerves to the submandibular ganglion, and postsynaptic fibers to the submandibular gland and sublingual gland. Therefore other symptoms in this patient will be reduced salivary secretion from submandibular and sublingual glands.

GAS 935; N 137-140; McM 56-58

227 **D.** The superior thoracic aperture is also referred to as the thoracic inlet because noncirculating substances (air and food) may only enter the thorax and not exit. Obstruction actually occurs outside the aperture in the root of the neck, and the manifestations of the syndromes involve the upper limb through this aperture. A supernumerary (extra cervical) rib or a fibrous connection extending from its tip to the first thoracic rib may elevate and place pressure on structures that emerge from the superior thoracic aperture, notably the subclavian artery or inferior trunk of the brachial plexus, and may cause symptoms. Other etiologies could include an elongated transverse process of the C7 vertebra and muscular abnormalities (e.g., in the scalenus anterior muscle, a sickle-shaped scalenus medius). Most common symptoms include discoloration of the hands, one hand colder than the other hand, weakness of the hand and arm muscles, and tingling.

GAS 31-33; N 109-112; McM 69-72

228 **C.** The superior paravertebral ganglion (the superior cervical ganglion of each sympathetic trunk) lies at the base of the cranium. It lies deep to the sheath of the internal carotid artery and internal jugular vein (carotid sheath), and anterior to the longus capitis muscle. It contains neurons that supply sympathetic innervation to a number of target organs within the head and also contributes to the cervical plexus. The postsynaptic sympathetic fibers stimulate contraction of the blood vessels (vasomotor) and erector muscles associated with hairs (pilomotor), and cause sweating (sudomotion). Postsynaptic sympathetic fibers in the cranium also innervate dilator muscle of the iris (dilator pupillae); therefore compression causes complete pupillary constriction. It also innervates the muscle that maintains elevation of the upper lid (holding the eye open); therefore compression causes partial ptosis (drooping of the upper lid). Paralysis of the CN III causes complete ptosis. (*GAS* Fig. 8-190).

GAS 1038-1040; N 74-76; McM 33

229 **A.** The lingual nerve is joined by the chorda tympani about 2 cm below the base of the skull, deep

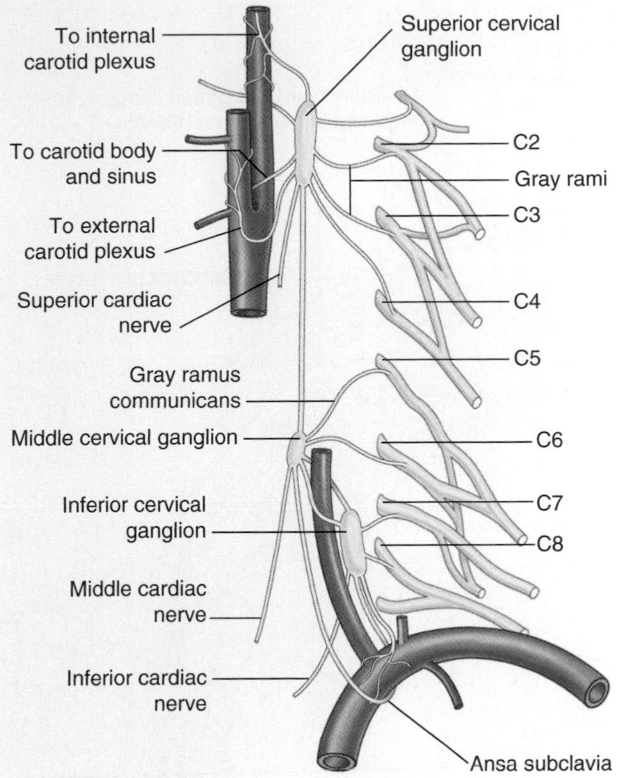

GAS **Fig. 8-190**

to the lower border of the lateral pterygoid muscle. It supplies the anterior two thirds of the tongue with common sensation and taste, the latter mediated by fibers in the chorda tympani. The secretomotor fibers of the chorda tympani are given off to the submandibular ganglion, which is suspended from the lingual nerve. They relay in the ganglion for the submandibular gland, and some postganglionic fibers rejoin the lingual nerve for transport to the salivary glands in the floor of the mouth. The lingual nerve also supplies all the mucous membrane of the floor of the mouth and the lingual gingiva (gums).

GAS 920, 1038-1040; N 80; McM 39-42

230 **E.** Perineural spread of a tumor (or spread of tumor along a nerve) is one of the more insidious forms of tumor metastasis. This form of spread is more commonly found in malignant rather than benign lesions. In this case tumor spreads along tissue at the jugular foramen, thus involving nerves glossopharyngeal (CN IX), vagus (CN X), and spinal accessory nerves (CN XI). Therefore in case of the pharyngeal reflex (gag reflex), sensory limb is mediated predominantly by CN IX (glossopharyngeal nerve) and motor limb by CN X (vagus nerve). Tongue, facial expression and sensation and hearing are mediated by cranial nerves XII, VII, V, and VIII respectively.

GAS 1042-1046; N 83; McM 49, 53

231 **A.** Extradural (epidural) hemorrhage is arterial in origin. Blood from torn branches of a middle meningeal artery (which passes through foramen spinosum) collects between the external periosteal layer of the dura and the calvaria. The extravasated blood strips the dura from the cranium. Usually this follows a hard blow to the head; an extradural (epidural) hematoma then forms. Typically, a brief concussion (loss of consciousness) occurs, followed by a lucid interval of some hours. Later, drowsiness and coma (profound unconsciousness) occur, and if the pressure is not relieved the patient will die (*GAS* Fig. 8-46).

GAS 133, 157, 172; N 208-210; McM 36-38

232 **A.** The oculomotor nerve (CN III) supplies the majority of the muscles controlling eye movements. Thus, damage to this nerve results in displaced outward and downward eye as a result of unopposed lateral rectus (innervated by the abducens nerve, CN VI) and superior oblique (innervated by the trochlear nerve, CN IV). The ciliary muscle within the ciliary body changes the shape of the lens. In the absence of nerve stimulation, the diameter of the relaxed muscular ring is larger, making the lens flatter for far vision. Parasympathetic stimulation via the oculomotor nerve (CN III) causes sphincter-like contraction of the ciliary muscle and the lens get thicker for near vision. These fibers also innervate the sphincter pupillae. Thus interruption of these fibers causes dilation of the pupil because of the unopposed action of the sympathetically innervated dilator pupillae muscle. Because the oculomotor nerve supplies the levator palpebrae superioris, a lesion there causes paralysis of the muscle; the patient cannot raise the superior eyelid (cannot open the eye). Ptosis is related more to paralysis of the superior tarsal muscle.

GAS 899-901; N 117-119; McM 35-37

233 **B.** Scalp lacerations are the most common type of head injury requiring surgical care. These wounds bleed profusely because the arteries entering the periphery of the scalp bleed from both ends owing to abundant anastomoses. The arteries do not retract when lacerated because they are held open by the dense connective tissue in the second layer two of the scalp. The scalp is composed of five layers, the first three of which are connected intimately and move as a unit. Each letter in the word SCALP serves as a mnemonic for one of its five layers, skin, connective

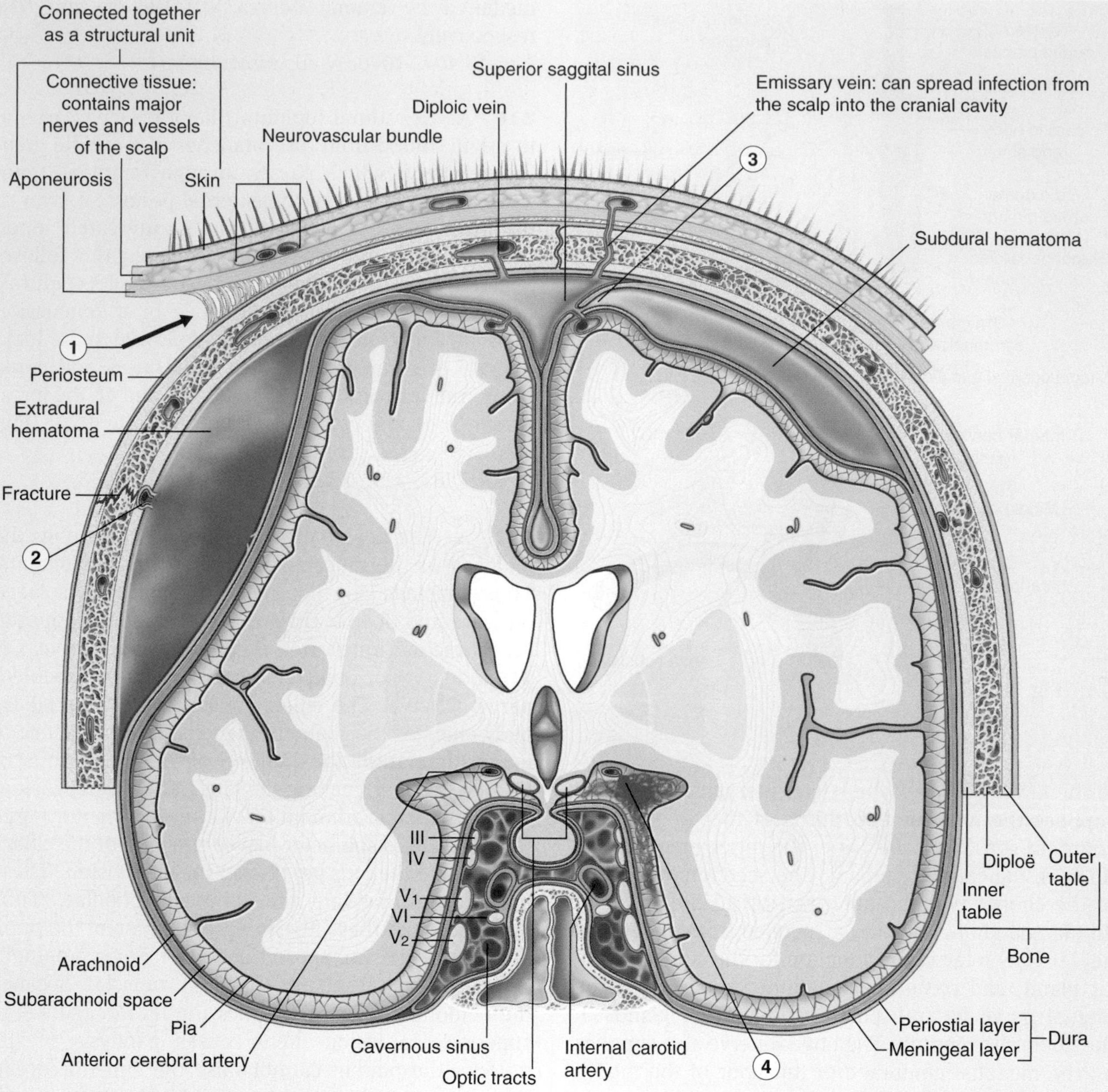

1 Loose connective tissue (danger area)
- In scalping injuries, this is the layer in which separation occurs.
- Infection can easily spread in this layer.
- Blunt trauma can result in hemorrhage in this layer (blood can spread forward into the face, resulting in "black eyes").

2 Rupture of the middle meningeal artery (branches) by fracture of the inner table of bone results in extradural hematoma. Under pressure, the blood progressively separates dura from the bone.

3 Tear to cerebral vein where it crosses dura to enter cranial venous sinus can result in subdural hematoma. The tear separates a thin layer of meningeal dura from that which remains attached to the periosteal layer. As a result, the hematoma is covered by an inner limiting membrane derived from part of the meningeal dura.

4 Aneurysm
- Ruptured aneurysms of vessels of the cerebral arterial circle hemorrhage directly into the subarachnoid space and CSF.

GAS **Fig. 8-46**

tissue, aponeurosis, loose areolar tissue, and pericranium. The loose connective tissue layer (fourth layer) of the scalp is the danger area of the scalp because pus or blood spreads easily in it. Infection in this layer can also pass into the cranial cavity through small emissary veins, which pass through parietal foramina in the calvaria and reach intracranial structures such as the meninges.

GAS 921, 969-971; N 124-127; McM 44, 62

234 **E.** The rima glottidis is the opening between the true vocal cords. The diameter of this opening is regulated by the laryngeal muscles to modulate pitch of sound. The piriform fossa is a shallow space found on the lateral side of the laryngeal orifice bounded laterally by the thyroid cartilage and medially by the aryepiglottic fold. While "vestibule" can mean any opening, in the head and neck it strictly is used to mean the anterior-most portion of the oral cavity, making B an incorrect option. In the head and neck region of the human body, the ventricles are cavities above the midbrain where the CSF is produced. The vallecula is a depression behind the root of the tongue that serves to hold saliva for lubrication and prevention of premature initiation of deglutition reflex.

GAS 881; N 20; McM 68

235 **D.** The mucosa of the piriform fossa receives sensory innervation from the internal laryngeal nerve. This nerve also supplies somatic sensory fibers to the larynx above the vocal cords, epiglottis, and valleculae. Owing to its superficial location in the mucosa of the piriform fossa, it could be damaged during procedures involving the piriform fossa with loss of sensation in the areas it innervates and loss of protective reflex of the larynx. The mandibular division of the trigeminal nerve (CN V3) supplies somatic sensation the lower face and motor innervation to muscles of mastication. It also sends sensory fibers to the meninges including the external acoustic meatus. The maxillary division of the trigeminal nerve (CN V2), although a sensory component of the trigeminal, does not innervate the piriform fossa. The glossopharyngeal nerve (CN IX) supplies special visceral efferent to the stylopharyngeus muscle, parasympathetic to the parotid gland, general visceral afferent to the carotid sinus and body, special sensory to the posterior one third of the tongue, and general somatic efferent to the external ear, internal part of the tympanic membrane, posterior tongue, and upper pharynx.

GAS 1078-1081; McM 54, 59

236 **D.** The first pharyngeal pouch gives rise to the tympanic recess, with its membrane giving rise to the tympanic membrane. The tympanic recess itself gives rise to the tympanic cavity and the mastoid antrum. The pharyngotympanic tube (eustachian), a part of the tympanic cavity, connects the tympanic cavity to the pharynx. Infections of the pharynx (pharyngitis) can spread from the pharynx to the middle ear through the pharyngotympanic tube. The second pharyngeal pouch usually obliterates with its tiny remains forming the tonsillar sinus with the remaining mesenchyme forming the lymphoid nodules of the palatine tonsil.

GAS 1104-1106; McM 44, 61, 80

237 **B.** The papillary light reflex is mediated by an afferent limb carried by the optic nerve (CN II) and the efferent limb carried by the oculomotor nerve (CN III). The pupil constricts when the light is shone because the optic nerve was able to pick up the light sensation while the oculomotor nerve mediates the contraction of the sphincter pupillae muscle of the iris that results in pupillary constriction. This muscle is specifically innervated by the parasympathetic component of the oculomotor nerve, which has its preganglionic cell bodies at the Edinger-Westphal nucleus and postganglionic fibers at the ciliary ganglion. The pupillary light reflex is not mediated by the combination of the other nerves.

GAS 954-956; McM 29-33

238 **A.** The oculomotor nerve (CN III) is the efferent limb of the pupillary reflex. It carries the parasympathetic nerve with preganglionic cell bodies in the Edinger-Westphal nucleus and postganglionic cell bodies in the ciliary ganglion and supplies the sphincter pupillae of the iris. The oculomotor nerve is found between the superior cerebellar artery and the posterior cerebral artery. Aneurysm of the superior cerebellar artery can therefore compress on the oculomotor nerve resulting in pupillary dilatation (due to unopposed sympathetic innervation of the dilator pupillae) and unresponsiveness of the affected eye. The trigeminal, facial, vagus, and abducens nerves do not participate in the pupillary light reflex.

GAS 134-136; McM 30

239 **C.** The superior orbital fissure is an opening in the skull found between the lesser and greater wings of the sphenoid bone and communicates with the orbit and maxillary sinus. Among other structures, it transmits the oculomotor nerve (CN III), branches of the ophthalmic division of trigeminal nerve (CN V1), abducens nerve (CN VI), and ophthalmic vein. Tumors around the superior orbital fissure can compress these

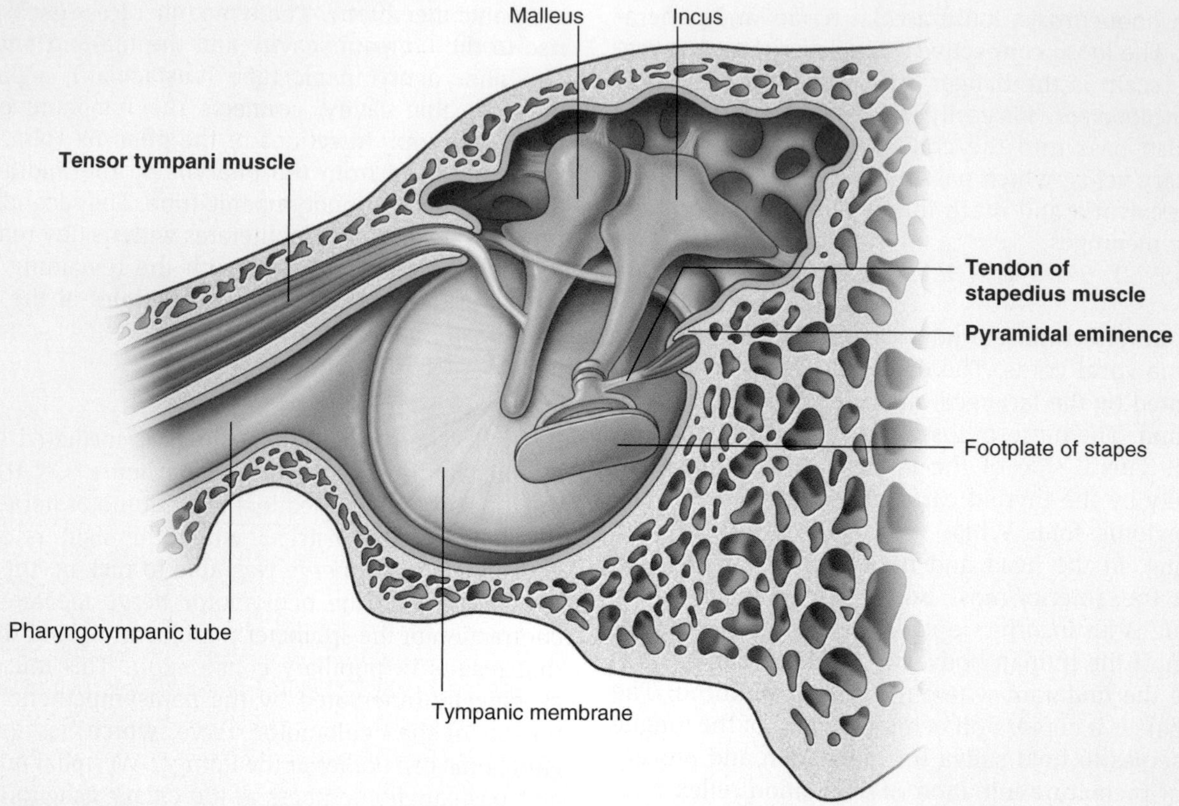

***GAS* Fig. 8-120**

structures. Abduction of the eye is done by the oculomotor nerve, and the ophthalmic nerve supplies sensation to the cornea and serves as the afferent limb of the corneal reflex. These functions were lost because of compression of these nerves. The optic canal is found in the anterior cranial fossa and transmits the optic nerve and ophthalmic artery. Similarly, the inferior orbital fissure is located inside of the orbit, transmitting the zygomatic branch of the maxillary nerve and branches of the pterygopalatine ganglion. The foramen rotundum and ovale are located in the middle cranial fossa.

N 131-133; McM 48, 79

240 B. Herpes zoster can affect spinal and cranial nerves. It usually follows reactivation of a dormant varicella infection, which resides in a sensory ganglion. Illness, stress or immunosuppression can reactivate the dormant virus, which may result in both motor and sensory dysfunction. In this case a dominant herpes infection in the geniculate ganglion of the facial nerve has been reactivated, resulting in dysfunction of the facial nerve branch that supplies the stapedius muscle (nerve to the stapedius). The stapedius muscle inserts in the neck of the stapes bone in the middle ear and functions to dampen the vibrations of the stapes by way of putting tension on the neck of the stapes. This results in loudness of sound in the ear (hyperacusis) (*GAS* Fig. 8-120).

N 46-48; McM 31, 34

241 B. The vagus nerve (CN X) is one of the major sensory nerves to the external auditory meatus and is the afferent limb of the cough reflex. The vestibulocochlear nerves mediates hearing and balance. Although the auriculotemporal branch of the trigeminal contributes in the innervations of the external acoustic meatus, it does not participate in the cough reflex. The facial nerve, which also contributes in the innervations of the external acoustic meatus, has no role in the cough reflex. The accessory nerve is motor to the sternocleidomastoid and trapezius nerves.

GAS 896-897, 900; N 127; McM 78

242 C. The recurrent laryngeal nerve, a branch of the vagus nerve (CN X), supplies motor innervation to all the intrinsic muscles of the larynx excluding the cricothyroid muscle and also supplies sensory fibers to the larynx below the vocal cord. Being two in number (right and left), the left recurrent laryngeal nerve upon emerging from the vagus nerve in the neck hooks (recurs) under the ligamentum arteriosum at the arch of aorta and then travels through the tracheoesophageal groove to the larynx. The right nerve hooks under the right subclavian artery. In the course of their recurrent path into the neck, these nerves are posterior to the middle part of the thyroid gland. Therefore, the recurrent laryngeal nerve may be inadvertently damaged during thyroidectomy. The internal laryngeal nerve, a branch of the superior laryngeal nerve, supplies sensory fibers to the laryngeal mucosa above the vocal cord. Injury to this nerve causes anesthesia in the larynx above the vocal cord. The external laryngeal nerve, also a branch of the superior laryngeal nerve, supplies the cricothyroid muscle. This muscle serves to tense the vocal cord. Paralysis of the external laryngeal nerve results in a monotonous voice because of inability to tense the vocal cord. Paralysis of the superior laryngeal nerve will also result in anesthesia above the vocal cord and loss of the protective reflex of the larynx (*GAS* Fig. 8-176).

GAS 1019-1020; N 76-78; McM 78

243 C. The pupillary light reflex is used to test the ability of the eyes to perceive light sensation. The afferent limb of this reflex arc is the optic nerve while the oculomotor is the efferent limb. By shining light into the eye from a penlight, each eye is tested individually for a direct constriction of the pupil on the ipsilateral side and then for a consensual reflex on the contralateral side. The startle reflex is a kind of acoustic reflex that occurs in reaction to sudden auditory stimulation. The blink or corneal reflex is a reflex that is produced in reaction to stimulation of the cornea of the eye. This reflex is mediated by the ophthalmic branch of the trigeminal (afferent limb) and the facial nerve (efferent limb). The H-test is a maneuver used to test the extraocular muscles, which are innervated by the oculomotor, trochlear, and abducens nerves. The vision test, also known as visual acuity test, is used to assess the ability of the eye to read or identify letters from different distances.

GAS 894-897; N 88, 122; McM 74

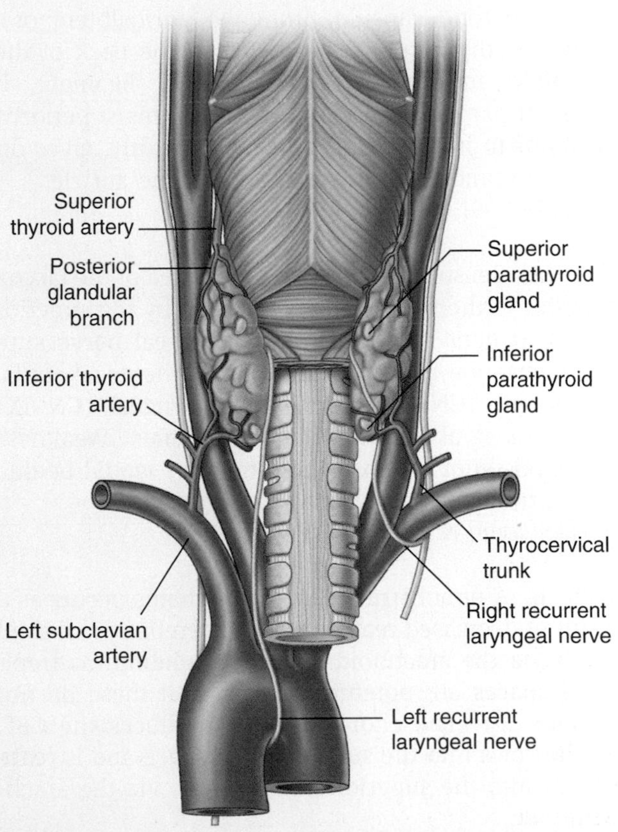

***GAS* Fig. 8-176**

244 D. The short ciliary nerves and ciliary ganglion is the correct answer option. It is clear from the vignette that the problem lies with accommodation, which involves pupil accommodation, lens accommodation, and convergence. Eye movements were not compromised and as such parasympathetic deficit is the likely cause of his condition. Preganglionic axons from the Edinger-Westphal nucleus are carried by the oculomotor nerve, which synapse at the ciliary ganglion. These parasympathetics then travel through the ciliary ganglion located in the posterior orbit and from here postganglionic axons, carried by the short ciliary nerves, go on to innervate the sphincter pupillae muscle, which constricts the pupil and the ciliary muscle. Contraction of the ciliary muscle relieves tension on the zonular fibers, allowing the lens to be more convex. Absence of action of the ciliary muscles and sphincter pupillae results in loss of the ability to focus on near objects. The trochlear nerve and abducens nerve is an incorrect option. These nerves innervate the superior oblique and lateral rectus muscles, respectively. Since eye movements were unaffected, this combination can be eliminated as an answer option immediately.

GAS 894-897; N 88, 122; McM 74

245 B. The herpetic infection of the forehead likely spread to supratrochlear veins, which join to form a single trunk that runs down near the middle line of the forehead parallel with the vein of the opposite side. The two veins are joined, at the root of the nose, by a transverse branch, called the nasal arch. At the medial angle of the orbit, it joins the supraorbital vein to form the angular vein and drains into the superior ophthalmic vein, which communicates with the cavernous sinus. The infection can also make its way to the inferior ophthalmic vein via facial and deep facial veins to spread to the cavernous sinus. The pterygoid venous plexus has communication with the anterior facial vein and communicates with the cavernous sinus but is not the danger area of the face since it does not drain directly into the pterygoid plexus. The superior petrosal sinus is located in the superior petrosal sulcus of the petrous part of the temporal bone. It drains the cavernous sinus and travels posterolaterally to drain into the transverse sinus. The basilar plexus is made up of multiple venous channels between the layers of the dura mater above the clivus, where it interconnects the two inferior petrosal sinuses. The parietal emissary vein connect the superior sagittal sinus with tributaries of the superficial temporal vein.

GAS 887-888; N 55, 74-74, 87; McM 47

246 C. The facial nerve is a mixed cranial nerve, which carries both motor and (special) sensory fibers. The motor component of the facial nerve arises from the facial nerve nucleus and forms the facial nerve proper, while the sensory and parasympathetic parts of the facial nerve emerge from the brain as nervus intermedius. The motor and sensory parts of the facial nerve enter the petrous part of the temporal bone via the internal auditory meatus, which is very close to the inner ear; it then courses through the facial canal, after which it emerges from the stylomastoid foramen and passes through the parotid gland, where it divides into five major branches. The facial nerve provides special sensory to the anterior one third of the tongue, motor to the muscles of facial expression and posterior belly of the digastric.

GAS 894-898; N 99, 125; McM 61

247 C. The internal acoustic meatus is a canal in the petrous part of the temporal bone. The facial nerve (CN VII) and VIII course through this canal. The vestibulocochlear nerve (CN VIII) consists of the cochlear nerve, carrying special sensory hearing, and the vestibular nerve, carrying signals for balance and equilibrium. The facial nerve (CN VII) carries special sensory taste to the anterior one third of the tongue and motor fibers that control the muscles of facial expression.

GAS 970-971; N 11, 13; McM 11, 50

248 E. The submental nodes are located between the anterior bellies of the digastric muscles. The central portions of the lower lip and floor of the mouth and the apex of the tongue drain into these nodes. Efferent lymphatic from these nodes go to the submandibular lymph nodes and partly to a gland of the deep cervical group of nodes. The occipital nodes drain the occipital region of the scalp. The parotid nodes drain the root of the nose, the eyelids, the frontotemporal region, and the external acoustic meatus, and a deep group drains the nasal part of the pharynx and the posterior parts of the nasal cavities. The retropharyngeal nodes are found in the buccopharyngeal fascia and drain the nasal cavities, the nasal part of the pharynx, and the auditory tubes. The jugulodigastric nodes drain primarily the tonsils (*GAS* Fig. 8-193).

GAS 920, 926; N 74-75; McM 32-34

249 D. Aneurysms of AICA cause direct impingement on the abducens nerve as it emerges from the brainstem at the pontomedullary junction between the labyrinthine artery above and the AICA below. Impingement of this nerve leads to loss of function to the lateral rectus muscle ipsilaterally, resulting in the inability to abduct the eye. The anterior communicating artery does not relate to the abducens nerve. Aneurysm of the posterior cerebral artery will likely affect the oculomotor nerve. Aneurysm of the superior cerebellar artery will also likely affect the oculomotor nerve. Vertebral artery aneurysm will likely affect the hypoglossal nerve.

GAS 881, 882; N 139-144; McM 68

250 B. The parotid gland receives visceromotor postganglionic parasympathetics and somatosensory (to the parotid capsule) from the auriculotemporal nerve. As the nerve passes between the neck of the mandible and the sphenomandibular ligament, it gives off parotid branches and then turns superiorly, posterior to its head and moving anteriorly, gives off anterior branches to the skin around the auricle.

GAS 911-913; N 135; McM 34, 39, 40

251 A. Sensory innervation to the area of the larynx superior to the vocal folds is supplied by the superior laryngeal nerve. The recurrent laryngeal nerve supplies sensation to the area inferior to the vocal cords. The vagus (CN X) and glossopharyngeal (CN IX) nerves bring about the swallowing reflex. Weakness to the posterior cricoarytenoid muscles would be due to recurrent laryngeal nerve damage.

GAS 1068; N 76-78; McM 45

252 B. A nonobstructive hydrocephalus occurs as a result of decreased reabsorption of cerebrospinal fluid (CSF) via the arachnoid villi. The subdural and epidural spaces are potential spaces, and these do not contain CSF. The choroid plexus produces the CSF, which flows into the subarachnoid space and is reabsorbed into the superior sagittal sinus via the arachnoid villi.

GAS 886, 888; N 101-105; McM 52-53

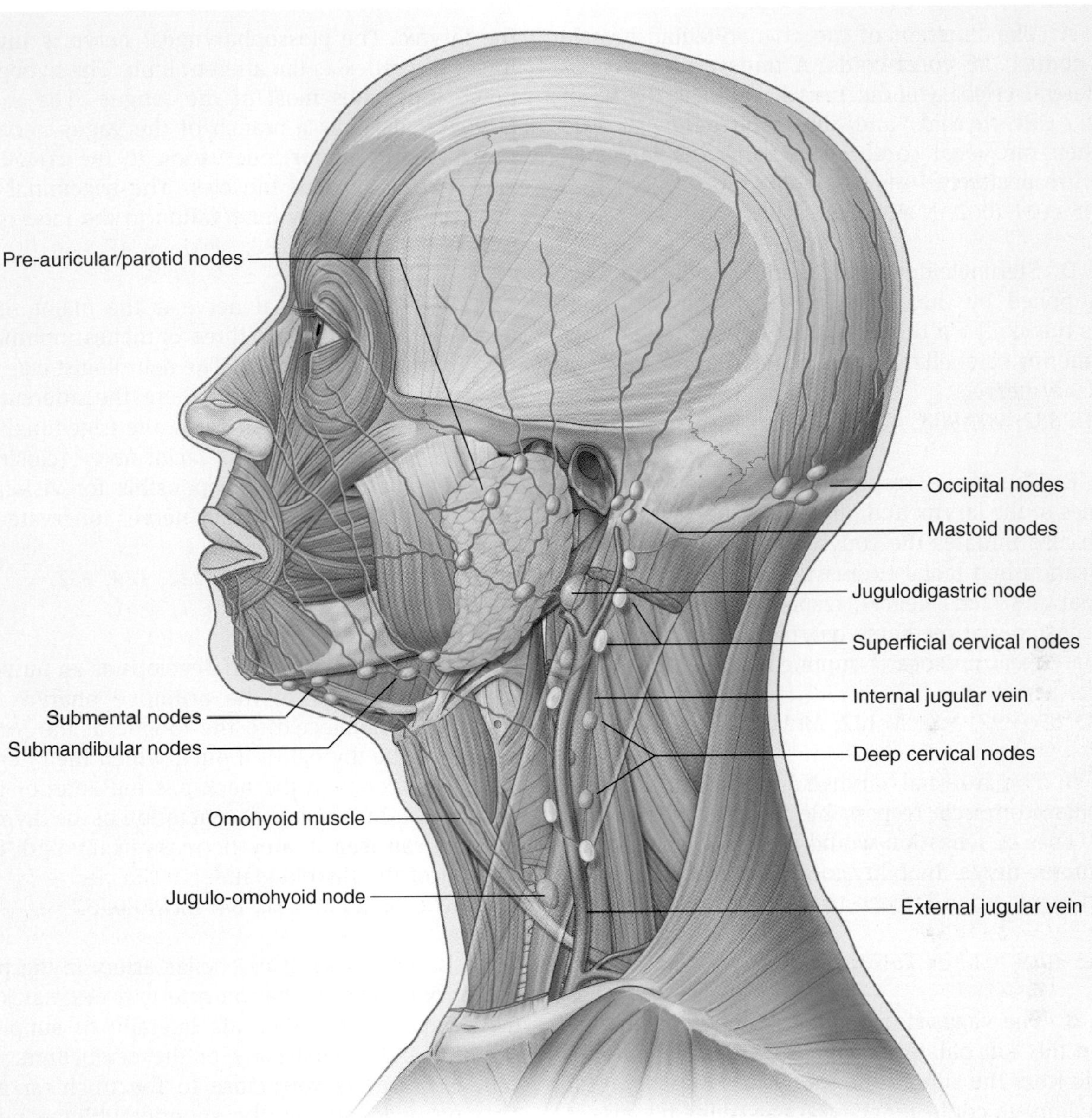

GAS **Fig. 8-193**

253 E. The location of the growing lump is close to the external acoustic meatus and is likely compressing on the facial nerve as it exits the stylomastoid foramen. The facial nerve is responsible for tight closure of the eyelids. Protraction of the tongue is due to innervation of the hypoglossal nerve and elevation of the mandible by the mandibular nerve. Pupillary constriction and partial ptosis result from damage to the oculomotor nerve.

GAS 898, 902; N 10, 99, 125; McM 61

254 D. Branches of the sphenopalatine, superior labial, and anterior ethmoidal anastomose anteriorly on the nasal septum are prone to bleeding. The descending palatine and ascending pharyngeal arteries are located posteriorly in the pharynx. The posterior superior alveolar artery travels within the maxilla and the accessory meningeal artery is found within the cranial cavity.

GAS 1083; N 40; McM 58

255 C. The glossopharyngeal nerve is located in the tonsillar bed as it runs with the stylopharyngeus muscle, which it innervates. The vagus nerve forms part of the pharyngeal plexus for supply of the pharynx and continues in the carotid sheath. The hypoglossal nerve is found inferior to the tongue. The external and internal laryngeal nerves are found in the neck.

GAS 899, 902-903; N 68, 69, 71, 126; McM 7

256 A. The function of the cricoarytenoid muscle is to abduct the vocal cords. A transverse arytenoid and lateral cricoarytenoid muscle adducts the vocal cords. Cricothyroid and thyroarytenoid muscles lengthen the vocal cords and narrow the laryngeal cavity, respectively.
GAS 1061-1062; N 80-82; McM 49

257 D. Sternocleidomastoid and trapezius muscles are supplied by the spinal accessory nerve, which enters the skull via the foramen magnum. The posterior inferior cerebellar artery is the artery nearest the accessory nerve.
GAS 882, 900-902; N 140, 142, 144; McM 50, 36

258 E. The nerve responsible for innervating the muscles of the larynx and pharynx is the vagus nerve, which also initiates the cough reflex. The muscles of mastication and facial expression are supplied by trigeminal and facial nerves, respectively. The vestibulocochlear nerve mediates hearing and balance. The oropharyngeal mucosa is supplied by the glossopharyngeal nerve.
GAS 896-897, 900; N 127; McM 78

259 B. The external laryngeal nerve supplies the cricothyroid muscle responsible for tensing the vocal cords. Loss of sensation would not result from injury to a motor nerve. Inability to abduct the vocal folds would result from damage to the recurrent laryngeal nerve.
GAS 1019-1020; N 76-78; McM 78

260 A. The vagus nerve is responsible for innervation to the soft palate; if damaged, the uvula would deviate from the side of the lesion. Glossopharyngeal nerve damage could reduce the gag reflex because it is the afferent limb but would not produce the other symptoms. Damage to the trigeminal nerve would not produce any of these symptoms.
GAS 846, 852, 853; N 126, 127, 61; McM 47, 52

261 B. The masseter muscle originates on the zygomatic bone and inserts on the lateral surface of the ramus of the mandible. It is a powerful elevator of the mandible. Grinding of the teeth can lead to hypertrophy of the muscles of mastication, especially the masseter. Patients will have difficulty in depressing the mandible due to spasms of this enlarged muscle.
GAS 977-978; N 48, 49; McM 32, 34, 75, 76

262 E. The vagus nerve mediates both the afferent and efferent limbs of the cough reflex: afferent to the mucus membranes and efferent to the muscles of the larynx. The glossopharyngeal nerve is involved in the gag reflex as the afferent limb. The hypoglossal nerve innervates most of the tongue. The external laryngeal nerve is a branch of the vagus nerve that provides only motor innervation to the cricothyroid and cricopharyngeus muscles. The trigeminal nerve does provide sensory innervation to the face.
GAS 900, 1014; N 127; McM 45, 47

263 C. The trigeminal nerve is the major sensory nerve of the face. It has three branches: ophthalmic, maxillary, and mandibular. The neurologist was trying to elicit the corneal reflex where the afferent limb (sensation on the eyeball) is via the trigeminal nerve and the efferent limb is the facial nerve (closing the eye). The optic nerve is responsible for vision, and the oculomotor and abducens nerves innervate extraocular muscles.
GAS 850, 898, 902; N 88, 122, 124, 132; McM 42, 44

264 D. The thyroid gland develops as an outpouching from the floor of the primitive pharynx. It is temporarily connected to the tongue at the foramen cecum by the thyroglossal duct, which then degenerates. It descends in the neck passing anterior to the hyoid bone. Incomplete degeneration of the thyroglossal duct can lead to a cystic mass in the path of the descent of the thyroid gland.
GAS 1018, 1019; N 60, 64; McM 30, 37

265 B. The superior cerebellar artery is the penultimate branch of the basilar artery. It originates from the basilar artery and runs laterally to supply the superior and medial parts of the cerebellum. In its course, it travels very close to the trochlear nerve. This nerve innervates the superior oblique muscle, which is responsible for depression of the eyeball when it is in the adducted state. This allows for proper vision when reading a newspaper or walking down stairs.
GAS 881, 882; N 139-144; McM 68

266 E. The aneurysm is located near the basilar artery between the left superior cerebellar and posterior cerebral arteries. This location is the origin of the oculomotor nerve, which innervates the extraocular eye muscles with the exception of the lateral rectus (innervated by the abducens nerve) and the superior oblique (done by the trochlear nerve). Compression of this nerve by an aneurysm will result in the eye being abducted (lateral rectus) and depressed (superior oblique).
GAS 881, 882; N 139-144; McM 68

267 B. The internal carotid is the artery that supplies the majority of the blood supply to the brain. It has several parts including the cervical, petrous, lacerum, cavernous, clinoid, ophthalmic, and communicating segments. The cavernous sinuses are paired dural sinuses that are located on the lateral wall of the sphenoid bone on either side of the sella turcica. The internal carotid artery and the abducens nerve run through it. Damage to this part of the internal carotid would affect the abducens nerve and the patient's ability to abduct the eye.
GAS 881, 887; N 105; McM 47, 68

268 E. The patient is suffering from an aneurysm of the anterior communicating artery. This artery connects the two anterior cerebral arteries across the beginning of the longitudinal fissure superior to the optic chiasm. An aneurysm in this area compresses the optic chiasm, resulting in blindness in the outer half of both right and left visual fields (bitemporal hemianopsia). An aneurysm of the anterior inferior cerebellar artery compresses the abducens nerve, which results in an inability to abduct the eye. Ptosis is as a result of compression to the oculomotor nerve, which can be compressed by an aneurysm in the superior cerebellar or the posterior cerebral arteries. An aneurysm of the superior cerebellar artery can also cause compression of the trochlear nerve and an inability to depress the adducted eye. Loss of corneal sensation is due to damage to the trigeminal nerve.
GAS 888; N 140-142; McM 47, 68

269 C. The CT scan shows an orbital (blow-out) fracture. The inferior rectus muscle originates from the inferior part of the common tendinous ring and inserts on the inferior anterior part of the eyeball. With an orbital fracture, an injury to the floor of the orbit results in entrapment of the inferior rectus muscle by a fragment of bone. This tethers the inferior rectus muscle to bone resulting in loss of function of the muscle. Patients experience diplopia when attempting upward gaze.
GAS 938; N 85-86; McM 54, 82

270 C. The area indicated by the arrow is the mastoid air cells of the mastoid process. The infection likely spread via mastoid emissary veins, which passed through the mastoid foramen of the temporal bone to the sigmoid sinus. The sigmoid sinus begins beneath the temporal bone and travels to the jugular foramen, at which point it joins the inferior petrosal sinus to form the jugular vein. The cavernous sinus does not have any direct relations to the mastoid process or mastoid air cells. The pterygoid venous plexus is located in the infratemporal fossa and communicates with the anterior facial vein and the cavernous sinus, by branches through the sphenoidal emissary foramen (of Vesalius), foramen ovale, and foramen lacerum. It has no relation to the mastoid process or mastoid emissary veins. The straight sinus is located within the dura mater, where the falx cerebri meets the midline of tentorium cerebelli. The superior petrosal sinus is located in the petrosal sulcus on the petrous part of the temporal bone. It receives blood from the cavernous sinus and passes backward and laterally to drain into the transverse sinus.
GAS 888, 964; N 99, 104, 105; McM 23, 69

271 C. The frontal sinuses are located in the frontal bone above the orbital margin. The maxillary sinus in the cheek region is within the maxillary bone. The ethmoid sinus is located between the nose and the eye. The sphenoidal sinus is within the sphenoid bone and cannot be palpated externally.
GAS 1074-1078; N 42, 44; McM 11, 16, 17

272 C. The temporal bone parts include mastoid, petrous, squamous, and tympanic portions. The mastoid process is part of the mastoid portion of the temporal bone.
GAS 972, 973; N 6, 10; McM 4, 7, 16

273 A. The central retinal artery is the major blood supply to the intima of the eye. It is a branch of the ophthalmic artery and travels with the optic nerve close to the eyeball to get to the intima or retina of the eye. The ciliary arteries arise from the ophthalmic artery and supply the sclera, choroid, conjunctiva, ciliary processes, and rectus muscles. The central retinal artery only rarely arises from the posterior ciliary arteries.
GAS 941; N 92; McM 73, 80

274 C. The auriculotemporal nerve, a branch of the mandibular division of the trigeminal nerve, passes posteriorly, deep to the ramus of the mandible and superior to the deep part of the parotid gland, emerging posterior to the temporomandibular joint to supply the skin anterior to the auricle and posterior two thirds of the temporal region. The nerve distributes to the skin of the tragus and adjacent helix of the auricle and therefore of the external acoustic meatus and skin of the superior tympanic membrane. The lesser occipital nerve, a branch of the cervical plexus, supplies the skin posterior to the auricle. The great auricular nerve, also a cervical plexus branch, supplies the skin overlying the mandible and the capsule of the parotid gland. The zygomaticotemporal nerve supplies the hairless patch of skin over the anterior part of the temporal fossa. The greater occipital nerve supplies the occipital part of the scalp.

GAS 985, 986; N 46, 50, 51, 71, 123; McM 39, 40, 75, 76

275 C. The two nerves found in the internal acoustic meatus are the facial nerve and vestibulocochlear nerve. Of the two, the facial nerve supplies facial muscles and can cause unilateral facial paralysis.

GAS 970-971; N 11, 13; McM 11, 50

276 D. The olfactory nerves arise from cells in the superior part of the lateral and septal walls of the nasal cavity. The processes of these cells (forming the olfactory nerve) pass through the cribriform plate and end in the olfactory bulbs, which lie on either side of the crista galli. Therefore a tumor here compresses the nerves, and the sense of smell will be affected. The optic tract and chiasm are not likely to be affected. Similarly, the vagus, vestibulocochlear, and facial nerves are not in close proximity.

GAS 896, 1085; N 39, 120; McM 43, 58

277 A. The butterfly-shaped middle cranial fossa has a central part composed of the sella turcica on the body of the sphenoid and large, depressed lateral parts on each side. The temporal bones are situated at the sides and base of the skull and consist of the squama temporalis, mastoid portion, petrous portion, tympanic part, zygomatic process, and styloid process. The occipital bone is situated at the back and lower part of the skull and is pierced by a large oval opening, the foramen magnum. The ethmoid and frontal bones are found in the anterior cranial fossa.

GAS 867; N 11; McM 4, 11, 12

278 E. The loose connective tissue layer (layer four) of the scalp is the danger area of the scalp because purulence or blood spreads easily in it. Infection in this layer can also pass into the cranial cavity through small emissary veins, which pass through foramina in the calvaria, and reach intracranial structures such as the meninges. The diploic veins are found in the skull and drain the diploic space. This is found in the bones of the vault of the skull and is the marrow-containing area of cancellous bone between the inner and outer layers of compact bone.

GAS 886, 890; N 3, 101, 103; McM 5, 81, 82

279 C. The muscles of facial expression are supplied by the facial nerve, which emerges from the stylomastoid foramen and passes through the parotid gland. The nerve gives off five major branches within the parotid gland from superior to inferior: temporal, zygomatic, buccal, marginal mandibular, and cervical. A fun mnemonic for these five branches is To Zanzibar By Motor Car. (This not only rhymes, but it's a geographical joke. You can't get to Zanzibar by motor car!). The lateral pterygoid and temporalis muscles are muscles of mastication and are supplied by the mandibular division of the trigeminal nerve (CN V3). The common carotid artery provides branches to supply the neck and the face while the vertebral artery supplies the spinal cord and the posterior part of the brain.

GAS 911-913; N 135; McM 34, 39, 40

280 D. The area behind the foramen magnum consists of the squamous part of the occipital bone. The foramen magnum is in the basilar part of the occipital bone (basiocciput). The dura mater is attached to the margins of the foramen as it sweeps down from the posterior cranial fossa. Within the tube of dura mater, the lower medulla with the vertebral and spinal arteries and the spinal roots of the accessory nerves traverse the foramen in the subarachnoid space. CN 1 passes through the cribriform plate of the ethmoid bone. The glossopharyngeal, vagus, and accessory nerves arise from the side of the medulla oblongata. The three nerves run laterally across the occipital bone and pass through the jugular foramen.

GAS 900, 902; N 13, 144; McM 11, 64, 65

281 A. The glossopharyngeal nerve emerges from the surface of the medulla and travels laterally in the pontine cistern to enter the anterior compartment of the jugular foramen. It gives off the tympanic nerve, which supplies the middle ear, a carotid branch to innervate the carotid body, the nerve to the stylopharyngeus, pharyngeal branches, a lingual branch and a tonsillar branch. The tonsillar branch provides afferent fibers for the tonsillar mucosa and the lingual branch conveys common sensation and taste from the posterior part of the tongue, as well as secretomotor fibers for lingual glands. Taste of the anterior two thirds of the tongue is innervated by the chorda tympani nerve and a branch of the facial nerve (CN VII). The vagus nerve (CN X) innervates the soft palate and the constrictor muscles of the pharynx.

GAS 846, 852, 853; N 126, 127, 61; McM 47, 52

282 E. The vocalis muscles lie medial to the thyroarytenoid muscles and lateral to the vocal ligaments within the vocal folds. The vocalis muscles produce minute adjustments of the vocal ligaments, selectively tensing and relaxing the anterior and posterior parts, respectively, of the vocal folds during animated speech and singing.

GAS 1061-1062; N 80-82; McM

283 B. Cricothyrotomy is an emergency airway procedure performed to ensure immediate airway ventilation in cases of laryngeal obstruction. It is performed by making an incision at the cricothyroid membrane, which is located between the thyroid cartilage and the cricoid cartilage. All the other options are incorrect because the cricothyroid membrane is located between the thyroid cartilage and the cricoid cartilage and this is where the incision is made.

GAS 1052, 1057; N 79; McM 48, 49

284 A. The larynx receives sensory innervation from the vagus nerve via the internal laryngeal nerve. The glossopharyngeal nerve does not innervate the epiglottis. The vestibulocochlear nerve mediates hearing and balance. The hypoglossal nerve supplies motor fibers to the tongue muscles. The facial nerve, while performing many functions including motor supply to muscles of facial expression and taste in the anterior two thirds of the tongue, does not supply sensory nerves to the epiglottis.

GAS 1068; N 82, 127; McM 78

285 D. An acoustic neuroma is an intracranial tumor that arises from the Schwann cell sheath investing the vestibulocochlear nerve. As this tumor grows, it eventually occupies a large portion of the cerebellopontine angle. Since cranial nerves VII and V are in close proximity to this location, these nerves are also usually affected, with subsequent manifestation of symptoms of impaired hearing, vertigo, loss of balance and nystagmus, paralysis of muscles of facial expression, hyperacusis, loss of taste sensation on the anterior two thirds of the tongue, loss of corneal reflex and sensation around the mouth and nose, and paralysis of muscles of mastication.

GAS 965; N 140, 144; McM 61

286 B. The patient described in the question has experienced vasovagal syncope after stimulation of his posterior external auditory canal by an otoscope speculum. In this form of syncope, parasympathetic outflow via the vagus nerve (CN X) leads to decreased heart rate and blood pressure. The posterior part of the external auditory canal is innervated by the small auricular branch of the vagus nerve. Most of the remainder of the external auditory canal, including the external portion of the tympanic membrane, is innervated by the mandibular division of the trigeminal nerve via its auriculotemporal branch. The inner surface of the tympanic membrane is innervated by the glossopharyngeal nerve (CN IX) via its tympanic branch.

GAS 850, 956; N 127; McM 23, 78

287 D. The superior thyroid artery, a branch of the external carotid artery, and the inferior thyroid artery, a branch of the thyrocervical trunk, provide the blood supply to the thyroid and parathyroid glands. The superior thyroid artery, superior thyroid vein, and external branch of the superior laryngeal nerve course together in a neurovascular triad that originates superior to the thyroid gland and lateral to the thyroid cartilage. Because the external branch of the superior laryngeal nerve courses close to the superior thyroid artery, it is at risk of injury during thyroidectomy.

GAS 1061, 1062; N 76, 82; McM 48, 49

288 D. The basilar artery is formed by the two vertebral arteries at the inferior part of the brainstem. At the medullopontine junction, the basilar artery gives two branches: the anterior inferior cerebellar artery first and then the labyrinthine artery. The abducens nerve (cranial nerve VI) emerges at the medullopontine junction and is usually found between the anterior inferior cerebellar and the labyrinthine arteries. The abducens nerve supplies the lateral rectus muscle, which abducts the eyes. This function of the nerve can be impaired if the nerve is compressed by a nearby aneurysm. If this condition occurs on the right side, it can result in weak abduction of the right eye.

GAS 881, 882; N 140, 142, 144; McM 68

289 B. The cranial nerve emerging anterolaterally at the junction of the pons and midbrain is the oculomotor (CN III). It passes between the superior cerebellar and posterior cerebral arteries (above). Both arteries are branches of the basilar artery. An aneurysm of the PCA could result in compression of the nerve and lead to oculomotor nerve palsy. This will result in the individual being unable to move the eye normally. The affected eye will be in a down and out position. The outward location of the eye is due to the lateral rectus (innervated by the sixth cranial nerve), which maintains muscle tone in comparison to the paralyzed medial rectus. The downward location is because the superior oblique muscle (innervated by the fourth cranial or trochlear nerve) is not antagonized by the paralyzed superior rectus, inferior rectus, and inferior oblique muscles.

GAS 881, 882; N 140, 142, 144; McM 68

290 D. The infratemporal fossa is a wedge-shaped region. It is positioned inferior to the temporal fossa and between the ramus of the mandibular laterally and the wall of the pharynx medially. The contents of the fossa include the temporalis, masseter, and lateral and medial pterygoid muscles. The pterygoid venous plexus and branches of the maxillary artery are also found in this fossa. Nerves passing through the fossa include the mandibular, inferior alveolar, lingual, buccal, and chorda tympani nerves. Tumors involving the infratemporal fossa present with a variety of symptoms depending on the structures involved.

GAS 972; N 71-74; McM 9

291 **E.** Due to the mass in the lumen of the parotid duct and distended parotid gland, nerves passing through the gland can be affected. The trunk of the facial nerve divides into temporofacial and cervicofacial divisions, which then further divide into temporal (supplies temple, forehead, and supraorbital muscles), zygomatic (infraorbital, lateral nasal, and upper lip muscles), buccal (upper lip and muscles at the corner of mouth), marginal mandibular (lower lip and chin muscles), and cervical branches (platysma muscle). Compression of any or all of the branches affects corresponding muscles and their functions. Pain sensation over the anterior auricle, tragus, and anterior helix is due to compression of the auriculotemporal nerve, which passes through the parotid gland and ascends just anterior to the ear, supplying the external acoustic meatus, surface of the tympanic membrane, and large area of the temple.

GAS 911-913; N 24, 46, 135; McM 34, 39, 40

292 **D.** The nerves involved are the lingual and buccal nerves, which are branches of the mandibular branch of the trigeminal nerve. These branches provide sensation to mucosa of the anterior two thirds of the tongue (general sensation), adjacent gums, cheek mucosa, and overlying skin.

GAS 985, 987, 988; N 50; McM 44, 75, 76

293 **C.** If the orbital rim is involved in the fracture, the patient may demonstrate a palpable bony "step-off" and complain of pain with palpation of the rim. Presentations of anterior cranial fossa fractures often include CSF rhinorrhea and bruising around the eyes.

GAS 896, 1072, 1085; N 11, 39, 120; McM 43, 58

294 **A.** The nerves that control lacrimal secretion pass through the superior orbital fissure, which is found in the orbit between the lesser and greater wings of the sphenoid. The superior orbital fissure is divided into three parts that are oriented from lateral to medial. The lateral part transmits the lacrimal nerve, which is well away from the fracture site at the apex of the orbit. Fracture at the base of the orbit will more than likely affect structures in the medial and middle parts of the fissure. Through the medial part courses sympathetics from the internal carotid plexus and the superior ophthalmic vein. The abducens nerve, the nasociliary nerve, and divisions of the oculomotor nerve all pass through the middle part of the fissure, which results in options B, C, D, and E being likely consequences of the injury as they are closer to the apex of the orbit.

GAS 934; N 13, 54, 85, 123; McM 11, 12, 74

295 **C.** The signals that regulate these functions are carried by the chordae tympani nerve, which then joins the lingual nerve. As the lingual nerve makes its way to the tongue it passes between the medial pterygoid muscle and the ramus of the mandible, where it was likely affected by the fracture. The elevation of the jaw or mandible is a function performed by the masseter, temporalis, and medial pterygoid muscles. The lateral deviation is performed by the medial and lateral pterygoid muscles.

GAS 987, 988; N 71; McM 40, 41, 60, 61

296 **B.** Coursing through the pterygoid canal are the artery, vein, and nerve of the pterygoid canal (Vidian canal). The Vidian nerve (nerve of the pterygoid canal) contains presynaptic parasympathetic fibers from the facial nerve via the greater petrosal nerve, which eventually go on to synapse in the pterygopalatine ganglion and postsynaptic sympathetic fibers from the deep petrosal nerve, which do not synapse in pterygopalatine ganglion (*GAS* Fig. 8-153B).

GAS 993, 997; N 39, 52, 53, 54; McM 25, 58

297 **E.** The nerves that control lacrimal secretion pass through the superior orbital fissure, which is found in the orbit between the lesser and greater wings of the sphenoid bone. Taste from the anterior two thirds of the tongue and secretions from the submandibular and sublingual glands were likely affected because their nerve signals are carried by the chorda tympani nerve, which joins the facial nerve in the facial canal located in the petrous part of the temporal bone. Movements of the right side of the face are also likely compromised or deficient because these muscles are innervated by branches of the facial nerve, which was likely impinged in the facial canal as a result of the fracture to the temporal bone.

GAS 994, 998; N 13, 54, 85, 123; McM 11, 72, 74

298 **D.** The fracture to the zygomatic bone, due to proximity, likely distorted the orbit resulting in damage to the structures running within the superior orbital fissure, where the nerves that transmit sensations from the lacrimal gland pass. It is divided into three parts, arranged from lateral to medial: the lateral part transmits the lacrimal frontal and trochlear nerves

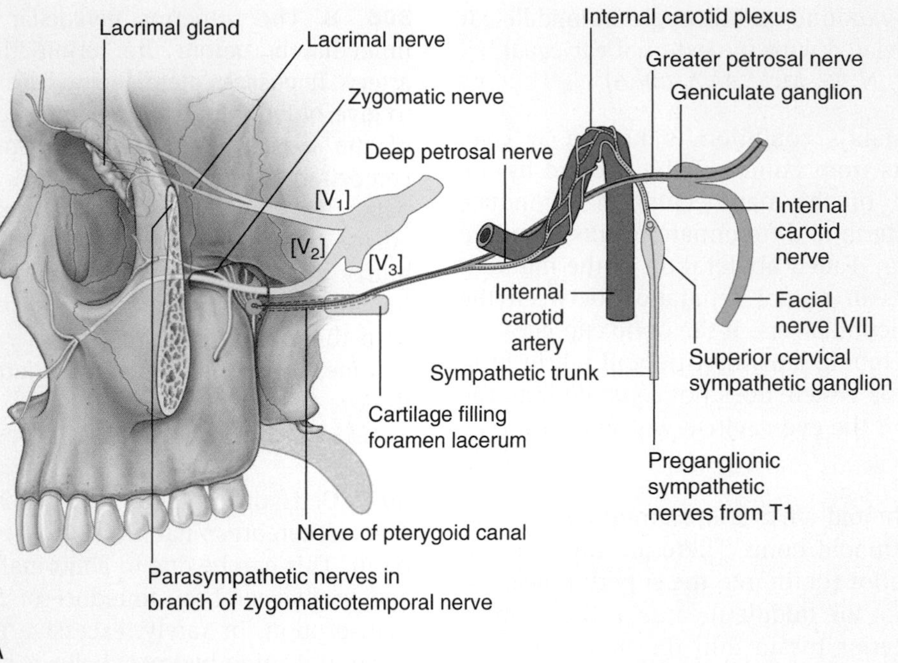

GAS **Fig. 8-153A**

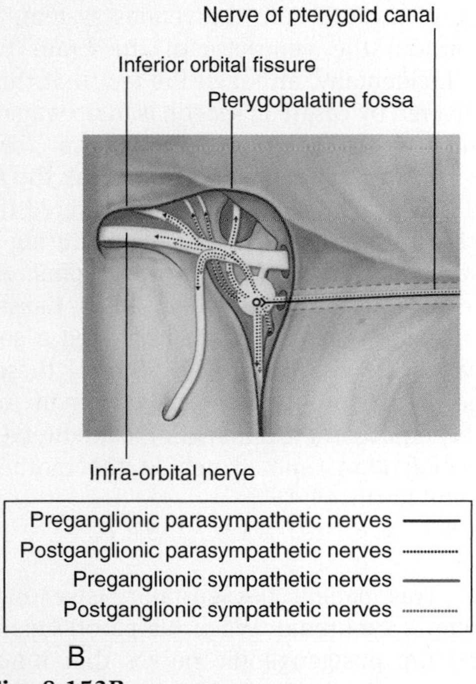

GAS **Fig. 8-153B**

and the meningeal branch of the lacrimal artery. The lacrimal nerve, being the structure closest to the fracture, will likely be the first to be injured.

GAS 938, 997; N 54, 5285-86; McM 54, 82

299 C. The patient suffers from either a damaged nerve or a trapped muscle; the inferior oblique muscle is defective. Complete or partial ptosis results from an inability to lift the upper eyelid and will not result from damage to the lower orbit. Inability to depress the abducted eyeball will result from damage to the superior oblique muscle. The nerve to the superior oblique and the muscle itself run superomedially and will therefore not be damaged in this patient. An inability to produce tears will result from parasympathetic damage and will only result from damage to the lacrimal nerve or the fibers traveling from the pterygopalatine ganglion (*GAS* Fig. 8-153A).

GAS 938, 940; N 85, 86; McM 54, 56

300 A. The petrous part of the temporal bone houses the middle and inner ear and has the facial canal with the facial nerve passing through it. Damage to the infratemporal fossa will not cause hearing loss or vertigo but will produce additional symptoms. The middle ear could account for the hearing loss, and the inner ear for hearing loss and vertigo, but not the facial palsy or lack of lacrimation.

GAS 1041; N 99; McM 37

301 B. The area of damage is in the external acoustic meatus, which is supplied by the facial, glossopharyngeal, and vagus nerves. The auriculotemporal and great auricular nerves supply the TMJ and external ear, respectively. The lesser occipital nerves supply the skin on the posterior aspect of the skull. The chorda tympani is responsible for taste to the anterior two thirds of the tongue and sensation to the middle ear. The lesser petrosal nerve and tympanic plexus carry autonomic innervation to and through the middle ear and are not associated with the external ear canal.

GAS 955, 957; N 96; McM 4, 7, 60, 61

302 C. The infant's condition is known as *coloboma* and results from failure of the choroid fissure to fuse. Failure of the neuroectoderm to induce the surface ectoderm to differentiate results in failure of the eye to form. Failed obliteration of the intraretinal space results in retinal separation between the pigmented and neural layers. If the optic cup does not overlap the developing lens, the iris will fail to form entirely. If the lens vesicle does not separate from the surface ectoderm, the eye cavities will not form.

N 91; McM 38

303 B. The ethmoid sinuses are groups of air cells located in the ethmoid bone. There are three groups of air cells: posterior (drain into the superior meatus), middle (drain into the middle meatus at the ethmoid bullae), and anterior (drain into the middle meatus by way of the ethmoid infundibulum at the semilunar hiatus). This can spread infections from the paranasal sinuses into the nasal cavity, leading to upper respiratory tract infections. The pharyngotympanic tube runs from the middle ear to the nasal cavity. The nasolacrimal duct indirectly drains the lacrimal gland, which is located on the lateral side of the orbit. The sphenoid sinus drains into the sphenoethmoidal recess.

GAS 1072; N 36, 37; McM 58

304 D. Oblique facial clefts are rare and often bilateral facial anomalies that extend from the upper lip to the medial margin of the orbit. In this condition, the nasolacrimal ducts are open grooves draining the tears from the lacrimal gland that lubricate the conjunctiva. This results from failure of the fusion of the mesenchyme of the maxillary process with the lateral nasal process. Failure of fusion of the medial nasal prominences results in a median cleft lip and palate, while failure of fusion of the intermaxillary segment with the maxillary processes results in a unilateral cleft lip.

N 25; McM 16

305 E. Treacher Collins syndrome (craniofacial dyostosis) is an autosomal disorder characterized by malar hypoplasia, underdeveloped mandible, downward slanting palpebral fissures, defects of the lower eyelids and external ears, and abnormalities of the middle and internal ears. This is a first arch syndrome due to failure of neural crest cells to migrate into the first arch during the fourth week of development.

N 54; McM

306 B. The superior cerebellar artery originates immediately before the termination of the basilar artery. It passes lateral below the oculomotor nerve to give blood supply to the anterior and medial parts of the cerebellum. An aneurysm of the superior cerebellar artery would result in oculomotor nerve palsy. This will affect the parasympathetics to the ciliary body and pupillary constrictor resulting in blurry vision, the levator palpebrae superioris resulting in ptosis, and the extrinsic muscles of the eye with the exception of the lateral rectus and superior oblique, resulting in lateral deviation (abduction) of the eye.

GAS 881, 882; N 140, 142, 144; McM 68

307 C. Hydrocephalus is an abnormal accumulation of cerebrospinal fluid in the ventricles of the brain. This can be due to abnormal flow (often blockage in the cerebral aqueduct of Sylvius), impaired reabsorption, or rarely, excessive production of CSF. Communicating hydrocephalus is caused by impaired reabsorption of CSF due to abnormal functioning of the arachnoid granulations, which are responsible for drainage of the CSF into the venous system. In this condition, all the ventricles of the brain become dilated. Incidentally, although the fact that this baby was delivered by cesarean section is in no way responsible for the hydrocephalus, the term "cesarean section" is interesting. Some people think the term is applied because Julius Caesar was delivered through an incision after his mother died during labor. However, that story is probably apocryphal. A more likely explanation is that when Julius Caesar was emperor of the Roman Empire he issued a series of rules called the Cesarean codes. One of these rules required somebody attending to a woman in labor (probably equivalent to a midwife) to attempt delivery of a viable infant immediately if the mother died during childbirth.

GAS 876; N 101-103; McM 52, 53, 62

308 C. This patient has gustatory sweating, also called Frey's syndrome. When his parotid gland was removed the postganglionic nerves that innervated the glandular epithelium of his parotid gland were cut, but the nerve cell bodies of those nerves, which are located in the otic ganglion, were undamaged and able to regenerate fibers. These fibers travel with the auriculotemporal nerve, and they "sought out" glandular epithelium. The closest glands are sweat glands in the skin of the face. Under circumstances that normally induce salivation (seeing appetizing food in this case), sweating occurs instead.

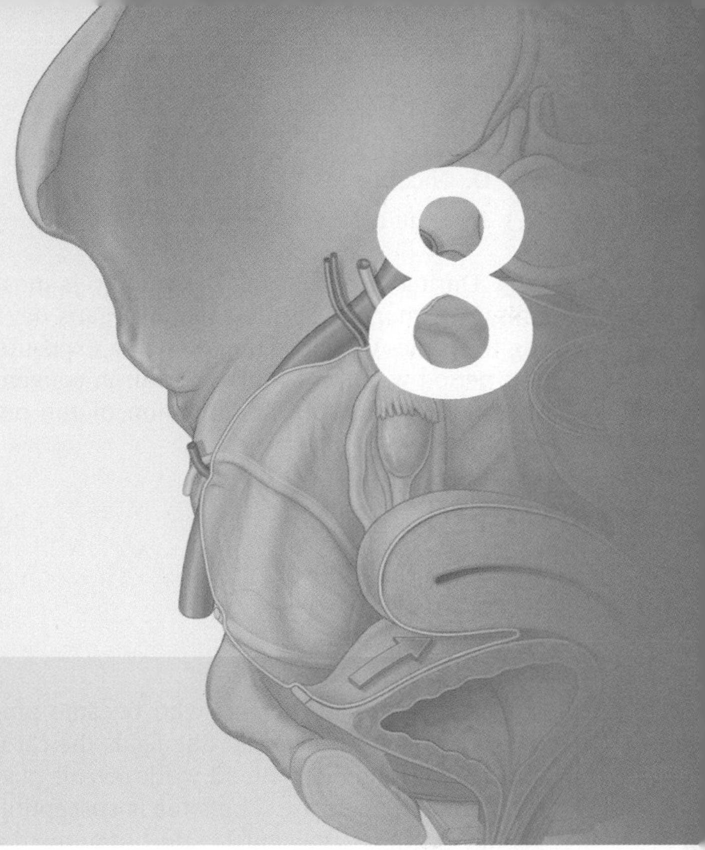

8

EMBRYOLOGY

QUESTIONS

1 A 32-year-old pregnant woman who is in the 30th week of her pregnancy visits her obstetrician for the first time (which is later in her pregnancy than usual). An ultrasound reveals that she is carrying twins. However, it is also revealed that one twin is surrounded by excessive amniotic fluid, while the other is surrounded by too little. A diagnosis of twin-to-twin transfusion syndrome is made. Which of the following types of pregnancy is most likely the cause of such a condition?

- ▢ **A.** Dichorionic, diamniotic twins
- ▢ **B.** Dichorionic, monoamniotic twins
- ▢ **C.** Monochorionic, monoamniotic twins
- ▢ **D.** Conjoined twins
- ▢ **E.** Monochorionic, diamniotic twins

2 An ultrasound of a 35-year-old pregnant woman reveals that she is carrying conjoined twins, a condition caused by incomplete division of embryonic discs. The most common location where conjoined twins (1/200 monozygotic conceptions) connects is:

- ▢ **A.** Thoracopagus
- ▢ **B.** Dicephalus
- ▢ **C.** Craniopagus
- ▢ **D.** Omphalopagus
- ▢ **E.** Rachipagus

3 A 27-year-old woman in a fishing town gives birth to an infant with severe neurologic symptoms of cerebral palsy including ataxia, numbness of hand and feet, and weakness of muscles. An evaluation of the infant reveals that he has Minamata disease. Which of the following teratogens/toxins consumed by the mother is the most likely cause of this congenital disorder?

- ▢ **A.** Lead
- ▢ **B.** Mercury
- ▢ **C.** Alcohol
- ▢ **D.** Cocaine
- ▢ **E.** Streptomycin

4 Between 1966 and 1969, seven out of eight girls whose mothers had taken a certain agent during pregnancy were diagnosed with clear cell adenocarcinoma of the vagina. As a result, the researcher who identified the cause for the rise of this condition performed a case-controlled study. Which of the following teratogens is the most likely agent that pregnant mothers took to cause this condition in their daughters?

- ▢ **A.** Alcohol
- ▢ **B.** Diethylstilbestrol (DES)
- ▢ **C.** Lithium

- ▢ **D.** Nicotine
- ▢ **E.** Folic acid

5 During weeks 3 to 8, the embryo is most susceptible to teratogens because major organs develop during this time. Which of the following exposures during this period would most likely result in congenital deafness, low birth rate, inflammation of the retina, and jaundice?

- ▢ **A.** Toxoplasmosis
- ▢ **B.** Heroin
- ▢ **C.** Mercury poisoning
- ▢ **D.** Alcohol
- ▢ **E.** Tetracycline

6 A 28-year-old woman who became pregnant 10 weeks ago has a house cat. She feeds the cat raw meat and handles the litter. Blood work reveals positive IgM for a zoonotic parasite. The fetus is susceptible to congenital deafness, low birth rate, inflammation of the retina, and jaundice. Which of the following teratogens can give rise to these findings?

- ▢ **A.** Toxoplasmosis
- ▢ **B.** Heroin
- ▢ **C.** Mercury poisoning
- ▢ **D.** Alcohol
- ▢ **E.** Tetracycline

7 An obstetrician has delivered a small-for-gestational age baby boy who is born 4 weeks too early. His mother is a 20-year-old chronic smoker who smoked a pack of cigarettes every day during her pregnancy. What teratogen most likely contributed to the low birth rate and premature delivery?

- ▢ **A.** Heroin
- ▢ **B.** Warfarin
- ▢ **C.** Rubella
- ▢ **D.** Tetracycline
- ▢ **E.** Nicotine

8 A pediatrician examines a newborn baby and finds a smooth philtrum, thin vermilion border (upper lip), and small palpebral fissures. These craniofacial abnormalities are mostly associated with which teratogen that can cross the placenta in utero and mammary glands during breastfeeding?

- ▢ **A.** Alcohol
- ▢ **B.** Warfarin
- ▢ **C.** Heroin
- ▢ **D.** Rubella
- ▢ **E.** Tetracycline

9 A couple hopes to start a family soon but the wife is currently taking medication for epilepsy. The obstetrician explains that exposure to this type of medication can cause serious birth defects, such as microcephaly, cleft palate, and congenital heart defects. Antiepileptic drug exposure during pregnancy will most likely cause which of the following?

- ▢ **A.** Fetal hydantoin syndrome
- ▢ **B.** Fetal alcohol syndrome
- ▢ **C.** Down's syndrome
- ▢ **D.** Treacher Collins syndrome
- ▢ **E.** DiGeorge's syndrome

10 A baby boy is born with a combination of congenital defects: atrial septal defect, patent ductus arteriosus, hypoplasia of the nasal bridge, and pectus carinatum (pigeon chest). The 35-year-old mother had not come in for any prenatal visits before parturition, and her medical history reveals that she had a heart surgery to repair a mitral valve defect secondary to rheumatic heart disease. She has been taking anticoagulant throughout her pregnancy. Which of the following teratogens will most likely explain the baby's congenital defects?

- ▢ **A.** Heroin
- ▢ **B.** Warfarin
- ▢ **C.** Rubella
- ▢ **D.** Tetracycline
- ▢ **E.** Nicotine

11 A 24-year-old woman visits an obstetrician and complains of not being able to get pregnant for the last 4 years. History reveals that she has been experiencing hot flashes, irregular periods, night sweats, and vaginal dryness. A diagnosis of premature ovarian failure is made. Estrogen replacement therapy is prescribed. What is the organ responsible for secreting estrogen?

- ▢ **A.** Anterior pituitary
- ▢ **B.** Posterior pituitary
- ▢ **C.** Hypothalamus
- ▢ **D.** Adrenal cortex
- ▢ **E.** Ovary

12 A 24-year-old overweight woman visits an obstetrician and complains of not being able to get pregnant for the last 4 years. History reveals irregular menstrual periods, decreased breast size, and hair growth on the chest and belly. Transvaginal ultrasound most likely reveals a thick band around which of the following reproductive organs?

- ▢ **A.** Ovary
- ▢ **B.** Posterior wall of the uterus

- ☐ **C.** Fimbriae of the uterine (fallopian) tube
- ☐ **D.** Isthmus of the uterine (fallopian) tube
- ☐ **E.** Ampulla of the uterine (fallopian) tube

13 A 28-year-old woman visits an obstetrician for in vitro fertilization. FSH-analogs are injected to stimulate follicles. Then hCG is injected to induce the final oocyte maturation. Lastly, the oocyte is retrieved via a procedure called transvaginal oocyte retrieval. Knowing the anatomic relationship between the ovary and the vagina, the physician will insert the needle through which space of the vaginal wall to reach the ovary?

- ☐ **A.** Posterior fornix
- ☐ **B.** Lateral fornix
- ☐ **C.** Pouch of Morison
- ☐ **D.** Retropubic space of Retzius
- ☐ **E.** Extraperitoneal space

14 A 28-year-old woman visits an obstetrician for in vitro fertilization. FSH-analogs are injected to stimulate follicles. Then hCG is injected to induce final oocyte maturation. Lastly, the oocyte is retrieved via a procedure called transvaginal oocyte retrieval. The retrieved oocyte is arrested at what stage of development?

- ☐ **A.** Prophase of meiosis 1
- ☐ **B.** Metaphase of meiosis 1
- ☐ **C.** Prophase of meiosis 2
- ☐ **D.** Metaphase of meiosis 2
- ☐ **E.** Prophase of meiosis 2

15 A 20-year-old pregnant woman in her third trimester visits an obstetrician complaining of periodic spotting. Ultrasound reveals implantation of the embryo near the internal os of the cervix. Despite periodic spotting, she experiences no pain during pregnancy. Which of the following describes this clinical symptom?

- ☐ **A.** Placenta previa
- ☐ **B.** Abruptio placentae
- ☐ **C.** Preeclampsia
- ☐ **D.** Leiomyoma
- ☐ **E.** Pelvic inflammatory disease

16 A 32-year-old woman visits an obstetrician complaining of significant bleeding in her first trimester and pain in the lower back. Ultrasound confirms the diagnosis of an abdominal pregnancy. Where is the most common place for an ectopic abdominal pregnancy?

- ☐ **A.** Pouch of Douglas
- ☐ **B.** Pouch of Morison
- ☐ **C.** Retropubic space
- ☐ **D.** Extraperitoneal space
- ☐ **E.** Retroperitoneal space

17 A 16-year-old boy visits the urologist with a lump in his left testis. Diagnosis of testicular teratocarcinoma is made. This tumor can be loosely referred to as "male pregnancy" because at an early stage the carcinoma contains all three primary germ layers: ectoderm, mesoderm, and endoderm. In normal embryologic development, which of the following processes give rise to these three primary germ layers?

- ☐ **A.** Morulation
- ☐ **B.** Gastrulation
- ☐ **C.** Cranio-caudal folding
- ☐ **D.** Cleavage
- ☐ **E.** Induction

18 A 20-year-old woman is trying to become pregnant. If she does, a blastocyst will form early in her pregnancy. Which of following statements accurately describes the formation of the blastocyst?

- ☐ **A.** Blastomere → morula → blastocyst
- ☐ **B.** Morula → zygote → blastocyst
- ☐ **C.** Blastomere → blastocyst
- ☐ **D.** Zygote → blastocyte → blastocyst
- ☐ **E.** Morula → blastocyte → blastocyst

19 A 29-year-old pregnant woman in her first trimester complains of preeclampsia and spotting. Ultrasound examination reveals an enlarged uterus and chorionic villi. Laboratory tests show elevated hCG levels. The physician suspects a hydatidiform mole, a condition characterized by gross edema of the chorionic villi surrounded by trophoblastic cells. The trophoblastic cell normally gives rise to which two cell layers?

- ☐ **A.** Ectoderm and endoderm
- ☐ **B.** Endoderm and mesoderm
- ☐ **C.** Hypoblast and epiblast
- ☐ **D.** Neural crest and neural tube
- ☐ **E.** Syncytiotrophoblast and cytotrophoblast

20 An obese 40-year-old woman is 33 weeks pregnant when she pays a visit to her obstetrician for her third trimester checkup. Physical exam reveals swollen hands. Her blood pressure (BP) is highly elevated, even though her BP throughout pregnancy has been normal. Laboratory tests reveal proteinuria. Because preeclampsia can develop into eclampsia (seizures) and put the baby and mother at risk, the physician immediately induces labor as treatment for the preeclampsia. Pain fibers from the uterus would follow which of the nerves below?

- ▢ **A.** Sympathetics (sympathetic pain line touching the peritoneum)
- ▢ **B.** Parasympathetics
- ▢ **C.** Somatic
- ▢ **D.** Somatic and sympathetics
- ▢ **E.** Sympathetics and parasympathetics

21 Nuchal translucency is used to screen for congenital defects during the 11th through 14th weeks of pregnancy. This procedure is recommended by an obstetrician for a 35-year-old pregnant woman who previously had a child with Down's syndrome (trisomy 21). Which of the following would be common to see in addition to a larger than normal accumulation of fluid at the back of the baby's head, indicating the possibility of another baby with Down's syndrome?

- ▢ **A.** Meromelia
- ▢ **B.** Hydrocephalus
- ▢ **C.** Anencephaly
- ▢ **D.** Atrioventricular septal defect
- ▢ **E.** Plagiocephaly

22 Genetic analysis of a 20-year-old, 6-foot-tall man reveals a mutation in the *FBN1* gene. He has unusually long and thin limbs, a hollowed chest, and severe nearsightedness (myopia). He is diagnosed with Marfan's syndrome. A computed tomography (CT) scan of the thorax revealed an unusual bulge anterior to the spinal cord and to the left of midline. Which condition will he be most susceptible to?

- ▢ **A.** Ruptured aorta
- ▢ **B.** Double inferior vena cava
- ▢ **C.** Portal hypertension
- ▢ **D.** Hydronephrosis
- ▢ **E.** Pyloric stenosis

23 A 3-year-old girl is brought to the emergency department for the fourth time in a year. The doctor suspects child abuse. Before social services is called, a genetics test is ordered and reveals that the patient has a mutation in the *COL1A1* gene. In addition to bone fragility and short stature, physical exam may discover which of the following?

- ▢ **A.** Pigeon chest
- ▢ **B.** Short limbs
- ▢ **C.** Yellow sclera
- ▢ **D.** Ruptured aorta
- ▢ **E.** Stiff joints

24 A pregnant mother is due in 2 weeks. Her body mass index (BMI) is in the overweight category and she has developed gestational diabetes. Pregnant women with gestational diabetes are more likely to have babies weighing 9 lb or more. During delivery, the obstetrician would be most concerned about which of the following for this expecting mother?

- ▢ **A.** Interspinous distance
- ▢ **B.** Distance of the pelvic inlet
- ▢ **C.** AP diameter
- ▢ **D.** Placenta previa
- ▢ **E.** Distance of the pelvic outlet

25 A 29-year-old, woman in her 27th week of pregnancy visits her obstetrician for a follow-up appointment. Ultrasound from a previous visit revealed a 4-cm mass growing at the base of the spine. What is the most likely diagnosis?

- ▢ **A.** Incomplete closure of the embryonic neural tube (lumbosacral myelomeningocele)
- ▢ **B.** Remnants of the primitive streak (sacrococcygeal teratoma)
- ▢ **C.** Swelling or growth of the endothelial cells that line blood vessels (hemangioma)
- ▢ **D.** Neuroendocrine tumor arising from any neural crest element of the sympathetic nervous system (neuroblastoma)
- ▢ **E.** Benign nerve sheath tumor of the peripheral nervous system (neurofibroma)

26 A 9-month-old male infant previously diagnosed with Down's syndrome is brought to the pediatrician by his parents because they observe a noticeable lump in the back of his neck. The physician learns that the infant has just recovered from a respiratory infection. Further analysis reveals the presence of fluid and white blood cells, an indication of embryonic lymphatic fluid. A differential diagnosis by the pediatrician is that there has been a failure of the jugular lymph sacs to join the lymphatic system, thereby preventing lymph drainage. Which of the following embryonic conditions could explain this case?

- ▢ **A.** Hemangioma
- ▢ **B.** Thyroglossal cyst
- ▢ **C.** Lingual cyst
- ▢ **D.** Cystic hygroma
- ▢ **E.** Squamous cell carcinoma of the larynx

27 A 28-year-old pregnant woman in her third trimester visits her obstetrician's office with her husband. The husband is short, with short limbs, bow legs, lumbar lordosis, and a large head with frontal bossing. Ultrasound revealed the baby to have a short humerus. As a precaution, genetic testing is ordered. Assuming the genetic test comes back positive for a mutation in the *FGF3* gene, what other features are more than likely to be present in their child?

- ☐ **A.** Pigeon chest (Marfan's syndrome)
- ☐ **B.** Brittle bones (osteogenesis imperfecta)
- ☐ **C.** Trident hand (achondroplasia)
- ☐ **D.** Cardiac abnormalities
- ☐ **E.** Mental retardation

28 A 25-year-old woman trying to have her first child has a spontaneous abortion due to failure of implantation. Under normal circumstances, at what stage of embryonic development will an embryo most likely implant into the endometrium of the uterus?

- ☐ **A.** Trilaminar embryo
- ☐ **B.** Zygote
- ☐ **C.** Morula
- ☐ **D.** Blastocyst
- ☐ **E.** Bilaminar embryo

29 Below are embryonic changes that occur during development of the upper limbs:

- ☐ **1.** Separate fingers
- ☐ **2.** Limb bud development
- ☐ **3.** Webbed fingers
- ☐ **4.** Digital rays

Which of the following most likely represents the correct order of developmental changes that occur in the upper limbs between weeks 5 and 8?

- ☐ **A.** 2-4-3-1
- ☐ **B.** 3-4-2-1
- ☐ **C.** 2-3-4-1
- ☐ **D.** 4-2-3-1
- ☐ **E.** 1-4-3-2

30 A researcher is studying the developmental origins of the arteries that supply blood to the brain. The investigation involves injecting contrast media into the hearts of fetal chicken eggs and studying the arteries that develop in the pharyngeal arches because blood vessels that develop bilaterally in several of these structures supply the cerebral arterial circle (of Willis). Which of the following pairs of pharyngeal arches most likely gives rise to arteries that contribute to the blood vessels in the circle of Willis?

- ☐ **A.** Pharyngeal arches 1 and 2
- ☐ **B.** Pharyngeal arches 2 and 3
- ☐ **C.** Pharyngeal arches 3 and 4
- ☐ **D.** Pharyngeal arches 4 and 5
- ☐ **E.** Pharyngeal arches 4 and 6

31 A 60-year-old man has been feeling "pins and needles" and some sharp pains over his right upper chest and back for several weeks. A rash of red erupted vesicles is seen at the right border of the sternum, a few centimeters above the nipple. Antiviral treatment is initiated to treat herpes zoster. The patient recovers, is free of pain, and his skin looks normal. Which of the following structures has the same embryologic origin as the location where the viral particles are still residing?

- ☐ **A.** Dorsal horn
- ☐ **B.** Ventral horn
- ☐ **C.** Dorsal root ganglion
- ☐ **D.** Conus medullaris
- ☐ **E.** Dura mater

32 A 63-year-old woman is admitted to the emergency department with severe pleuritic chest pain radiating to the bottom portion of her scapula. The pain is relieved by bending forward and worsened by lying down or during inspiration. During physical examination the patient exhibits a friction rub sound auscultated at the lower left sternal border. Which of the following embryonic structures will most likely give rise to the affected structure?

- ☐ **A.** Splanchnopleuric mesoderm
- ☐ **B.** Somatopleuric mesoderm
- ☐ **C.** Septum transversum
- ☐ **D.** Oropharyngeal membrane
- ☐ **E.** Coelomic cleft

33 A 51-year-old man visits the emergency department with high fever, left lower quadrant pain, and blood in his urine (hematuria) for the past 3 days. A CT scan reveals the presence of a thrombus in the left inferior vena cava (IVC). Which of the following structures is most likely responsible for the presence of a left IVC?

- ☐ **A.** Right anterior cardinal vein
- ☐ **B.** Right vitelline vein
- ☐ **C.** Left vitelline vein
- ☐ **D.** Left supracardinal vein
- ☐ **E.** Left anterior cardinal vein

34 A cyanotic 9-year-old boy is brought to the emergency department, coughing up blood and complaining of severe chest pain. Examination by the physician reveals a heart arrhythmia and a heart murmur. Looking at the patient's history, the physician diagnoses the boy with Eisenmenger's syndrome, a left-to-right shunt converted into a right-to-left shunt secondary to elevated pulmonary artery pressure. Which of the following disorders could be the initial congenital defect (left-to-right shunting) causing this syndrome?

- ▢ **A.** Ventricular septal defect
- ▢ **B.** Ebstein's anomaly
- ▢ **C.** Underdeveloped left ventricle (hypoplastic left heart syndrome)
- ▢ **D.** Common atrioventricular canal
- ▢ **E.** Large foramen secundum

35 A neonate with marked cyanosis in the lower extremities, cardiomegaly, harsh heart murmurs, and dyspnea is diagnosed with a patent ductus arteriosus. This condition is due to faulty migration of neural crest cells that leads to partial development of which of the following embryologic structures?

- ▢ **A.** Right subclavian artery
- ▢ **B.** Aorticopulmonary septum
- ▢ **C.** Tricuspid valve
- ▢ **D.** Inferior vena cava
- ▢ **E.** Left subclavian artery

36 A 1-year-old female infant was brought to her pediatrician because of a small "strawberry" like swelling on her scalp that has been growing rapidly. A diagnosis of hemangioma is confirmed. Which of the following embryologic layers gives rise to this vascular tumor?

- ▢ **A.** Mesoderm
- ▢ **B.** Endoderm
- ▢ **C.** Ectoderm
- ▢ **D.** Trophoblast
- ▢ **E.** Syncytiotrophoblast

37 A 55-year-old man with severe mitral regurgitation is scheduled for minimally invasive mitral valve repair. A percutaneous coronary sinus catheter is placed to deliver retrograde cardioplegia. During the procedure, the catheter stuck in an enlarged thebesian valve. Which of the following embryonic structures gives rise to the coronary sinus?

- ▢ **A.** Primitive ventricle
- ▢ **B.** Bulbus cordis
- ▢ **C.** Truncus arteriosus
- ▢ **D.** Left horn of the sinus venosus–left common cardinal vein
- ▢ **E.** Primitive atria

38 Oxygenated blood that reaches the heart in fetal circulation from the IVC passes through which of the following valves formed by a portion of the septum secundum?

- ▢ **A.** Foramen ovale
- ▢ **B.** Ductus arteriosus
- ▢ **C.** Foramen primum
- ▢ **D.** Ductus venosus
- ▢ **E.** Truncus arteriosus

39 Ultrasound of a 20-year-old pregnant woman in the 20th week of pregnancy revealed abnormal limb development of her fetus, showing one arm to be shorter than the other. Which of the following most accurately describes this condition?

- ▢ **A.** Meromelia
- ▢ **B.** Central digit ray deformity
- ▢ **C.** Talipes equinovarus
- ▢ **D.** Polydactyly
- ▢ **E.** Syndactyly

40 A male infant is born with cleft hand, also known as "lobster-claw hand." This abnormality is caused by the apical ectodermal ridge (AER) failing to properly develop. Which of the following best describes the principal function of the AER?

- ▢ **A.** Establishes the anteroposterior axis of the limb bud
- ▢ **B.** Stimulates blood vessel growth into the limb bud
- ▢ **C.** Stimulates cartilage differentiation in the limb bud
- ▢ **D.** Stimulates nerve growth into the limb bud
- ▢ **E.** Stimulates outgrowth of the limb bud

41 A 42-year-old woman gave birth to an 8 lb baby girl with two additional toes to the right of her left big toe. Which of the following best describes this limb anomaly?

- ▢ **A.** Amelia
- ▢ **B.** Cleft foot
- ▢ **C.** Club foot
- ▢ **D.** Polydactyly
- ▢ **E.** Syndactyly

42 A 40-year-old alcoholic man visits his physician's office for the fourth time this year complaining of abdominal and back pain. Abdominal CT scan shows a pancreas containing two separate duct systems emptying into the duodenum. The main pancreatic duct is very short and drains only a small portion of the head of the pancreas, while the remainder of the pancreas is drained via the other duct. The gastrointestinal (GI) specialist diagnosed the patient with pancreas divisum. Which of the following accurately describes the embryologic abnormality?

- ▢ **A.** Formation of a bifid ventral bud
- ▢ **B.** Formation of a bifid dorsal bud
- ▢ **C.** Failure of the dorsal and ventral buds to fuse
- ▢ **D.** Fusion of the dorsal and bifid ventral bud
- ▢ **E.** Nonrotation of the midgut

43 A 6-year-old child was brought into the emergency department with vomiting and abdominal pain. He complains that pain is radiating down his back and is worsened when he lays flat on his back. Physical exam reveals abdominal tenderness. Lab results show elevated serum pancreatic enzymes. Abdominal CT scan shows a pancreas containing two separate duct systems emptying into the duodenum. The main pancreatic duct is very short and drains only a small portion of the head of the pancreas, while the remainder of the pancreas is drained via the other duct. The GI specialist diagnosed the patient with pancreas divisum. Which of the following accurately describes the embryologic anomaly?

- ▢ **A.** Formation of a bifid ventral bud
- ▢ **B.** Formation of a bifid dorsal bud
- ▢ **C.** Failure of the dorsal and ventral buds to fuse
- ▢ **D.** Fusion of the dorsal and bifid ventral bud
- ▢ **E.** Nonrotation of the midgut

44 A 3-day-old male infant was brought into the emergency department. The parents complained that their son cried constantly, especially hours after feeding. History revealed chronic diarrhea, fatigue, foul smelling stools, and inability to gain weight. The infant had not passed meconium and was also small for his age. Abdominal CT revealed obstruction of a small segment of the bowel due to the superior mesentery artery wrapping itself around the segment. A GI specialist diagnosed this intestinal deformity as a type IIIb intestinal atresia (also known as Christmas tree or apple peel deformity). Which of the following arteries is also affected?

- ▢ **A.** Middle colic/right colic/ileocecal artery
- ▢ **B.** Splenic artery
- ▢ **C.** Inferior mesenteric artery
- ▢ **D.** Left renal artery
- ▢ **E.** Left gastric artery

45 A 32-year-old man presents to the emergency department with severe abdominal pain. Physical exam reveals rebound tenderness localized below the edge of the liver. Lab tests reveal a high white blood count, and CT scan shows an abnormal mass anterior to the right kidney. The physician suspects appendicitis due to an inflamed subhepatic appendix. Which of the following will cause the appendix to develop subhepatically?

- ▢ **A.** Rubella infection
- ▢ **B.** Malrotation of the midgut
- ▢ **C.** Failure of migration of the neural crest cells
- ▢ **D.** Meckel's diverticulum
- ▢ **E.** Failure of lateral folds to close

46 A 6-hour-old female newborn is assessed in the neonatal intensive care unit (NICU). Medical records show cyanosis, an APGAR score of 0, pulmonary edema on radiograph, and a tetralogy of Fallot confirmed by echocardiography. Which of the following conditions is most likely associated with this clinical picture?

- ▢ **A.** Pulmonary edema
- ▢ **B.** Hepatosplenomegaly
- ▢ **C.** Cardiomegaly
- ▢ **D.** Anal atresia
- ▢ **E.** Meckel's diverticulum

47 A 4-hour-old infant boy with respiratory distress is examined in the NICU. His symptoms are alleviated when placed in the prone position. Which of the following will most likely explain his symptoms?

- ▢ **A.** Down's syndrome
- ▢ **B.** Treacher Collins syndrome
- ▢ **C.** Pierre Robin sequence
- ▢ **D.** Patent ductus arteriosus
- ▢ **E.** Bronchopulmonary dysplasia

48 A 5-year-old boy is brought to a plastic surgeon's office. He has a small jaw, large mouth, flat cheekbones, and malformed pinna. He had a cleft palate at birth, which was surgically corrected shortly afterward. The parents complain that sometimes he does not respond when they talk to him. What correctly describes this boy's embryologic defect?

- ▢ **A.** Trisomy 13
- ▢ **B.** Defect in *FBN1* gene
- ▢ **C.** Failure of fusion of medial nasal prominences
- ▢ **D.** Failure of rostral neuropore to close
- ▢ **E.** Failure of neural crest migration into the first arch

49 A 47-year-old homeless man presents to the emergency department with a severe toothache. He has a large facial swelling that had previously been painless until this admission. The physician diagnoses an ameloblastoma, a benign tumor of ameloblasts. During normal development, what develops from the ameloblasts?

- ▢ **A.** Enamel
- ▢ **B.** Alveolar bone
- ▢ **C.** Cementum
- ▢ **D.** Periodontal ligaments
- ▢ **E.** Pulp

50 During an eye examination of a 6-year-old boy, an ophthalmologist sees a wormlike structure projecting from the optic disc. The diagnosis is the persistence of the distal portion of the hyaloid artery. What does the proximal portion of the hyaloid vessels eventually become?

- ▢ **A.** Optic artery and vein of the retina
- ▢ **B.** Optic artery and vein of the lens
- ▢ **C.** Central artery and vein of the retina
- ▢ **D.** Central artery and vein of the lens
- ▢ **E.** Supra-orbital vessels

51 A 14-month-old boy is brought to the ophthalmologist's office. His parents noticed that when photos of their child were taken, his eyes appeared white instead of red from the camera flash. Eye exam revealed poor vision in the right eye and CT scan showed calcifications within the right intraorbital mass. The boy is diagnosed with retinoblastoma. Which of the following structures share the same embryologic origin as the retina?

- ▢ **A.** CN II
- ▢ **B.** Lens
- ▢ **C.** Sclera
- ▢ **D.** Sphincter pupillae muscle of the iris
- ▢ **E.** Vitreous body

52 A young mother brings her 3-year-old daughter to the pediatrician with concerns of developmental delay. The pediatrician orders a CT scan, which shows partial atresia of the cerebellum. What is the embryologic origin of the cerebellum?

- ▢ **A.** Telencephalon
- ▢ **B.** Diencephalon
- ▢ **C.** Mesencephalon
- ▢ **D.** Metencephalon
- ▢ **E.** Myelencephalon

53 A 55-year-old man visits his primary care provider complaining that he can no longer go bike riding without getting breathless and having chest pains. Upon examination, the physician detects a heart murmur. Echocardiography confirms aortic stenosis. What is the embryologic origin of the aorta?

- ▢ **A.** Bulbus cordis
- ▢ **B.** Truncus arteriosus
- ▢ **C.** Sinus venosus
- ▢ **D.** Ductus arteriosus
- ▢ **E.** Ductus venosus

54 A 25-year-old woman in her 28th week of pregnancy visits her obstetrician for a routine check-up. Her doctor explains that her baby's lungs are starting to produce surfactant, a necessary component for respiration. Surfactant is produced during which of the following periods of lung development?

- ▢ **A.** Pseudoglandular period
- ▢ **B.** Canalicular period
- ▢ **C.** Terminal sac period
- ▢ **D.** Bronchiole period
- ▢ **E.** Alveolar period

55 The parents of a 2-week-old infant bring their child to the emergency department complaining of poor feeding, wheezing, coughing, and a hoarse cry in the child. Imaging confirms a double arched aorta resulting in a ring around the trachea and esophagus. What is the embryologic origin of this condition?

- ▢ **A.** Failure of the distal part of the right aorta to disappear
- ▢ **B.** Failure of the fifth aortic arch to disappear
- ▢ **C.** Failure of the first aortic arch to disappear
- ▢ **D.** Failure of the second aortic arch to disappear
- ▢ **E.** Failure of the sixth aortic arch to disappear

56 A woman in her first trimester visits her obstetrician for a routine ultrasound examination. Imaging reveals increased amniotic fluid surrounding the fetus. Which of the following is most likely to increase amniotic pressure?

- ▢ **A.** Renal hypoplasia
- ▢ **B.** Esophageal atresia
- ▢ **C.** Ureter obstruction
- ▢ **D.** Potter's syndrome
- ▢ **E.** Down's syndrome

ANSWERS

1 E. In monochorionic diamniotic twins, the single placenta (due to as yet unknown factors) develops blood vessel connections between the umbilical vessels of the twins. These connections result in an unbalanced blood supply known as twin–twin transfusion syndrome (TTTS). In TTTS, the donor twin does not get enough blood and the recipient twin becomes volume overloaded. In an attempt to reduce its blood volume, the recipient twin increases urine production, eventually resulting in polyhydramnios. At the same time, the donor twin produces less than the usual amount of urine leading to oligohydramnios. As the disease progresses, the donor produces so little urine that its bladder may not be seen on ultrasound. The twin becomes wrapped up by its amniotic membrane (known as a "stuck" twin). Often the polyhydramnios of the recipient twin is the first thing noticed by the patient due to a sudden increase in the size of the uterus. This condition is only possible when twins share a single chorion but have separate amniotic sacks.

See Moore KL, Persaud TVN, Torchia MG: *Before We Are Born,* ed 8, 2013, pp. 85-87*

2 A. Failure of complete division or fusion of adjacent embryonic discs leads to conjoined twins. These are always monozygotic and share a single chorion, placenta, and amniotic sac. The most common site of attachment is an anterior union of the thoracic regions called thoracopagus, with the second most common being omphalopagus, where the twins are joined at the anterior abdominal wall. The original "Siamese twins" were of this latter type.

87-88

3 B. Minamata disease is a severe neurologic syndrome caused by methylmercury poisoning. It can be acquired or congenital, following maternal mercury ingestion as in this case. Accumulation of methyl mercury from maternal ingestion of fish and shellfish or pork (due to certain pesticide contamination) is the primary cause. Lead poisoning can cause permanent learning and behavioral disorders, and alcohol exposure can result in fetal alcohol syndrome, which has a wide spectrum including mental and growth retardation plus morphogenetic disturbances. Cocaine exposure can cause microcephaly, neurobehavioral disturbances, spontaneous abortion, and urogenital disturbances. Streptomycin exposure can result in vestibulocochlear (CN VIII) nerve defects.

309

4 B. Diethylstilbestrol (DES) is a synthetic nonsteroidal estrogen once commonly used in pregnant women to prevent breast engorgement, among many other uses. Prenatal exposure increases risk of multiple conditions including vaginal clear cell adenocarcinoma and reproductive tract malformations. It has since been proven to be toxic and teratogenic. Fetal alcohol syndrome from maternal alcoholism has a wide spectrum including mental and growth retardation plus morphogenetic disturbances. Lithium causes heart and great vessel abnormalities in utero. Nicotine causes premature delivery, conotruncal defects, and urinary tract abnormalities (Table 8-1).

304-305

5 A. Infectious teratogens include toxoplasmosis, which causes jaundice, intracranial calcifications and chorioretinitis, microcephaly, microphthalmia, and hydrocephalus. Congenital syphilis can lead to abnormal teeth and bones, congenital deafness, hydrocephalus, and mental retardation. Herpes simplex exposure can result in microcephaly, microphthalmia, spasticity, and mental retardation. Cytomegalovirus infection may result in cerebral palsy, mental retardation, intrauterine growth retardation, microphthalmia, blindness, deafness, and hepatosplenomegaly. Congenital rubella syndrome presents with cataracts, cardiac defects, and deafness. Alcohol exposure can result in fetal alcohol syndrome, which has a wide spectrum including mental and growth retardation plus morphogenetic disturbances. Cocaine exposure can cause microcephaly, neurobehavioral disturbances, spontaneous abortion, and urogenital disturbances. Streptomycin causes vestibulocochlear nerve defects. Methadone and heroin are behavioral teratogens and present with small birth weight, central nervous system dysfunction, and small head circumference. Tetracycline causes tooth and bone defects including yellow discoloration and hypoplasia.

304-305, 310

6 A. Infectious teratogens include toxoplasmosis, which can result in jaundice, intracranial calcifications, chorioretinitis, microcephaly, microphthalmia, and hydrocephalus. Congenital syphilis can result in the formation of abnormal teeth and bones, congenital deafness, hydrocephalus, and mental retardation. Herpes simplex can also result in spasticity and mental retardation. Cytomegalovirus infection may result in cerebral palsy, mental retardation, intrauterine growth

*Subsequent cross-references to *Before We Are Born* list page numbers only.

Table 8-1 Some Teratogens Known to Cause Human Birth Defects

Agents	Most Common Congenital Anomalies
Drugs	
Alcohol	Fetal alcohol syndrome (FAS); intrauterine growth restriction (IUGR); mental deficiency; microcephaly; ocular anomalies; joint abnormalities; short palpebral fissures; fetal alcohol spectrum disorders (FASDs); cognitive and neurobehavioral disturbances
Androgens and high doses of progestogens	Varying degree of masculinization of female fetuses; ambiguous external genitalia (labial fusion and clitoral hypertrophy)
Methotrexate	IUGR; skeletal and renal defects
Cocaine	IUGR; prematurity; microcephaly; cerebral infarction; urogenital anomalies; neurobehavioral disturbances
Diethylstilbestrol	Abnormalities of uterus and vagina; cervical erosion and ridges
Isotretinoin (12-cis-retionic acid)	Craniofacial abnormalities; neural tube defects such as spina bifida cystica; cardiovascular defects; cleft palate; thymic aplasia
Lithium carbonate	Various anomalies, usually involving the heart and great vessels
Methotrexate	Multiple anomalies, especially skeletal, involving the face, cranium, limbs, and vertebral column
Misoprostol	Abnormal development of the limbs, ocular defects, cranial nerve defects, and autism spectrum disorders
Phenytoin (Dilantin)	Fetal hydantoin syndrome; IUGRl microcephaly; mental retardation; ridged metopic suture; inner epicanthal folds; eyelid ptosis; broad, depressed, nasal bridge; phalangeal hypoplasia
Tetracycline	Stained teeth; hypoplasia of enamel
Thalidomide	Abnormal development of the limbs; meromelia (partial absence of limb) and amelia (complete absence of the limb); facial anomalies; systemic anomalies (e.g., cardiac and kidney defects and ocular anomalies)
Trimethadione	Abnormal development of the limbs; V-shaped eyebrows; low-set ears; cleft lip and/or palate
Valproic acid	Craniofacial anomalies; neural tube defects; often hydrocephalus; heart and skeletal defects; poor postnatal cognitive development
Warfarin	Nasal hypoplasia; stippled epiphyses; hypoplastic phalanges; eye anomalies; mental deficiency
Chemicals	
Methylmercury	Cerebral atrophy; spasticity; seizures; mental deficiency
Polychlorinated biphenyls	IUGR; skin discoloration
Infections	
Cytomegalovirus	Microcephaly; chorioretinitis; sensorineural loss; delayed psychomotor and mental development; hepatosplenomegaly; hydrocephaly; cerebral palsy; brain (periventricular) calcification
Herpes simplex virus	Skin vesicles and scarring; chorioretinitis; hepatomegaly; thrombocytopenia; petechiae; hemolytic anemia; hydranencephaly
Human parvovirus B19	Fetal anemia; nonimmune hydrops fetalis; fetal death
Rubella virus	IUGR; postnatal growth retardation; cardiac and great vessel abnormalities; microcephaly; sensorineural deafness; cataract; microphthalmos; glaucoma; pigmented retinopathy; mental deficiency; neonatal bleeding; hepatosplenomegaly; osteopathy; tooth defects
Toxoplasma gondii	Microcephaly; mental deficiency; microphthalmia; hydrocephaly; chorioretinitis; cerebral calcifications; hearing loss; neurologic disturbances
Treponema pallidum	Hydrocephalus; congenital deafness; mental deficiency; abnormal teeth and bones
Varicella virus	Cutaneous scars (dermatome distribution); neurologic anomalies (e.g., limb paresis, hydrocephaly, seizures); cataracts; microphthalmia; Horner syndrome; optic atrophy; nystagmus; chorioretinitis; microcephaly; mental deficiency; skeletal anomalies (e.g., hypoplasia of limbs, fingers, and toes); urogenital anomalies
High levels of ionizing radiation	Microcephaly; mental deficiency; skeletal anomalies; growth retardation; cataracts

From Moore KL, Persaud TVN, Torchia MG: *Before We Are Born*, ed 8, Philadelphia: Elsevier, 2013, p. 303.

retardation, microphthalmia, blindness, deafness, and hepatosplenomegaly. Congenital rubella syndrome presents with cataracts, cardiac defects, and deafness among other defects. Alcohol exposure can result in fetal alcohol syndrome, which has a wide spectrum including mental and growth retardation plus morphogenetic disturbances. Cocaine use can cause microcephaly, neurobehavioral disturbances, spontaneous abortion, and urogenital disturbances. Streptomycin can cause vestibulocochlear (CN VIII) nerve defects. Methadone and heroin exposure can result in small birth weight, central nervous system dysfunction, and small head circumference. Tetracycline exposure can result in tooth and bone defects including yellow discoloration and hypoplasia.

304-305, 310

7 E. Nicotine can cause premature delivery, low birth weight, and poor physical growth due to its constrictive effect on uterine blood vessels. It also causes conotruncal defects and urinary tract abnormalities. Tetracycline exposure can cause tooth and bone defects including yellow discoloration and hypoplasia. Heroin is a behavioral teratogen and presents with small birth weight, central nervous system dysfunction, and small head circumference. Congenital rubella syndrome presents with cataracts, cardiac defects, and deafness among other defects.

306

8 A. Fetal alcohol syndrome (FAS) is associated with intrauterine growth restriction (IUGR), mental deficiency, microcephaly, ocular anomalies, joint abnormalities, and small palpebral fissures. Warfarin can be associated with nasal hypoplasia, stippled epiphyses, hypoplastic phalanges, eye anomalies, and mental deficiency. Tetracycline exposure can be associated with stained teeth and hypoplasia of enamel. Rubella virus is associated with various anomalies such as IUGR, postnatal growth retardation, cardiac and great vessel abnormalities, microcephaly, sensorineural deafness, cataract, microphthalmos (also referred to as microphthalmia), glaucoma, pigmented retinopathy, mental deficiency, neonate bleeding, hepatosplenomegaly, osteopathy, and tooth defects. Women who use heroin during pregnancy greatly increase their risk of serious pregnancy complications. These risks include poor fetal growth, premature rupture of membranes, premature birth, and stillbirth.

304-307

9 A. Fetal hydantoin syndrome occurs in 5% to 10% of children born to mothers treated with phenytoin or hydantoin anticonvulsants. The usual pattern of defects consists of IUGR, microcephaly, mental deficiency, ridged frontal suture, inner epicanthal folds, eyelid ptosis, broad depressed nasal bridge, nail and/or distal phalangeal hypoplasia, and hernias. Fetal alcohol syndrome (FAS): intrauterine growth restriction (IUGR), mental deficiency, microcephaly, ocular anomalies, joint abnormalities, and short palpebral fissures. Trisomy 21 (Down's syndrome), the most common numerical abnormality resulting in birth defects (intellectual disability, abnormal facies, heart malformations), is usually caused by nondisjunction. The risk of meiotic nondisjunction increases with increasing maternal age. Treacher Collins syndrome is characterized by craniofacial deformities, such as absent cheekbones. Infants with DiGeorge syndrome are born without a thymus and parathyroid glands and have defects in their cardiac outflow tracts.

304-308

10 B. Fetal alcohol syndrome (FAS) is associated with intrauterine growth restriction (IUGR), mental deficiency, microcephaly, ocular anomalies, joint abnormalities, and short palpebral fissures. Warfarin is associated with nasal hypoplasia, stippled epiphyses, hypoplastic phalanges, eye anomalies, and mental deficiency. Tetracycline is associated with stained teeth and hypoplasia of enamel. Rubella virus is associated with various anomalies like IUGR, postnatal growth retardation, cardiac and great vessel abnormalities, microcephaly, sensorineural deafness, cataract, microphthalmos, glaucoma, pigmented retinopathy, mental deficiency, neonate bleeding, hepatosplenomegaly, osteopathy, and tooth defects. Women who use heroin during pregnancy greatly increase their risk of serious pregnancy complications. These risks include poor fetal growth, premature rupture of the membranes, premature birth, and stillbirth.

304-307

11 E. The ovaries are almond-shaped reproductive glands located close to the lateral pelvic walls on each side of the uterus that produce oocytes. The ovaries also produce estrogen and progesterone, the hormones responsible for the development of secondary sex characteristics and regulation of pregnancy. Follicle stimulating hormone (FSH) is produced by the anterior pituitary gland, which stimulates the development of ovarian follicles and the production of estrogen by the follicular cells. Luteinizing hormone (LH) serves as the "trigger" for ovulation (release of secondary oocyte) and stimulates the follicular cells and corpus luteum to produce progesterone. Gonadotropin releasing hormone (GnRH) is secreted from

the hypothalamus and stimulates the production and secretion of FSH and LH from the anterior pituitary.
10, 14-17

12 A. Polycystic ovary syndrome (PCOS) is a syndrome of ovarian dysfunction along with the cardinal features of hyperandrogenism and polycystic ovary morphology. Its clinical manifestations include menstrual irregularities, signs of androgen excess (e.g., hirsutism), and obesity. The ultrasound criteria for the diagnosis of a polycystic ovary are eight or more subcapsular follicular cysts <10 mm in diameter and increased ovarian stroma.
14-18

13 A. Each ovary is oval shaped, and is attached to the back of the broad ligament by the mesovarium. The position of the ovary is, however, extremely variable, and it is often found hanging down in the rectouterine pouch (pouch of Douglas). The posterior wall of the vagina is longer than the anterior wall and the posterior fornix is deeper than the other fornices. The posterior fornix is covered by peritoneum of the front of the rectouterine pouch (of Douglas) (*GAS* Fig. 5-58).
14-18

14 A. Primary oocytes begin the first meiotic divisions before birth, but completion of prophase in meiosis 1 does not occur until adolescence. The follicular cells surrounding the primary oocytes secrete a substance, oocyte maturation inhibitor, which arrests the meiotic process of the oocyte.
14-19

15 A. Placenta previa is defined as a placenta that has implanted into the lower segment of the uterus. It is now classified as either major, in which the placenta is covering the internal cervical os, or minor, when the placenta is sited within the lower segment of the uterus, but does not cover the cervical os. The mother will present with painless bleeding, often recurrent in the third trimester, and ultrasound scans will demonstrate the abnormal location of the placenta. The bleeding occurs due to separation of the placenta as the lower segment develops in the third trimester. A placental abruption is separation of a normally positioned placenta from the uterine wall. Preeclampsia is a serious disorder that occurs during pregnancy, usually after the 20th week of gestation. Maternal hypertension, proteinuria, and edema are essential features of this condition. Leiomyoma is a benign tumor of smooth muscle (fibroid). Pelvic inflammatory disease is characterized by inflammation and infection arising from the endocervix leading to endometritis, salpingitis, oophoritis, pelvic peritonitis and subsequently, formation of tubo-ovarian and pelvic abscesses.
81-82

16 A. Ectopic pregnancy is the existence of a pregnancy outside the normal confines of the uterus or abnormally in the uterus. Although the uterine (fallopian) tube is the most common site of an ectopic pregnancy, it can also occur in the abdominal cavity, and when that is the case, the pouch of Douglas in the most common site. The pouch of Morison is the space between the liver and the right kidney and is not usually a site for ectopic pregnancy. The retropubic space is an extraperitoneal space between the pubic symphysis and the urinary bladder. It is a very unlikely site for ectopic pregnancy. Ectopic pregnancies rarely exist at the other sites listed (Fig. 8-1).
32-33

17 B. Gastrulation occurs in early embryogenesis and is the process by which the blastula is reorganized into a three-layered structure, that is, ectoderm, mesoderm, and endoderm. Morulation involves the cleavage or division of the fertilized ovum usually into a 16-cell structure that resembles a ball. Cranio-caudal folding is a process that occurs with lateral folding of the embryo that transforms it from a flat disc into a three-dimensional tube within the body. Cleavage is the process of division of the fertilized ovum. Induction is the physiologic and chemical signal to stimulate cells to differentiate.
35-38

18 A. After fertilization of the ovum, cleavage commences with the formation of blastomere and then a 16-cell morula. Fluid would then enter the cavity of the morula with the formation of a blastocyst. The blastocyst will then invade the endometrial wall.
21-24

19 E. Upon trophoblastic invasion of the endometrium, the trophoblastic cells produce two cell layers: the syncytiotrophoblast is the outer layer that is related to the endometrial wall while the cytotrophoblast is the inner layer, which usually gives rise to the chorionic villi. The ectoderm, endoderm, and mesoderm are body germ layers produced during gastrulation. Hypoblast and epiblast cells are derived from the inner cell mass of the blastocyst, and the epiblast will ultimately, under gastrulation, form the germ layers. Neural crest cells do not give rise to

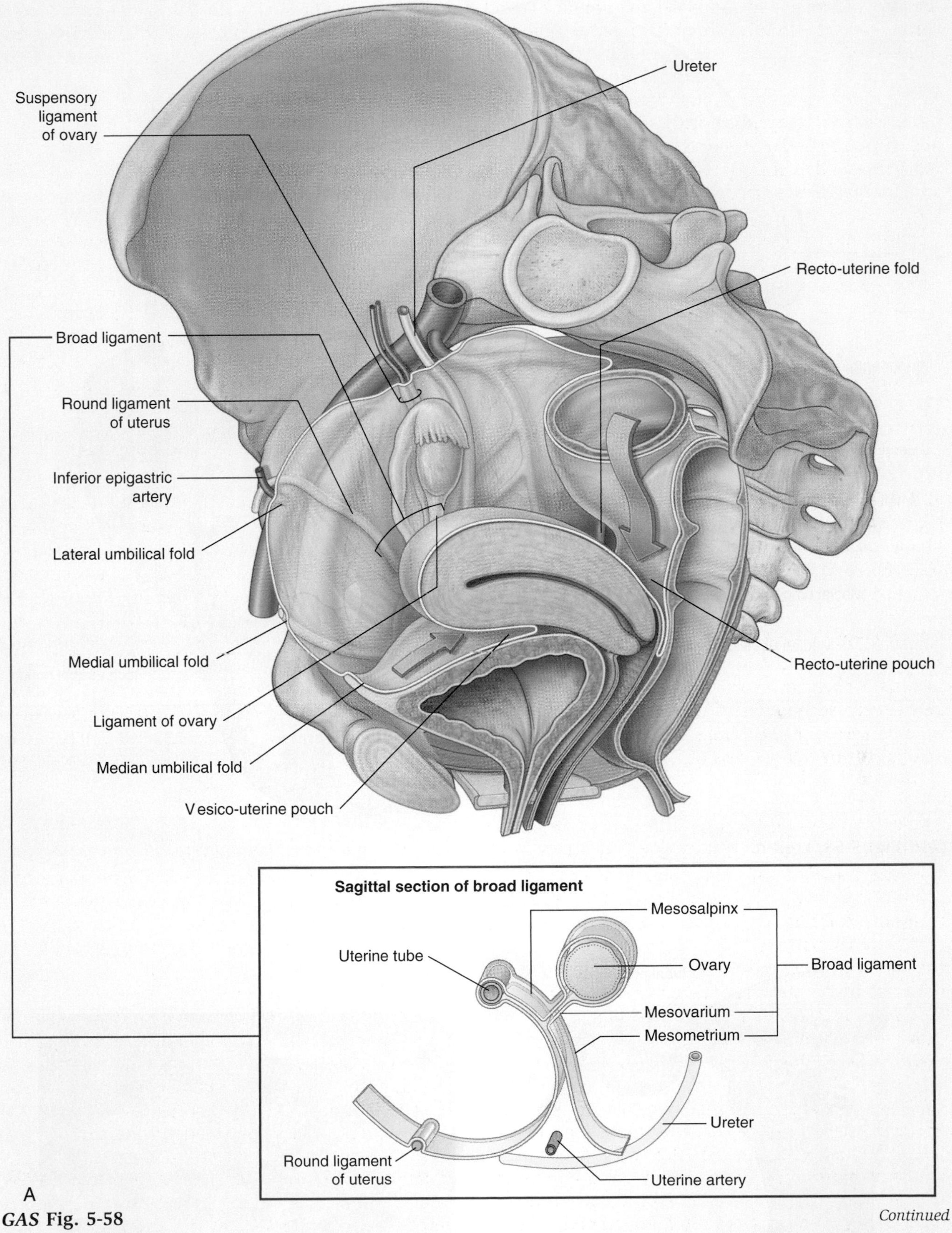

Ureter
Suspensory ligament of ovary
Recto-uterine fold
Broad ligament
Round ligament of uterus
Inferior epigastric artery
Lateral umbilical fold
Medial umbilical fold
Recto-uterine pouch
Ligament of ovary
Median umbilical fold
Vesico-uterine pouch
Sagittal section of broad ligament
Mesosalpinx
Uterine tube
Ovary
Broad ligament
Mesovarium
Mesometrium
Ureter
Round ligament of uterus
Uterine artery
A

GAS Fig. 5-58

Continued

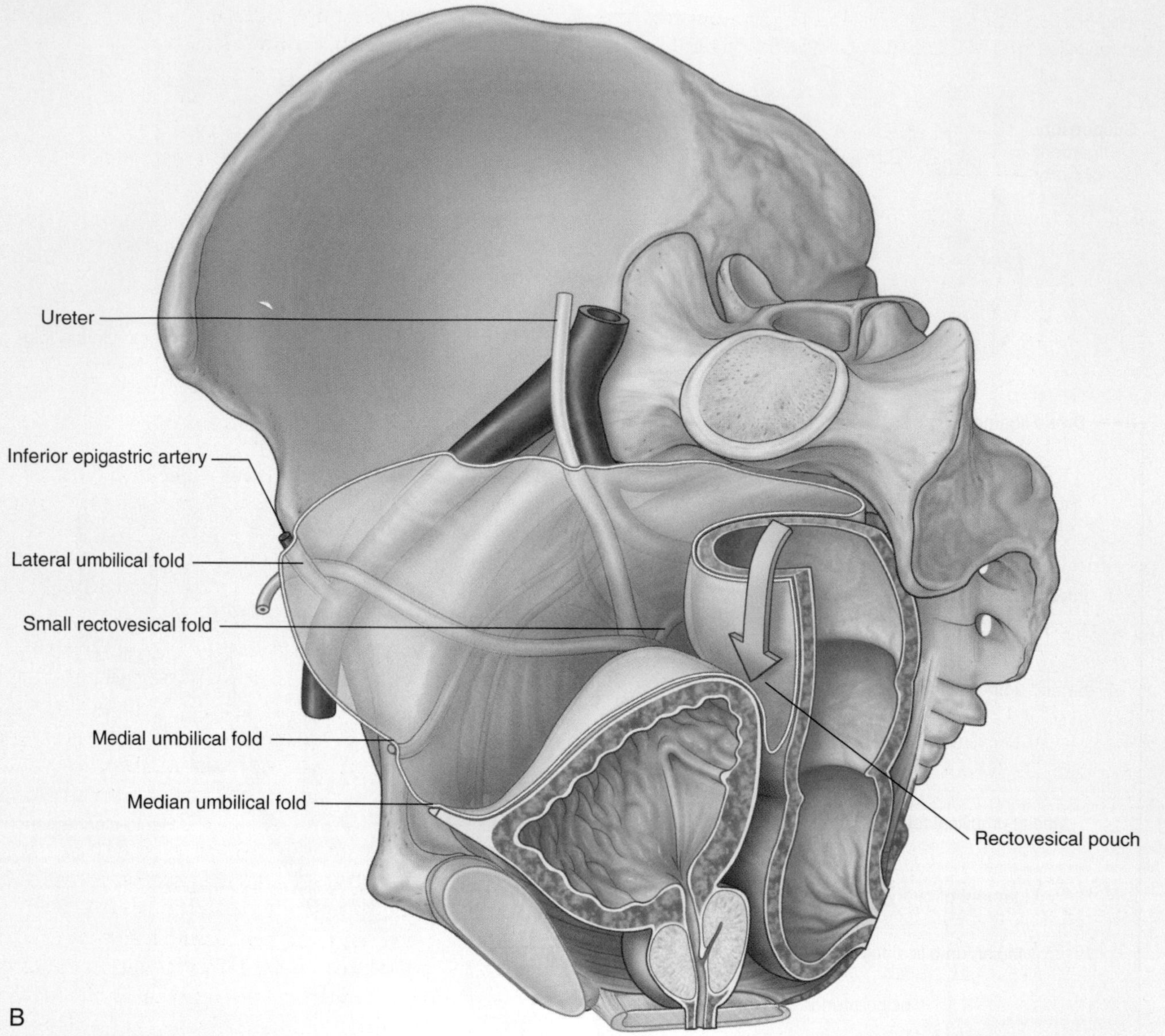
Ureter
Inferior epigastric artery
Lateral umbilical fold
Small rectovesical fold
Medial umbilical fold
Median umbilical fold
Rectovesical pouch
B

GAS **Fig. 5-58, cont'd**

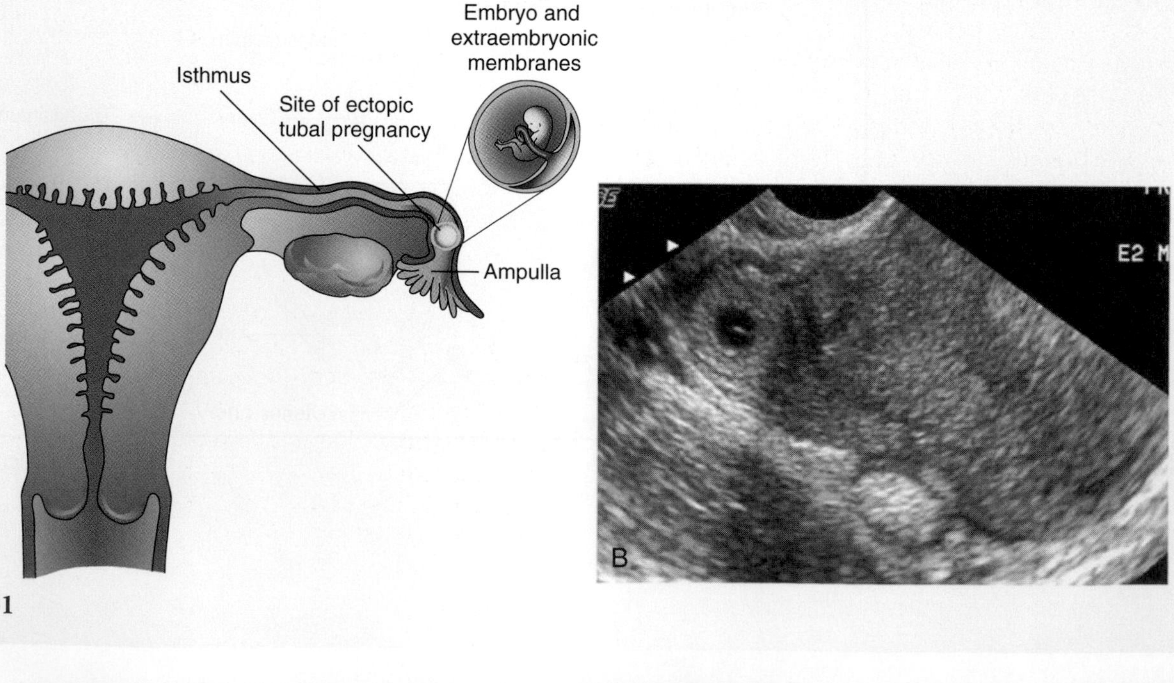
Embryo and extraembryonic membranes
Isthmus
Site of ectopic tubal pregnancy
Ampulla
A
B

Fig. 8-1

the syncytiotrophoblast and cytotrophoblast; the neural tube forms the central nervous system.
24-25, 45

20 B. Pain fibers from organs and structures above the pelvic pain line will follow the sympathetic nerve fibers. Recall that the uterine fundus and body are located above the most inferior part of the pelvic peritoneal reflection, which is known as the pelvic pain line. Pain fibers from structures below the pelvic pain line will follow the parasympathetic nerves: the uterus is above the pelvic pain line. The uterus is a visceral organ and as such will not have somatic innervations. Pain fibers from the uterus are visceral afferent fibers and will only run with sympathetic fibers.
9-10

21 D. Down's syndrome is a congenital abnormality involving a triplication of chromosome 21. It is more common in children of women who become pregnant at 35 years or older (advanced maternal age is a risk factor). Down's syndrome is associated with various abnormalities including congenital heart defects. The most common congenital heart defect in Down's syndrome is endocardiac cushion type of atrial septal defect (40%) followed by ventricular septal defects (35%).
68, 298, 329

22 A. Marfan syndrome affects the connective tissue supporting the body's joints and organs (e.g., heart, aorta, and eyes). Abnormalities in the connective tissue are due to mutations in a single protein building block (amino acid) in the fibrillin-1 protein. This leads to a severe reduction in the amount of fibrillin-1 available to form microfibrils, and elasticity in many tissues is decreased. In Marfan's syndrome elastic fibers are significantly reduced, eventually leading to aortic aneurysm and rupture. The thoracic aorta is contained in the posterior mediastinal cavity. It begins at the lower border of the fourth thoracic vertebra, where it is continuous with the aortic arch, and ends in front of the lower border of the twelfth thoracic vertebra at the aortic hiatus, where it becomes the abdominal aorta.
225-229

23 B. The *COL1A1* gene produces a component of type I collagen called the pro-α1(I) chain. Mutation of the gene leads to reduced production of pro-α1(I) chains and future reduced type I collagen. A shortage of this critical protein underlies the bone fragility and other characteristic features of osteogenesis imperfecta. Osteogenesis imperfecta has 4 types (I, II, III, and IV). In addition to more severe bone problems (fractures), features of these conditions can include blue sclerae, hearing loss, short stature, respiratory problems, and a disorder of tooth development. Discoloration of the sclera gives the appearance of a blue or blue gray color. This is due to the thinning of the sclera caused by a defective type I collagen; as a result the choroidal veins are evident, giving the appearance of a blue color.
225-229

24 A. During embryogenesis, poorly controlled diabetes mellitus in the mother is associated with a 2- to 3-fold increase in the incidence of birth defects such as macrosomia, which is diagnosed as birth weight greater than 8 pounds 13 ounces (4000 grams), regardless of gestational age. Fetal macrosomia makes vaginal delivery difficult and puts the baby at risk of injury during birth. Therefore, cesarean section is recommended, during which epidural anesthesia is given. Hence, the interspinous distance is of concern. Other common anomalies with maternal diabetes mellitus include holoprosencephaly (failure of the forebrain to divide into hemispheres), meroencephaly (partial absence of the brain), sacral agenesis, congenital heart defects, and limb anomalies.
311

25 B. Remnants of the primitive streak (a thick linear band of epiblast at the beginning of week 3) may persist and give rise to a large tumor known as a sacrococcygeal teratoma. Because it is derived from pluripotent primitive streak cells, the tumor contains tissues derived from all three germ layers in incomplete stages of differentiation. Sacrococcygeal teratomas are the most common tumors in newborn infants and have an incidence of approximately 1 in 27,000. These tumors are usually surgically excised promptly and the prognosis is good (Fig. 8-2).
45, 47

26 D. Cystic hygromas are large swellings that usually appear in the inferolateral part of the neck and consist of large, single or multilocular, fluid-filled cavities. Hygromas may be present at birth, but they often enlarge and become evident during later infancy. Hygromas are believed to arise from parts of a jugular lymph sac that are pinched off, or from lymphatic spaces that do not establish connections with the main lymphatic channels, whereas a thyroglossal cyst is a fibrous cyst that forms from a persistent thyroglossal duct. Lingual cysts in the tongue may be derived from remnants of the thyroglossal duct. They may

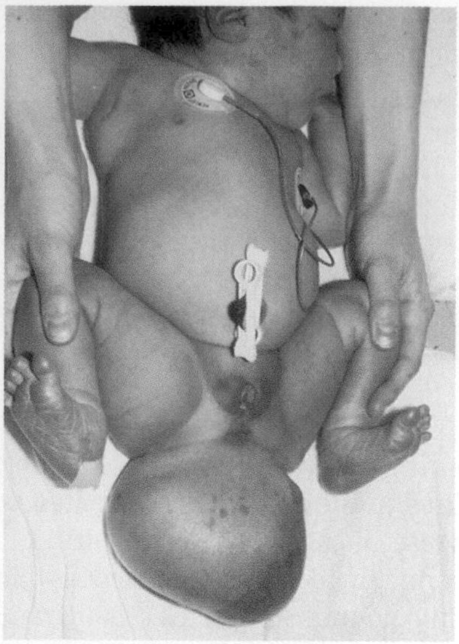

Fig. 8-2

enlarge and produce pharyngeal pain, dysphagia (difficulty in swallowing), or both.
222, 285

27 C. The *FGFR3* gene provides instructions for making a protein called fibroblast growth factor receptor 3. These proteins play a role in several important cellular processes, including regulation of cell growth and division, determination of cell type, formation of blood vessels, wound healing, and embryo development. Mutations in the *FGFR3* gene cause more than 99% of cases of achondroplasia. In achondroplasia (autosomal dominant disorder) the problem is not in forming cartilage but in converting it to bone (endochondral ossification at the epiphysial cartilage plates), particularly in the long bones of the limbs. Other features include an average-size trunk, short arms and legs with particularly short upper arms and thighs, and limited range of motion at the elbows. The head is enlarged (macrocephaly) with a prominent forehead and a "scooped out" nose (flat nasal bone). Fingers are typically short and the ring finger and middle fingers may diverge, giving the hand a three-pronged (trident) appearance. Also, lordosis and kyphosis of the vertebral column may be present.
235, 236, 302

28 D. Implantation of the blastocyst begins at the end of the first embryonic week and normally occurs in the endometrium of the uterus, usually superiorly in the body of the uterus and slightly more often on the posterior than on the anterior wall. The blastocyst begins to implant on approximately the 6th day of the luteal phase.
29

29 A. Development of the upper limb begins at 26 to 27 days after fertilization with the appearance of the upper limb buds; at 33 to 36 days the hand plates are formed and the digital rays are present; at 44 to 46 days notches form between digital rays, and at 49 to 51 days webbed fingers are distinct. Separate fingers appear at 52 to 53 days.
58-60

30 C. Pharyngeal arches 3 and 4 give rise to the common carotid artery, internal carotid artery, the aortic arch, and subclavian artery. The cerebral circle of Willis is formed by arteries that take their origin from these structures. Arches 1 and 2 give rise to the maxillary artery, external carotid artery, stapedial artery, and hyoid artery, which do not contribute to the cerebral circle of Willis. Although Arch 3 participates in the formation of the circle of Willis, second arch structures do not. Arch 5 is rudimentary (if present) and has no derivatives. Arch 6 gives rise to the aortic arches, pulmonary artery, and ductus arteriosus but does not contribute to the circle of Willis (Fig. 8-3).
104, 211-212

31 C. The herpes zoster virus after initial infection can remain latent in the dorsal root ganglion until the body becomes immunocompromised or stressed, and then reappears as a vesicular rash along one of the dermatomes, in this condition called shingles. The dorsal root ganglion sensory neurons are derivative of neural crest cells. Other neural crest cell derivatives include the pia mater, chromaffin cells of the adrenal medulla, thyroid parafollicular cells, Schwann cells, melanocytes, cranial nerves, connective tissue, and some bones of the skull and face. There are usually 21 pairs of denticulate ligaments, which take their origin from the pia mater and attach to the dura mater. As the pia mater is derived from neural crest cells the denticulate ligaments take their origin from the pia mater, which dictates that they share the same embryologic origin. The dorsal horn, ventral horn, and conus medullaris are all part of the spinal cord and are notochord derivatives. The dura mater is of mesenchymal origin.
252-253, 266

32 B. The structure involved is likely the parietal pleura, a derivative of the somatopleuric mesoderm.

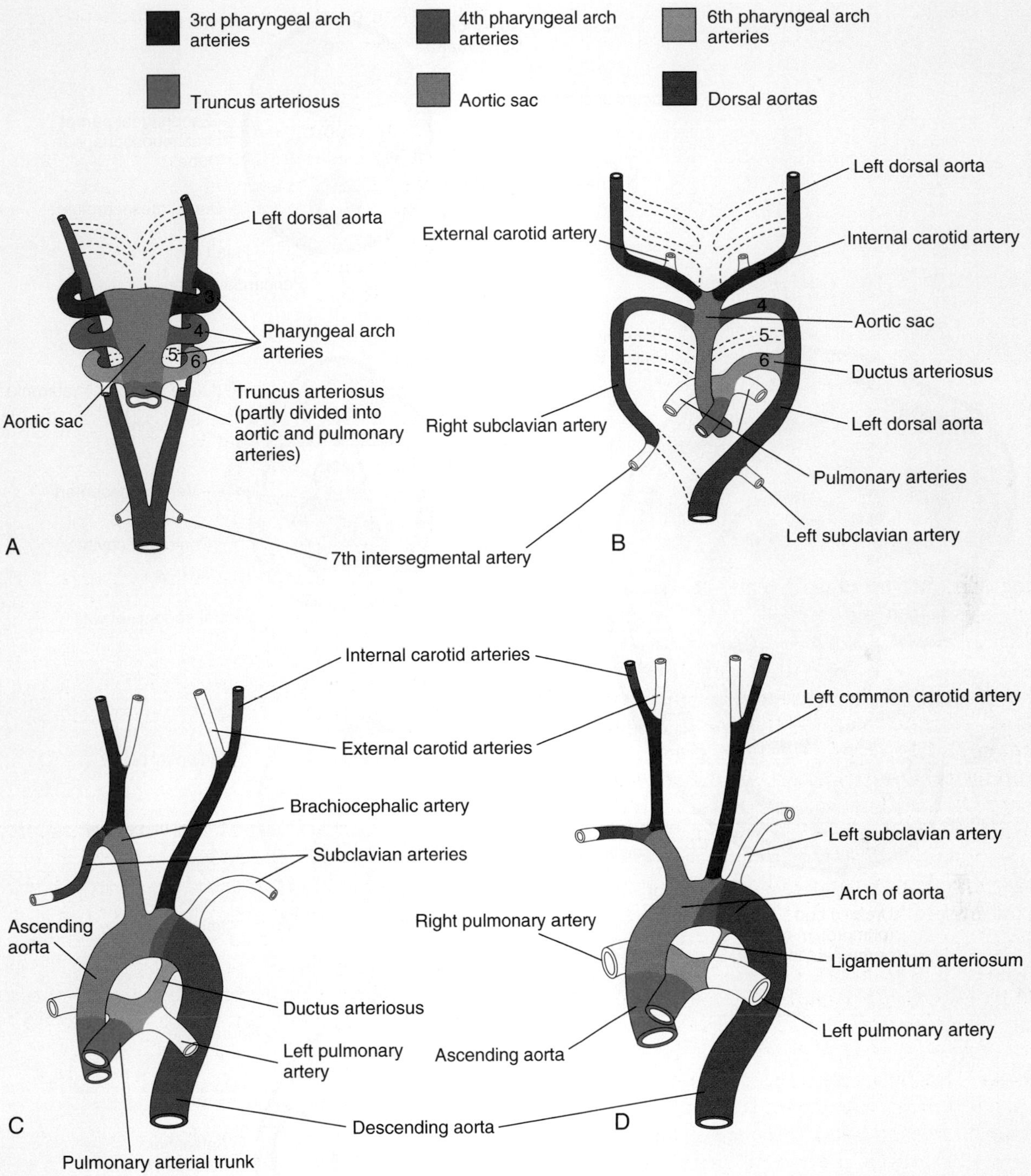

Fig. 8-3

The lateral plate mesoderm gives rise to somatopleuric mesoderm and splanchnopleuric mesoderm. The somatopleuric mesoderm is the dorsal layer that is associated with ectoderm, which forms the body wall lining and dermis. The splanchnopleuric mesoderm, the ventral layer of the lateral mesoderm, is associated with endoderm; this forms the viscera and heart. The septum transversum forms the central tendon of the diaphragm. The oropharyngeal membrane forms a septum between the primitive mouth and pharynx. The coelomic cleft is formed during the division of the coelomic cavity and does not relate to the development of the pleura (Fig. 8-4).

39, 41, 53

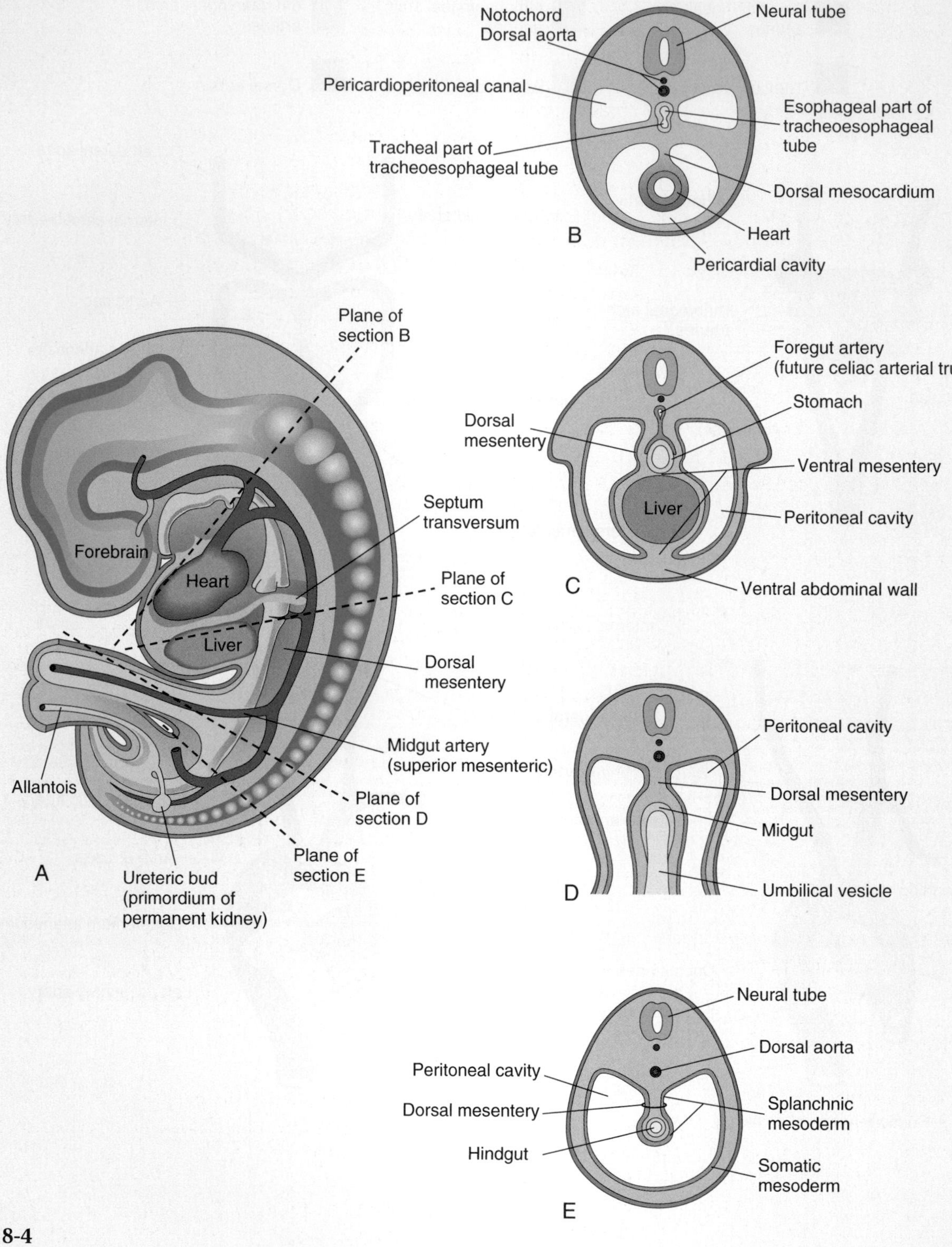

Fig. 8-4

33 D. The left inferior vena cava results from regression of the right supracardinal vein while the left supracardinal vein persists. The right anterior cardinal vein and left cardinal veins contribute to the formation of the internal jugular veins and superior vena cava (with the common cardinal veins). The vitelline veins, during development, drain the yolk sac; they contribute to the formation of the hepatic veins, portal vein, and distal part of the inferior vena cava.

147, 192

34 A. Eisenmenger's syndrome or tardive cyanosis is the process in which a left-to-right shunt caused by a congenital heart defect causes increased flow through the pulmonary vasculature, causing pulmonary hypertension. This in turn causes increased pressure in the right side of the heart and reversal of the shunt into a right-to-left shunt. Eisenmenger's syndrome is a cyanotic heart defect characterized by a long-standing intracardiac shunt caused commonly by ventricular septal defects. In Ebstein's anomaly the septal leaflet of the tricuspid valve is displaced toward the apex of the right ventricle of the heart. There is subsequent atrialization of part of the right ventricle (which is now contiguous with the right atrium). This causes the right atrium to enlarge and the anatomic right ventricle to be small. Here there is an initial right-to-left shunt that results in a cyanotic baby. With the underdeveloped left ventricle, both the aorta and left ventricle are underdeveloped before birth, and the aortic and mitral valves are each too small to allow sufficient blood flow. As blood returns from the lungs to the left atrium, it must pass through an atrial septal defect to the right side of the heart. In this defect babies appear cyanotic. In the common atrioventricular canal defect the heart has one common chamber due to defects in the formation of its septae. Patients develop pulmonary hypertension by the second year of life. In a large foramen secundum (foramen ovale) the atrial septal defect (ASD) does lead to pulmonary hypertension but has a much slower progression. Symptoms usually appear after the third decade of life.

208, 211-212

35 B. Aorticopulmonary septum is the correct answer. The cardiac neural crest cells are involved in the development of the muscle and connective tissue walls of large arteries, parts of the cardiac septum, and parts of the thyroid, parathyroid, and thymus glands. The aorticopulmonary septum is derived specifically from the cardiac neural crest cells; once formed it separates the aorta and pulmonary arteries and fuses with the interventricular septum within the heart during development. The right subclavian artery takes its origin from the fourth pharyngeal arch. The tricuspid valve is formed from proliferation of tissue around the atrioventricular canal. The inferior vena cava takes its origin from the vitelline veins.

209, 211-212

36 A. A hemangioma is a benign endothelial cell tumor. It is characterized by an increased number of normal or abnormal vessels filled with blood. Hemangiomas usually appear in the first weeks of life and grow most rapidly over the first 6 months. Hemangioblast is the common precursor for blood vessels and blood formation induced by vascular endothelial growth factor secreted by surrounding mesoderm. The endoderm forms the epithelial lining of the primitive gut, respiratory tract, tympanic cavity and auditory tube, and the allantois and vitelline duct. The ectoderm gives rise to the central nervous system, the peripheral nervous system, the sensory epithelium of the ear, nose, and eye, the epidermis, hair, and nails, the subcutaneous, mammary, and pituitary glands, and the enamel of the teeth. Trophoblast become cells that form the outer layer of a blastocyst and that provide nutrients to the embryo and later develop into a large part of the placenta. They are the first cells to differentiate from the fertilized egg. Syncytiotrophoblast is the epithelial lining of the placental villi, which will penetrate the walls of the uterus to establish maternofetal circulation.

285

37 D. The left horn of the sinus venosus gives rise to the coronary sinus. The primitive atria and ventricles will give rise to the atria and ventricles, respectively. Bulbus cordis and truncus arteriosus gives rise to the smooth parts of the right and left ventricles and their corresponding arteries.

190-194

38 A. In the fetal heart the left and right atria communicate with each other by an opening in the septum secundum, referred to as the foramen ovale. Ductus arteriosus is a vessel that connects the pulmonary artery and the aortic arch in the fetus. Foramen primum is the perforation in the inferior septum primum, which is closed off as it fuses to the endocardial cushion. Ductus venosus is the vessel that connects the left umbilical vein to the inferior vena cava. Truncus arteriosus will give rise to the aorta and pulmonary trunk (Fig. 8-5).

196-202

39 A. Meromelia is the partial absence of a limb (amelia is total absence). Syndactyly refers to fused digits, and polydactyly is an excess in the number of digits. Central digit ray formation is the underlying mechanism for syndactyly, and talipes equinovarus is a malrotation of the foot, more commonly referred to as clubfoot.

245, 304

40 E. The AER secretes growth factor, which initiates outgrowth of the limb mesenchyme that initiates formation of the limb bud.

235, 239

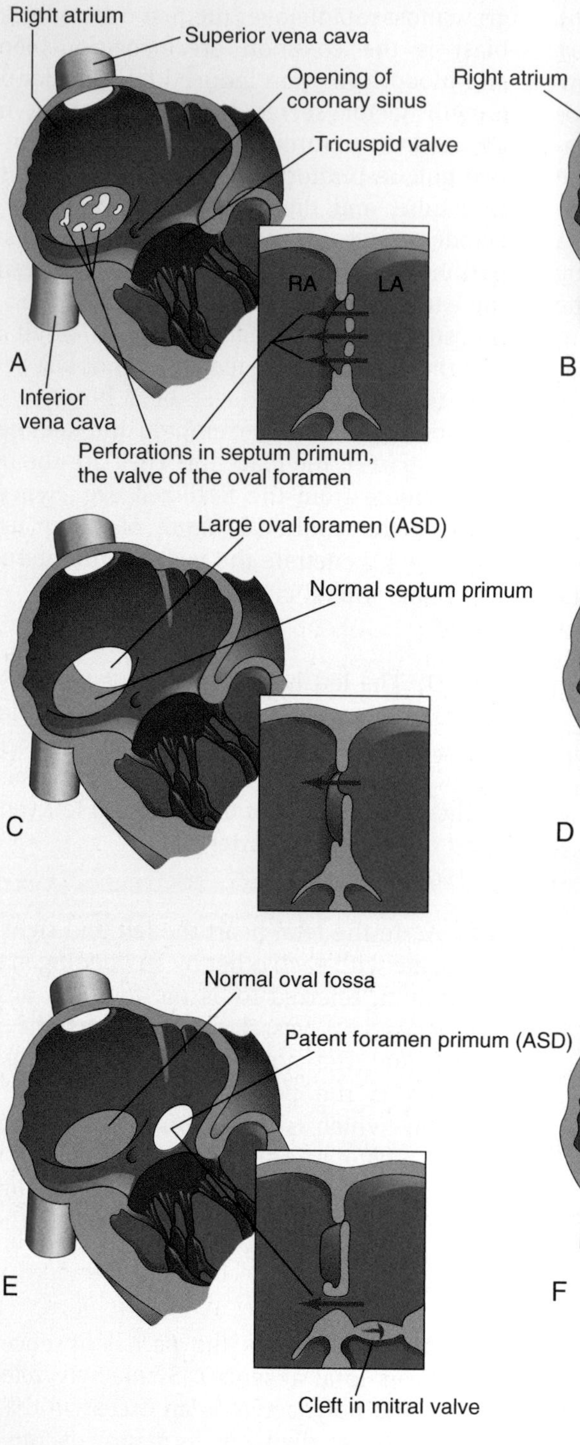

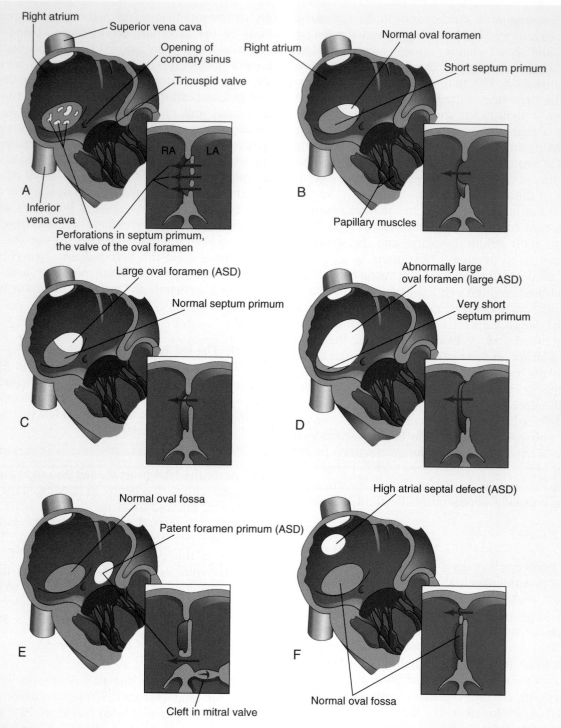

Fig. 8-5

41 D. Polydactyly describes the presence of supernumerary digits of the hands and feet. Cleft foot occurs when one or more digital rays fail to develop, causing absence of the central digits. Clubfoot is a malrotation of the foot around the axis, and amelia is complete absence of a limb. Syndactyly is absence of digits either due to failure of digital rays to form or incomplete apoptosis.

244

42 C. The dorsal and ventral buds normally fuse to form the adult pancreas. The ventral duct, although smaller, becomes the terminal portion of the main duct. A bifid ventral bud, when fusing to the dorsal bud, typically leads to the formation of an annular pancreas, which is a band of pancreatic tissue that wraps around the duodenum. Nonrotation of the midgut would result in displacement of the entire pancreas.

144

43 **C.** The dorsal and ventral buds normally fuse to form the adult pancreas, the ventral duct although smaller becomes the terminal portion of the main duct. A bifid ventral bud, when fusing to the dorsal bud, typically leads to annular pancreas, which is a band of pancreatic tissue that wraps around the duodenum. Nonrotation of the midgut would result in displacement of the entire pancreas.

144

44 **A.** The superior mesenteric artery is closely related to the duodenum and gives rise to the middle colic, right colic, and ileocecal arteries. Therefore, any of these vessels may be affected. The splenic and left gastric arteries are branches of the celiac artery and lie superior to the intestines. The inferior mesenteric artery branches of the abdominal aorta are located too inferiorly. The left and right renal arteries branch from the aorta retroperitoneally and are not related to the intestinal tract.

141-159

45 **B.** Misplacement of a normally formed appendix is due to malrotation of the midgut. Rubella infection leads to a myriad of birth defects including cataracts and cardiac problems but not GI problems. Neural crest cells do not directly contribute to the formation of the GI tract and failure of the lateral folds to close will form neural tube defects. Meckel's diverticulum is an outpouching of the ileum and may become infected, mimicking the symptoms of appendicitis, but would not be found subhepatically.

149

46 **D.** VACTERL syndrome is a cooccurrence of birth defects. It commonly occurs in mothers who are 13 to 19 years of age who have taken progesterone-estrogen birth control pills during the critical stage of development. The acronym stands for Vertebral, Anal, Cardiac, Tracheal, Esophageal, Renal, and Limb anomalies. Tetralogy of Fallot is a common heart defect seen with the VACTERL association, as in anal atresia.

307

47 **C.** Pierre Robin sequence (also called Robin sequence) is an autosomal recessive congenital disorder due to failure of neural crest cells to migrate to the first arch. It is initiated by a hypoplastic mandible, which results in posterior displacement of the tongue and obstruction to the closure of the palatine plates leading to bilateral cleft palate. Respiratory symptoms are common in patients with Robin sequence particularly when the baby is placed on his/her back (supine). The small, recessed mandible (micrognathia) causes the tongue to fall backward and obstruct the airway when babies are placed in the prone position. Down's syndrome is a result of trisomy 21; patients present with slanted palpebral fissures, cardiac anomalies, and impaired cognitive function. Although Treacher Collins is also a first arch syndrome, it also includes other craniofacial anomalies, disfigured external ears, and impaired hearing. Patent ductus arteriosus is a cardiac anomaly due to failure of closure of the ductus arteriosus at birth that usually presents with a holosystolic murmur. Bronchopulmonary dysplasia is a respiratory syndrome seen in newborns and characterized by lung inflammation and scarring. Patients will have respiratory distress when lying in any position (Fig. 8-6).

108

48 **E.** Treacher Collins syndrome (craniofacial dysostosis) is an autosomal disorder characterized by malar hypoplasia, downward-slanting palpebral fissures, defects of the lower eyelids and external ears, and sometimes abnormalities of the middle and internal ears. This is a first arch syndrome due to failure of neural crest cells to migrate to the first arch during the fourth week of development. Trisomy 13, also called Patau syndrome, is a chromosomal condition associated with severe intellectual disability and physical abnormalities in many parts of the body including microphthalmia, cleft lip and palate, and brain and spinal cord anomalies. Defect in the fibrillin 1 (*FBN1*) gene leads to Marfan's syndrome. Failure of fusion of the medial nasal prominences leads only to cleft lip and palate, while failure of closure of the rostral neuropore leads to meroencephaly or anencephaly.

108

49 **A.** Tooth development (odontogenesis) usually begins in the sixth to eighth week. This development occurs in three stages: bud stage, cap stage, and bell stage. The enamel usually develops in the advanced bell stage when cells of the inner enamel epithelium develop into ameloblasts, which produce and deposit enamel in the form of rods over the dentine.

288-289

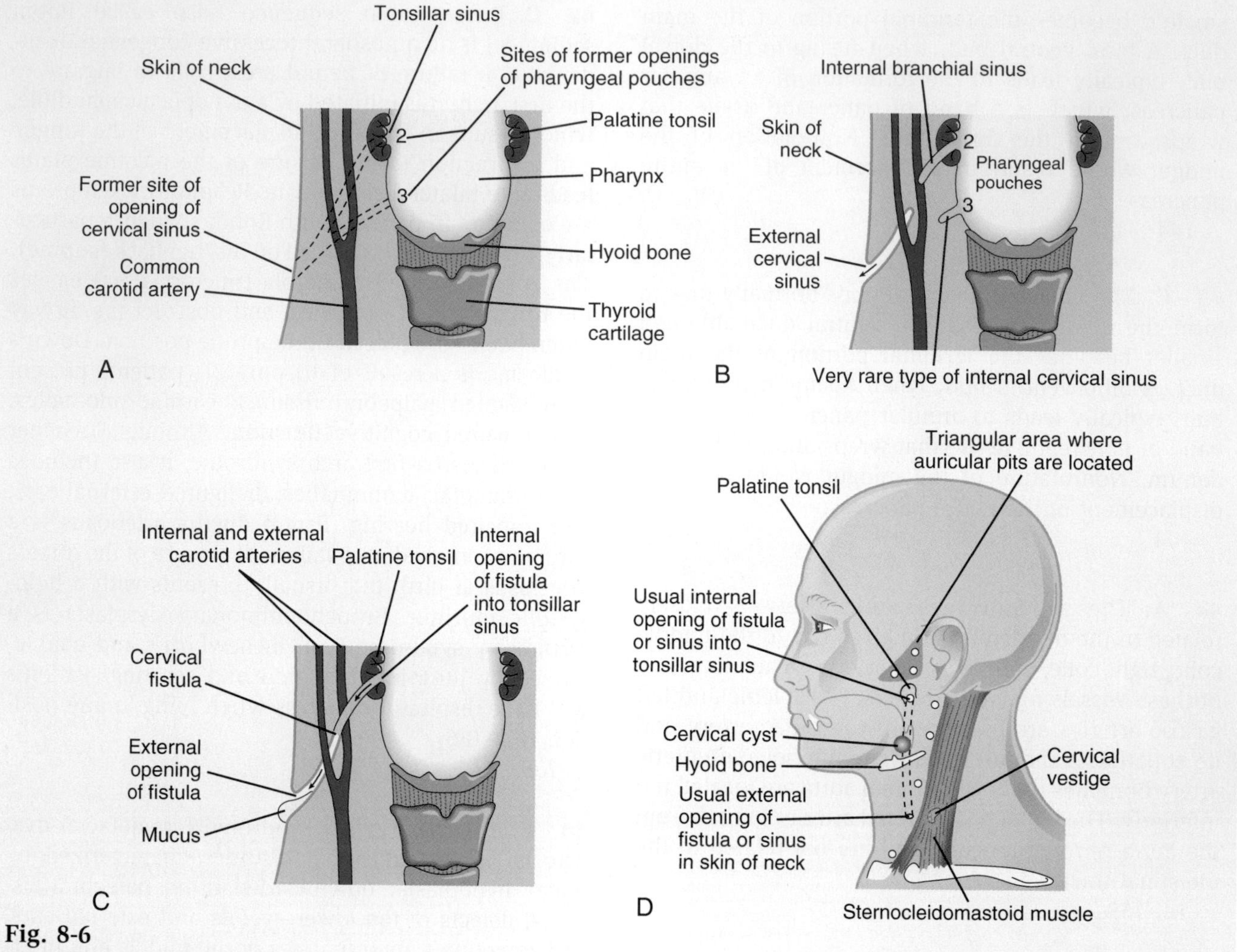

Fig. 8-6

50 C. In the area of the embryo that becomes the eyes, the optic cup (an invagination of the neuroectoderm) is formed. This is connected to the developing brain by the optic stalk. Linear grooves called retinal fissures develop in the optic cups and along the optic stalks. These fissures contain vascular mesenchyme, which develop into the hyaloid artery and vein. The hyaloid vessels supply the optic cup and lens. As the retinal fissures fuse, these vessels are enclosed within the primordial optic nerve. The distal portion usually degenerates but the proximal portion becomes the central artery and vein of the retina.

271-277

51 D. Retinoblastoma is a malignant carcinoma of the retina. The retina develops from the inner and outer layers of the optic cup, which is an invagination of the neuroectoderm. The outer thin layer becomes the inner pigment epithelium of the retina, while the inner layer becomes the light sensitive neural retina. The sphincter pupillae muscle of the iris develops from the neuroectoderm of the optic cup. CNII develops from the optic stalk. The lens develops from surface ectoderm. The sclera and the vitreous body develop from the mesoderm.

272-273

52 D. The brain develops from the neural tube. By the 28th week the caudal and rostral neuropores close, leading to the development of three primary brain vesicles: prosencephalon (forebrain), mesencephalon (midbrain), and rhombencephalon (hindbrain). By the fifth week, the forebrain subdivides into the telencephalon, which becomes the cerebral hemispheres, and a diencephalon, which becomes the thalamus, hypothalamus and epithalamus. The midbrain remains as the midbrain. The hindbrain subdivides into a metencephalon, which becomes the pons and cerebellum, and the myelencephalon, which becomes the medulla oblongata.

38, 254

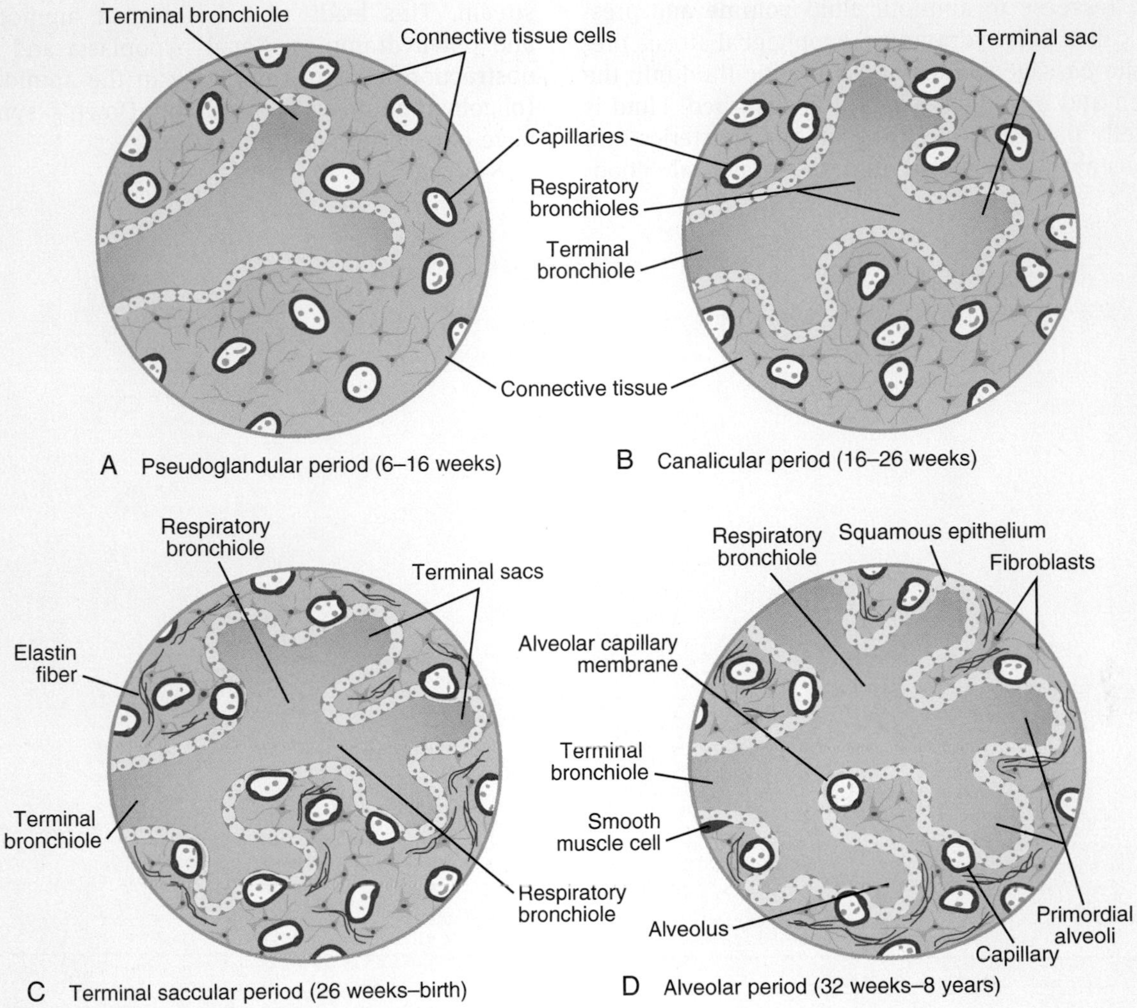

Fig. 8-7

53 B. The arch of the aorta develops from the truncus arteriosus, which is the cranial part of the primitive heart tube. It also gives rise to the pulmonary trunk. The bulbus cordis develops into the conus arteriosus of the right ventricle. The sinus venosus has two horns: a right horn that develops into the smooth sinus venarum of the right atrium and a left horn that develops into the coronary sinus. The ductus arteriosus connects the fetal pulmonary trunk to the aorta allowing for blood to bypass the pulmonary circulation. The ductus venosus connects the umbilical vein to the inferior vena cava allowing blood to bypass the hepatic circulation in the fetus.

204-205, 211-214

54 C. The development of the lungs occurs in four stages: the pseudoglandular stage (6 to 16 weeks), where the lungs resemble exocrine lungs. The parts of the lung involved in gaseous exchange have not yet formed. The canalicular stage (16 to 26 weeks) involves maturation of the bronchioles and development of a few primordial alveoli. The terminal sac stage (26 weeks to birth) is when the alveoli begin maturing, the blood gas barrier is formed, and surfactant is secreted by type 2 pneumocytes. The final stage is the alveolar stage (32 weeks to 8 years); alveoli continue to develop as the lungs prepare for the transition to autonomous gas exchange (Fig. 8-7).

130-135

55 A. A double arch of the aorta is a rare cardiac anomaly. There is the formation of a right and left arch of the aorta, which occurs due to a persistence of the distal part of the right dorsal aorta. This creates a vascular ring around the trachea and esophagus with resulting compression of these structures. Babies present with wheezing aggravated by crying, feeding, and flexion of the neck.

211-214

56 B. Increase in amniotic fluid volume and pressure is called polyhydramnios. Esophageal atresia prevents the passage of excessive amniotic fluid into the stomach and intestines where it is absorbed. Fluid is eventually passed through the umbilical arteries into the placenta for removal into the maternal bloodstream. This leads to a buildup of amniotic fluid and polyhydramnios. Renal hypoplasia and ureteric obstruction lead to a decrease in the amniotic fluid (oligohydramnios). Potter's and Down's syndromes have other associated anomalies.
84, 130, 138

CREDITS

Chapter 1

Fig. 1-1

From Bogart BI, Ort VH: *Elsevier's Integrated Anatomy and Embryology*, Philadelphia: Elsevier, 2007, Fig. 9-18, p. 260.

Fig. 1-4

Courtesy of A.E. Chudley, MD, Children's Hospital and University of Manitoba, Winnipeg, Manitoba, Canada. From Moore KL, Persaud TVN, Torchia MG: *Before We Are Born*, ed 8, Philadelphia: Elsevier, 2013, Fig. 16-10, p. 253.

Fig. 1-5

From Manaster BJ, May DA, Disler DG: *Musculoskeletal Imaging: The Requisites*, ed 4, Philadelphia: Elsevier, 2013, Fig. 9-9, p. 146.

GAS Fig. 2-20, *GAS* Fig. 2-21, *GAS* Fig. 2-31, *GAS* Fig. 2-34, *GAS* Fig. 2-46, *GAS* Fig. 2-49

From Drake RL, Vogl AW, Mitchell AWM: *Gray's Anatomy for Students*, ed 3, Philadelphia: Elsevier, 2015.

Chapter 2

Figs. 2-10 to 2-12

From Moore KL, Persaud TVN, Torchia MG: *Before We Are Born*, ed 8, Philadelphia: Elsevier, 2013, Fig. 14-10, p. 199

GAS Fig. 3-9, *GAS* Fig. 3-16, *GAS* Fig. 3-34, *GAS* Fig. 3-46, *GAS* Fig. 3-71, *GAS* Fig. 3-75, *GAS* Fig. 3-77, *GAS* Fig. 3-88, *GAS* Fig. 3-102, *GAS* Fig. 3-108

From Drake RL, Vogl AW, Mitchell AWM: *Gray's Anatomy for Students*, ed 3, Philadelphia: Elsevier, 2015.

Chapter 3

Fig. 3-9

From Jazayeri SB, Shahlaee A: A 2.5-month-old infant with refractory vomiting and failure to thrive, *Gastroenterology* 144:e3–e4, 2013.

GAS Fig. 4-22, *GAS* Fig. 4-27, *GAS* Fig. 4-29, *GAS* Fig. 4-38, *GAS* Fig. 4-41, *GAS* Figs. 4-47 to 4-50, *GAS* Fig. 4-57, *GAS* Fig. 4-63, *GAS* Fig. 4-64, *GAS* Fig. 4-66, *GAS* Fig. 4-79, *GAS* Fig. 4-80, *GAS* Fig. 4-83, *GAS* Fig. 4-86, *GAS* Fig. 4-93, *GAS* Fig. 4-97, *GAS* Fig. 4-100, *GAS* Fig. 4-102, *GAS* Fig. 4-104, *GAS* Fig. 4-106, *GAS* Fig. 4-107, *GAS* Fig. 4-121, *GAS* Fig. 4-122, *GAS* Fig. 4-126, *GAS* Fig. 4-127, *GAS* Fig. 4-132, *GAS* Fig. 4-139, *GAS* Fig. 4-140, *GAS* Fig. 4-155, *GAS* Fig. 4-157

From Drake RL, Vogl AW, Mitchell AWM: *Gray's Anatomy for Students*, ed 3, Philadelphia: Elsevier, 2015.

Chapter 4

GAS Fig. 5-7, *GAS* Fig. 5-12, *GAS* Figs. 5-15 to 5-17, *GAS* Fig. 5-34, *GAS* Fig. 5-46, *GAS* Fig. 5-54, *GAS* Fig. 5-57, *GAS* Fig. 5-58, *GAS* Fig. 5-65, *GAS* Fig. 5-69, *GAS* Fig. 5-75, *GAS* Fig. 5-78

From Drake RL, Vogl AW, Mitchell AWM: *Gray's Anatomy for Students*, ed 3, Philadelphia: Elsevier, 2015.

Chapter 5

Fig. 5-3

From Weir J, Abrahams P: *Imaging Atlas of Human Anatomy*, ed 3, Philadelphia: Elsevier, 2003.

GAS Fig. 6-16, *GAS* Fig. 6-30, *GAS* Fig. 6-38, *GAS* Fig. 6-41, *GAS* Fig. 6-50, *GAS* Fig. 6-98, *GAS* Fig. 6-99, *GAS* Fig. 6-105, *GAS* Fig. 6-110, *GAS* Fig. 6-119

From Drake RL, Vogl AW, Mitchell AWM: *Gray's Anatomy for Students*, ed 3, Philadelphia: Elsevier, 2015.

Chapter 6

Fig. 6-10

From Neligan PC, Chang J: *Plastic Surgery*, ed 3, vol 6, *Upper Extremity*, Philadelphia: Elsevier, 2013, Fig. 34.23, p. 761.

Fig. 6-14

From Preston DC, Shapiro BE: Median neuropathy. In *Electromyography and Neuromuscular Disorders: Clinical-Electrophysiologic Correlations.* Boston: Butterworth-Heinemann, 1998.

GAS Fig. 7-22, *GAS* Fig. 7-24, *GAS* Fig. 7-39, *GAS* Fig. 7-50, *GAS* Fig. 7-52, *GAS* Fig. 7-57, *GAS* Fig. 7-69, *GAS* Fig. 7-72, *GAS* Fig. 7-73, *GAS* Fig. 7-83, *GAS* Fig. 7-86, *GAS* Fig. 7-87, *GAS* Fig. 7-90, *GAS* Fig. 7-103, *GAS* Fig. 7-109

From Drake RL, Vogl AW, Mitchell AWM: *Gray's Anatomy for Students*, ed 3, Philadelphia: Elsevier, 2015.

Chapter 7

Fig. 7-23

From Netter F: *Atlas of Human Anatomy*, ed 6, Philadelphia: Elsevier, 2014, All rights reserved. www.netterimages.com.

GAS Fig. 8-33, *GAS* Fig. 8-35, *GAS* Fig. 8-38, *GAS* Figs. 8-44 to 8-46, *GAS* Fig. 8-65, *GAS* Fig. 8-66, *GAS* Fig. 8-72, *GAS* Fig. 8-84, *GAS* Fig. 8-103, *GAS* Fig. 8-116, *GAS* Fig. 8-120, *GAS* Fig. 8-121, *GAS* Fig. 8-146, *GAS* Fig. 8-153, *GAS* Fig. 8-159, *GAS* Fig. 8-169, *GAS* Fig. 8-176, *GAS* Fig. 8-190, *GAS* Fig. 8-192, *GAS* Fig. 8-193, *GAS* Fig. 8-217, *GAS* Fig. 8-235, *GAS* Fig. 8-239, *GAS* Fig. 8-257

From Drake RL, Vogl AW, Mitchell AWM: *Gray's Anatomy for Students*, ed 3, Philadelphia: Elsevier, 2015.

Chapter 8

Figs. 8-1 to 8-7

From From Moore KL, Persaud TVN, Torchia MG: *Before We Are Born*, ed 8, Philadelphia: Elsevier, 2013, p. 32.

GAS Fig. 5-58

From Drake RL, Vogl AW, Mitchell AWM: *Gray's Anatomy for Students*, ed 3, Philadelphia: Elsevier, 2015.

INDEX

G

H

M

N

O

P